DOCTOR'S
GUIDE

TO
Natural Medicine

DOCTOR'S GUIDE

TO
Natural Medicine

The Complete and
Easy-to-Use Natural Health Reference
from a Medical Doctor's Perspective

PAUL BARNEY, M.D.

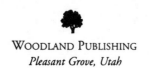

WOODLAND PUBLISHING
Pleasant Grove, Utah

©1998
Woodland Publishing, Inc.
P.O. Box 160
Pleasant Grove, Utah
84062

NOTE: The information contained in this book is not intended as medical advice, but is solely for educational purposes only. It is not intended to diagnose, treat, or prescribe, and does not replace the services of a trained physician. It is assumed that the reader will consult a medical or health professional if you know or suspect you have a serious health problem. Neither Woodland Publishing nor the author directly or indirectly dispenses medical advice or prescribes the use of herbs, supplements, or other forms of treatment for illness without medical approval.

Cover design by Cord Udall

PRINTED IN THE UNITED STATES OF AMERICA

CONTENTS

Preface viii
Acknowledgment viii
Introduction: How To Effectively Use This Book ix

Part 1: A Course on the Essential Components of Wellness

WHY I BELIEVE IN SUPPLEMENTATION 11

How to Select Effective, Pure, and Superior
Supplements 12

The Profound Importance of Guaranteed
Potency 13

**A DISCUSSION OF DIET: WHAT WE EAT
PROFOUNDLY DETERMINES HOW WE FEEL** 14

Typical American Eating Habits 14

Why do Medical School Courses Ignore the
Health Implications of Diet? 15

Why the RDA Needs Revision 15

Proper Digestion: A Major Problem in This
Country 15

The Neglected Role of Digestive Enzymes 16

Hydrochloric Acid Deficiency 16

Fiber 16

Autointoxication: Fact or Fiction? 20

Colon Cleansing 20

Fasting 21

Food Allergies 21

Soy-Based Foods 24

Food Additives 24

Sugar and Artificial Sweeteners 24

Dietary Guidelines for Good Health 26

Weight Loss 27

The Exercise Component 29

Macronutrients: Carbohydrates, Fats
and Proteins 30

Micronutrients: Vitamins and Minerals 33

Amino Acids and Their Actions 41

Free Radicals 43

Antioxidants 44

Water 45

**PREVENTION: HOW TO BOOST OUR
IMMUNE SYSTEM** 46

A Brief Overview of Immune Function 46

Immune System Dysfunction 47

Causes of Immune System Impairment 47

Diet and Immunity 48

Herbs and Herbal Combinations That Boost
Immune Function 49

**EXERCISE: THE MANY BENEFITS OF
MOVING THE BODY** 49

**THE BODY-MIND-SPIRIT CONNECTION
AND HEALING** 50

Stress: Public Health Enemy Number One 50

Stress Test: Personality and Events 51

Visualization Therapy 52

Spiritual Healing: Linking Back to Our Creator 52

Part 2: Alternative Therapies

MAINSTREAM MEDICINE AND ALTERNATIVE THERAPIES: MY STORY 53

EDUCATION IN NATURAL MEDICINE IS CRUCIAL TO EFFECTIVE HEALING 54

WHY ARE MORE DOCTORS EXPLORING ALTERNATIVE THERAPIES? 54

SCIENTIFIC DOCUMENTATION OF NATURAL TREATMENTS 55

Cranberry and Urinary Tract Infections: Magic or Science? 55

Phytomedicinals: Herbal Medicine 55

Herbs vs. Drugs: A Comparison 56

Are Herbs Safe? 57

Incorporating Herbs into Your Meals 58

Chinese Herbal Medicine 58

The Theory of Yin and Yang 58

MAJOR HERBS AND THEIR APPLICATIONS 59

AN OVERVIEW OF OTHER NATURAL SUPPLEMENTS 81

LEARNING ABOUT OTHER NATURAL PROTOCOLS 91

Part 3: Individual Ailments and Their Recommended Treatments

Acne 97

AIDS/HIV 101

Allergies 106

Alzheimer's Disease 110

Angina 114

Anxiety 119

Arteriosclerosis 123

Arthritis 123

Asthma 128

Athlete's Foot 132

ADD/Hyperactivity 134

Autism 137

Back Pain 140

Bad Breath 143

Bedwetting 145

Bee Stings 147

Bladder Infections 147

Boils 151

BPH (Benign Prostatic Hypertrophy) 153

Bronchitis 153

Bulimia 156

Burns 159

Bursitis 163

Cancer 166

Canker Sores 174

Carpal Tunnel Syndrome 176

Cataracts 179

Chicken Pox 182

Chronic Fatigue Syndrome 184

Colic 188

Colitis 190

Coronary Heart Disease 194

Crohn's Disease 198

Cysts, Breast 198

Dermatitis 198

Diarrhea 198

Diverticulitis 202

Dysmenorrhea 206

Earache 206

Ear Infection 209

Eczema 209

Endometriosis 213

Epilepsy 216

Fever 220

Fibrocystic Breast Disease 223

Fibromyalgia 227

Gall Disease 231

Gallstones 231

Gingivitis 234

Glaucoma 234

Gout 237

Halitosis 241

Headaches 241

Heart Attack 241

Heartburn 245

Heart Disease 248

Hemorrhoids 248

High Blood Pressure/High Cholesterol 252

Hypertension 257

Hypoglycemia 257

Impotence 260

Infertility 263

Inflammatory Bowel Disease 267

Insect Bites 267

Insomnia 269

Kidney Stones 273

Lupus 276

Meningitis 280

Menopause 283

Menstrual Cramps 287

Migraine Headaches 290

Mononucleosis 294

Motion Sickness/Nausea 297

Multiple Sclerosis 300

Obesity 304

Osteoporosis 308

Panic Disorder 312

Parkinson's Disease 312

Periodontal Disease 316

PMS 319

Pneumonia 323

Pregnancy-Related Complications 326

Prostate Disease 330

Psoriasis 333

Rheumatic Fever 337

Shingles 339

Sinusitis 342

Skin Disorders 346

Sleep Disorders 346

Sprains/Strains 346

Stress 349

Stroke 353

Sunburn 357

Temporomandibular Joint Syndrome (TMJ) 360

Tooth Grinding 364

Ulcers 367

Urinary Tract Infections 371

Vaginitis 371

Varicose Veins 375

Visual Disorders 378

Warts 382

Weight Control 385

Wrinkles 385

Yeast Infections 388

Appendix A: Resource Information 389

Appendix B: Glossary 395

Index 401

Preface

As a medical doctor who sincerely wants his patients to get well, I offer this book as a complete guide to natural healing. This book is based on the individual experiences of my own patients. I currently treat 80 to 85 percent of my patients with alternative therapies, so I have come to understand which nutritional supplements work best for a whole host of ailments and diseases. I hope that you, the reader, will be the beneficiary of years of schooling in the role that alternative medicine can play in restoring and maintaining health not only in the doctor's office, but at home as well.

In writing this book, I have collected years' worth of data concerning alternative therapies, their physiological mechanisms, and how to apply them correctly. It is my hope that this information will help to dispel the confusion that sometimes surrounds natural health practices—especially now, when all kinds of information bombards us concerning health supplements. Frequently, that information is contradictory, causing us to become more perplexed than ever, a situation which often prompts us to abandon potentially valuable therapies.

Not only does this manual discuss the proper use of alternative therapies for over 100 diseases and ailments, it includes the latest scientific documentation supporting specific herbs, supplements, etc. In addition to reference material and terminology defining the role of vitamins, mineral, herbs, amino acids, acupuncture, and scores of other supplements and treatments, this book guides you, as an interested consumer, in how to choose potent, pure products, the best delivery systems for those products, and how to apply them for maximum benefit.

It is essential that my patients understand how much of a suggested herbal treatment to take and how long to continue treatment. In addition, issues of safety and success rates are also reviewed and how to prevent disease is individually addressed. I have determined that successfully implementing new treatments depends on the patient's willingness to not only utilize these therapies, but to understand how they work as well.

Moreover, to ignore the spiritual aspect of healing is to overlook one of the most powerful forces intrinsically linked to health and happiness. The more sickness I see, the more I am convinced that one's spiritual health is intricately woven into the notion of total wellness and contentment. As I continue to practice medicine and teach medical students, I am more convinced than ever that true medicine must incorporate a "holistic" approach to disease. In other words, people cannot be treated in slices, they must be cared for as multifaceted, whole beings in terms of the physical, intellectual and the spiritual. In so doing, medical practitioners will finally learn to heal in the way Hippocrates intended. As a medical doctor, it has only been after considerable study and application that I have seen first hand the value of alternative therapies for my patients.

Paul Barney, M.D.

Acknowledgment

I express many thanks to Rita Elkins, whose seemingly endless hours of writing and research pulled this project through. Without her work, insight, and perseverance, this book would not be a reality.

Introduction: How To Effectively Use This Book

I believe that this is the most comprehensive reference guide available concerning the maintenance of optimal health and the natural treatment of disease. It is based on years of experience and boils down the glut of health information floating around out there, to the latest and the most reliable data available. Because I believe in integrating alternative medicine with orthodox practices, I have written this guide to efficiently cover virtually every area of wellness, giving you, as the patient, a ready-reference of viable health options with scientific validation whenever possible. Ideally, I would like to see patients taking this guide with them when they visit their physicians. It will undoubtedly spark some fascinating conversation.

In addition to the initial sections, which act as easy-to-read tutorials on virtually every natural supplement and health discipline, the best natural treatments for over 100 diseases and disorders are delineated and just about every pertinent fact you may need to know has been addressed. Symptoms, causes, dietary guidelines, conventional treatments, herbal and nutritional supplements, precautions, product recommendations and prevention guidelines are supplied. The most effective supplements are listed in insets under the primary heading with secondary nutrients inventoried. I have included a section called "Doctor's Notes" in which I share with you my own personal experience with the natural treatments of the disease referenced. Helpful and practical suggestions that one can implement at home are also described for each ailment.

The mind/spirit link to achieving health, which is equally important and frequently excluded from other professional health guides, is also included. I am a staunch believer that in our quest to get to the bottom of disease, we must talk about both the spiritual and psychological factors which profoundly influence the lives and well-being of our patients. Stress management is also examined and after years of dealing with the health implications of stress, I have included the most effective approaches.

A number of glossary sections with easy-to-find definitions will help you as the consumer walk into a health food store feeling more confident about your choices. Bioactive compounds, practices from homeopathy to aroma therapy, and a comprehensive listing of just about any nutritional supplement are all defined. New compounds such as CMO, CLA, glucosamine, pyruvate, etc., are all evaluated. Natural products can take the form of herbs, vitamins, minerals, amino acids and a wide variety of other substances which have impressive therapeutic credentials. Instead of simply defining these compounds, I have added my own comments concerning their use.

The key to using these products correctly is education. No one wants to spend money on worthless products. On the other hand, most of us need to become much more health aware and self-guided in order to heal. It is my intention that this reference book will supply you with information on what are the latest, up-to-date natural treatments, their applications and safety issues. I hope you will find it not only useful, but enlightening.

PART 1

A Course on the Essential Components of Wellness

"It is often the scientist's experience that he senses the nearness of truth when connections are envisioned. A connection is a step toward simplification, unification."

—MAHLON HOAGLAND

Why I Believe In Supplementation

Simply stated, the medical establishment has not been particularly enthusiastic about using supplements. I can see that attitudes are in the process of changing somewhat; however, the change is much too slow. Scientific evidence supporting supplementation is overwhelming and can no longer be considered quackery as it once was. Numerous scientific studies support the fact that basic supplementation of what we would call a one-a-day vitamin can improve our overall health. Study after study tells us that many of us are deficient in calcium, magnesium, zinc and manganese. Zinc is involved in at least 80 to 90 metalo-enzymatic reactions; many of which determine immune function. Obviously a zinc deficiency means that the immune system will be compromised. Taking all the herbs in the world cannot make up for this deficiency because, without zinc, our response to even the most potent herb would be faulty.

Keeping our bodies supplied with minerals is absolutely essential, and if we grew our own food, perhaps we could forego supplements. We don't grow our own food, and com-mercial farming practices have severely depleted our soils of vital minerals, especially trace minerals. If we want to take certain minerals into our bodies, we had better turn to good supplements. If we only needed nitrogen and potassium to survive, our current supply of artificially fertilized, farm-grown produce would do nicely. Trace mineral supplements can keep us supplied with these important minerals.

My view on the importance of supplementation is based on years of my own clinical experience. I consider my patient's dietary habits initially and have continually discovered that most of them are not eating properly. Eating on the run, choosing sweet, fatty foods as meal replacements, and using caffeine for energy are more the rule than the exception. Unquestionably, the majority of Americans are not getting the nutrient levels set by RDA standards. Moreover, RDA standards are often too low. Using a good multivitamin supplement only makes good sense. In addition, learning to add other single micronutrients according to specific need and gender makes for a much better health scenario. Our eating habits can improve; however, if we're going to take a realistic approach, they will probably never be good enough. Women are especially prone to nutrient deficiencies in that they continually restrict calories, lose iron through their periods and frequently take birth control pills which can lower certain nutrient levels.

At this writing, statistics which are randomly emerging show significant deficiencies in the B-vitamins, chromium, iron, selenium, calcium, etc. In the area of cancer alone, deficiencies in vitamins A, C, and E have all been linked to increased risk. Copper and zinc depletions profoundly impact immunity and low chromium levels are thought to be responsible for cholesterol escalation and many blood sugar disorders. A lack of selenium can predispose us to heart disease, low magnesium significantly contributes to PMS, and so on. Data strongly suggests that using nutritional supplements early on could avoid millions of dollars in health care services later. For example, making sure that we get adequate and absorbable amounts of calcium/magnesium in our younger years could help prevent the high incidence of hip fractures we see in our older populations. Simply stated, taking supplements is wise. The notion of using supplements to treat disease conditions rather than just maintaining health is another ball game entirely.

Professor Linus Pauling, who won the Nobel Prize twice for his work, coined the term "orthomolecular" psychiatry, which refers to the treatment of mental disease by providing the most optimal molecular environment for the mind through certain concentrations of substances normally present in the body. Administering extra large doses of vitamin C was Pauling's specialty and he has some engaging theories concerning vitamin megadose therapy. The use of these naturally occurring compounds is usually considered much safer than drug therapy. There are countless accounts of people who have died or been injured by medicinal drugs. Dying from a nutrient overdose is extremely rare. Dr. Zoltan P. Rona, M.D., points out that there has never been a death as a result of any supplemented vitamin or mineral. By contrast, he emphasizes that something as commonly used as the birth control pill has 200 known and potentially dangerous side effects.

Psychiatrists are typically skeptical of the orthomolecular approach to treating any mental disorder. Pauling firmly believed that nutrition is crucial in the treatment of most mental disorders. He openly condemned the medical establishment's bias against vitamin therapy for mood disorders and pointed out that various studies conclusively demonstrate that people suffering from schizophrenia experienced clear and undeniable benefits by improving their nutritional habits. By taking optimum amounts of niacin, ascorbic acid, thiamine, pyridoxine and other nutrients, their mental outlook improved.

Unfortunately, in their zeal to protect us from quackery, some medical doctors tend to ignore what can be of real value. There is plenty of good scientific evidence that using vitamins and amino acids can successfully treat behavioral disorders, schizophrenia, depression and many other ailments. Sadly enough, the immovability of some health care professionals concerning this subject can create a great deal of prejudice and a lack of objectivity.

My basic philosophy concerning supplementation is that everyone should be taking a good, basic multimineral, multivitamin supplement daily. Moreover, they should augment that supplement with a broad spectrum antioxidant formula. During periods of disease or other forms of stress, vitamin and mineral supplementation should be increased. Recent studies have found that in some diseases like breast cancer the aggressive use of nutritional antioxidants, essential fatty acids and coenzyme Q10 has resulted in significant remission. Concerning the use of supplements for diseases like cancer, B. Levin, in the Winter 1995 *Quarterly Review of Natural Medicine*, states: ". . . this study should help convince us that serious health compromise can increase the need for certain nutrients. This study also suggests a primary role for aggressive nutritional supplementation in the treatment of breast cancer."

Yes, it is true that we can go overboard and no one wants to take a handful of pills everyday. On the other hand, I believe that if most of us were truly aware of the powerful health roles supplements can play, we would never be without them. Learning what to buy and why enables us to make wise choices based on the individual needs of our bodies. We need to read up and make educated purchases designed to augment our diets and counteract the detrimental effects of our modern world.

HOW TO SELECT EFFECTIVE, PURE AND SUPERIOR SUPPLEMENTS

One of the pitfalls of purchasing a guidebook to natural therapies is that too often the author neglects to give the reader specific direction about what to look for when shopping. Most of us who wander down the aisles of a health food store often feel as though we need the services of a health "translator." Hundreds of strange sounding compounds fill countless shelves and even deciding on which vitamin C supplement or what kind of calcium is best can be difficult and frustrating. Through my practice and personal research, I have come to believe in the profound value of guaranteed potency, the importance of the proper delivery system and the notion that all compounds are not created equal. In other words, a vitamin or antioxidant compound that has been chemically synthesized in the laboratory may act very differently inside the human body than those extracted from natural sources.

In general, you want to look for vitamins and minerals extracted from natural sources, when possible and practical, herbs that have a guaranteed percentage of their active ingredients (they usually cost a bit more), and supplements that come from reputable companies. In addition, all minerals are not created equal as far as assimilation goes. In other words, a zinc lozenge can be more effective than a zinc tablet. Certain forms of calcium are better absorbed than others. Many over-the-counter forms of calcium come from inexpensive inorganic sources such as calcium oxide or carbonate which is often found in antacid products. These forms of calcium are not well absorbed, therefore, you may be faithfully taking what you think is an adequate calcium supplement and still become calcium deficient. Enteric coatings enable certain nutrients to bypass the stomach and dissolve in the intestinal tract, where they will be of much more value for diseases like irritable bowel disorder. Enteric garlic, for example, would be more effective as a treatment for colon disorders than regular garlic capsules. Some organic vitamins are also better assimilated than synthetic varieties. For example, organic vitamin E derived from soy is much more effective than its artificially synthesized counterpart. It's also important to know that much of vitamin B12 is lost through the digestion process; therefore, a sublingual form is preferable. Beta carotene converts to vitamin A; thus, taking beta carotene may be preferrable to vitamin A supplementation in that large doses of vitamin A can be toxic, especially for pregnant women. In general, look for the following:

- Chelated minerals or plant-derived trace minerals with no aluminum additives.
- Vitamins and minerals from organic sources where possible. NOTE: Many natural products contain a combination of naturally and synthetically derived nutrients. In the case of vitamin C, for example, ascorbic acid may be used rather than just rose hips due to the high cost of the natural source.
- Free-form amino acids.
- Calcium (gluconate, citrate, aspartate, lactate). NOTE: Carbonate is acceptable if combined with other sources. Citrate has a good track record for absorbability and assimilation.
- Zinc and chromium picolinate or, GTF chromium; these forms are much more desirable. ·
- Enteric-coated peppermint oil capsules for bowel applications.
- B12 and B6 in sublingual tablets.
- Vitamin E with selenium.
- Calcium with magnesium.
- Wild yam for progesterone in cream/topical forms.
- Shark cartilage in powdered bulk form for practicality in treating tumors.
- Proteolytic enzymes (can also be enteric coated to dissolve in bowel only).
- Iron from natural sources such as ferrous gluconate or certain botanicals.
- Acidophilus in liquid or capsule form that guarantees bacterial count and includes bifidobacteria (check expiration date).
- Glucosamine sulfate with chondroitin sulfate (without chondroitin present, glucosamine's action is limited).
- Protein from soy or other vegetable sources.
- Guaranteed potency herbs.
- Broad spectrum antioxidant blends using vitamin E, selenium, germanium, lipoic acid, vitamin C, vitamin A, beta carotene, bioflavonoids, or grape seed extract
- Multiple vitamins with strong potency for each nutrient and a good array of trace minerals.
- Bee pollen that is freeze dried and comes from local plants, if possible.
- Be wary of products that contain sugar, starch, salt, coal tars, yeast, corn, milk or artificial colorings or flavorings.

Just because a product is found on the shelves of a health food store does not mean that it is necessarily good for you or without side effects. Hormonally based compounds such as DHEA, melatonin, pregnenolone, etc., are just beginning to emerge as therapeutic agents, therefore, no one really knows what their long term usage will cause. While some of their properties are impressive, they should be used with caution.

Buying products from reputable manufacturers who believe in purity, potency and have high quality control, is essential. Companies that have in-house research and development departments are also recommended. Learn to read labels, look for percentage of active ingredients and ask lots of questions. Never hesitate to make a phone call to a particular distributor and find out all you can about a certain product. The health of your body as well as your pocketbook depends on it.

THE PROFOUND IMPORTANCE OF GUARANTEED POTENCY

While I wholeheartedly support the use of various natural therapies, I caution my patients to purchase natural products from distributors who guarantee the potency of their active ingredients. Virtually every clinical study performed on herbs or other natural substances works with the active ingredients which must be taken in certain dosages to achieve desired results. It's not enough to learn that cascara sagrada effectively remedies constipation. Research results which support the use of various herbs and other natural substances are based on a certain percentage of active ingredient. Not every herbal product guarantees potency. As a result, you might be wasting your money and time, not to mention the fact that if you neglect to see any desired result, you may conclude that natural therapies are worthless.

Learning to recognize good herbal blends is very helpful. Over time I have learned the value of herbal formulas and have incorporated them into my practice. As a physician, I feel confident suggesting guaranteed potency products for my patients. I liken these medicinal agents to "herbal prescriptions" in that they are standardized and subject to rigorous quality control. When I consult clinical studies which use natural products, I am struck with the notion that often we are not getting what a label may claim to contain. Diluted, inert, or inactive forms of herbs will not initiate the physiological reactions we desire. We need to look for guaranteed potency in capsules, extracts and tinctures.

Make sure when you purchase an herbal formula that it contains the right proportion of each herbal component. Here is where reputability and expertise of the manufacturer comes into play. I can honestly say that if the products are good, herbal treatments in combination with other therapies such as acupuncture can achieve remarkable results.

A Discussion of Diet: What We Eat Profoundly Determines How We Feel

Diet should be the first thing we look at in diagnosing and treating disease. Often, just changing one's dietary habits immediately promotes better health. Ironically, nutrition is usually the last thing most physicians address. I have found that the majority of people who go on a good nutritious diet find that not only good health results, but the unexpected benefit of a heightened sense of well-being. Moreover, in many cases, ailments that often do not respond to drug therapy disappear when diet and lifestyle are changed.

In spite of the profound roles nutrients play in maintaining wellness, we are still rather oblivious when it comes to making wise food choices. If you don't believe that how you choose to satisfy your hunger can have far reaching health implications, think again. What we nonchalantly pop into our mouths sets off a series of complex chemical reactions that impact virtually every organ and every body system. Just look at the effects of caffeine consumption, for example. Caffeine stimulates the release of norepinephrine which can create a temporary energy surge. What is not commonly known is that it also inhibits the body's ability to absorb vitamin B1, causes the body to lose magnesium, agitates the nervous system, stresses the adrenal glands and is 100 percent addictive.

The use of food to prevent or even treat disease is nothing new. Johns Hopkins University uses a ketogenic diet to successfully treat pediatric epilepsy; a treatment protocol that is rarely suggested by most physicians. While this diet has existed for decades, only a small percentage of parents who have an epileptic child know anything about it. Typically, soon after the child's first seizure, harsh anticonvulsant drugs are employed and no other alternative therapies are discussed. For many children, something as simple as producing ketones in the body, which the ketogenic diet accomplished, can decrease seizures and even cure a significant number of children. It becomes clear that food profoundly affects brain function, not to mention the rest of the body's mechanisms.

According to the American Institute for Cancer Research, approximately 40 percent of all cancer in men and 60 percent in women is associated in one way or another with diet. Our choice of diet can either contribute to diseases like stroke, diabetes, cardiovascular disorders, heart attack, colon disease, cancer, etc., or it can help protect us from these potentially fatal afflictions. The first thing anyone should do who wants to maintain their health is to look at what they're eating. Checking out the contents of your grocery cart can be very revealing. If all you see is processed, instant, sugary, fatty, snacky foods like yellow cheeses, bacon, red meat, high-fat milk, sour cream, hot dogs, crackers, chips, cookies, white rice, jello, instant potatoes, highly sweetened cereals and soda pop, things need to change. Instead, try to fill your cart with fresh fruits and vegetables, whole grain cereals and flours, dried beans of all varieties, brown rice, millet, lean white meats, olive oil, semolina pastas, part skim mozzarella cheese, low-fat active yogurts, tofu, etc. While it may take some doing, making the change from the first cart to the second is possible. To help you understand the necessity for such a change, let's look at our eating traditions and how they are ruining our health.

TYPICAL AMERICAN EATING HABITS

Over the last three decades, we have witnessed dramatic changes not only in what we eat, but also when and how we eat. One of the biggest changes is that modern technology has created new "edibles" which have undergone countless chemical processes. We routinely consume new crop varieties that have been genetically engineered; beef, poultry and pork are commonly filled with hormones given to animals for quick fattening; and high-tech processing techniques inhibit the natural deterioration of processed meats like sausage or salami. New foods and synthetic food substitutes like aspartame and newly emerging "fake fats" are rapidly dominating our selection of grocery store foods. Another change is that, unlike our grandparents, we no longer eat foods in season. Fruits and vegetables are shipped trans-continentally and are often packed in dry ice or cold storage for extended periods of time. And, of course, millions of gallons of sugary or artificially sweetened soda pop are consumed annually.

In many ways the diets of our ancestors and of many third world countries far surpass the nutritive value of our own. Primitive cultures who dine on beans, seeds, fibery vegetables, brown rice and little meat have had the right idea all along. Sadly, many of these cultures have begun to adopt Western eating habits and are now experiencing diseases like diabetes, never a problem before. The Pima Indians of Arizona's Sonora desert are a good example. For thousands of years they gathered food from their land. While food variety was scarce, they were able to single out nutrient-rich pods, cacti, and seeds. By adding tepary beans and corn, they had a health-promoting diet that kept them relatively healthy and free from what we refer to as Western diseases.

Unfortunately, this is not the case today. According to available statistics, more than 50 percent of Pimas over the age of 35 suffer from type-2, adult-onset diabetes. Why? Because these people gave up their traditional diet for one that we should all recognize: a diet high in fat, sugar, and processed foods. As a result diabetes has become more rampant and obesity common. Apparently the Pimas are particularly susceptible to adult-onset diabetes but it had remained dormant during the generations when a low-fat, high-fiber, low-sugar diet was consumed. What this implies is that all of us have certain predispositions to disease which can be triggered by our eating habits.

We might be able to get away with some of our deplorable eating habits if we exercised the way our great-grandparents did. But the reality is that we eat more, consume more fat, smoke, use alcohol and caffeine and then sit at a desk all day. While many of us have become more exercise-aware, we are still considered a sedentary society. Our dietary goals should be 1) to move away from animal-based protein to plant sources; and 2) to decrease saturated fats and sugar and increase fresh fruits, vegetables, whole grains and legumes. It's a simple formula that is possible to incorporate into daily life—especially if we realize its profound health impact. If we become diet conscious we will inevitably become health conscious as well. Simple dietary modifications enhanced by supplement use can dramatically improve our health and lower the risk of diseases many of us now accept as inevitable.

WHY DO MEDICAL SCHOOL COURSES IGNORE THE HEALTH IMPLICATIONS OF DIET?

Medical schools need to re-evaluate their curriculums and begin to address the incredible effect of diet on health. Doctors need to ask their patients questions like: "What do you normally eat for breakfast? Do you experience food-related symptoms? How do you feel about keeping a food journal for a week and then going over it together?" Learning to recognize the effects of conusmption of sugar, processed foods, and not enough fiber is tantamount to achieving not only an accurate diagnosis, but to getting to the root of the problem.

Doctors need to be more aware of the fact that a vitamin B12 shot can often help a depressed or fatigued person more than any prescription drug. They must come to realize that some muscle cramping can be alleviated with a simple calcium/magnesium supplement. Recommending vitamin E supplementation for women with fibrocystic breasts should be routine, and talking about natural sources of progesterone with every middle-aged woman should be the rule rather than the exception. These are just a few isolated examples of the role supplementation can play in medicine. Unfortunately, many doctors haven't investigated this area of disease treatment or health maintenance. I have a feeling the doctors of the future will be infinitely more well-versed on the profound role of natural remedies.

WHY THE RDA NEEDS REVISION

RDA requirements set by the government provide the minimum daily allowance of vitamins and minerals necessary to prevent illnesses caused by deficiencies, but these amounts are not necessarily the dosages needed to maintain optimal health. While it is fine to presume that food should supply us with all the nutrients we need, it is foolhardy to believe that our diets are all that nutritious. The average American diet is commonly lacking in the B vitamins, folic acid, vitamin E, vitamin C and iron. Ideally, if we routinely consume a diet comprised of unrefined, unprocessed natural foods, our nutritional needs would be met.

Unquestionably, in order to receive the maximum nutritional benefit from foods that we consume, our diet would typically have to consist of several portions of whole grain products, several servings of fresh, raw fruits and vegetables, legumes, nuts, or other protein sources and adequate, absorbable sources of calcium. Who eats like this every day?

Several studies that analyze diet have discovered that it is common to find at least three to four nutrient deficiencies even by RDA standards and significantly more by ideal set point charts. As mentioned, in a perfect world, we should get what we need from our diet. In reality, this is rarely the case.

Clearly, RDA standards for dietary nutrients designed by the government are too low in many instances and do not take into account the needs of the body when exposed to stress, pollution, toxins or disease. Many of today's foods are considered antinutrient in that they destroy or inhibit the assimilation of nutrients. Phosphorus found in soft drinks causes the body to leech out calcium and sugar and caffeine depletes the body of B-vitamins and other essential nutrients. In addition, scores of drugs can cause nutrient deficiencies, a fact which is rarely addressed by physicians who prescribe them freely. The fact is that the RDA requirements must undergo some form of revision to meet our needs.

The *Journal of Clinical Nutrition* reported that less than 10 percent of those surveyed eat a balanced diet. Dr. James Scala, Ph.D., points out that the price of supplementation is cheap considering we consume more than 60 cents worth of soft drinks per day per capita.

PROPER DIGESTION: A MAJOR PROBLEM IN THIS COUNTRY

If we were eating the right foods in the right way, we would not have to rely on gallons of the pink stuff, scores of antacids or acid inhibitors, or enormous amount of laxative medications. In other words, we need chemicals to help us digest our food, assimilate its contents and eliminate its waste byproducts. It is rather ironic that we have been designed with magnificent digestive systems that far surpass the most efficient machine ever created by man, but we still suffer from mechanical breakdowns such as abdominal cramping, inordinate amounts of gas, sluggish colons and an overall lousy feeling after ingesting a meal. Red flags go up everywhere and many of us still remain oblivious to possible problems.

Clearly, we are not eating the right foods. We consume an incredible amount of soda, drugs, caffeine, and alcohol, which impede normal digestive processes so that when we do eat, we suffer the consequences. Adding stress and eating on the run creates a combination of factors which can lead to heartburn and indigestion and may develop into ulcers and colon disease.

Simply stated, the process of digestion includes chewing our food and combining it with saliva which contains enzymes designed to begin breaking down starches. Food then travels to the stomach, an expandable pouch which secretes hydrochloric acid and other biochemicals designed to break down proteins. In the stomach is where the food is broken down into a mixture called chyme. The chyme then proceeds to the small intestine, the scene of additional digestion, absorption and the transportation of nutrients. Pancreatic and liver secretions are brought into this portion of the intestine to augment the process. It is here that the majority of nutrient absorption takes place.

Malabsorption results when part of the small intestine becomes impaired as a result of disease, injury or infection. The pancreas supplies vital enzymes which make the digestion and absorption of nutrients possible. The large intestine or colon is responsible for the absorption of water and electrolytes and provides a "holding tank" for waste storage until elimination. This reservoir of waste provides the perfect habitat for bacteria and can either serve to enhance our health or contribute to its breakdown. (It's important to remember that not all bacteria are bad.)

Surprisingly, many of us suffer from a lack of both hydrochloric acid and pancreatic enzymes, which causes us to poorly digest our food and worse yet, to poorly assimilate its nutrients. In addition, our low-fiber diets have created a veritable colon crisis where constipation and poor elimination are the rule rather than the exception.

THE NEGLECTED ROLE OF DIGESTIVE ENZYMES

As mentioned earlier, pancreatic enzymes are responsible for the proper digestion and absorption of our food. Pancreatic juices which are transported to the small intestine make it possible for us to utilize the life-giving nutrients found in the food we eat. There are three basic categories of digestive enzymes: 1) amylases, which break down starches; 2) lypases, which break down fats; and 3) proteases which are designed to break down proteins.

A lack of any of these enzymes can result in malabsorption. The proteases are especially important because they break down proteins into amino acids. Anytime a deficiency of protease exists, bits of undigested protein will stay in the body. These protein parts are thought to be responsible for the development of allergies, autoimmune diseases, and autointoxication. Proteases also keep the intestines protected from parasites and other organisms that may weaken the intestinal system. More and more evidence suggests that certain individuals have increased permeability of the digestive tracts allowing macro nutrient "bits" to pass through the walls of the stomach and subsequently end up in the bloodstream. Severe problems may result, so it is vital that we do not look at symptoms of indigestion as inconsequential.

Digestive Enzyme Supplementation

Anyone who suffers from gas, bloating, heartburn, or constipation should add digestive enzymes to their meals. The most effective are pancreatin, bromelain and papain. These can be combined with other enzymatic compounds to promote better food break down. Try to find full-strength potency products that have not been weakened by the addition of filler substances. Chewable tablets and gums are available and should be taken just prior to eating, although they can be taken after a meal. Taking digestive enzymes can make all the difference when it comes to making the most of the food we eat. In addition, these enzymes are useful in treating other seemingly unrelated diseases which further confirms the far-reaching effects of properly breaking down the nutrient content of our foods. Carry them around in your pocket or purse and get accustomed to using them. Take them just before and right after a meal. These enzymes can make all the difference and can help to lower our risk of diseases which may be caused by faulty digestion.

HYDROCHLORIC ACID DEFICIENCY

While most of us are all too aware of the plight of excess stomach acid, few of us realize that not having enough stomach acid can be a major problem. If we do not produce enough gastric acid, we can become susceptible to many unpleasant symptoms and diseases. Many of the symptoms we normally associate with indigestion could signal a deficiency of hydrochloric acid (HCL). Bloating, gas, belching, constipation or diarrhea can all indicate a lack of HCL. Some diseases which have been linked to a lack of stomach acid include diabetes, gallbladder disease, lupus, rheumatoid arthritis, and osteoporosis. The incidence of low stomach acid is common in people over the age of 60, a factor that may help explain why elderly people typically suffer from malnutrition. If you suspect you may have a HCL deficiency, take a hydrochloric acid pill with each meal. Continue to up the dose by one capsule until you feel a warm sensation in the stomach region. Stop at this point and try to take this amount throughout the meal.

FIBER

Hippocrates, the father of medicine, recommended eating whole wheat "for its salutary effects upon the bowels." Roman athletes took his admonition to heart and ate whole grains, believing that their endurance and strength would be enhanced. Ever since ancient times, whole grains were considered diet staples and were typically consumed by lower class societies who could not afford the fatty, sweet, high protein diets of their king's table.

Fiber, often called roughage, is technically a food component that remains undigested as it is processed through the gastrointestinal tract. Because it readily absorbs water, fiber helps to form the bulk required to form a good bowel movement.

Technically, fiber is a complex carbohydrate consisting of a polysaccharide and a lignin substance that gives structure to the cell of a plant. Insoluble fiber has the ability to pass through the intestines intact and virtually unchanged. Unlike fats, carbohydrates and proteins, fiber does not provide the body with nutrients or fuel for energy. It usually has no caloric value. Dietary fiber is found only in plant components such as vegetables, fruits and whole grains. There are primarily two categories of fiber: soluble and insoluble. Some foods contain both types.

Kinds of Fiber

There are seven forms of fiber (insoluble and soluble), each with its own specific function.

1. Pectin

Pectin slows the absorption of food after meals, and is recommended for anyone with hypoglycemia or diabetes because blood glucose levels rise more gradually. Pectin also has the ability to help remove toxins and metals, reduce blood cholesterol levels, and reduce the risk of heart disease and gallstones. It can also bind bile acids to keep our gallbladders healthy.

how much fiber do we need?

A good diet should include 25 to 35 grams of fiber or at least one ounce of dietary fiber each and every day. Some health practitioners are recommending up to 50 grams of fiber per day. Two thirds of that fiber should be insoluble. Adding wheat bran to your diet is the easiest way to boost your fiber intake. The average American eats from 9 to 13 grams of fiber per day. The ideal barometer of determining if you're getting enough fiber is whether you have a good bowel movement at least every 24 hours. Your transit time is very important. Unless you suffer from certain bowel conditions like Crohn's disease or ulcerative colitis, some experts believe that you can't get too much fiber. Note: Make sure you're not hypersensitive or allergic to grain and certain high fiber legumes. An intolerance to gluten can result in gas, diarrhea, and abdominal cramping, which can result in celiac disease and mal-absorption of nutrients.

Sources of pectin: Carrots, beets, cabbage, citrus fruits, apples, grapes, bananas, cabbage, okra and dried peas, green beans, onion skin and sugar beet pulp.

2. Cellulose

Cellulose, an insoluble source of fiber, is a carbohydrate that is the main structural component in the outer covering of vegetables and fruits. It is the fibrous part of the cell walls of these plants. Cellulose helps to nourish the blood vessels so it is beneficial for varicose veins, colitis, constipation and hemorrhoids. Cellulose also has the proven ability to rid the colon of carcinogenic substances and significantly increase fecal weight. It binds up water impressively. Make sure to check what kind of cellulose you may be getting when you buy certain food items.

Sources of cellulose: Wheat bran, beets, peas, broccoli, carrots, lima beans, pears, apples, Brazil nuts, whole grains and green beans.

3. Hemicellulose

Like cellulose, hemicellulose is not digestible and is considered a complex carbohydrate. It comprises the matrix of cell walls of plants which are filled with cellulose fibers. This type of cellulose is chemically broken down through the action of certain friendly bacteria in the bowel and can cause gas in some individuals. Hemicellulose has a remarkable ability to retain water. It is recommended for weight loss, colon cancer, constipation and for removing cancer causing substances which can inhabit the bowel.

Sources of hemicellulose: Psyllium seeds, oat bran, apples, pears, bananas, beans, corn, cabbage, whole grains, peppers, and green vegetables.

An example of hemicellulose is psyllium seed, a hardy botanical whose seed husk is an excellent intestinal cleaner and stool softener. It is commonly used in several over-the-counter laxatives. Psyllium thickens very quickly, as anyone whose mixed up a glass of Metamucil knows. Psyllium seeds are covered with mucilage that swells when it comes in contact with water. For this reason it bulks up the stool and promotes bowel movements. Mucilage can also help soothe inflamed tissue. The value of psyllium for keeping blood cholesterol levels down has recently been confirmed. Even the American Heart Association recommends adding psyllium to our diet for its cholesterol-lowering properties.

The typical dose of psyllium is one to two rounded teaspoons in a full glass of water taken after a meal. Psyllium is safe for children and can be taken consistently with few or no side effects. Familiar laxatives which use psyllium include Metamucil, Correctol and Fiberall. Many natural health advocates recommend using natural laxatives with psyllium that do not also contain artificial colors or metals like aluminum. Also be aware that many of the psyllium products sold in the United States have been diluted with rice hulls.

4. Lignin

Lignin is a non-carbohydrate cell wall material that is made up of chemical polymers and aromatic alcohols. Lignin contributes to the rigidity of plant cell walls and inhibits cell wall digestion by intestinal bacteria. Lignin has shown its ability to help lower blood serum cholesterol levels and to prevent the formation of gallstones. It does this by binding with bile acids that can ultimately contribute to the formation of stones. It is also transformed by intestinal bacteria into a type of lignin that helps inhibit the action of estrogens which have been linked to the development of breast cancer. Lignin is recommended for anyone with diabetes, breast cancer, or colon cancer.

Sources of lignin: Flaxseed, wheat, potatoes, apples, cabbage, peaches, tomatoes, strawberries, Brazil nuts, carrots, peas and green beans.

5. Gums

Gums are complex polysaccharides that are water soluble. Their role in plants is to repair damaged areas. Various gums and mucilagees are used in fat-free foods to create that gooey, creamy texture. Most of the gums in the following list are extruded from the stems or seeds of tropical or sub-tropical trees and shrubs. They can form gels in the small intestine and bind with acid and other organic waste material.

Guar gum (guar flour): Comes from a plant native to India and is tasteless, odorless and completely water soluble. It serves as a protective colloid, a thickener, and is primarily used in very thick viscous liquids or spreadable foods.

Gum Arabic: Comes from the acacia tree and consists of a variety of sugars. It is commonly used to maintain food product flavor and lengthen shelf life.

Flaxseed Gum: Used as a substitute for gum arabic, this gum is used in similar applications. The whole flaxseed is sometimes added to cereals for its laxative action.

Karaya Gum (Indian Tragacanth): A white, slightly acidic gum with a mild acidy odor, karaya serves as a texturizer, thickener and food emulsifier.

Locust Seed Gum (Carob Flour): Swells in cold water and goes clear in hot. It has a legume-like flavor and serves as a binder and thickener. It has been used as a substitute for cocoa, chocolate and coffee.

Psyllium Seed Gum: Psyllium seeds are one of the best natural laxative promoters. As a gum, psyllium has a very high level of soluble dietary fiber and is added to some cereal products for this reason.

Xanthin Gum: Usually sold as a potassium salt, xanthin gum is a microbial gum. It serves to form a film, has good heat resistance, and can stabilize and thicken food products.

6. Mucilages

Mucilages are routinely obtained from seed and seaweeds and are used as thickening and stabilizing agents. They effectively hold water and can be excellent bulking agents.

Sources of mucilages: Legumes, psyllium, guar.

Agar: A sweet mucilage that can remain stable in high temperatures and is often used for thickening dairy products and confections.

Alginate: Extracted from brown seaweed, it gives foods a creamy texture and inhibits the formation of ice crystals. (This is one of the mystery ingredients often listed on ice cream cartons.)

Carrageenan: Another seaweed mucilage that is typically used to gel and emulsify certain foods.

Bran Fibers

The word bran refers to the fibrous covering that surrounds certain whole grains. Bran is technically referred to as a cereal fiber and is the portion of the grain discarded from whole wheat as waste in modern milling processes. Bran has excellent stool-bulking capacities and can significantly reduce transit time. To a great degree, bran was not much consumed after the introduction of refined flours. It's no coincidence that as bran consumption dwindled the incidence of certain so-called Western diseases escalated. Bran has the ability to hold water better than any other source of fiber. Different cereal brans have different chemical construction so their ability to retain water can vary, but they all hold more water than other fibers.

Oat Bran

Oat bran is made by grinding the inner husk of the whole oat grain. Over the last decade, oat bran has enjoyed a high level of publicity—some good, some not so good. When original scientific findings on the benefits of oat bran hit the media, an oat bran frenzy resulted. While eating oat bran may not get rid of cellulite, it can help to lower blood cholesterol, thereby preventing heart disease. Study after study has confirmed that consistently eating oat bran can lower high blood serum cholesterol as much as 20 percent or more. Even already low blood cholesterol can be reduced by 5 percent when consuming daily doses of oat bran. It is the soluble fiber found in oat bran that makes it an impressive fiber source. Remember that oatmeal, the ground version of the whole oat grain, contains about one third less fiber than the bran.

Can You Get Too Much Fiber?

Some health care experts believe that eating more than 35 grams of fiber per day may adversely affect vitamin and mineral absorption. While this is technically true, rarely does anyone eat near that amount of fiber. Most of us don't eat even the small amount we need. While it is true that some fibers may absorb calcium, zinc, iron and magnesium, and while the presence of fiber in the intestines may inhibit the absorption of certain nutrients, these effects are present only under extreme conditions. In other words, don't let the fear of becoming nutrient deficient stop you from boosting you fiber intake. This particular phenomenon does not pose a significant threat. The marvelous benefits of fiber far outweigh the remote possibility that you will eat quantities large enough to pose any problem.

Remember to add fiber gradually, drink plenty of water and chew your food thoroughly so that the necessary digestive enzymes will be activated in the saliva. Some people believe that taking supplemental digestive enzymes right before eating fiber can cut down on the formation of gas.

In her book, *The Complete Fiber Fact Book*, Rita Elkins lists some simple ways to increase fiber intake:

- Take a good fiber supplement every morning with breakfast or 30 minutes before any meal.
- Grab a handful of oat cereal when you need to snack.
- Add bran, millet, barley etc. to your meatloaves, casseroles, pancakes, cake and cookie batters, stuffings, and compotes.
- Use crunchy granola cereals or barley nuts as a topping for ice cream, yogurt, baked potatoes, fish, salads, etc. Adding whole wheat that has been soaked to salads is delicious. Always add seeds or fresh raw fruit to make yogurt more fiber acceptable, and only buy active culture yogurts.
- Eat fresh, raw fruit and vegetables with their peelings whenever possible.
- Reach for prunes, dates, or figs when you need to appease your sweet tooth instead of cookies, candies or juice.
- Look for fiber-rich foods offered in salad bars and add them liberally (broccoli, carrots, red beans, garbanzo beans, sunflower seeds, etc.)
- Get in the habit of sprouting your own legumes. Peas, lentils, mung beans, garbanzo beans, lentils, soybeans and wheat can all be sprouted and make delicious additions to tossed green salads.
- Buy canned, precooked beans of all kinds and add them to salads, soups, casseroles and stews.
- Keep a good supply of grains on hand that you can add to any recipe to make it more "fibery." Good grains are millet, barley, brown rice, whole oats and whole wheat.

Faulty Fiber Sources

Several misconceptions exist about certain foods that are thought to be high in fiber. One of the most common is that if you eat a lot of lettuce salads, you're getting plenty of fiber. Lettuce, tomatoes and even celery are not good fiber sources. They are, in fact, much lower in fiber than legumes and whole grains. So while these veggies provide some fiber, by themselves they are an insufficient source.

Another misconception is that a food is high in fiber just because the label says wheat, wheatberry, multigrain, natural, fortified, etc. None of these terms means the whole grain has been used. In fact, many products labeled with such terms are mostly comprised of white flour. Even the term "whole wheat" doesn't necessarily mean that all of the flour used has been milled from the whole grain. Caramel coloring is frequently added to food products to make them appear more natural.

Watch out for high-fat baked goods that are disguised as fiber rich foods. Oat-bran doughnuts, cookies or even tortilla chips are commonly high in fat and sugar and notoriously low in oat bran. A *New York Times* survey showed that some so-called oat bran muffins contain so little oat bran they are virtually useless as a source of fiber. Also, a single bran muffin can contain as much fat as three lunch-size bags of potato chips. Just because it has bran in it doesn't necessarily make it good for you.

Fiber—Elimination and Disease

We've already discussed the types of diseases which seem to specifically target western cultures. High-fat, high-protein, low-fiber diets exact a devastating toll on our health and will cause thousands of premature deaths and an enormous amount of physical infirmity. Dr. Arbuthnot Lane served as surgeon to the King of England in the early 1900s and spent several years specializing in bowel problems. He noticed that after he removed diseased sections of the bowel, his patients were remarkably and unexpectedly cured of completely unrelated diseases such as arthritis and goiter. From such observations he concluded that there is a causal relationship between a toxic colon and other organs of the body. His advice was to care for the bowel through good nutrition. Dr. Lane's work is receiving validation as scientists today are beginning to understand and accept that the condition of the colon is intrinsically related to all body systems and can potentially affect numerous chronic diseases, including cancer. Zolton P. Rona, M.D., MSc., has stated:

". . . many degenerative diseases are brought about by toxins generated in the large bowel. Bacterial flora imbalance, putrefaction of undigested foods, parasitic and yeast infections may be at the bottom of many diseases."

Burkitt and Trowell, two doctors famous for their work on the health implications of fiber, express the simple importance of fiber in the following hypothesis: A diet rich in foods which contain fiber or plant cell walls (legumes, whole grains, fruits and vegetables) can protect the human body against a wide variety of serious diseases which have specifically attacked western cultures. A diet low in fiber or plant cell walls can cause the incidence of these western diseases.

Fiber: The Single Best Nutrient to Prevent Autointoxication

Intestinal toxemia or autointoxication is linked to what you eat because what you eat determines the kind of bacteria that will inhabit your bowel. For example, if you eat a lot of complex carbohydrates, which are usually fiber-rich, and little protein, your intestinal flora will primarily consist of bacteria designed to metabolize carbohydrates. On the other hand, if your diet is high in protein and low in complex carbohydrates, bowel bacteria will be of the proteolytic type that breaks down and decomposes protein. This type of bacteria releases harmful gases and toxins that often remain in the colon and find their way back onto the body. Unhealthy intestinal flora also create adverse chemical reactions which can result in the production of powerful toxins.

Eating refined foods, a lot of meat and little fiber causes delayed elimination. Consequently, poisons, such as phenols, form in the colon. Some health experts believe that the presence of phenol in the body can be linked to a whole host of diseases ranging from allergies to arthritis to cancer, back pain and even mental illness. The unexplained incidence of autoimmune diseases like lupus may be linked to this phenomenon.

Boosting your fiber intake while reducing animal protein and fats can decrease the amount of proteolytic bacteria in the colon which contribute to the putrefaction of food waste. Any food material which enters the colon is subject to breakdown by the bacterial flora of the colon. Dietary fiber reaches the colon intact and provides a major source of energy for intestinal bacteria. In addition, studies have shown that in as little as two weeks, intestinal micro flora can be altered by increasing your intake of dietary fiber. Because dietary fiber affects several vital metabolic processes, eating enough of it is crucial to maintaining good health and preventing disease. Diseases which are specifically impacted by the consumption of dietary fiber include

- ◆ appendicitis
- ◆ breast cancer
- ◆ colitis
- ◆ colon and colorectal cancer
- ◆ constipation
- ◆ coronary heart disease/cholesterol
- ◆ Crohn's disease
- ◆ dental carries
- ◆ diverticular disease
- ◆ duodenal ulcers
- ◆ gallstones
- ◆ hemorrhoids
- ◆ hiatal hernia
- ◆ hypertension
- ◆ irritable bowel syndrome
- ◆ kidney stones
- ◆ obesity
- ◆ periodontal disease
- ◆ pernicious anemia
- ◆ prostate cancer
- ◆ rheumatoid arthritis
- ◆ varicose veins

While these diseases are certainly serious enough, a lack of fiber has also been linked with gout, autoimmune disorders, multiple sclerosis and various skin disorders.

AUTOINTOXICATION: FACT OR FICTION?

This section addresses the role of pathogenic bacteria in the colon. Most of us are aware that maintaining healthy intestinal flora (bacteria) is absolutely essential for health preservation. Unfortunately, if our diets are poor and we suffer from a sluggish colon, harmful bacteria flourish and contribute to putrefaction and toxicity. Today, to make matters worse, we rarely replenish friendly flora by eating good sources of acidophilus (live bacteria). Moreover, we routinely kill our own friendly bacteria by using antibiotics, other drugs, alcohol, etc. What we end up creating is the perfect habitat for pathogenic bacteria to flourish. Consequently, our colon becomes nothing more than a toxic waste dump.

One of the best ways to keep your colon healthy is to eat a high-fiber diet. Unfortunately, diets high in fiber faded away with the advent of "new and improved" foods: refined, artificially synthesized, soft, white and without character. In other words, the fiber famine we are experiencing now is a result of decades of consuming rice that has had its brown fibrous coat removed, flour that has been bleached and its bran removed, and the exchange of fibery legumes like beans and lentils for greasy hamburgers and fries.

What is Transit Time?

"Transit time" simply refers to how long it takes food to travel from your mouth to your stomach to your small intestine to your colon. Western nations that eat diets low in fiber have longer transit times than third world countries. It is commonplace for an American to have a transit time of three days to two weeks (in cases of severe constipation) while in cultures where whole grains, fruits and plants are routinely consumed, 8 to 35 hours is the usual transit time.

Normally, adults who eat from 35 to 45 grams of fiber every day have an average transit time of approximately 36 to 48 hours. Transit time can vary from person to person and can be 24 percent slower for women than for men. Changes in transit time from one day to the next are also common, but it is not normal to have three bowel movements a day and then go without one for a week.

You can test your transit time by eating beets, taking two tablespoons of liquid chlorophyll, or ingesting charcoal tablets which can be purchased at your pharmacy. Record when you ate the beets or took the tablets and watch for either the purple or the black to show up after a bowel movement. Ideally, the trip should take less than 36 hours. If it takes longer, look at your diet and beef up on fiber. Increasing the fiber content of your diet is the one most important thing you can do to decrease your transit time. In *Eating Right for a Bad Gut*, Dr. James Scala writes, "Adding guar gum to food increased the transit time by 75 minutes, pectin by 15 minutes, and cellulose had no effect. This tells us that the largest amount of time that food spends in our body is its residence in the large intestine. But it also tells us that passage through the small intestine is influenced by fiber."

Summary

1. The longer waste material stays trapped in the colon, the more the risk of potentially harmful situations increases. When putrefaction occurs, toxic compounds are created. They often find their way back into the bloodstream and the liver has to filter them out again. This process is referred to as autointoxication by some health care practitioners. Some of the toxic compounds include

- bile salts
- volatile fatty acids
- heavy metals
- pigments and preservatives
- phenol
- cadaverine
- butyric acid
- botulin
- putrescine
- ammonia
- creosol
- sepsin

2. Long transit times are usually associated with poorly formed stool that lacks water. People who have to strain to have a bowel movement put additional pressure on the intestines and may be prone to developing hemorrhoids and diverticula.

3. Long transit times can result in chronic intestinal gas and even in diarrhea, which can actually be a form of constipation.

COLON CLEANSING

As I have studied acupuncture and its philosophy, the notion of cleansing the bowel began to make a lot of sense to me. I have seen some impressive results from bowel cleansing One of my patients, a 54-year-old woman, came to see me for fatigue. She had a high cholesterol count in the 350 range and her triglyceride level was approximately 1200. She was also chronically tired due to a metabolic derangement that stressed her liver and digestive system. Under my direction she went through a bowel cleanse along with an herbal and supplement regimen. At the end of the cleanse, her cholesterol and triglyceride levels had fallen considerably and she was amazed that she had regained about 90 percent of her energy.

Now, this doesn't mean that all people with chronic fatigue syndrome will be cured by cleansing their bowels, but it does mean that we could benefit from a bowel cleanse at least yearly, if not twice a year. Colon cleansing is an often overlooked therapy when designing a treatment program for disease. When you follow a colon cleansing regimen based on a specific herbal blend, you will notice increased urine production, more bowel movements and, for some people, an enhanced feeling of well-being. Cleansing your colon can improve overall physiologic function. Herbs designed to augment liver function should be added to your cleansing blend in combination with blood purifiers. When the bowel is functioning well, all other organs benefit. The intestines more efficiently absorb nutrients, the liver detoxifies the blood and our defense mechanism functions more effectively.

Colon Cleanse Herbal Formula

Generally speaking a good colon cleanse combination will include herbs to stimulate colon muscles, herbs to prevent gas and cramping, blood purifying botanicals and a fiber source. NOTE: Cascara sagrada should be the primary herbal constituent of blends designed to promote elimination. A typical colon cleansing formula can include a combination of some of the following herbs:

- acidophilus
- aloe vera
- black walnut
- buckthorn
- burdock
- butternut
- capsicum
- cascara sagrada
- fennel
- garlic
- ginger
- Irish moss
- peppermint
- psyllium hulls
- pumpkin seeds
- red clover
- senna
- slippery elm

The purpose of blends that use the herbs listed is to provide nutritive support while stimulating intestinal cleansing and detoxification. Ridding the intestines of parasites, cleansing the blood and strengthening the liver and gallbladder are also involved in optimal colon cleansing. Frequently, seemingly unrelated health problems can be traced to a sluggish or congested colon. Harboring toxic waste in the large intestine can pose a significant health risk. Carcinogens, altered hormones and other poisonous chemical compounds can be reabsorbed into the body if not eliminated properly. In addition, disorders like chronic constipation attest to poor dietary habits and a lack of colonic health. These herbs provide the optimal blend for colon function which will, inevitably, improve overall health.

Most herbal blends are comprised of what might be called dominant, more active plants that are usually responsible for primary therapeutic actions. These are combined with more passive herbs that serve to soothe, support and potentiate. Stimulatory herbs are usually of the bitter variety and are very nicely complemented by aromatic, carminative and demulcent herbs. For example, senna is a stimulatory herb which initiates colon muscle contraction. Adding ginger, a carminative, to senna soothes the stomach and prevents gripping which may occur if senna was taken alone. The addition of capsicum to any herb formula acts as a catalyst, increasing the efficiency of each individual herb.

A colon cleanse usually starts with a fast that is followed by a juice diet and herbal supplementation. Eating only raw foods for a short period of time is also recommended, combined with as many glasses of pure water as you can sustain. Drinking hot water with fresh squeezed lemon juice upon arising is recommended for stimulating the liver. Certain tea formulations can be used instead of capsulized herbs to stimulate colonic muscle and initiate bowel emptying. If you feel nauseated use ginger supplements and clear soups.

FASTING

Fasting may seem like a rather drastic measure to take to help the body rid itself of toxic substances, yet it is considered a safe and very effective method. The idea of fasting is based on the belief that abstaining from food affords the body a chance to rest from the work of digestion, assimilation and elimination. Instead of having to spend energy on these processes, the body can concentrate on flushing out toxins and other harmful substances that accumulate over time. It is always a good idea to make your doctor or other health care professional aware that you are fasting. If you have any kind of a serious condition, such as diabetes, hypoglycemia, or if you take any medication, make sure to check with your physician before you begin a fast.

Advocates of fasting suggest that we make it a regular monthly event and usually suggest a fast of one to three days. Also, if you feel yourself becoming ill, it helps to stop eating solid food. When you fast, remember that supplementation and the use of good, nutritious food after the fast is completed will extend its therapeutic benefits.

There are several different types of fasts. Juice fasts consist of eating nothing but freshly squeezed or extracted fruit and vegetable juices. Green drink fasts utilize spirulina, chlorophyll and other green food supplements. Drink only pure water or diluted juices with no added sweeteners. Stay away from citrus juices. Cabbage, beet, carrot, celery, grape, and apple juice are recommended. Raw cabbage juice is good for ulcers, cancer, and colon problems.

Using herb teas while fasting can also be effective. Pau d'arco and echinacea herb teas help to boost immunity. Dandelion, red clover, alfalfa, and chamomile teas detoxify the blood and settle the stomach. Vegetable broths are also good. Liquid mineral supplements or garlic extracts can also promote healing. Continue to take your vitamin and mineral supplements while fasting. Don't chew gum. It will only serve to stimulate gastric juices, making the fast uncomfortable.

FOOD ALLERGIES

What is a food allergy exactly? Food allergies or sensitivities do not trigger the same kind of symptoms we normally associate with allergies such as sneezing, wheezing, hives, runny nose, etc. A food allergy is based on some type of immune malfunction, which has its origins in the digestive system. Because of this reason, some scientists are slow to recognize the reality of food allergies nevertheless, their far reaching symptoms and very marked effects on certain susceptible people cannot be ignored. What we eat can and does affect how we feel, both physically and emotionally.

A great number of health care experts support the notion that food allergies can cause hyperkinetic behavior in children. For this reason hyperactive children or those diagnosed with Attention Deficit Disorder (ADD) are immediately taken off of sugar, wheat and chemical additives. While the evidence is not totally conclusive, enough data suggests that hyperactivity is related to food choices. In other words, certain foods initiate a cascade effect in susceptible individuals causing a dramatic change in mood and behavior.

Elisa Lotter, Ph.D., relates the story of Henry, a mentally disturbed seventeen year old who had been on tranquilizers, electric shock treatments, and psychotherapy for several years with no significant improvement. He was subsequently placed on a strict fast in which he was given only spring water. After four days he experienced a complete reversal of symptoms, until the fifth day, in which he was given a meal consisting of only wheat. Within an hour, he began to experience negative, paranoid thoughts. Further testing confirmed that when certain foods were withheld from Henry, his symptoms disappeared; when they were added back, he became mentally disturbed once again. Doctors Philpott and Kalita, in their book *Brain Allergies*, discuss the very significant mental impact that dairy products and cereal grains have in some schizophrenics. The implication is that hidden food sensitivities and intolerances may be responsible for a number of emotional disorders in certain susceptible people.

The very nature of what we eat is often unknown to us. In other words, we open microwaveable dinners, brightly colored boxes, and gladly ingest a number of mystery ingredients and chemicals. Marshall Mandell, M.D., has written two books and numerous scientific papers on the subject of food intolerance. He says, "Contemporary mass-production strips food of many valuable nutrients that, were they left intact, would provide protective benefits." When humans tamper with natural food substances they can become contaminants rather than nutrients to the body. Such contaminants can trigger a change in mood or other physiological response. During an allergic reaction, for example, the body leaks histamine from the capillaries, which can cause edema or swelling around them. Dr. Mandell believes that the same reaction can take place in brain cells when you eat a culprit food, causing a disruption in brain chemistry. In addition, in the same way that muscle spasms cause the bronchiole tubes to constrict during an allergic asthma attack, Dr. Mandell proposes that similar spasms in the small arteries of the brain can reduce the flow of glucose, oxygen and other nutrients to brain tissue. Both of these scenarios would naturally precipitate a change in behavior or mood.

Regardless of the mechanisms, sensitivities to certain foods can make us feel mentally and physically depressed. This is the reason some people feel unusually good when they fast. Food sensitivities have been linked to autoimmune diseases, inflammatory bowel diseases, and a number of mental disorders.

Symptoms of Food Sensitivities

Multiple symptoms are typical of food intolerances and should be watched for. In her book, *Depression and Natural Medicine*, Rita Elkins talks about golfer Billy Casper, who complained for years of weight gain, stomach aliments, sinus congestion, backaches, headaches and bad temper. Apparently, after some investigation and testing, he was found to be sensitive to beet sugar, lamb, apples, pork, eggs, citrus fruit, wheat and any fruits or vegetables fertilized with nitrates or sprayed with chemicals. Billy Casper changed his lifestyle and diet, and as a result, his health and moods significantly improved. The most common symptoms of a food allergy in adults are depression, headaches and fatigue. Mood changes can range from mild forms of anxiety to feeling seriously depressed. Manic outbursts of uncontrollable anger are also possible. The relationship between food allergies and even schizophrenia has been proposed.

Two types of reactions can occur if you eat something you are sensitive to. One, there can be an immediate reaction characterized by symptoms that quickly occur and are easy to recognize. If you eat shrimp and break out in hives or develop an unusual headache, you know the shrimp is probably responsible. It's the second type of reaction to a food that is more difficult to identify because it may not occur for a day or two. If you eat a large meal and various foods on Sunday, you may feel overly fatigued, lethargic and depressed on Tuesday. In such a case, connecting your symptoms to a meal you ate two days ago is unlikely.

Several medical journals in the 1980s published articles proposing that delayed food allergies cause nearly all cases of migraine headaches. In addition, reports in the *Journal of Arthritis and Rheumatism* disclosed that many cases of rheumatoid and osteoarthritis cleared up when certain offending foods were removed from the diet. In fact, when some test groups fasted, their arthritic symptoms all but disappeared. What this suggests is that a major malfunction causes food particles to trigger a series of biochemical events, causing them to act as inflammatory agents and affecting joints, creating what appears to be arthritis. For this reason, perhaps calling this phenomenon a food allergy is not totally accurate because the same kind of immune processes that occur with a typical allergy are not found in these situations.

Foods Commonly Associated with Allergic Reactions

The following foods are commonly associated with allergic reactions:

- all dairy products
- wheat products
- yeast
- corn and corn by-products (corn syrup, sweeteners, oil, etc.)
- chocolate
- shellfish
- eggs
- nuts
- berry fruits or fruit peelings
- food additives and preservatives

Sulfite Food Allergies

Many of the foods we buy contain sulfides, additives designed to preserve and prevent discoloration. Sulfides are typically added to dehydrated foods, some canned foods such as tuna, and some frozen foods. Anyone who suffers from unexplained allergic symptoms may be sulfite-sensitive. Sulfite allergies can create a wide variety of reactions in certain individuals. The most common symptoms of sulfite sensitivity include dizziness, hot flashes, runny nose, headaches, stomach cramps, and irritability. The symptoms of a sulfite reaction usually occur soon after consumption. If you experience any of these or other symptoms, check for sulfite content. If you suffer from severe allergic reactions or asthma, sulfites can pose a significant risk to your health and may cause you to go into labored breathing or even anaphylactic shock.

Foods that commonly contain sulfites include canned sea food, dried fish, fresh shell fish, shrimp, scallops, oysters, and lobster. Sulfites can be listed on a product label as potassium bisulfite, sodium sulfite, sodium bisulfite, sulfur dioxide, or any ingredient that ends in "sulfite." Make sure to get into the habit of checking ingredient labels. Ask your pharmacist about this home test kit. For more information write to: Sulfitest Center Laboratories, 35 Channel Drive, Port Washington, NY 11050, or call (800) 645-6335.

What To Do if You Suspect a Food Allergy

One of the easiest ways to determine if you are suffering from a food allergy is to keep track of your pulse rate after eating. Sit quietly and count the number of beats that occur in a minute. A normal pulse ranges between 50 to 70 beats per minute. After you have recorded your pulse, eat the food in question. Wait 20 minutes and then take your pulse. If you find that your pulse rate has increased within 10 beats, omit the food from your diet for a time and later try the test again. Keep the foods that you test in their purest and most simple form.

Keeping a food journal in which you list everything you eat and how your feel afterwards is also recommended. This record enables you to eliminate individual foods for certain time periods and assess your symptoms. It is somewhat time consuming, but it can help to pinpoint culprit foods. Remember that what you eat on the weekend can determine how you feel Monday morning. You can also purchase special testing strips to help determine the presence of sulfites.

How to Determine If You are Food Sensitive

Discovering if foods are causing allergies is rather tricky. Typically, we continue eating foods which initiate sensitivity reactions in our bodies, creating a vicious cycle of symptoms we can't trace to one source or time. For this reason, going on an elimination diet is probably the most effective way to pinpoint those foods which cause adverse responses. It's a simple premise: When you stop eating certain foods, you will feel markedly better. Generally speaking, each food you eliminate should not be eaten for at least a week to make sure that no trace of that food remains in the body. Eliminating foods for two to six weeks is even better.

While elimination is far from an exact science, it will be up to you to make a list of foods that you think are likely to be a problem. You can begin rather slowly by eliminating all

examples of food additives recognized as safe by the FDA

Cysteine	Butylated hydroxy toluene	Sodium carbonate
Disodium phosphate	Linoleic acid	Propyl gallate
Magnesium hydrochloride	Sodium pyrophosphate, tetra	Methionine
Sodium hexametaphosphate	Methylparaben	Chondrus extract
Nitrous oxide	Manganese glycerophosphate	Sodium citrate
Ascorbic acid	Acacia (gum arabic)	Propylparaben
Inositol	Sodium acetate	Sodium ascorbate
Sodium metaphosphate	Potassium bisulfite	Niacin
Papain	Manganese hypophosphite	Guar gum
Ascorbyl palmitate	Agar-agar	Methylcellulose
Iron, reduced	Sodium acid pyrophosphate	Sodium benzoate
Sodium phosphate	Potassium metabisulfite	Glycocholic acid
Phosphoric acid	Manganese sulfate	Tocopherols
Benzoic acid	Ammonium alginate	Mono and diglycerides
Isoleucine	Sodium aluminum phosphate	Tocopherol acetate
Histidine	Potassium sorbate	Bentonite
Sodium potassium tartrate	Manganous oxide	Aconitic acid
Potassium acidtartrate	Calcium alginate	Butane
Butylated hydroxy anisole	Sodium bicarbonate	Anethole
Leucine	Propionic acid	Tyrosine
Sodium pyrophosphate	Mannitol	Benzaldehyde
Potassium bicarbonate	Carob bean gum	Magnesium carbonate

From G.O. Kermode, Food Additives in Human Nutrition: Readings from Scientific American, W.H. Freeman and Co., San Francisco, 1978.

fish, nuts, white bread, white sugar and citrus fruits and going on a diet of just chicken and rice to assess your physiological response. A better approach would be to exclude foods that you eat the most often. What is challenging about this type of test is to eat only food items with no hidden ingredients. Drugs, supplements, etc., may also contribute to allergic reactions and must be taken into consideration. Just be sure to never discontinue a medication without your doctor's approval.

While you want to be aware of your body and any changes, keep in mind that people who try an elimination diet will often go through an adjustment period when they actually become worse. This usually happens within a day of beginning the program. Some people feel downright sick. What this strongly suggests is that the foods excluded are indeed problem foods. In time, if you don't break down and eat the foods again, you will start to feel 100 percent better. Then you will be able to slowly reintroduce single foods into your diet. Watch your symptoms and don't introduce foods too quickly. Try one every five days. Keep a journal of what you eat, when you eat it and how you feel afterwards. Try to find patterns or consistencies with certain foods and subsequent symptoms over time.

SOY-BASED FOODS

I often tell my patients that the consumption of soy-based foods such as tofu or soy-based drinks can help decrease the incidence of breast and prostate cancer. Significant scientific evidence supports this particular effect. In addition, soy-based foods also help to lower total cholesterol levels while raising "good" HDL levels. The isoflavones found in soy are very impressive and should be consumed by every woman. They have the distinct ability to block the effects of bad estrogen in breast tissue and have multiple anticarcinogenic properties as well. I would advise everyone to add tofu to their recipes. My experience with tofu has been that it can be easily added to soups, salads, and many cooked foods.

FOOD ADDITIVES

Most of us would agree that as a nation we eat an enormous amount of processed and preserved foods. In fact what we refer to as "food" sometimes constitutes a real stretch of the imagination. Michael Jacobson, in the April 1975 edition of *Smithsonian*, stated, "The United States, not surprisingly, has been the leader in the genetic engineering of food crops and in the laboratory creation of new foods. Benjamin Franklin and Abraham Lincoln, if they could visit us, would probably have some difficulty distinguishing between a toy store and a super market. They would not even recognize as foods such products as artificial whipped cream in its pressurized can, or some breakfast 'cereals' that are almost half sugar and bear little resemblance to cereal grains. . . . Many of the new foods do save us time and trouble, but they are often costly, in terms of both dollars and, ultimately, health."

SUGAR AND ARTIFICIAL SWEETENERS

The average American eats over 125 pounds of white sugar every year. It has been estimated that sugar makes up 25 percent of our daily caloric intake, with soda pop supplying the majority of that intake. Desserts and sugar-laden snacks constantly tempt us and our taste for rich desserts escalates as we consume more and more. Americans eat an average of 15 quarts of ice cream per person per year. In excess amounts, sugar can be toxic. Sufficient amounts of B-vitamins are actually required to metabolize and detoxify sugar in our bodies. When we overload our bodies with sugar, we can inhibit the assimilation of nutrients from other foods. In other words, our bodies are not designed to cope with the high quantity of sugar we routinely ingest. Too much sugar can generate a type of nutrient malnutrition which, according to a number of experts, can affect the way we behave and feel. In addition, too much sugar can predispose us to yeast infections, aggravate some types of arthritis and asthma, cause tooth decay, and may elevate the level of blood lipids.

Why Do We Crave Sugar?

Considering how potentially damaging sugar can be, why do we eat so much of it? Our extraordinary craving for sugar stems from a complex mix of physiological and psychological components. Even the most brilliant scientists fail to totally comprehend this intriguing chemical dependence which, for the most part, hurts our health. A sweet tooth can contribute to PMS, osteoporosis, coronary artery disease, diabetes, obesity and depression.

Ironically, most of our children don't think of sugary foods as special treats anymore. For some, they are a dietary staple. Twenty years ago, candy was only available to most American children at Christmas or Halloween. A fresh orange in the Christmas stocking was considered a wonderful and sweet delicacy. Today, however, our homes, schools and workplaces are loaded with candy, cookies, cakes, sugar cereals, and soda. The fact that sweets often serve as a reward for good behavior compounds the problem further.

Some experts believe that sugar is physically addictive. In his book *Sugar Blues*, William Dufty writes, "The difference between sugar addiction and narcotic addiction is largely one of degree." Perhaps it would be more accurate to refer to sugar as a substance that has drug-like properties. In and of itself, a moderate amount of sugar consumed now and then may be perfectly harmless to most people. But because of sugar's easy access, over-indulging occurs all to often.

Hypoglycemia: A Sign of the Times

It is rather disturbing to learn that statisticians estimate that almost 20 million Americans suffer from some type of faulty glucose tolerance. Hypoglycemia and diabetes are the two major forms of blood sugar disorders and are deservedly called modern-day plagues. Much controversy has surrounded hypoglycemia within the medical establishment. Unfortunately, the majority of physicians shake their heads when you mention the term hypoglycemia. Most doctors believe that this condition is extremely rare or is directly related to diabetics who may get too much insulin. Because hypoglycemia is rarely understood by the medical community, it is often brushed off as a bogus malady. One reason for this denial is the inadequacies of the five-hour glucose tolerance test (GTT) as an effective diagnostic tool.

In reality, hypoglycemia is believed to cause a great deal of misery. Moreover, new studies are revealing that certain psychological disorders are directly linked to disturbed glucose utilization in brain cells. One study in particular showed that depressed people have overall lower glucose metabolism. The truth is that many normal and otherwise healthy people experience dramatic swings in their blood sugar levels. Low blood sugar, in fact, can initiate a number of troublesome symptoms.

Hypoglycemia involves a domino effect. If carbohydrates are eaten in excess, more insulin than usual is secreted in order to compensate. As a result blood sugar drops dramatically. Glucagon, cortisol and adrenalin are then poured out into the system to help raise blood sugar back to acceptable levels. This can inadvertently result in the secretion of more insulin and the vicious cycle goes on. Achieving proper blood sugar balance is tricky business and eating the wrong things can throw the system into extreme responses. High insulin secretion can cause substantial changes in brain chemistry and wreak havoc with our blood lipids. It is also true that ingesting caffeine can adversely affect blood sugar levels. Eating sugary foods can propel the pancreas, pituitary, and adrenal glands into a highly complex chemical reaction based on a feedback loop. The irony of this hypoglycemic cycle is that when blood sugar drops, we run for more sugar and perpetrate the disorder.

If you suspect that you are hypoglycemic emphasize the following foods: white meats, fish, nuts and seeds, whole grains including whole grain pastas, unsweetened yogurt, vegetable juices and eggs, low carbohydrate vegetables such as celery, beet greens, chives, cucumbers, lettuce, parsley, radishes, asparagus, broccoli, cabbage, cauliflower, mushrooms, onions, peppers, tomatoes, squash, spinach and zucchini.

Fruits should be limited to two servings per day and should be eaten as part of a meal rather than a separate snack. Recommended fruits include: berries, cantaloupe, coconut, muskmelon, cranberries, casaba melon, lemons, and limes.

Avoid all processed or enriched foods like white flour or sugar, quick cooking grains, artificial sweeteners, caffeine, alcohol, and high fat, empty calorie foods like doughnuts, pastries, cakes, and soda pop.

Eat small meals throughout the day supplemented with protein snacks. A snack or mini-meal every two hours is recommended. Raw almonds are excellent. Supplementing any hypoglycemic diet with B-complex vitamins, vitamin E, pantothenic acid, and vitamin C is desirable. Dr. Ross also adds L-glutamine, an amino acid that appears to boost brain nutrition to the mix.

Keep in mind that when you first start to eat this way, you will probably feel less than well. You may feel weak, dizzy, nauseous and depressed. This is particularly true if you have been eating a diet high in white sugar and fat. Give the diet a chance. Your body takes time to adjust and results will not be seen overnight. If you persevere, the next phase typically brings a dramatic improvement in feelings of physical well-being and mental elevation. Within three to five weeks, things should really be looking up.

Artificial Sweeteners: Too Good to be True?

It could be assumed that in order to avoid the risks of sugar, artificial sweeteners would be the ideal alternative. Ironically, switching to a sugar substitute to enhance health is one of the worst things we can do. Among some of the most troubling food additives routinely consumed are artificial sweeteners, also referred to as non-nutritive sweeteners. Having received the FDA stamp of approval, they are liberally ingested with little thought to what their actual health risks may be. Andrew Weil, M.D., in his book, *Natural Health, Natural Medicine*, writes:

"Recently, aspartame (NutraSweet) has become enormously popular. The manufacturer portrays it as a gift from nature, but, although the two component amino acids occur in nature, aspartame itself does not. Like all artificial sweeteners, aspartame has a peculiar taste. Because I have seen a number of patients, mostly women, who report headaches from this substance, I don't regard it as free from toxicity. Women also find that aspartame aggravates PMS (premenstrual syndrome). I think you are better off using moderate amounts of sugar than consuming any artificial sweeteners on a regular basis. A natural sweetener that may cause some people problems is sorbitol, originally derived from the berries of the mountain ash tree. Sorbitol tastes sweet but is not easily absorbed form the gastrointestinal tract and is not easily metabolized. It is a common ingredient of sugarless chewing gums and candies. If you eat a lot of it, you will probably get diarrhea. People with irritable bowel syndrome or ulcerative colitis should avoid sorbitol."

While thousands of Americans continue to consume aspartame in unprecedented amounts, controversy surrounding its safety lingers. Dr. Richard Wurtman of the Massachusetts Institute of Technology (MIT) has reported that abnormal concentrations of neurotransmitters developed when he fed laboratory animals large doses of aspartame. He believes that the phenylalanine content of the sweetener actually manipulates and alters certain brain chemicals, a process that could initiate behavioral changes and even seizures. He also purports that while small quantities of aspartame may be safe, the cumulative effects of the compound could be serious, particularly if consumed with high-carbohydrate, low-protein snacks. But in spite of serious concerns, saccharine and aspartame packets sit in restaurant sugar bowls all over our country.

The FDA and Current Noncaloric Sweeteners

Though white sugar, turbinado, fructose, honey and corn syrup all qualify as natural sweeteners, none of these are calorie-free nor can they be used by people who suffer from blood sugar disorders. They can encourage weight gain and tooth decay, raise blood sugar quickly, and can also predispose certain individuals to yeast infections. These sugars can also contribute to indigestion, bowel disorders and, possibly, hyperactivity or ADD in children.

caffeine: the acceptable addiction?

Our society is becoming so caffeine dependent that psychiatrists have coined a new phrase for their diagnostic manual: "caffeinism." Our obsession with caffeine consumption has made it the most widely used drug in the world. It is found in a number of foods, medications and beverages, and the average American consumes 150-225 mg of caffeine each day. And alarmingly, the intake of caffeine has been positively correlated with the degree of mental illness in psychiatric patients.

Caffeine stimulates the release of norepinephrine and other neurotransmitters in the brain. This explains the immediate lift you experience after you drink a cup of coffee. Consistent overuse of caffeine results in a lack of these same brain amines which affect mood, not to mention its adverse effects on vitamin B1, iron and magnesium absorption. Remember, caffeine activates the sympathetic nervous system and can make us feel jittery, anxious or even fearful. Caffeine continually stimulates the nervous system, and it artificially creates energy. Cocaine and amphetamines work the same way as caffeine.

Pharmaceutical sweeteners like aspartame and saccharin qualify as calorie-free but come with significant limitations and health risks. Saccharin has been labeled with a warning that it has caused the development of cancer in laboratory animals. In 1970, cyclamates, another class of artificial sweeteners were banned because of the strong possibility that they are, in fact, carcinogenic. Aspartame has been marketed as a safe substance for the general public except for those few individuals who suffer from PKU (phenylketonuria), a relatively rare disorder. Aspartame is comprised of phenylalanine, aspartic acid, and methanol (wood alcohol). Despite the protest of various organizations and health professionals, these pharmaceutical sweeteners have been approved by the FDA and are recognized as safe.

DIETARY GUIDELINES FOR GOOD HEALTH

I tell my patients that in order to enjoy good health, there are a few simple things they can do. First, consume more whole grains and vegetables, with special emphasis on the cruciferous variety. Along with that, the intake of red meats, sugar and saturated fats needs to be reduced.

We also need to eat more foods in their whole and natural state. Some of our children, and some of us, for that matter, would not even recognize certain foods in their whole, unchanged states. For the most part, whole foods from the plant kingdom offer us significant dietary fiber. Even if food producers and manufacturers add natural and synthetic fibers to foods, they cannot improve on Mother Nature's creations.

Whole Foods

Eating whole grain foods intact and unaltered may be one of the best things we can do for our health. Like medicinal plants, whole grains have been intrinsically designed with a wide array of inherent compounds which potentiate and complement each other. We got in trouble when we isolated certain chemicals from herbs to create synthetic drugs and threw away the rest, causing a whole host of various bad side effects to result. Separating grain constituents may not be as desirable as eating the whole food, the way Mother Nature intended. Annmarie Colbin, in her book *Foods and Healing*, writes:

". . . instead of eating a vegetable in the shape in which it grows, we consume it in fragmented form, its separate components split apart, and we are not following the natural scheme of things. When we consume wheat germ, white flour and bran separately, it is not the same as eating them in their natural, integrated and properly balanced state as whole wheat. . . . A hundred or so years ago, it was discovered that stripping the bran and germ off the wheat made the flour not only whiter and fluffier, but also longer-lasting . . . soon we were eating white bread and putting wheat germ in the meat loaf . . . Noting that almost half the Western world is constipated, food reformers, following Dr. Burkitt's lead, identified bran as the bowel saving element."

Current data strongly suggest that we look at the value of whole foods very carefully. When we eat bran or fragmented flours separately, our living systems react to them differently than a whole, integrated food. When cereal grains, fruits, vegetables, beans, nuts and seeds are altered or fragmented, they become artificial foods to some extent. Of course, it would be bettter to use bran separately than to not get it at all. But just by refining wheat flour into white flour, not only are the bran and germ removed, but over 15 nutrients are lost or compromised as well. The notion that artificially enriching white flour will return it to its original nutritive state is a fallacy. Annmarie Colbin compares this to, ". . . cutting off your arm and then fitting you with a prosthetic one—it may have the same form and fulfill some of the same functions, but it is hardly as good as the original."

The notion of consuming foods in their original states also applies to fruits and vegetables. When you juice fruits and vegetables, their fibrous components are often discarded as pulp. While apple, carrot, grape and other juices have nutritive value, when their fiber is either screened out or altered, they are assimilated differently. Altered fruits and grains can make us get hungrier quicker, which may contibute to weight gain. We need to remember to reach for whole, unpeeled fruits rather than fruit juices. It is also beneficial to keep vegetables "dressed," eating them peeling and all whenever feasible. Finally, we need to try to always purchase foods in their original whole states, looking to brown rice, whole wheat, and whole barley.

Cruciferous Vegetables (Indoles)

Cruciferous vegetables include cauliflower, cabbage, broccoli, and Brussels sprouts. The word *cruciferous* refers to a cross-shaped pattern found on the underside of the central stalk or core of these vegetables. Consuming cruciferous vegetables has been associated with a decreased risk of colon, breast and prostate cancer. The specific compounds in these vegetables that are thought to be of value are indoles. Indoles belong to a class of phytonutrients which have been scientifically shown to benefit the body in a number of important ways.

Like so many other nutrients, ancient physicians were well aware of the remarkable curative power of the indoles found in certain vegetables. Two thousand years ago, Roman practitioners prescribed cabbage leaves to cure an ulcerated breast. Today, science has confirmed that certain phytochemicals contained in cabbage are considered breast cancer preventative agents. Indole-3 carbinol can actually help decrease C16 estrogen and increase C2 estrogen, which is believed to decrease a woman's risk of getting breast cancer. Indole-3 carbinol also assists in detoxifying human tissues, promotes hormone balance, and provides excellent cellular nourishment.

Indoles are part of a large class of plant-based compounds called phytonutrients. They include allyl sulfides found in onions and garlic, indoles found in vegetables belonging to the cabbage family, and dithiolthinones found in broccoli and other cruciferous vegetables. New phytochemicals are currently emerging and we are beginning to glimpse their extraordinary therapeutic potential as health protectants. These remarkable nutrients can boost the production of certain enzymes which inhibit the formation of malignant tissue, they can block carcinogens from mutating DNA, they can neutralize the effects of bad estrogen, and they work hand in hand with antioxidants to prevent free radical damage.

Unfortunately only 9 percent of the American population eats an adequate amount of vegetables and fruits. Typically only one in five Americans eats a fibrous or cruciferous vegetable in a day, and only 28 percent eat a fruit or vegetable at all. Remember that to keep C2 estrogen levels elevated consistently, phytonutrients—including indole-3 carbinol—must be continually consumed. Clearly, supplementation of phytonutrients is warranted and can enhance longevity and improve the quality of life. It is important to remember that if you can't eat broccoli and cabbage every day, there are other options. Taking cruciferous vegetable extracts as part of a balanced supplement can provide as many indoles as several servings of raw cruciferous vegetables.

Isoflavones

Isoflavones found in some cruciferous vegetables have some extraordinary health benefits. In particular, they have the ability to act as a phytoestrogens to protect against the development of hormonally linked cancers. One specific isoflavone called genistein actually acts to reduce the growth of breast cells. A 1993 study demonstrated its ability to limit blood supply to tumors. These are impressive credentials and more than adequately support the use of phytonutrients in supplement form. The nutritional and antioxidant properties of indoles greatly contribute to sustained health and cellular nourishment.

The Case for Cruciferous Supplementation

I have found that even patients who are convinced of the necessity of increasing their intake of cruciferous vegetables frequently find it difficult to consistently eat these foods. While I admit that initially I was not particularly enthusiastic about the notion of "vegetables in a capsule," I believe that cruciferous supplements can be valuable for people who fail to eat enough of these vital, health-promoting foods. Ideally, vegetables of all varieties should be consumed in their whole state, either raw or slightly steamed. However, vegetable supplements in the form of capsules or "green" foods offered as powders or in tablets are certainly worth taking.

Summary

Our dietary objectives should focus on

- Increasing our consumption of whole grain cereals and breads and fruits and vegetables (especially cruciferous varieties).
- Reducing our intake of refined and processed sugars.
- Reducing our consumption of animal and plant foods high in fats, especially saturated fats.
- Switching to monounsaturated oils like olive oil and using flaxseed oil or taking an essential fatty acid supplement.
- Reducing our intake of high-cholesterol foods such as eggs, fatty meats, and staying away from hydrogenated fats altogether (corn oil, margarines, etc.).
- Reducing our intake of salt and salty foods.

WEIGHT LOSS

If you are overweight, even by as little as 10 or 20 pounds, getting rid of excess fat stores can be incredibly beneficial. Did you know that cholesterol synthesis is elevated in overweight subjects? By reducing fat tissue, cholesterol is targeted and transported to the liver for removal. If an ideal weight is maintained, fasting blood sugar levels decline, serum cholesterol drops, and glucose tolerance improves.

Unfortunately, trying to initiate weight loss by dieting has consistently resulted in compromising health and diminishing self esteem. Why do 97 percent of all diets ultimately fail? Why are 33 billion dollars spent on weight loss programs that don't work? Why are we more overweight now than we've ever been before? The average American has gained eight pounds over the last 10 years. Statistics tell us that two out of three people who go on a diet regain the weight in one year or less. Ninety-seven percent will regain the weight in five years. Most troubling of all, obesity in children has more than doubled since the 1950s and average weights for males and females is continually escalating.

In reality, there is no diet that can cure obesity and there never will be. The business of losing weight has become more of a recurring syndrome rather than a health promoting activity. Health is frequently sacrificed in exchange for burning fat, a fact that only serves to compound weight problems and compromise vitality as well. Ironically, calorie restriction, which is the basis of dieting, only serves to force the body to protect itself against the threat of a diminished supply of fuel. This protective mode inhibits the body's ability to release and burn fat. In addition, increased production of enzymes known as lipoprotein lipase (LPL) assist fat cells in scavenging for any lipids present in the blood stream. Drastic weight reduction diets can put this enzyme into overdrive. Months after dieting is stopped, this enzyme can remain abnormally active, making it more difficult to return to eating normal quantities of food without gaining weight.

Because the body is engineered toward self-preservation, when it is threatened through starvation diets, fat is conserved for future energy reserves. As a result of this nutrient hoarding, hunger is produced, prompting more eating, and the malicious cycle continues. Typically, most weight loss programs expect the body to respond to a drastic alteration of diet and activity with no prior physiological preparation. Being overweight is frequently "treated" as a disease. Consequently, the symptoms of obesity are targeted rather than addressing and correcting the cause of obesity.

The notion that only powerful, expensive and potentially dangerous drugs can suppress the appetite and create successful weight loss is not true. For every synthetic or pharmaceutical drug, an alternative compound exists in nature. As more attention is focused on safer, natural compounds, weight-loss formulas will continue to improve. The role of hormones like DHEA and melatonin are only now beginning to surface and their therapeutic implications are profound. If you feel like pharmaceutical agents like phen-fen are your only hope, think again. Mother Nature has provided a vast array of safe and effective compounds that can significantly contribute to healthy and permanent weight loss.

Prescription for Weight Loss

Today, we know that just lowering fat content and exercising may work in theory. State-of-the-art research in the area of weight loss, however, has discovered that through the addition of certain supplements and nutrients, the process of decreasing the amount of fat we process in the stomach and boosting the amount of fat we burn can be expedited. For those of us who suffer from a "fat imbalance," a condition where we store more fat than we burn, it is often a matter of life or death to lose fat in order to protect our arteries and hearts.

Most doctors will advise us to cut our fat intake to 20 grams per day and to boost our exercise time. Unfortunately, for those of us who fall into the "obese" category, even a very small amount of exercise can be an extremely taxing thing to pull off. The extra poundage that taxes the skeletal and cardiovas-cular systems can create labored breathing, excess sweating, joint pain. Obesity inhibits the transport of oxygen to the cells of the body. When we exercise, we need more oxygen. When we don't get it, a whole host of unpleasant symptoms arise. When heart muscle becomes robbed of oxygen, angina can occur, or in serious cases, a heart attack can develop.

Ideally, a sensible weight loss program should employ a nutritional strategy that works in tandem with body systems to maximize fat burning capabilities. Successful weight management depends on fully understanding human biochemistry, and in so doing targeting those physiological processes that expedite weight reduction. When given the proper tools, the human body has an inherent ability to effectively manage its weight. The key to boosting this ability lies in creating a biological equilibrium between all body systems by integrating nutrition, exercise and the proper supplementation.

What To Look For in Natural Weight Loss Products

Fiber Supplements

Psyllium-based products are the most common type of fiber supplement to which guar gum and other fiber sources are often added. Italian studies have found that in a reducing diet for women who averaged about 60 percent overweight, weight loss was greater when plantain or psyllium was added to the diet. It appears that psyllium promoted weight loss by limiting caloric intake due to its appetite-satiating effect and by reducing the intestinal absorption of lipids. Good formulas combine different types of fibers and often add various herbs to tone the colon and promote better elimination and digestion.

Liquid Protein Supplements

Several protein replacement drink powders and liquids exist that can help to facilitate the creation of lean muscle mass and the burning of fat. Spirulina-based and soy-based products are an excellent source of usable proteins and when other nutrients, fat emulsifiers and dietary aids are added to the formula, these products can serve as good meal replacements. Good supplements include a complete array of amino acids, enzymes, antioxidants, vitamins, minerals and specific herbs that facilitate weight loss and promote regularity.

Fat-Burning Formulas

The most effective fat-burning combinations include 1) ephedra, 2) a natural caffeine-containing plant such as kola nut or guarana, and 3) some source of salicylic acid such as white willow or aspirin. Adding *Garcinia cambogia* (citrin), chromium picolinate, chitosan or amino acids such as carnitine or methionine can further potentiate the mix. Taking ephedra alone is not recommended as dosages must be too high to be effective. Any thermogenic formula designed to burn calories off as heat can create some unpleasant side effects and should not be used by pregnant or nursing women, or by anyone suffering from hypertension, heart disease, adrenal or thyroid disorders or prone to anxiety attacks.

Natural Appetite Suppressants

The best natural appetite suppressants include phenylalanine and tyrosine combined with *Garcinia cambogia* (citrin) or glucomannan and calcium. Other ingredients such as herbs which discourage eating and minerals such as manganese or potassium citrate help to make the formula even more effective. Chromium picolinate is also used in supplements designed to fight food cravings, stabilize blood sugar, and promote the creation of lean muscle mass. Pyruvate is also emerging as a viable weight loss enhancer and should be investigated.

Valuable and Practical Weight Loss Suggestions

Exercise regularly. Exercise is considered by far the best method to control weight. Begin slowly. Take a 10- to 15-minute walk every other day to start and then slowly increase your distance and your pace. Light exercise right after eating is recommended to burn calories that have just been consumed. If you feel that you cannot walk every other day, to begin with go out two times a week and take it from there.

- Don't become constipated. Drink six to eight glasses of water a day.
- Don't chew gum. Chewing gum can activate the flow of gastric juices and make you feel like eating.
- Eat only when you are truly hungry. Often thirst can be mistaken for hunger. Drink when you feel the urge to eat.
- Take a good strong vitamin and mineral supplement that will help to balance out your nutrients and prevent food cravings.
- Eating a diet that is high in fiber can automatically increase chewing time and slow the eating process. People who eat too fast can often become hungry again soon after eating.
- Don't eat when you are depressed, lonely or angry.
- Avoid fad diets. They can make your body feel as if it's starving and actually lower your metabolism, which slows the burning of fat stores.
- Do not use diuretics or laxatives to induce weight loss. These can be potentially hazardous to your health and result in temporary weight loss only.
- Join a support group like Weight Watchers that takes a sensible and healthful approach to losing weight. Be wary of diet organizations that are costly or limit you to their own foods.
- Be patient. More permanent results will be obtained if weight loss is gradual. Remember that it takes time for the body to readjust to a new programmed weight set point.
- Some studies indicate that when there is an inadequate intake of essential nutrients, fat is not burned efficiently.
- Do not eat too little. Any diet that is less than 1200 calories is not sufficient to maintain good health and promote permanent weight loss. In addition, all diets should contain some percentage of desirable fat which can be ingested in the form of olive or safflower oil. Supplementing your diet with 1 to 2 teaspoons of these oils is thought to actually improve the burning of fat.

- Use digestive enzymes before every meal.
- Do not consume alcohol. All alcoholic beverages are high in calories.
- Fiber supplements can be taken in the form of guar gum or glucomannan.
- Avoid artificial sweeteners. There is some evidence that artificial sweeteners can actually increase appetite and result in weight gain.
- Omit all substances thought to be appetite stimulants such as salt, hot spices, coffee, tea, tobacco and sugar.
- Avoid any fad diets that are designed around a high-protein, low-carbohydrate diet. This combination, if eaten over a long period of time, poses some significant health hazards.
- Emphasize the following foods: lentils, beans, plain baked potatoes, baked squash, brown rice, whole grain breads (low fat or nonfat), white fish, white chicken, skim milk, low or nonfat cottage cheese, nonfat yogurt, turkey, fresh fruits and vegetables. Restrict your intake of the following: avocados, figs, bananas, white rice, sweet potatoes, coconut and corn.
- Avoid the following foods: high fat dairy products (cheese, sour cream, ice cream, butter, whole milk, rich dressings), soda pop, mayonnaise, fried foods, red meats, gravies, custards, pastries, cakes, peanut butter, and junk foods.
- Weigh yourself regularly and record your weight on a chart. If you go up three pounds from your ideal weight, adjust your diet and exercise to lose those three pounds. It is so much easier to lose three pounds than to lose 20.
- Stay off the diet roller coaster of overeating and then crash dieting. Keep a consistent healthy lifestyle centered around sensible eating and regular exercise.
- Keep your kitchen stocked with healthy low fat, low sugar snacks.

THE EXERCISE COMPONENT

Simply restricting calorie intake to lose weight is not a good idea. Exercise must be added to the mix to promote permanent weight loss and metabolic adjustment. Exercise increases energy expenditure while it serves to protect against extreme caloric restriction. In other words, if you exercise, you can eat more and not gain weight. Weight-loss programs that rely solely on caloric restriction end up perpetuating a starvation cycle that only contributes to malnutrition and even more weight gain in the future. Even just a little exercise has tremendous health benefits. New studies are suggesting that breaking up exercise times into divided periods such as 10 minutes here or there is just as effective as a sustained 30 minute work out. While it is true that even strenuous exercise burns relatively small amounts of calories, it is the impact exercise exerts on our metabolic processes that is of so much value. Exercising helps us to burn calories more efficiently rather than to store them as fat. It helps us to eliminate waste material, improve cardiovascular function, builds strength and endurance, and releases endorphins that make us feel happier and help to keep us looking good.

MACRONUTRIENTS: CARBOHYDRATES, FATS AND PROTEINS

Carbohydrates, fats and proteins comprise a category of compounds called macronutrients. Over the last few decades much controversy has arisen regarding how much of these macronutrients we should consume as part of our daily diet. Presently, most of us eat a diet which is comprised of 12 percent protein and approximately 42 percent fat and 46 percent carbohydrates. Our obsession with fatty, sugary foods has created a new war on fat, which is not necessarily all good in its health implications. It is vital for us to realize that it is the type of carbohydrate, fat and protein that we choose which in many ways determines whether it is good or bad for us.

All macronutrients are not equal, although food manufacturers would have us believe so. For example, a piece of whole grain bread is not the same as a piece of artificially enriched white bread. When fiber and bran are removed, nutrients are assimilated differently. It's the same with protein sources. Protein from soybeans is not the same as protein from a marbled piece of meat. Again, while amino acid content may be similar, the way these two sources of protein are digested and assimilated are determined by factors such as fat content and digestibility. Fats are an especially good example of the inequality of macronutrients. Corn oil and linseed oil are not the same as olive or flaxseed oil. They are all lipids, but their health implications are very different and can result in either good or bad biological consequences.

We must eat a balance of all three macronutrients in order to function at optimal levels. For some of us that may mean more protein than for others. If we suffer from any kind of blood sugar disorder, we may need to eat less carbohydrates. When it comes to fats, we must realize that some fats are very good for us if eaten in moderation.

Carbohydrates: The Body's Glucose Suppliers

Plants create carbohydrates as a by-product of the photosynthetic process. Carbohydrates are considered the most abundant organic compound found in nature. Dietary carbohydrates consist of sugars or simple carbohydrates found in white sugar, fructose, honey, and molasses; and complex carbohydrates found in whole grains, legumes, vegetables and fruits. Chemically speaking, carbohydrates are organic compounds composed of carbon atoms attached to hydrates such as water molecules. Dietary carbohydrates supply the primary source of energy for all physiological processes including the digestion and assimilation of all macronutrients. They are by far, the body's favorite energy source and provide glucose for the body which is its primary fuel source.

Eating an excess of simple carbohydrates is one of the single most destructive dietary habit of Western societies. Diabetes, obesity, tooth decay, hypoglycemia and nutritional depletion have all been linked to eating too much sugar or simple starches. While we absolutely must have carbohydrates, the type of carbohydrates we choose to eat makes a profound difference in how our bodies will react. The key to health lies in how much and what kind we choose to eat.

Carbohydrate Categories

Carbohydrates are classified according to their chemical structure. Monosaccharides are single (or simple) sugars; ogligosaccharides are multiple sugars; and polysaccharides are complex molecules made of several simple sugars. Monosaccharides have three to seven carbon atoms each. It is the hexoses or six carbon atoms sugars that we are most interested in. Listed below are different hexose sugars or simple sugars that we ingest on a daily basis.

Monosaccharides

Fructose (levulose, fruit sugar) is found in honey, ripe fruits and some vegetables. It has a much sweeter taste than cane sugar, easily dissolves without crystallization and cannot be absorbed directly into the bloodstream. This may help to explain why people who are sugar sensitive may get the sugar shakes after eating a bowl of frosted corn flakes (sucrose) but not after eating a whole apple.

Glucose (also called dextrose, corn sugar, or grape sugar) is the chemical form of sugar after it has entered the bloodstream. Glucose is another name for blood sugar and is the carbohydrate used on a cellular level to drive virtually every metabolic process. Dietary glucose is water soluble, crystalizes readily and is less sweet than cane or white sugar.

Galactose is a monosaccharide sugar that is produced during the digestion of lactose (milk sugar).

Mannose, xylose and arabinose are all pentose (five) carbohydrate compounds that are produced when certain meats and fruits are digested. Ribose is another pentose produced during digestion; it is also synthesized by the human body. Ribose is a constituent of riboflavin (a B-complex vitamin), ribonucleic acid (RNA) and deoxyribonucleic acid (DNA).

Oligosaccharides

Lactose (milk sugar) is the only nutritionally significant carbohydrate that comes from an animal rather than plant source. Cow's milk has a significant amount of lactose.

Sucrose (common table sugar) is derived from sugar cane, sugar beets, molasses, maple sugar or sorghum. Some vegetables and many fruits contain at least some sucrose. Sucrose is consumed in excessive amounts in typical Western diets because of its addition to prepackaged foods, pop, and candy.

Maltose (malt sugar) is found in malted snacks, beer and some breakfast cereals.

Polysaccharides

Starch is a polysaccharide composed of long chains of glucose units. It is commonly found in a number of plants like potatoes.

Dextrins are shorter chains of glucose units that are the intermediate products of the hydrolysis of starch.

Glycogen, also called animal starch, is produced in the liver and muscle from glucose. Glycogen comprises a very important alternative energy source for our bodies if our blood sugar dips too low.

The term "indigestible polysaccharides" refers to a group of saccharides that comprise fiber. In addition to cellulose,

fat and cholesterol: facts to know

Cholesterol is an essential body lipid compound made by the liver. It can also be supplied from the diet by eating meat and dairy products. Dietary cholesterol is only found in animal products and by-products. Excess cholesterol consumption may raise blood cholesterol levels and lead to heart disease. Cholesterol is transported through the bloodstream via lipo-proteins. The fact that Eskimos eat a diet high in cholesterol from fish lipids and yet have a low incidence of cardiovascular disease suggests that perhaps we should concentrate more on the lipids we are lacking in our diet rather than on cholesterol consumption alone.

HDLs (high-density lipoproteins) are also called "good cholesterols" because they transport cholesterol away from artery walls and back to the liver for storage.

LDLs (low-density lipoproteins), called "bad cholesterols," promote the circulation of cholesterol in the bloodstream, predisposing the arteries to plaque buildup and eventual blockage.

Triglycerides are fats that contain three groups of fatty acids: saturated, polyunsaturated, and mono-unsaturated.

Saturated fats are the only lipids capable of raising blood cholesterol levels. Butter, margarine, whole milk, and fats found in meat are high in saturated fat. Eating too much sugar which can create excess insulin response can also raise blood cholesterol.

Monounsaturated and polyunsaturated fats do not raise blood cholesterol levels. Two recommended monounsaturated oils are canola and olive oil. Safflower and corn oil are highest in polyunsaturated fats. Current research suggests that cooking with monounsaturates is preferred.

hemicellulose and lignin, this category also includes agar, alginate and carrageen.

Carbohydrate derivatives are produced when sugars undergo a chemical reaction and produce amino sugars, glycosides, uronic acid, and sugar alcohols. For example, sorbitol is a sweet sugar alcohol found in berries and ripe cherries.

How Much of Our Diet Should Be Made Up of Carbohydrates?

The dietary requirements for carbohydrates have not been set by RDA standards. The general consensus is that we eat too many simple carbohydrates and not enough complex ones. Generally speaking, our over-emphasis on protein and simple sugars has resulted in a deficit of consumption of fresh fruit, vegetables, whole grains and legumes. Many nutritionists recommend increasing our dietary intake of complex carbohydrates to promote good health and for the therapeutic management of various diseases. Americans generally receive approximately 46 percent of their dietary calories from carbohydrates. By contrast, Asian societies eat a diet that is 70 to 80 percent carbohydrate. Again, the type of carbohydrates consumed is very important.

One third of the carbohydrates we consume as a nation are comprised of refined and processed sugar products. Refined sugars or white sugar come from cane and beet sources. Processed sugars include corn sugar, corn syrup, molasses and honey. Natural sugars are found in fruits, fruit juices and vegetables. Remember that all sugars are not metabolized in the same way by the body. While all carbohydrates may eventually raise blood sugar as glucose, the speed in which they are assimilated can have far-reaching health effects when it comes to insulin disorders or diseases like hypoglycemia and diabetes.

Dietary carbohydrates are the body's preferred source of energy, and once in the body they are either burned as fuel or stored as glycogen reserves in the muscle and liver. Though it is true that over the last few decades nutritionists have advised us to eat more carbohydrates and less fats and protein, eating a "fatless" diet that is high in simple sugars can initiate significant weight gain, predispose us to elevated blood cholesterol and defeat the entire reason we cut down on fats to begin with. Nonfat or low-fat foods high in sugar calories can be even more fattening and less satisfying than some fat-containing foods. Moreover, we must have a certain percentage of lipid consumption to be healthy and slender.

Fats: Essential for Life

While it is true that fats have taken a beating in the media and are frowned upon for their negative biological impact, they are absolutely essential for life. I want to strongly reiterate here that it is not so much the quantity of fat we consume as what type of fats we eat.

Lipids are considered a group of fats and fat-like compounds that are insoluble in water. Technically speaking, this category of macronutrients includes fats, fatty acids, oils, waxes, sterols, and esters of fatty acids. Much like carbohydrates, lipids are chemically comprised of carbon, hydrogen and oxygen atoms. They serve as a source of energy which is either 1) converted to other essential tissue components, 2) burned off, or 3) stored as fat in adipose tissue.

Keep in mind that the macronutrient category of fats does not refer to body fat—which ideally accounts for around 10 percent of the body weight of a normal adult. The more we learn about fats, the more convinced we all should be that bad dietary fats are really bad and good ones are absolutely vital and should be consumed in the proper proportion. Dietary lipids in the form of olive oils, flaxseed oils, and canola oil are an excellent source of nutrition and can actually discourage cardiovascular disease rather than contribute to it. Lipids provide us with a high-energy food source, facilitate digestive processes, help to metabolize other nutrients and contribute to the absorption and transport of the fat-soluble vitamins (A, D, E, K). In addition, they comprise the sheaths that protect our nerves and help to make up fat stores to protect our vital organs.

If lipids are missing from our diets, the body will synthesize some fatty acids from other macronutrients; however, linoleic acid is considered an essential fatty acid which means that it cannot be synthesized and can only be obtained from food or supplement sources. For example, flaxseed oil is a very good source of this essential fatty acid. We are just beginning to understand the profound health implications of this acid which serves as a precursor to a series of hormone-like substances called prostaglandins. It would be wise to mention here that as Americans, the majority of fats we eat are saturated and hydrogenated varieties. Many of these artificially manipulated fats (such as we see in vegetable margarines) produce dangerous fat compounds and are completely lacking in essential fatty acids. Because we do not consume fish routinely and typically do not use olive, flaxseed or evening primrose oils in our diets, supplementation is very much warranted. Deficiencies in these essential fatty acids have been linked with all kinds of autoimmune diseases, including multiple sclerosis and lupus.

Triglycerides are considered the major form of fat and make up the majority of fat found in foods and in the body. What we need to know about triglycerides is that the length and degree of their saturation as chemical compounds determines the way they behave in the body. Fatty acids are chemically comprised of carbon atoms. If each carbon atom is connected to each of its hydrogen neighbors, it is called *saturated*. If two adjacent carbon atoms are linked in a double bond and could bind to additional hydrogens, the fat is called monosaturated. If more than one locality on a carbon chain is able to accept additional hydrogen atoms, the fat is called polyunsaturated. Linoleic acid is a polyunsaturated fatty acid and oleic acid is an example of a monounsaturated fatty acid.

An easy way to recognize some unsaturated fats is that they are usually more liquid at room temperature than a saturated fat. For example, sunflower oil, high in polyunsaturated fatty acids, is liquid at room temperature, while lard or butter, high in saturated fats, is solid.

Proteins: Building Blocks of our Cells

Unless we are consuming enough protein, our bodies will not be able to function optimally. For this reason, vegetarians need to be particularly careful that they consume a full range of proteins from non-animal sources. Time and time again, studies have shown that a poor protein intake can have serious consequences on immune function. Eating fish several times a week is an excellent source of protein, as is tofu. Chicken and turkey eaten occasionally are also good sources of protein.

Protein is considered one of the most abundant substances found in our bodies and is second only to water. Our skin, muscles, hair, nails, eyes and enzymes are essentially comprised of protein. Unless we supply our bodies with protein, we cannot create infection-fighting antibodies, regenerate our tissues or grow. Protein is chemically composed of carbon, hydrogen oxygen and nitrogen. Its primary function is to build and repair body tissues. Protein molecules are made up of organic compounds called amino acids. These amino acids are linked end to end and create a structure resembling long, sphere-like chains. The individual attributes of each protein are determined by the nature and shape of these amino acid chains. Twenty amino acids are required to synthesize protein and half of these are produced by the human body. Essential amino acids, which must be obtained from the diet include isoleucine, leucine, lysine, methionine, phenylalanine, threonine, tryptophan, and valine. Arginine and histidine are considered semi-essential.

The most common dietary sources of protein are meat, fish, seafood, eggs, dairy products, grain products, and legumes (which include beans and peas). As we mentioned earlier, as a nation, we consume much more meat than we require. Excess protein consumption can tax the kidneys, contribute to obesity and create colon toxicity. NOTE: New studies suggest that some people actually need to increase their protein consumption and lower their carbohydrate intake. Remember, it's the type of protein you eat that counts. The properties of specific proteins vary depending on the number and arrangement of individual amino acids.

Proteins are classified as being nutritionally complete or incomplete. Complete proteins such as eggs are able to initiate cellular growth. Partially complete protein, such as the gluten found in wheat, contributes to physiological function but is missing specific amino acids necessary to promote growth. Incomplete proteins found in corn, for example, cannot sustain life in and of themselves. However when combined with beans, they form a complete protein.

For our purposes, it is important to learn which foods contain the essential amino acids our bodies cannot produce. Meat and dairy products are the most common sources of essential amino acids in western nations. While plant sources of protein can be lacking in some of these amino acids, mixing certain foods together can create a complete protein food as mentioned in the example of corn and beans. A dietary mix of whole grains and beans can satisfy the body's amino acid needs.

The Biological Function of Proteins

Proteins are the major constituents of every living cell and body fluid except bile and urine. It is not difficult to see that cellular replacement and therefore, tissue regeneration hinges on providing our bodies with a continuous supply of complete proteins. Moreover, some enzyme and hormone components are made of protein also. Hormones and enzymes are what drive virtually every mechanism of the human body. Hemoglobin is an iron-bearing protein and carries blood nutrients and oxygen via every red blood cell to our body systems. Plasma proteins regulate osmotic pressure and water balance, and blood proteins maintain our acid/alkaline balance. Antibodies are considered proteins that arm our immune systems with the ability to fight disease invaders.

When we fail to eat enough protein or eat only incomplete proteins, very serious developmental abnormalities occur. Children in third-world countries frequently lack sufficient protein and suffer from a variety of maladies from stunted growth to kidney failure. Pregnant women need to be particularly vigilant in eating enough protein, or they can miscarry or have premature births.

The Importance of Protein: A Word to Vegetarians

Depending on the type of metabolism you have, you should be careful of going on a strict vegetarian diet because it can result in a protein deficiency which can leave some people feeling very fatigued, weak, unfocused and susceptible to sickness. Make sure you throughly acquaint yourself with vegetable foods that are protein-rich and eat enough of them to sustain your body on a cellular level. This is particularly important if you have eliminated eggs and dairy products from your diet as well. Because protein synthesis is hindered by the deficiency of specific amino acids in the diet, it's important for any vegetarian to recognize plant foods that lack certain amino acids.

PLANT SOURCE	AMINO ACID DEFICIENCY
Corn	Tryptophan, Threonine
Grain cereals	Lysine
Legumes	Methionine, Tryptophane
Peanuts	Methionine, Lysine
Rice	Tryptophan, Threonine
Soybeans	Methionine

The body will produce protein only until it runs out of amino acid stores.

MICRONUTRIENTS: VITAMINS AND MINERALS

Vitamins supply us with the building blocks of life. They are remarkable micro-compounds designed to initiate and assist in myriads of biochemical processes which sustain life. Technically, vitamins fall into the category of micronutrients in that only minute amounts are needed by the body. Vitamins are intrinsically linked to enzymes, which are catalysts that activate the chemical chain reactions required by every body system. For this reason, vitamins may also be referred to as coenzymes.

Two types of vitamins exist: fat soluble and water soluble. It is important to continually replenish water-soluble vitamins in that they are continually excreted and cannot be stored. They include vitamin C and B-complex vitamins. Fat-soluble vitamins can be stored in liver and fatty tissue; however, these vitamins also need continual replacement. These include vitamins A, D, E and K. Ideally, our diets should provide us with adequate supplies of vitamins. Realistically, this is far from the case. RDA requirements may be enough to ward off deficiency symptoms, but they rarely address disease, stress, environmental toxins, etc. For this reason, vitamin supplementation is recommended, especially for those who suffer from ill health or require extra endurance.

Today, a vitamin revolution is underway. Vitamins are now being intensely studied for their role in not only the prevention of disease but treatment as well. Amidst controversy, more and more data is emerging suggesting that vitamin therapy may play an integral role in the treatment of disease. Combining certain vitamins with herbs and other natural compounds can be very effective in the treatment of various diseases and disorders. Moreover, taking a good, powerful vitamin and mineral supplement on a daily basis is the first health practice we should incorporate into our daily routine.

All Vitamins Are Not Created Equal

While the debate continues over synthetic versus natural vitamins, it is important to keep in mind that vitamins derived from inorganic chemicals may be combined with undesirable substances such as sugar, artificial colors, preservatives, and coal tars. There is substantial scientific evidence that vitamins derived from natural sources are more readily absorbed and assimilated by the human body. Protein-bonded vitamins have been shown to have some advantages much in the same way as "chelated" minerals do (see mineral section). Always read label breakdowns and purchase vitamins that come in protective, dark, containers. Gel-capsulized vitamins or tablet forms that breakdown in the stomach are also recommended. Remember, more is not always better and use reliable sources for vitamins that are pure and potent.

Fat-Soluble Vitamins

Vitamin A

Applications: Antioxidant, acne, night blindness, immune weakness, skin disorders, gastric ulcers, tissue repair.

Scientific Data: Vitamin A depletion may play a significant role in diseases like cancer, Crohn's disease and gastric ulcers.[1]

Depleting Agents: Antibiotics, sulfa drugs, contraceptive drugs, alcohol, cortisone, estrogen, mineral oil, coffee, some types of indoor lighting, air pollution.

Sources: Butter, whole milk, liver, fortified low-fat and skim milk, dark green leafy vegetables (such as spinach) and yellow and orange vegetables (such as yams and squash)

Safety: Excess consumption of vitamin A in either supplement form or in cod liver oil may result in toxicity. Pregnant women should not take over 10,000 IU, and children should avoid over 18,000 IU. Taking beta carotene cannot result in a vitamin A overdose. NOTE: Anyone with diabetes or hypothyroidism should not take beta carotene as it cannot be converted to vitamin A.

Interactions: A lack of zinc, vitamin C, vitamin E or protein can inhibit the proper absorption and function of vitamin A in the body.

Recommendations: Use a high quality form of vitamin A with beta carotene. If you use fish oil sources, take vitamin E with your supplement. You can purchase natural vitamin A as retinol or retinyl-palmitate. If the product is emulsified or micellized, absorbtion will be enhanced.

Vitamin D

Applications: Cancer prevention, Crohn's disease, epilepsy, high blood pressure, kidney disease, liver disease, osteoporosis, skin ailments.

Scientific Data: Recent research suggests that elderly people may be deficient in this vitamin due to a lack of sunlight exposure and dietary depletion.[2] Studies have found that women are consistently low in vitamin D which may predispose them to osteoporosis.[3]

Depleting Agents: Mineral oil, smog, barbituates, cholesterol lowering drugs, antacids, prednisone, anticonvulsive drugs (dilantin), sedatives, intestinal disorders, liver and gallbladder disease.

Sources: This vitamin is produced in the body when we are exposed to sunlight. It is naturally supplied in cod liver oil, coldwater fish, egg yolks, and butter. Dark green leafy vegetables also contain some vitamin D.

Safety: Toxicity can occur, and dosages over 500 IU per day are not recommended unless supervised by your physician. Calcium should always be taken with vitamin D.

Interactions: This vitamin plays an integral role in the proper metabolism of calcium.

Recommendations: Vitamin D can be taken singularly but is usually included in multiple formulas or with vitamin A. Vitamin D2 is the most common supplement form. Calcitrol is the prescription version of vitamin D and is only used in cases where certain diseases prohibit the conversion of vitamin D in the body.

Vitamin E

Applications: Aging, atherosclerosis, fibrocystic breast disease, cholesterol, blood clots, scar tissue, infertility, cardiovascular disease, hypertension, burns, headaches, wound healing, lupus, PMS. NOTE: Taking vitamin E with fish oils and other lipids affords antioxidant protection from free radicals associated with rancidity and oxidation and protects essential fatty acids from molecular damage.

Scientific Data: Studies have shown that vitamin E has a relationship to elevated risks of certain kinds of cancers, fibrocystic breast disease and certain neurologic disorders.[4]

Depleting Agents: Estrogen, birth control pills, mineral oil, chlorine, food processing, inorganic iron, rancid fat.

Sources: Seeds, nuts, polyunsaturated oils, whole grains, asparagus, avocados, tomatoes, green leafy vegetables, berries.

Safety: Very few side effects have been observed with this vitamin even in high doses; however, taking more than 400 IU should be cleared with your doctor. Do not take iron at the same time as vitamin E. Anyone with hypertension, diabetes or rheumatic heart disease should not take excessive doses and begin with smaller doses.

Interactions: Vitamin E should be taken with selenium and vitamin C. It also improves the utilization of vitamin A. Vitamin E may potentiate anticoagulant drugs such as Coumadin or Warfarin and may also boost the function of vitamin K. It is also thought to boost the anticoagulant effect of aspirin.

Recommendations: Use organic sources of vitamin E which are better assimilated than synthetic varieties. They are designated by a *d* as in d-alpha tocopherol and synthetic products begin with a *dl*. Water soluble forms of vitamin E are very expensive and not necessarily worth it.

Vitamin K

Applications: Osteoporosis, hemorrhaging, heavy periods, energy demands, post-surgery, colitis, gallstones.

Scientific Data: A study found that a significant number of women who suffered from osteoporosis were also deficient in vitamin K.[5]

Depleting Agents: Antibiotics.

Sources: Green leafy vegetables such as spinach, dark lettuce, broccoli, asparagus, whole wheat, whole oats, fresh peas.

Safety: Large doses of synthetic vitamin K should not be taken during pregnancy. Excessive doses can cause reddening of the skin and sweating. The development of hemolytic anemia may indicate a vitamin K overdose. NOTE: If you are taking any medication, especially anticoagulant drugs, check with your physician before taking a vitamin K supplement.

Interactions: Vitamin K can interfere with the action of anticoagulant drugs.

Recommendations: Fat-soluble chlorophyll is an excellent source of vitamin K and is recommended. Make sure you look for fat-soluble varieties as water soluble chlorophyll will not provide the same biological benefits.

Water-Soluble Vitamins

Vitamin B1 (thiamine)

Applications: Alcoholism, anemia, depression, diarrhea, mental illness, stress, beriberi, shingles, infections.

Scientific Data: Thiamine deficiencies have been linked to mental illness.[6] Geriatric patients who have surgery may experience a thiamine loss which may explain their postoperative confusion and mental deterioration.[7] Antibiotics, oral contraceptives and sulfa drugs may also decrease thiamine levels. Eating a diet high in carbohydrates increases the need for thiamine.

Depleting Agents: Stress, caffeine, surgery, excess carbohydrate consumption (sugar), tobacco, raw fish and shellfish, antibiotics, oral contraceptives, sulfa drugs, muscle relaxants.

Sources: Sunflower seeds, soybeans, brown rice, whole wheat, peanuts.

Safety: Thiamine would have to be taken in inordinately large doses to produce any toxicity. There have been no reports of toxicity in humans with oral supplements of vitamin B1.

Interactions: Adequate supplies of magnesium must be present in order for thiamine to convert to forms the body can use. In addition, a full array of the other B-vitamins must also be supplied in order for all of them to be utilized correctly.

Recommendations: Thiamine hydrochloride is the most common source of this vitamin in nutritional supplements.

Vitamin B2 (riboflavin)

Applications: Anemia, arteriosclerosis, baldness, bladder infections, carpal tunnel, cataracts, hypoglycemia, immune system disorders, mental disorders, muscle diseases, morning sickness, obesity, sickle cell anemia, stress, depression, trembling.

Scientific Data: Riboflavin deficiencies have been linked to cataract formation, psychiatric and emotional disorders, sickle cell anemia, and esophageal cancer.[8] Some studies suggest that riboflavin therapy may help to alleviate carpal tunnel syndrome.[9] Testing of 42 adolescent boys found that 38 percent of them were riboflavin deficient.[10]

Depleting Agents: Alcohol, dieting, tobacco, oral contraceptives, coffee, cooking, radiation, ultraviolet light, white sugar, estrogen, exercise, certain antimalarial drugs.

Sources: Almonds, organ meats, whole grains, mushrooms, soybeans, green leafy vegetables.

Safety: Riboflavin has no known toxicity.

Interactions: Thiamin has a synergistic effect with riboflavin.

Recommendations: Most supplements will use riboflavin as a simple compound or what is referred to as activated riboflavin or riboflavin-5-phosphate.

Vitamin B3 (niacin, niacinamide, nicotinic acid)

Applications: Cancer prevention, epilepsy, high cholesterol levels, high blood pressure, mental illness, migraines, leg cramps, poor circulation, stress, poor memory, senility.

Scientific Data: Several clinical tests have confirmed the ability of niacin to lower blood cholesterol and triglycerides by up to 50 percent or more.[11] It has also proven its effectiveness at preventing cancer after exposure to carcinogens.[12] Niacin may also be very useful for epilepsy and can be used in conjunction with anticonvulsant drugs.[13]

Depleting Agents: Antibiotics, caffeine, alcohol, estrogen, sleeping pills, sulfa drugs, excessive consumption of white sugar.

Sources: Organ meats (especially liver), eggs, fish, peanuts, legumes, milk, avocados, whole grains with the exception of corn.

Safety: After taking vitamin B3 a "niacin flush" may occur which is a redness of the skin, usually in the face and neck region. Time-released products can help to reduce this effect; however, they are not recommended. A tingling sensation may also be experienced. Both of these reactions are considered harmless. High doses of vitamin B3 should not be used by pregnant women or anyone with diabetes, gout, peptic ulcers, glaucoma, or liver ailments. Take niacin with meals.

Interactions: Niacin needs adequate supplies of all the other B-vitamins to function properly. Niacin is also thought to potentiate the action of cholesterol-lowering drugs.

Recommendations: This vitamin can be purchased as niacin (nicotinic acid or nicotinate) or niacinamide (nicotinamide). These forms are used for different applications. Inositol hexaniacinate is a specific kind of niacin which does not cause flushing and has been used in Europe to treat high cholesterol and impaired blood flow for decades.

Vitamin B5 (pantothenic acid)

Applications: Alcoholism, anxiety, depression, allergies, anemia, arthritis, asthma, diabetes, Addison's disease, diarrhea, joint inflammation, mental illness, muscle cramps, respiratory infections, hair loss, premature aging, stress.

Scientific Data: Data reveals that some people suffering from rheumatoid arthritis have decreased levels of pantothenic acid. Using this vitamin therapeutically has resulted in the alleviation of typical arthritis symptoms in some people.[14]

Depleting Agents: Insecticides, alcohols, coffee, cooking, sulfa drugs, estrogen, sleeping pills.

Sources: Organ meats, milk, fish, poultry, whole grains, yams, broccoli, cauliflower, oranges, strawberries, legumes

Safety: It has no known toxicity.

Interactions: No drug interactions have been noted. Carnitine, an amino acid, and coenzyme Q10 work together with pantothenic acid to promote proper fatty acid utilization.

Recommendations: Pantothenic acid is usually found as calcium pantothenate. Pantetheine is another form which is considered more bioactive.

Vitamin B6 (pyridoxine)

Applications: Anxiety, carpal tunnel, depression, epilepsy, headaches, kidney disease, anemia, mental illness, hypoglycemia, epilepsy, arthritis, asthma, insomnia, Parkinson's disease, pregnancy, lactation, cataracts, eczema, high cholesterol, immune deficiency.

Scientific Data: A vitamin B6 deficiency has been profoundly linked to a number of mental disorders, including clinical depression and schizophrenia.[15] Pyridoxine therapy has been successfully used to treat childhood epilepsy, for enhanced cardiovascular health, and to inhibit melanoma in test animals.[16] Vitamin B6 depletion has also been connected to immune deficiency, kidney diseases, asthma, sickle cell anemia and diabetes.

Depleting Agents: Antidepressant drugs, alcohol, oral contraceptives, estrogen, most drugs, stress.

Sources: Bananas, yeast, seeds, nuts, whole grains, potatoes, cauliflower, Brussels sprouts, legumes.

Safety: Long term use of appropriate doses is considered safe and nontoxic. Extremely high doses may produce nervous system-related side effects.

Interactions: Magnesium and riboflavin play an integral role in converting this vitamin to a chemical form useable in the human body. In addition, vitamin B6 may potentiate the concentration of magnesium and zinc.

Recommendations: Look for pyridoxine hydrochloride or pyridoxal-5-phosphate. Injections of this vitamin are also available if liver disease is present.

Vitamin B12 (cyanocobalamin)

Applications: Mental disorders, fatigue, debilitated states, smokers, post-surgery, pernicious anemia, cancer prevention, insomnia, depression, shingles, neuritis, hepatitis, stress, multiple sclerosis, bursitis.

Scientific Data: Several studies support the notion that a vitamin B12 deficiency in the elderly and others may account for psychiatric disturbances.[17]

Depleting Agents: Anticoagulant drugs, antigout medication, laxatives, alcohol, aspirin, antibiotics, diuretics, antacids, caffeine, estrogen, sleeping pills, contraceptives, cooking temperatures.

Sources: Liver, organ meats, eggs, dairy products, fish, meat.

Safety: Considered safe. NOTE: Prolonged exposure to nitrous oxide may result in a type of anemia caused by a lack of vitamin B12. Elderly people and vegetarians are susceptible to vitamin B12 deficiencies and should use a B12 supplement.

Interactions: A lack of vitamin B12 can result in folic acid and melatonin depletion.

Recommendations: You will see this vitamin most commonly sold as cyanocobalamin. Methyl cobalamine and adenosylcobalamin are also sources of B12. Some experts consider methyl cobalamine to be more bioactive. Look for sublingual tablets for adequate absorbability. Injections of vitamin B12 are also available.

Biotin

Applications: Baldness, depression, dermatitis, eczema, leg cramps.

Scientific Data: New research has found that people on dialysis saw significant improvement in neurological disorders they suffered as a result of the treatment by using biotin supplementation.[18]

Depleting Agents: Raw egg whites, sulfa drugs, saccharin, rancid fats, refined foods, estrogen, white sugar, alcohol. NOTE: The presence of seborrheic dermatitis in infants may indicate a biotin deficiency.

Sources: Organ meats, soybeans, cheese, mushrooms, eggs, cauliflower, nuts, whole wheat.

Safety: Biotin is considered nontoxic.

Interactions: This vitamin works in tandem with other B-vitamins as well as with carnitine and coenzyme Q10.

Recommendations: You can obtain this vitamin as biocytin from yeast sources or as simple biotin. If you suspect food or other type of allergies, stay away from yeast sources.

Choline

Applications: Parkinson's disease, high cholesterol, arteriosclerosis, baldness, multiple sclerosis, glaucoma, eczema, alcoholism, muscular dystrophy, hypertension, diseases of the nervous system.

Scientific Data: Lecithin is a common source of choline. Studies have shown that taking lecithin can decrease cholesterol levels and may be an effective way to treat atherosclerosis.[19]

Depleting Agents: Water, sulfa drugs, estrogen, food processing, alcohols, excess sugar consumption.

Sources: Legumes, grains, egg yolks, cauliflower, whole grains, liver, soybeans.

Safety: No known side effects; however, very large doses may produce nausea, dizziness or diarrhea.

Interactions: The proper function and availability of folic acid depends on the contribution of choline.

Recommendations: Choline is available as choline bitartrate, choline citrate, choline chloride or as a compound found in lecithin called phosphatidylcholine.

Folic Acid

Applications: Alcoholism, anemia, arteriosclerosis, baldness, diarrhea, depression, mental illness, mental retardation, immune system, birth-defect prevention, fatigue, ulcers, stress, blood disorders.

Scientific Data: Various studies support the use of folic acid supplementation during and after pregnancy to prevent birth defects and post-partum depression.[20]

Depleting Agents: Oral contraceptives, high heat, alcohols, stress, coffee, sulfa drugs, tobacco, estrogen, barbiturates, dilantin, oral pancreatic extracts. NOTE: A tongue that is red and sore may indicate a folic acid deficiency.

Sources: Green leafy vegetables such as spinach, kale, chard and beet tops, legumes, broccoli, cabbage, asparagus, oranges, whole grains, root vegetables.

Safety: Anyone with hormonally related cancers or with convulsive disorders should not use excessive amounts of folic acid for extended periods of time. Because folic acid supplementation lowers plasma zinc levels, women who are also taking oral contraceptives, which also lower zinc, may become zinc deficient.

Interactions: Folic acid works in tandem with choline, vitamin B12 and B6.

Recommendations: Folate is the most common form of this vitamin. Folinic acid is also a source and is considered by some experts to be the most bioavailable type.

Inositol

Applications: Baldness, eczema, psoriasis, cardiovascular disease, arteriosclerosis, cirrhosis of the liver, glaucoma, obesity, gallbladder disease, multiple sclerosis.

Scientific Data: Inositol helps to remove fats from the liver and is vital in the formation of lecithin and the proper maintenance of cholesterol levels.

Depleting Agents: Caffeine, alcohols, insecticides, sulfa drugs.

Sources: Citrus fruits, nuts, seeds, legumes, whole grains.

Safety: Considered safe if it is not used in excess.

Interactions: None known to date.

Recommendations: Inositol monophosphate is the commercial compound found in nutritional supplements.

PABA (para-aminobenzoic acid)

Applications: Eczema, nervous disorders, baldness, hyperthyroidism, stress, infertility. NOTE: PABA supplements have been known to restore grey hair to its original color in animals; however, this effect in humans has not been substantiated.

Scientific Data: PABA is included in sunscreens for its ability to block UV rays. Taking PABA orally cannot prevent sunburn.

Depleting Agents: Coffee, alcohols, estrogen, sulfa drugs, food processing.

Sources: Brewer's yeast, molasses, liver, kidney, whole grains.

Safety: Generally considered safe and nontoxic. Very high doses may cause malaise, liver ailments, fever or low white blood cell count.

Interactions: PABA is required for the synthesis of folic acid within the body and contributes to the proper metabolism of protein. It has the ability to block against the UV rays of the sun and is commonly used in sunscreen preparations.

Recommendations: The usual dose of PABA is between 25 and 300 mg for adults. PABA is usually included in multivitamin and B-complex formulas; however, it is available as an individual supplement.

Vitamin C (ascorbic acid)

Applications: Infections, bruising, colds and flu, sinusitis, earaches, sore throats, smokers, blood clots, atherosclerosis, high blood pressure, physical and mental stress, weak immune system, cholesterol levels, liver toxicity.

Scientific Data: Numerous studies have proven the ability of vitamin C to help open constricted bronchiole tubes, accelerate wound healing, scavenge free radicals and help prevent cardiovascular disease.[21] Its role in cancer prevention is also thought to be significant.

Depleting Agents: Aspirin, alcohol, antidepressant drugs, analgesics, oral contraceptives, anticoagulants, steroids, cooking, food processing, diuretics, air pollution, smoking, acetaminophen toxicity. NOTE: Even fresh vegetables and fruits can quickly lose their vitamin C content if left standing.

Sources: Peppers, potatoes, broccoli, Brussels sprouts, citrus fruits, melons, berries.

Safety: Vitamin C is considered nontoxic. Some studies suggest that taking it in large doses depletes vitamin B12 stores. Anyone who has a history of kidney stones should take vitamin C only with physician approval. Unusually excessive doses may cause intestinal upset, gas or diarrhea. Pregnant or nursing mothers should not use amounts larger 5,000 mg daily.

Interactions: Vitamin C is intrinsically involved with vitamin E, selenium and beta carotene. For this reason, taking vitamin C with any antioxidant array is recommended. Vitamin C also increases the absorption of iron, decreases the absorption of copper and can alter blood tests measuring vitamin B12 levels.

Recommendations: Ascorbic acid is the least expensive and most common form of vitamin C. Adding adequate levels of bioflavonoids enhances absorption. Buffered vitamin C is for individuals with sensitivity to acid foods, and time-released products are also available. Ester-C has recently emerged and is thought by some to have better absorption and bioavailability, although some experts debate this claim. If you need to use large quantities of vitamin C, powdered ascorbic acid is the most practical form. Chewables can be appealing for children.

Vitamin P (bioflavonoids)

Applications: Bruising, varicose veins, spider veins, arthritis, hemorrhaging, cholesterol levels, herpes, cataracts, inflammation, phlebitis, bleeding gums, blood clots, colds, scurvy, hemorrhoids, edema, hypertension, hemophilia.

Scientific Data: The profound value of bioflavonoids is beginning to emerge in scientific circles. While technically not vitamins, over 64 varieties are found in the white portion of citrus fruit peel and in pine bark and grape seeds. Bioflavonoids act as antioxidants and natural anti-inflammatory agents. They should be taken with vitamin C as they increase its absorbability.[22]

Depleting Agents: Aspirin, alcohol, cortisone, antibiotics, smoking, some pain killing drugs.

Sources: Citrus fruits, onions, parsley, berries, green tea, legumes, grape seed extract.

Safety: It is considered nontoxic.

Interactions: Naringin can interfere with the action of caffeine, coumarin and estrogens and can enhance the effect of nifedipine, varapramil, felodipine and terfenadine. This flavonoid is found in grapefruit juice.

Recommendations: Bioflavonoids refer to compounds such as quercitin, naringin, rutin, hesperidin, grape seed extract, etc. Proanthocyanidins, which are found in pine bark or grape seed extract, are also flavonoid compounds and have some impressive therapeutic effects. Look for quality pure products which offer a combination of bioflavonoid types without fillers.

Endnotes

1. Hepatogastroenterology, January-February, 1985, 32: 34-38. The New England Journal of Medicine, April 19, 1984, 310: 1023-31. Lancet, Oct. 16, 1982, 876.
2. Journal of Clinical Nutrition, 1982, 36: 1225-33. Journal of the American College of Nutrition 1983, 2: 173-99.
3. Clinical Science, 1984, 66: 103-07. Journal of Bone and Joint Surgery, 1982, 64 B: 542-60. Lancet, Feb. 9, 1985, I: 307-09.
4. Canadian Journal of Neurological Science, November, 1984, II: 561-64. Journal of Nutrition, April, 1986, 116: 675-81. British Journal of Dermatology, July, 1984, III: 125-26. Lancet, January, 29, 1983, 225-28.
5. Journal of Clinical Endocrinology and Metabolism, June, 1985, 60: 1268-69.
6. Age and Aging, 1982, II: 101-07. Journal of the American College of Nutrition, 1988, 7: 61-67. British Journal of Psychiatry, 1982, 111: 271.
7. Age and Aging, 1982, II: 101-07.
8. American Journal of Opthamology, 1931, 14: 1005-09. Journal of the National Cancer Institute, April, 1984, 72: 941-48. Proceedings of the National Academy of Science, November, 1984, 81: 7076-78. American Journal of Clinical Nutrition, Dec. 1983, 38: 884-87.
9. Proceedings of the National Academy of Science, Nov. 1984, 81: 7076-78.
10. American Journal of Clinical Nutrition, May, 1984, 39: 787-91.
11. Drug Therapy, August, 1984, 62-70.
12. Journal of the National Cancer Institute, September, 1984, 73: 767-70.
13. Byolleten Eksperimental Noi Biologii I Meditsiny, 94 (9), 61-64.
14. Shari Liebermann and Nancy Bruning, The Real Vitamin and Mineral Book, (Avery Publishing, New York, 1990), 106.
15. Biological Psychiatry, 1984, 9(4): 613-16.
16. Annals of Neurology, Feb. 1985, 17: 117-20. Atherosclerosis, June, 1985, 55: 357-61. Nutrition and Cancer, January-June, 1985, 7: 43-52.
17. British Journal of Psychiatry, August, 1988, 153: 266-67.
18. Nephron,1984, 36: 183-86.
19. Biochemical and Medical Metabolism and Biology, Jan-Feb 1986, 31-39.
20. Lancet, July 24, 1982, 217.
21. American Review of Respiratory Disease, Feb 1983, 127: 143-47. Oral Surgery, March 1982, 231-36. Annals of Nutrition and Metabolism, 28, May-June, 1984, 186-91.
22. Liebermann, 122.

Minerals

Minerals, like vitamins, enable the body to carry out virtually every biochemical reaction needed to sustain life. Minerals are considered naturally occurring elements that come from soil, rock, water, animal and plant sources. Minerals can be classified as macro or bulk minerals and micro or trace minerals. Bulk minerals, which are needed in more substantial amounts include calcium, magnesium, potassium phosphorus and sodium. Trace minerals which are only needed in tiny amounts include zinc, copper, iron, manganese, chromium, selenium, and iodine.

Today more than ever before we need to be taking mineral supplementation. Agricultural practices have resulted in minerally depleted foods which look beautiful but can be significantly mineral deficient. Intensive farming methods have depleted nutrients from our soils which suggests that a diet rich in fresh foods does not guarantee a diet high in minerals and vitamins. Remember that a vegetable cannot be rich in minerals if it grew in low-mineral soil. Estimates indicate that farm soils in most of the world's agricultural regions are deficient in almost 85 percent of all minerals. Chemical fertilizers such as nitrogen phosphors and potassium can make plants grow rapidly; however, they do not replace the full array of minerals which should be present in good soil.

In an issue of *August Celebration*, Linda Grover made a very enlightening and somewhat alarming comment. She said:

"In 1948 you could buy spinach that had 158 milligrams of iron per hundred grams. But by 1965, the maximum iron they could find had dropped to 27 milligrams. In 1973, it was averaging 2.2 milligrams. That's down from a hundred and fifty. That means today you'd have to eat 75 bowls of spinach to get the same amount of iron that one bowl might have given you back in '48. That's when Popeye was really big, right?"

We need to replenish these vital minerals in supplement form. We not only need nitrogen and potassium to survive but chromium, calcium, magnesium, copper, iron, molybdenum, cobalt, iodine and many other trace minerals as well. Commenting on the current mineral situation of our produce supply, Dr. Michael Colgan, who wrote *The New Nutrition*, stated, "Unfortunately, the human body cannot create minerals, so it has to get them through dietary means. Hence, deficient food produces deficient bodies (which culminates in sickness and disease)."

The Meaning of Chelated Minerals

Minerals that are attached to a molecule of protein that enhances their transportation into the bloodstream are called chelated. Chelated minerals are thought to be more absorbable and are recommended for any mineral supplementation. As with vitamins, a balanced array of minerals should be taken in order to achieve optimal results. Taking minerals with meals also helps to make them more absorbable.

NOTE: A large increase in dietary fiber can deplete mineral supplies. Make sure to take a good mineral supplement at a different time than the fiber in order to avoid this effect.

Individual Minerals

Boron (trace mineral)

Applications: Needed for calcium uptake and may be depleted in the elderly. Can help prevent and treat osteoporosis and arthritis.

Sources: Fresh fruits, vegetables (boron content depends on soil amounts available).

Safety: Taking more than 9 mg per day is not recommended. Possible side effects have been observed only when very high levels of boron are ingested.

Interactions: None known to date; however, low levels of boron can cause urinary excretion of calcium and magnesium.

Recommendations: Look for sodium borate or borate chelates.

Calcium

Applications: Vital for strong bones and teeth and to maintain regular heartbeat. Calcium also lowers the risk of colon cancer and protects against osteoporosis. Calcium also helps to prevent muscle cramping and calms the central nervous system. Organic forms are recommended for maximum absorption.

Sources: Dairy products, tofu, spinach, kale, turnip greens, cabbage, collards, mustard greens.

Safety: It is considered safe; however, anyone with kidney disease, kidney stones, cancer or hyperparathyroidism or who takes calcium channel blocking drugs should not take calcium without the consent of their physician.

Interactions: Taking high doses of magnesium, zinc, or oxalates can interfere with calcium absorption. If doses are balanced, calcium works synergistically with magnesium, vitamin D and vitamin K. Aluminum containing antacids can boost calcium excretion and are not recommended.

Recommendations: Some calcium supplements have been associated with high lead content. In general using supplements which combine calcium citrate, gluconate and carbonate can be effective. Calcium carbonate is found in over-the-counter antacids; however, by itself, it is not the most absorbable variety. Calcium chelates are absorbed more readily. Calcium citrate, lactate, aspartate and orotate are assimilated better than calcium carbonate or calcium from oyster shells or bone meal.

Chromium

Applications: Involved in glucose metabolism and synthesis of cholesterol, proteins and fats. The average American diet can be chromium deficient, a fact which has been linked to high rates of hypoglycemia and diabetes.

Sources: Whole grains, meats.

Safety: Take as directed. If you suffer from low blood sugar, you may experience symptoms of hypoglycemia if chromium is taken in excess.

Interactions: Eating diet high in refined and processed foods can result in a chromium deficiency. Taking antacids and calcium carbonate may interfere with chromium absorption.

Recommendations: Picolinate and GTF forms of chromium are thought to be more absorbable and effective.

Copper

Applications: Contributes to healing, the synthesis of hemoglobin and hair and skin color. Copper is essential for collagen formation, for the prevention of cardiovascular disease and to treat arthritis.

Sources: Shellfish, legumes, copper pipes carrying drinking water.

Safety: Copper can create nausea and stomach upset, and as little as three grams can be fatal if taken by a small child. Excess copper ingestion from copper pipes can be dangerous.

Interactions: An excess of copper can create a vitamin C and zinc deficiency. NOTE: Taking high amounts of zinc or vitamin C can lower copper levels. Take as directed.

Recommendations: Use gluconate or picolinate varieties.

Germanium (trace mineral)

Applications: Recently discovered by Japanese scientists, germanium is an effective antioxidant that can improve rheumatism, arthritis, high cholesterol, infections, food allergies and pain. Organic germanium can increase tissue oxygenation.

Sources: Garlic, comfrey, sushi, ginseng, aloe and chlorella.

Safety: No known side effects, although doses larger than 2 grams can cause skin rash and stool softening. Large doses are not recommended. Extended ingestion has been associated with kidney problems in some individuals. Check with your doctor before taking germanium for extended periods of time.

Interactions: None known to date.

Recommendations: Doses range from 30 to 150 mg per day. Germanium dioxide is more potent and can lead to kidney dysfunction if taken in doses over 50 mg per day.

Iodine

Applications: Thyroid health, proper metabolism, endocrine system disorders. Note: Iodine deficiencies have been linked to mental retardation and breast cancer.

Sources: Seafood (including kelp), iodized salt.

Safety: Only small amounts of iodine are needed to help breakdown excess fat and contribute to thyroid health. Excess iodine can produce mouth sores, metallic taste, diarrhea, swollen salivary glands and possible vomiting.

Interactions: None known to date.

Recommendations: Organic sources are much more preferable than inorganic ones. Look for iodine caseinate and kelp.

Iron

Applications: Essential for the production of hemoglobin and red blood cell oxygenation, iron is essential for anemia, stamina, and healthy immune systems. An iron deficiency can cause pallor, hair loss, brittle nails, dizziness and anemia. Rheumatoid arthritis and cancer can contribute to iron depletion causing anemia. Excessive menstrual bleeding, ulcer, and poor digestion can result in iron depletion.

Sources: Animal products contain heme iron which is much more useful than plant sources of iron which contain the nonheme iron compound. Meat and dairy products are the best heme sources. Dark green leafy vegetables contain nonheme iron.

Safety: Excess iron can produce free radicals and stomach upset. Children should not be given iron unless prescribed by a physician for a particular disorder or malnutrition. Iron can be fatal to children if taken in an overdose.

Interactions: Taking an excess of calcium, zinc or magnesium can interfere with the absorption of iron. Vitamin C enhances absorbtion. Several herbal compounds can also interfere with iron absorption.

Recommendations: Ferrous sulfate and fumarate are non-heme iron supplements and are not absorbed as well as heme iron, although ferrous succinate is a better choice.

Magnesium

Applications: Essential for calcium and potassium assimilation, magnesium contributes to proper nerve and muscle impulses and enzyme reactions, and it plays a role in the formation of bone and carbohydrate metabolism. It is used for anxiety, depression nervousness, muscle weakness, heart disease, dizziness, high blood pressure, and PMS. NOTE: alcohol, diuretics, diarrhea, fluoride, digitalis, refined sugar and excess vitamin D are magnesium depletors. The typical American diet which is low in whole grains and high in processed foods is magnesium poor.

Sources: Legumes, seeds, nuts, whole grains and green leafy vegetables.

Safety: No side effects if it is used as directed.

Interactions: Magnesium should be taken in a balanced formula with other minerals. A high intake of calcium or vitamin D fortified products can interfere with magnesium absorption. Magnesium also works together with vitamin B6.

Recommendations: Look for magnesium citrate, malate, fumarate or citrate that are chelated. Magnesium carbonate, chloride or oxide are inorganic forms and are less absorbable.

Manganese (Trace Mineral)

Applications: Only trace amounts required for blood sugar regulation and fat and protein metabolism. Manganese is vital for proper bone growth and works in tandem with B-complex vitamins. It is recommended for lactation, diabetes, asthma, muscle and mental fatigue, epilepsy, PMS, and digestion.

Sources: Dried fruits, whole grains, nuts and green leafy vegetables.

Safety: There are no known side effects.

Interactions: Antacids can interfere with manganese absorption as can excess magnesium, calcium, copper, zinc or iron. Too much manganese can also interfere with the assimilation of these same minerals.

Recommendations: Look for chelated types, such as manganese picolinate or gluconate.

Molybdenum

Applications: Very tiny amounts of this mineral are needed for nitrogen metabolism. Low levels of molybdenum have been linked to mouth and gum disease, impotence, and some cancers. It is used to treat anemia.

Sources: Whole grains and legumes. NOTE: Soil content determines food content of this mineral.

Safety: High amounts of this mineral can cause gout and may interfere with copper utilization.

Interactions: This mineral can react with copper and fluoride blocking their absorption.

Recommendations: Sodium molybdate is the most common source of this mineral and it has a good absorption rate.

Phosphorus

Applications: It is essential for bone and tooth development, heart muscle contraction and proper kidney health. Phosphorus also contributes to the utilization of food for energy. Good for tooth and gum disease, sterility, impotence, equilibrium, muscle disorders, and bone formation.

Food Sources: Meat, dairy products, carbonated beverages.

Safety: Taking excessive amounts of phosphorus can interfere with calcium absorption.

Interactions: If phosphorus is taken in supplement form it must be balanced out with proper amounts of calcium. Excessive consumption of phosphorus can inhibit calcium uptake. Vitamin D enhances the action of phosphorus.

Recommendations: Most of us need to reduce rather than enhance our phosphorus levels.

Potassium

Applications: Works in tandem with sodium for proper electrolyte balance and contributes to heart muscle health, changes glycogen to glucose and promotes healing. In cases of diarrhea, excessive perspiration, laxative or diuretic use, potassium depletion can occur which can cause heart irregularities. It is used for stress, diabetes, heart problems, high blood pressure, hypoglycemia and arthritis.

Sources: Fresh fruits and vegetables (especially bananas, apricots, avocados and dates), meat, and dairy products.

Safety: Considered nontoxic. Use as directed; however, people with kidney disease cannot handle potassium normally and should not take it unless supervised by their physician.

Interactions: Anyone taking digitalis, diuretics and angiotensin type hypertension drugs should not take potassium unless under the direct orders of their physician. Potassium/sodium ratios must be balanced in order for both to function properly. Too much sodium can disrupt the action of potassium and cause its excretion.

Recommendations: Potassium citrate or aspartate or any other chelated form is recommended.

Selenium (Trace Element)

Applications: As an impressive antioxidant, selenium works well with vitamin E to scavenge free radicals, helping to prevent cellular mutation, cancers and the effects of aging. It is used for premature aging, cardiovascular disease, sexual dysfunction, menopause and skin ailments.

Sources: Grains, fruits, vegetables. The content in food is wholly dependent on the selenium content of the soil in which the food was cultivated. Foods high in selenium include wheat germ, nuts, oats, chard, brown rice, and bran. NOTE: Typical American diets are notoriously low in whole grains and fresh produce. Coupled with selenium-depleted soils, a selenium deficiency is much more common than one would expect.

Safety: No known side effects if taken in small amounts. The body cannot tolerate large doses of selenium therefore

orthomolecular medicine: megavitamin therapy

In 1968, Nobel Prize winner Linus Pauling, Ph.D., coined the term "orthomolecular," which he used to describe a nutritional therapy which involves the use of naturally occurring substances, normally present in the body in large doses, to treat disease. The idea was to try to correct nutritional compound imbalances, which are the root of biological dysfunction. The use of nutrients in therapeutic doses still sparks considerable debate, although evidence is mounting that these compounds can act as powerful medicines. Moreover, they advocate the notion that each person is different; therefore, their nutrient requirements can vary according to their particular biological type. Moreover,

orthomolecular physicians believe that biochemical individuality can play a crucial role in health maintenance and that RDA levels of nutrients are not adequate when disease conditions are present.

Although meeting the RDAs for nutrients may prevent the occurance of deficiencies that lead to disease, orthomolecular physicians believe that these levels do not provide for optimal health. In other words, people need much more than the suggested RDA levels to maintain health or fight disease. Animal studies have shown that vitamin C needs in animals can vary as much as 200 percent in different members of the same species. When it comes to humans, evidence suggests that older individu-

als need more vitamin B12, that women may need more folic acid than previously thought and men need more zinc. Orthomolecular medicine is based on the notion that nutrition must be the first variable considered in coming to a diagnosis before attempting to treat the disease. If the disease is linked to a nutrient imbalance, it can be cured nutritionally. This discipline also advocates the idea that no one set standard of nutritional amounts applies to everyone universally. Genetics, personality, stress, environmental factors, age, sex, etc., all determine individual nutrient needs. In addition, drugs should be used judiciously, and blood tests to determine nutrient levels are not always accurate.

it should not be taken in amounts over 200 mcg unless under the supervision of a physician.

Interactions: Selenium works best when combined with other antioxidants like vitamin E and glutathione. A high intake of trace minerals can interfere with selenium absorption. Zinc and heavy metals can inhibit its activity. Many drugs, including chemotherapeutic agents, can increase the body's selenium requirements.

Recommendations: Look for organic forms which include selenomethionine and yeasts which are high in selenium.

Silicon

Applications: Necessary for bone and collagen formation, it maintains the flexibility of arteries, counteracts the toxic effects of aluminum and contributes to preventing cardiovascular disease. It may play a role in the prevention of Alzheimer's disease.

Sources: Brown rice, whole oats, root vegetables.

Safety: No known side effects. It is considered nontoxic in recommended amounts.

Interactions: None known to date.

Recommendations: Horsetail is a rich natural source of silicon. It is also sold as trace silicic acid and sodium metasilicate. Some experts recommend the trace form for enhanced bioavailability.

Sodium

Applications: Essential for proper water and blood pH balance, stomach and nerve function, sodium can be lost during periods of excessive perspiration, vomiting or diarrhea. Inorganic sodium, which is found in table salt can be detrimental if used in excess.

Sources: Processed, salty foods (such as cheeses, bacon, lunch meats, canned entrees and some soda pop) contain high amounts of sodium. Salt reduction is a good way to reduce sodium intake.

Safety: Taking too much sodium can result in water retention, hypertension, liver and kidney dysfunction and potassium depletion.

Interactions: In order to properly assimilate sodium, calcium, potassium, sulfur and vitamin D need to be present.

Recommendations: Like phosphorus, most of us need to reduce our sodium intake rather than boost it.

Sulfur

Applications: Vital for cellular protection, sulfur has anti-aging properties and is needed for the formation of collagen. It is good for blood purification, dandruff, acne, hair, and irregular menstrual cycles.

Sources: Meat, poultry, eggs and fish and in small amounts in thiamine and biotin. NOTE: Sulfur is found in some of the amino acids of high protein foods. Garlic is particularly high in sulfur, which contributes to its therapeutic actions.

Safety: Take as directed. Safe dosage ranges have not been established for this mineral.

Interactions: Sulfur can react with some prescription drugs and should not be taken as a single supplement under normal conditions. To be assimilated properly, adequate amounts of vitamin B1, B5 and biotin need to be present.

Recommendations: Sulfur is usually found as part of total supplemental formulas. For some individuals, sulfur intake should be reduced.

Vanadium

Applications: Required for good circulation and proper cholesterol levels, vanadium deficiencies have been linked to kidney and heart disease. Vanadium is difficult to absorb. It is used for goiter, high cholesterol and heart disease.

Sources: Fish, olives, dillweed, radishes, vegetable oils, whole grains, snap beans.

Safety: Vanadium should be taken in balance with other minerals and preferably not with chromium therapy. It should not be taken in excess amounts as side effects can occur. Dosages over 100 mcg are not recommended.

Interactions: Food processing and tobacco can interfere with the uptake of vanadium. If you are taking lithium, you should not use vanadium unless directed to do so by your physician.

Recommendations: Vanadium is not easily absorbed and at this point is not considered a single dietary supplement. It is usually found as vanadyl sulfate in nutritional supplement formulas.

Zinc

Applications: The profound role of zinc in prostate gland disease is emerging. It is also essential for other reproductive organs and for strong immune function. Zinc is also involved in taste and smell and protects the liver from toxins. Zinc therapy is used for prostate disease, infections, sterility, diabetes, wound healing and ulcers. Kidney disease, diarrhea, liver disease, excess fiber and diabetes can lower zinc levels.

Sources: Oysters, shellfish, seafood, red meat, whole grains, legumes, nuts, seeds. NOTE: Zinc from plant sources is not as bioavailable as zinc from animal foods.

Safety: Excessive doses of zinc can actually impair the immune system. Doses should be kept to under 100 mg per day unless supervised by a physician. Zinc supplements can cause nausea if taken on an empty stomach, and zinc lozenges can dry out the mouth.

Interactions: Zinc and copper compete for assimilation and calcium and iron can interfere with zinc absorbtion. High fiber foods can also interfere with zinc absorption.

Recommendations: Zinc picolinate, acetate, citrate, and monomethionine are recommended. Zinc chelates and zinc lozenges are also good.

AMINO ACIDS AND THEIR ACTIONS

As we discussed in the protein section, amino acids are the building blocks of proteins and are vital to life. Protein is the nutrient that gives structure to virtually every living thing. For a protein to be considered a whole unit it must contain all of its amino acid array. Linking different amino acids together can create over 50,000 types of proteins and 20,000 known enzymes. Each protein has its specific amino acid signature. Approximately 20 commonly known amino acids exist. Within the human body, it is the liver which produces 80 percent of the amino acids we need to sustain life.

The remaining 20 percent must be obtained from the diet and are therefore referred to as essential amino acids. These have been marked with an asterisk. Amino acids enable vitamins and minerals to act properly within our biosystems. If any of these amino acids are missing, the assimilation and utilization of other nutrients will be impaired.

Today, amino acid therapy is emerging as an exciting source of therapeutic treatment. Recent studies confirm that certain amino acids when taken singly or in combination can exert the same types of medicinal effects as some prescription drugs.

Amino Acid Deficiencies Can Easily Occur

Once again, the common assumption may be that the majority of Americans get plenty of amino acids through their diets due to their high meat consumption. Just the opposite, however, may be the case. Diets that are not balanced and high on empty carbohydrates can become protein deficient. Balance is the key here. While we are well aware of the perils of a diet that is too high in protein, most of us do not eat quality protein foods. High fat red meats are not the only source of amino acids. Other protein foods, including nuts, beans, soy products, fish and eggs, are excellent sources of protein. Unfortunately the majority of Americans eat diets that are deficient in the total amino acid array we need to maintain our health.

Commercial Amino Acid Preparations

Amino acid supplements are available in single or combination form and are often part of a complete multivitamin or protein supplement formula. They come in capsules, powders or tablets and are usually derived from soy, egg or yeast protein. The term crystalline free form refers to amino acids which are extracted from grain sources such as brown rice bran. Free form amino acids are recommended in that they are rapidly assimilated.

Single Amino Acids and Their Physiological Actions

Essential amino acids—those that must be obtained from dietary sources—are marked with an asterisk (*).

L-Alanine: Involved in the metabolism of glucose and recommended for hypoglycemia.

L-Arginine:* Retards tumor growth, increases sperm count and promotes the formation of lean muscle mass and the proper formation of scar tissue. Do not take if pregnant or lactating.

L-Asparagine: Helps nourish the central nervous system to promote emotional stability.

L-Aspartic Acid: Boosts energy and endurance by enhancing liver toxin removal.

L-Carnitine: Helps to prevent fatty buildup and boosts fatty acid utilization.

L-Citrulline: Promotes energy and helps detoxify ammonia from cells.

L-Cysteine: Detoxifies cells and is an excellent free radical scavenger which also promotes muscle mass.

L-Cystine: Protects against copper toxicity, promotes healing and contributes to insulin formation.

Gamma-Amino Butyric Acid: Considered a natural tranquilizer, it decreases neuron activity.

L-Glutamic Acid: Metabolizes sugars and fats and helps to fight brain and mental disorders.

L-Glutamine: Good for treating alcoholism, sugar cravings, epilepsy, mental disorders and ulcers.

L-Glutathione: A powerful antioxidant which helps protect against radiation, smoke, x-rays and alcohol.

L-Glycine: Used for bipolar depression, prostate gland, and central nervous system health.

L-Histidine:* Repairs tissue and is good for rheumatoid arthritis, anemia and allergies.

L-Isoleucine:* Essential for hemoglobin formation and regulates blood sugar and energy levels.

L-Leucine:* Decreases blood sugar and boosts tissue healing, including bone. Recommended for post-surgery convalescence. An excess of this amino acid can cause hypoglycemia.

L-Lysine:* Inhibits virus infections and is recommended for *Herpes simplex,* cankers and cold sores.

L-Methionine:* Breaks down fats, detoxifies tissue and assists with choline production.

L-Ornithine: When combined with carnitine and arginine, it breaks down excess body fat.

L-Phenylalanine:* Needed to make neurotransmitters, aids in depression, memory and migraines. Can also act as an appetite suppressant.

DL-Phenylalanine: Suppresses appetite and helps control arthritic pain. Do not use if pregnant, have high blood pressure or diabetes.

L-Proline: Contributes to the production of collagen and strengthens joints and tendons.

L-Serine: Contributes to strong immune functions and works to metabolize fats and promote muscle mass.

L-Taurine: A key component of bile, good for cholesterol levels, hyperactivity, epilepsy and brain function.

L-Threonine:* Helps to control epilepsy and aids in formation of elastin and collagen.

L-Tryptophan:* Contributes to serotonin production, stabilizes moods, promotes sleep and stress control. NOTE: In 1989, all tryptophan was taken off the market due to a batch contaminated with EMS, a blood disorder. The FDA has recalled all products containing tryptophan; however, new modified forms of tryptophan are emerging as marketable.

L-Tyrosine: Important for brain function and can help with depression, headaches, anxiety and food cravings.

L-Valine:* Acts as a natural stimulant and is involved in tissue regeneration and nitrogen balance.

Amino Acid Products: Recommendations

◆ Amino acid preparations are readily available at health food stores in the form of capsules, powders, and liquids. Their sources are usually animal, yeast or vegetable proteins. Brown rice, milk protein and yeast sources are also utilized. More and more companies are offering amino acid supplements. Some simple guidelines to follow include the following:

free radicals and cancer

Numerous research studies support the fact that many cancers, breast cancer in particular, are diet related. Moreover, the risks of certain kinds of cancer can be significantly reduced with dietary changes. While most of us are aware of the wonders of a low-fat diet, a tremendous amount of data conceding other cancer preventative nutrients never reaches the average consumer. For example, recent studies suggest that just reducing dietary fat may not be enough to prevent certain cancers. In light of this notion, perhaps research should focus on why some cultures that eat fat still have low cancer rates? Perhaps it's not so much a question of what we eat, but what we don't eat. More and more research suggests that it is a lack of certain protective nutrients which appear to originate from dietary sources that increase our risk of cancer and other degenerative diseases.

The role of certain bioflavonoid compounds as exceptional free radical scavengers is just beginning to emerge, and the protective-potential of these flavonoids is impressive, to say the least. It's only a matter of time before overwhelming scientific confirmation supports the fact that this family of nutrients is far more valuable as antioxidants than previously assumed.

- Look for USP (U.S. Pharmacopoeia) or pharmaceutical grade products that are denoted by the letter L and by the word crystalline. NOTE: Phenylalanine comes in the DL form.
- Look for free form products which are much easier to digest and assimilate and are considered less allergenic. Capsulized, powdered forms are best.
- Take amino acids either singly or in combinations on an empty stomach with a little fruit juice. If you take them with meals, the other nutrients you have ingested will compete with the amino acids for absorption. Make sure that you do not eat for at least 30 minutes before or after taking an amino acid supplement.
- Amino acid therapy should be short term, rather than indefinite. Large doses are discouraged and going off and on them is preferable. For example, two months on, two months off seems to work best. Children should not be given these supplements unless under the supervision of their physician.

FREE RADICALS

A free radical is nothing more than a molecular structure which contains an unpaired electron. Electrons tend to stay in pairs. Electron pairs make up the chemical bond which keep molecules from flying apart. An unpaired electron is driven by a potent chemical force which compels it to find a mate. This molecular instinct to merge with another electron is so powerful that the searching molecule behaves erratically, moving about much like a weapon within cellular structures. Its random and wild molecular movements within cellular material can create cellular damage, which can eventually result in degeneration or mutation.

Why Are Free Radicals So Dangerous?

A free radical can destroy a protein, an enzyme or even a complete cell. To make matters worse, free radicals can multiply through a chain reaction mechanism resulting in the release of thousands of these cellular oxidants. When this happens, cells can become so badly damaged that DNA codes can be altered and immunity can be compromised. Contact with a free radical or oxidant on this scale can create cellular deterioration, resulting in diseases like cancer. Tissue breakdown from this oxidative stress can also occur, which contributes to aging, arthritis and a whole host of other degenerative conditions. Our constant bombardment with free radicals has been likened to being irradiated at low levels all the time.

Unfortunately, because of the damage free radicals cause within our cellular structures, the sad fact is that many of us will die prematurely from one of a wide variety of degenerative diseases. Free radical damage has been associated with over 60 known diseases and disorders. An important fact to remember is that the act of breathing oxygen activates these reactive chemical structures known as free radicals. To make matters worse, because our generation more than any other, is exposed to a number of potentially harmful environmental substances, free radical formation can reach what has been referred to as epidemic proportions. Some of the more dangerous free radical producing substances include:

- cigarette smoke
- herbicides
- high fats
- pesticides
- smog
- car exhaust
- certain prescription drugs
- diagnostic and therapeutic x-rays
- ultra-violet light
- gamma radiation
- rancid foods
- certain fats
- alcohol
- some of our food and water supplies
- stress
- poor diets

Even exercising, as beneficial as it is, can initiate the release of free radicals within our cellular systems. Aerobic exercising produces damaging oxidation by-products. Many of these are not completely neutralized by internal safety mechanisms and an overload can occur. Supplementing the diet with effective antioxidant compounds is highly recommended for everyone, but especially for those who exercise on a regular basis. V. Singh, in his article "A Current Perspective on Nutrition and Exercise," states:

"Several human and animal studies suggest that strenuous exercise may promote free radical production leading to lipid peroxidation and tissue damage. . . . concordance between the heath benefits of exercise and nutrition and a compensatory role of antioxidant nutrients against the potentially harmful effects of exercise suggest that nutrition and exercise should form important components of any regimen for prevention of chronic disease and/or promotion of optimal health."

ANTIOXIDANTS

Twentieth-century life gave us a myriad of new and stunning technological advances that served to not only reduce our work load but to expose us to a whole host of new and potentialy harmful toxins. Virtually every day most of us are exposed to countless pollutants which cause the formation of damaging oxidants in our bodies. Auto exhaust, tobacco smoke, UV rays, pollution, preservatives, and food and water additives continually assault our bio-cellular systems and may cause physiological damage. As a result, our risk of developing a degenerative disease is significantly increased. Moreover, our constant exposure to oxidizing agents can even accelerate premature tissue breakdown causing us to age more rapidly.

Inevitably, regardless of where or how we live, we will find ourselves vulnerable to these dangerous substances. While this declaration sounds ominous at best, mother nature has provided us with some very impressive defense compounds called antioxidants, which have the capability to protect us from the perils of oxidants or free radicals as they are also called.

While supplementing our diets with vitamins and minerals is strongly recommended, certain remarkable, natural substances exist which have recently come to the forefront of scientific research. These compounds are referred to as antioxidants, and they aroused interest in the scientific community.

Determining what substances provide the most optimal antioxidant capabilities and making those nutrients available to the public must be first and foremost in our quest for health and disease prevention. In addition, making sure that the nutrient compounds selected are bioavialable is vital. Frequently, supplements we believe are assimilated within the cellular structures of our bodies, do little more than just pass through them.

Antioxidants: Nature's Best Defense Against Free Radicals

Potent substances called antioxidants afford us the best prospect for disease prevention, toxin protection and sustained longevity and vigor. In light of this fact, making sure we arm our cellular systems with adequate supplies of antioxidants should become one of our first health priorities. It has now been established that more than 60 human diseases involve free-radical damage, including cancer and heart disease. Several natural protectants against free radicals, which are also called free radical scavengers, have the chemical ability to donate electrons to free radical molecules, thereby making them more stable and less dangerous. Some of the most common of these free radical scavengers or antioxidants include vitamin E, vitamin C, vitamin A and beta carotene, coenzyme Q10, selenium, proanthocyanidins, glutathione, alpha lipoic acid, superoxide dismutase, bioflavonoids, melatonin, bilberry (herb), and *Ginkgo biloba* (herb).

Each of the antioxidant compounds listed are discussed in more detail in the appropriate reference sections of this book. At this point, we will discuss the role of bioflavonoids.

Bioflavonoids

Recently, the profound effect of phytochemicals, which are derived from plant-based foods in the form of Indole-3 carbinol, quercetin, hesperidin, and naringin, have been investigated. Certain types of bioflavonoids have been found to significantly surpass other known antioxidants in their ability to scavenge free radicals. One group of bioflavonoids, specifically known as proanthocyanidins, have extraordinary antioxidant capabilities. The term *bioflavonoid* refers to a large family of chemicals found throughout the plant world. Bioflavonoids are sometimes called vitamin P; however, they are not technically vitamins. So what exactly is a bioflavonoid? Bioflavonoids are phytochemicals or plant derivatives which can have remarkable effects on biochemical pathways in human physiology. There are over 20,000 known bioflavonoids registered in chemical abstracts and over 20 million structures that fit into their chemical classification. Obviously not all flavonoids are the same.

For this reason, selecting the most biologically valuable compounds is extremely important when designing any supplement which utilizes bioflavonoid compounds. Bioflavonoids occur naturally in fruits and vegetables but they are subject to rapid decomposition and degradation during storage and cooking. Bioflavonoids are considered synergists to vitamin C and must be combined with vitamin C (ascorbic acid) for optimal benefit.

Naringen, Hesperitin and Rutin

These three bioflavonoids are also efficient antioxidants and work synergistically with vitamin C and the proanthocyanidins to scavenge free radicals. Moreover, this particular trio of flavonoids has significant antiallergenic properties. Studies have indicated that these compounds can inhibit the release of histamine, which is the chemical cause of a whole host of miserable allergic symptoms. We hear so much about anti-inflammatory drugs today and they are routinely prescribed for a number of disorders. Several laboratory tests support the fact that these flavonoids can significantly decrease inflammation by preventing histamine from permeating vessel walls. Obviously, any allergic condition, edema or other inflammatory diseases would substantially benefit from this vascular action. In addition, if you bruise easily, this group of bioflavonoids is particularly desirable. Naringin and hesperitin significantly prevent capillary fragility and interstitial bleeding.

Quercetin

Quercetin is another remarkable flavonoid. Its particular antioxidant activity has been found to help reduce the risk of coronary heart disease. Quercetin helps to dilate and relax blood vessels and has a protective effect against certain types of arrhythmias. It is the major active component of *Ginkgo biloba* and may be responsible for the beneficial effects that ginkgo has on brain neurons. Quercetin has demonstrated its ability to reduce tumor incidence which attests to its ability to neutralize oxidants within cellular material. Its antiviral activity is particularly significant today, as we face new viral diseases capable of adjusting to various pharmacological treatments. Quercetin is a remarkable bioflavonoid which can help to protect the body against viral or bacterial invasion if given before an infection progresses. It is invaluable as an immune system booster and a protectant against disease. For anyone who suffers from asthma, quercetin may effectively treat and help to prevent asthmatic symptoms.

Seven Chinese herbal drugs were screened for their ability to inhibit certain enzymes which cause several of the complications associated with diabetes. Quercetin was among the compounds tested and exhibited a potent action against these destructive enzymes. Anyone who suffers from diabetes should be aware of quercetin's potential benefits.

Another exciting result of laboratory tests on quercetin was its ability to help normalize hormone levels in both males and females. The effect that quercetin demonstrated on female estrogen and male testosterone levels suggests that the flavonoid is valuable in treating women with high estrogen related problems and men who suffer from prostate disorders. While quercetin has not been clinically tested for its ability to treat migraine headaches, its activity as a mast cell stabilizer suggests that it may indeed be useful.

How To Use Antioxidants

Taking a broad spectrum antioxidant is the best way to go. Antioxidants work in the body at different sites or cellular metabolism; therefore, relying on one particular antioxidant is not as effective as a broad spectrum. A person needs a nice variety of free radical scavengers in both vitamin and herb form. Look for formulas that use some or all of the following: grape seed extract, bioflavonoids, vitamin E, selenium, glutathione, lipoic acid, vitamin C, beta carotene and herbs like *Ginkgo biloba*. Sometimes other vitamins and minerals that enhance each other may be added to the mix.

WATER

We've all heard over and over that we should be drinking between six and eight glasses of water per day to ensure optimal health. It is also true that most of us could survive without food for over a month, but would perish without water for longer than five days. Today, while we may be more aware of the importance of drinking more water, much confusion abounds regarding purity issues, especially the value of purchasing water and if fluoridation poses a health threat.

Where does the water come from that flows from our household taps? This water is generally collected in reservoirs from surface water, which has run off from creeks, streams, rivers etc., or from ground water which has filtered down through soil and rock layers to the water table and is supplied through a well.

Water can harbor a multitude of undesirable compounds depending on its source, purification processes and even the plumbing it runs through. Some of these compounds include arsenic, iron, lead, copper, fluoride and radon. Unfortunately, water is susceptible to contamination by other substances like asbestos, cyanides, fertilizers, herbicides, pesticides, and industrial chemicals which can easily leach into ground water in various ways. Most of our purification plants add a number of potentially harmful chemicals to our water supply to purify and freshen it. Some of these include chlorine, phosphate, lime and aluminum sulfate. These additives perform a number of functions such as regulating pH, killing microorganisms and getting rid of cloudiness and contributing to aeration.

New statistics tell us that much of our water supply contains biological contaminants, such as viruses, bacteria and parasites, some of which escape destruction even when exposed to powerful chemicals like chlorine. The notion of boiling what we have assumed is safe drinking water is becoming more prevalent, especially when it comes to certain very resistant parasite organisms. As far as chlorine is concerned, the potential long-term effects of chlorine ingestion are still being debated with emphasis placed on the fact that some of the by-products of chlorine are considered carcinogenic. At this writing EPA officials are looking to reduce public water chlorine levels.

Can we tell if our water supply is poor? Some of the warning signs of undesirable water include visible floating particles, cloudiness or murkiness that does not clear up when water stands for a few minutes, foaming (may signal bacterial contamination), soapiness, strange smell, or an odd taste (metallic or foul). NOTE: Remember that many potentially dangerous substances like pesticides and herbicides will not present any odor or visible change to drinking water.

Some microbiologists advocate boiling all of our tap water supplies just to be safe. Bacteria can be destroyed by boiling water for at least five minutes. While none of us want to take an alarmist position concerning our water supplies, many cities dispense water that cannot really be called "completely health promoting."

To Fluoridate or Not to Fluoridate?

Regardless of the hype we may have heard in the past, scientific evidence conclusively proving that fluoridated water results in stronger bones and teeth has been controversial and rather inconclusive. I must admit that the potential risks of fluoridation seem to outweigh its possible benefits. It must be understood that the inorganic forms of fluoride used in drinking water are totally different from the naturally occurring fluoride called calcium fluoride which is considered nontoxic. Fluoride ingestion has been linked to osteoporosis and osteomalacia and in some cases can actually cause damage to tooth enamel. Sodium fluoride and fluorosalicic acid are the two compounds used in public water supplies and are both considered inorganic industrial by-products. These chemicals can be toxic in the right amounts and are added to some insecticides. Over 50 percent of the cities in our country fluoridate their public water supplies regardless of the controversy which surrounds the practice. In these areas, purchasing pure drinking water is recommended. The potential hazards of fluoride far outweigh any of its proposed advantages.

Bottled Water and Filtration Systems

One must be somewhat careful when purchasing bottled water in order to ensure that you are getting what you think you are buying. Bottled water can come from spring water; it can be called spa water, mineral water, etc. Remember that distilled forms of water will have had certain minerals removed. Demineralization, or a process called deionization, removes the nitrites, calcium, magnesium and other heavy metals from the water. For water to be accurately labeled mineral water, it must come from a free flowing source and be bottled at its location. The mineral content of these waters will vary according to their location. For this reason, they often provide a poor source of minerals in that their content is in question. Natural or spring waters only refer to water that has not been artificially altered in any way; however, their source and any filtration processes they may have undergone remain unknown. Distilled water is created by boiling the water, and then condensing it back to a liquid form. This method leaves behind a residue of minerals, microorganisms, contaminants, etc. This type of water is the safest variety but becomes rather tasteless in the process. It can also sometimes fail to satisfy thirst unless a bit of salt, lemon juice or vinegar is added. Using liquid mineral supplements to enhance distilled water is also recommended, and this allows the consumer an exact knowledge of what minerals are included.

Filtration systems are based on three methods: (1) microfiltration systems: forces water through filters with very small pores designed to screen out contaminants, (2) absorbent filtration: forces water through absorbent materials such as carbon to catch impurities, and (3) ion/exchange systems: chemically removes heavy metals from water.

Some systems use reverse osmosis which can be effective also. It is important to keep in mind that any system must be continually kept in good working order and then many of these systems cannot filter out all viruses or parasite organisms. Our best alternative concerning water it to purchase distilled water and add to it if possible. Water filtration systems can be beneficial but must be bought with caution so as to obtain the best possible system.

For more information on how to assess the quality of your drinking water contact:

Water Quality Association
4151 Naperville Rd.
Lisle, Il 60532
(708) 505-0160

Prevention: How to Boost Our Immune Systems

Another area of dramatic contrast between natural medicine and orthodox practices is in the prevention of disease or simply reacting to it. Many conventional medical practitioners do little to educate their patients on prevention. It's simply not a priority in their medical school training. Jack Stobo, a senior physician at Johns Hopkins, has said:

"The way we educate physicians is out of sync with the problems they have to face when they go into practice. . . . [Of the] number of the problems that end up in the hospital . . . somewhere around half are preventable."

Contrastingly, natural medicine has always stressed the prevention of disease through diets rich in whole grains, legumes, fresh fruits and vegetables and by using supplements for heightened health. Meditation and stress management are also thrown in the mix as integral factors in determining our total well being. One of the best things we can do for ourselves is to enhance our immunity. In order to do so, we need a basic understanding of how our immune system works to defend us against invading microorganisms and carcinogens.

A BRIEF OVERVIEW OF IMMUNE FUNCTION

The immune system consists of various body organs and processes: the main ones are the thymus gland, spleen, tonsils, adenoids and lymph nodes, and a variety of white blood cells designed to protect the body. The thymus gland is an intregal part of our immune defenses. It produces T-lymphocytes, which are a special kind of white blood cell that plays a profound role in creating cell-based immunity. Immunity on a cellular level is what protects us against fungi, viruses, bacteria, and yeast infections.

Today, more and more evidence suggests that all basic immune functions also play a vital role in protecting us from allergies and malignancies. All of us have tumor cells which our immune systems recognize and destroy. When a person does develop cancer, this immune function has failed to provide the body with protection. For some reason, it does not recognize malignant cells, and they are allowed to reproduce.

As we grow older, our spleen ages and shrinks. It is particularly vulnerable to the kind of oxidative injury caused by free radicals. It is also very sensitive to radiation and infection. For this reason, it is crucial that we make sure to supply our diet with thymic building nutrients. These include vitamin C with bioflavonoids, selenium, vitamin E, beta carotene, zinc, and alpha lipoic acid. Recent clinical data supports the notion that many of us become zinc deficient as we grow older. This may help to explain why elderly people become so much more susceptible to disease. Herbs which support the thymus gland include astragalus, echinacea, and pau d'arco.

The lymph system is responsible for collecting lymph fluid and draining waste from the tissues. This fluid must be purified by white blood cells which are responsible for destroying infections microorganisms and cellular waste. Our lymph nodes also help to produce antibodies which comprise armies of special cells designed to kill specific organisms. The lymph system can be supported by using herbs, such as ginseng and echinacea, and by making sure we get enough exercise each day.

The body's defense mechanisms are complex and incredibly marvelous. In some cases, a virus must penetrate several lines of defense in order to cause a problem. Some of our best defenses are things we can do like washing our hands to prevent the spread of germs and by properly storing and preparing food to prevent food-borne illness.

The body's defenses include the skin, mucus layers covering infection-susceptible tissues, white blood cells (leukocytes), and interferon. Leukocytes are divided into two classes called granulocytes and agranulocytes. These two classes are further divided into smaller groups. Granulocytes are primarily phagocytic, which mean they have the ability to ingest particulate substances, a process called phagocytosis. Granulocytes include juvenile neutrophils, segmented neutrophils, basophils, and eosinophils. Each of these perform a specific task. Neutrophils neutralize bacteria and small particles by ingesting them. Basophils are believed to deliver anticoagulants to facilitate blood clot absorption. Eosinophils increase in numbers with asthma and during certain infections.

The agranulocytes include monocytes· and large and small lymphocytes. Monocytes are able to ingest large particles such as foreign proteins and peptides, while lymphocytes produce antibodies and are important to cellular immunity. Interferon is a protein formed when cells are exposed to viruses. Noninfected cells will become immune to the virus when exposed to interferon. Interferon inhibits with the virus's ability to reproduce.

If the body's ability to properly produce interferon or leukocytes is impaired, the health of the body may be successfully challenged by invading disease-producing microorganisms. It is· therefore, easy to understand why maintaining a healthy immune system is so critical.

IMMUNE SYSTEM DYSFUNCTION

With the emergence of so many diseases and syndromes with unknown causes, we must turn our attention to the immune system and why it is failing to function properly in so many individuals. Before effectively treating whatever malady someone might suffer from, the cause of why he or she became ill in the first place must be addressed. What is the root cause? Autoimmune diseases, new diseases like fibromyalgia and chronic fatigue syndrome are all associated with immune dysfunction, whether primary or secondary. Conceivably, if we continue to discover new illnesses which originate from faulty immune response, we can be sure that immune system dysfunction will become one of the major disease categories of the 21st century.

CAUSES OF IMMUNE SYSTEM IMPAIRMENT

Stress

Studies of the National Institutes of Health in a meeting on alternative medicine reported that they had studied a group of people caring for elderly Alzheimer's patients as compared to another test group who were not. You can imagine the stress involved in the day to day care of anyone with Alzheimer's. They inflicted a cut or wound on both test groups and observed the healing process and how long it took to complete. Healing is a direct manifestation of immune system function and efficiency. Those caring for the Alzheimer's patients took 25 percent longer to heal. The conclusion is that stress directly inhibits the healing process. Anyone who approaches a health care expert with stress complaints and asks for medicine to alleviate stress is probably suffering from immune dysfunction to some degree. For this reason, it is always important to provide that person with immune building nutrients and herbals in combination with stress-relieving agents to improve function or stop degradation.

Another study observed an adult care facility where people came to participate in social activity only. These were ambulatory elderly. This group was assessed for immune function, some changes implemented and several months later, was reevaluated. A marked improvement in immune function was noted. Why? Because this group had been given a simple multivitamin and mineral supplement. This daily supplement greatly improved their immune function. For the elderly, who typically suffer from immune weakness, this was a simple yet profoundly beneficial addition. While this is a relatively easy step we can take to boost our immunity, there are other activities which can significantly combat the deleterious health effects of stress in our lives.

Dr Herbert Benson, a cardiologist trained at Harvard University who wrote *The Relaxation Response*, proved through his research that people who meditated for 15 to 20 minutes per day reacted differently to stress. While it may be true that under stressful conditions their blood pressure would rise, it would only stay elevated for 20 or 30 minutes rather than for hours at a time. The effects of stress were markedly reduced for people who meditated regularly.

Nutrient Deficiencies

Deficiencies of virtually any single nutrient can negatively impact the immune system; however, certain compounds are vital to immune function. One of these is zinc. Zinc as a single deficiency can cause severe immune impairment. Zinc deficiencies are rather common; a fact which certainly has very important health implications for all of us. It is involved in at least 90 metallienzymatic reactions in the body many of which are immune-related. Any individual who is complaining of disease susceptibility or "catches everything that comes along," may want to turn to immune-building herbs like astragalus or echinacea. While those are certainly beneficial, if this person is lacking in zinc or any other nutrient, that concern must be addressed first. Unquestionably, immune-building herbs will work much better if certain nutrients are supplied to the body. If a zinc deficiency exists, herbal therapy will not be very effective. In addition, iron, manganese, copper and selenium must also be supplied for optimal immune response. Selenium is emerging as a much more important nutrient than previously assumed and has significant cancer-protective properties. Becoming depleted in any of these nutrients can predispose us to all kinds of illnesses including cancer. Current research has found that if we lack EFAs (essential fatty acids), immune function can become deranged. By deranged, we mean that it can overreact or respond inappropriately causing a number of autoimmune diseases—where it sets out to destroy our own tissue, a phenomenon we see in diseases like lupus or multiple sclerosis. Supplementing with EFAs for autoimmune disease is crucial. The first thing we need to do in boosting our immunity is to add a potent vitamin and mineral supplement.

DIET AND IMMUNITY

Ironically, while we may be considered the most prosperous nation in the world, we eat food items that can leave us seriously lacking in certain vitamins and minerals. Studies confirm that becoming depleted in even one nutrient can cause us to suffer a variety of ailments and can certainly predispose us to infection, allergies, and even cancer. Our adolescent and elderly population are especially at risk. Following the basic diet suggestions outlined in our food section will supply the types of foods that enhance immunity. In addition, if we find that we or members of our family are prone to recurring infections such colds, strep throat, flu, earaches, supplementation with vitamins and herbs is strongly recommended.

Diet Guidelines for Enhancing Immunity
- Limit intake of white sugar/refined flour products.
- Drink plenty of pure water.
- Use whole grains.
- Limit intake of fatty dairy products.
- Increase consumption of fresh fruits, vegetables and legumes.

Vitamins and Herbs To Boost the Immune System
- vitamin E: 400 IU
- vitamin K: 60 mcg
- vitamin C: 1200 mg
- vitamin B1: 100 mg
- vitamin B2: 50 mg
- niacin: 50 mg
- niacinamide: 150 mg
- vitamin A (fish liver oil): 10,000 IU
- beta carotene: 15,000 IU
- vitamin D (fish liver oil): 100 IU
- pantothenic acid: 400 mg
- vitamin B6: 50 mg
- folic acid: 800 mcg
- vitamin B12: 100 mcg
- biotin: 300 mcg
- choline: 150 mg
- calcium (citrate or gluconate): 500 mg
- magnesium: 99 mg
- copper: 2 mg
- manganese: 20 mg
- zinc: 20 mg
- iodine (kelp): 150 mcg
- chromium GTF or picolinate: 200 mcg
- selenium: 200 mcg
- PABA: 50 mg
- citrus bioflavonoids: 100 mg

choosing the best exercise program for you

You won't find any fancy charts with all sorts of exercises listed and projected times and heart rates in this section. The following easy-to-use plan focuses on walking and begins at the most rudimentary level and works up. Begin where you feel comfortable and gradually increase your exercise from there. Remember, if you take on too much at the beginning you will end up doing nothing at all. Do not look to exercise as a way to lose weight. In fact, expect absolutely no results at all. Do it as an "exercise in faith" (excuse the pun) and you will eventually reap many benefits.

At first, (depending on your conditioning) you may seem tired, and even a simple and easy walk may seem overwhelming. Take it slow and adjust your speed if you need to, but keep going!

If you make walking a priority in your life, it will happen. If you do it only as something you plan to do temporarily or when it's convenient, you will not reach your goals because other things may distract you.

- Walk for ten minutes twice a week.
- Walk for ten minutes three times a week.
- Walk for fifteen minutes three times a week.
- Walk for twenty minutes five times a week

If you feel you cannot go outside, use a treadmill, go to an indoor track or even walk around the room if you have to. No excuses allowed. Even if you never progress to the next level, keep with the level you can live with. Try, however, to work up to walking for 20 minutes three to five times a week at a brisk pace. At first, keep your tempo slow until your stamina and endurance increases. Always remember to check with your doctor if you have any medical condition before you start any kind of exercise program.

NOTE: Take a strong multiple vitamin and mineral supplement daily and a good antioxidant array product. Herbs listed below can also significantly enhance immunity should also be used appropriately.

HERBS AND HERBAL COMBINATIONS THAT BOOST IMMUNE FUNCTION

As a general rule, I use herbs that have astragalus as their main component, with adaptogenic mushrooms such as reishi, shitake, and mitake. Echinacea should be used at the start of an infection, but should not be taken indefinitely just to boost immunity. Remember, no herbal therapy will be able to strengthen the immune system if you are deficient in zinc, magnesium, calcium or any of the B vitamins. Basic supplementation is of utmost importance.

Astragalus: This herb is almost always found in Chinese herbal formulas designed to enhance immunity, or deal with any immune-related diseases. Astragalus improves phagocytosis, the process where foreign invaders are literally devoured by phagocytes.

Schizandra and Dong Quai: Although dong quai is known for its use as a female tonic herb, it is traditionally used in Chinese formulas as a general tonic to augment the immune system.

Shitake, Reishi and Mitake Mushrooms: These mushrooms contribute to increased cellular immunity and to promote the conversion of cancer cells to normal cells. Chinese research supports the use of these mushrooms to stimulate immune function. These mushrooms contain betaglucans that are proven immuno-stimulants. Betaglucans can be purchased as isolated compounds or can be taken in the whole mushroom form. Anyone with impaired immunity or suffering from cancer can take betaglucan in 3 to 6 mg doses two to three times a day, while also taking whole medicinal mushrooms to maximize the amount of active ingredient they are ingesting.

Echinacea and Goldenseal: These herbs can help to boost immunity by enhancing white blood cell activity, but they should not be taken for indefinite periods of time.

Exercise: The Many Benefits of Moving the Body

The psychological benefits of regular exercise cannot be overemphasized. Any kind of exercise can help you to balance your body systems. Moreover, exercise can naturally give us what some drugs try to accomplish, elevating certain brain amines that make us feel happier and more energetic. Most of us are aware of studies that prove brain endorphins are released after a certain amount of sustained exercise, creating a feeling of invigoration and well-being. (Marathon runners seem particularly susceptible, experiencing euphoric, altered states of consciousness while they run.)

The subject of exercise spawns all kinds of controversy and seemingly contradictory information. Ten years ago we were told that exercise was only effective if you exercised for 30 to 40 minutes, 3 to 4 times a week at 70 to 80 percent of your maximum heart rate. We are discovering that for sedentary people, minimal exercise such as a leisurely stroll or gardening can be very beneficial and should be strongly encouraged. Views are also emerging on how much time we should spend exercising. Research now indicates that three ten minute bursts of exercise can be just as good as a thirty minute session.

Exercise and Depression

In light of its connection to the biochemical makeup of the brain, exercise can be an effective tool for fighting depression. Simply exercising will help lift your spirits. Learning to walk briskly every day or to jog at a moderate pace not only eases the blues, it provides untold physical benefits as well. Vigorous regular exercise can help releive insomnia, poor appetite, irritability and anxiety, all symptoms that usually accompany depression. In her book, *Depression and Natural Medicine*, Rita Elkins writes:

"Two of the basic requirements for a healthy and happy life are fresh air and exercise, to which the benefit of sunlight exposure is also added. If we were smart, we would view exercise as crucial to our survival. Unfortunately, even when we feel relatively happy, its hard for us to make time to exercise. If we're depressed, we have to fight our way out of a force that can paralyze us."

We need to get out of our houses into the fresh air, even on an overcast day. A cloudy day still gives us a light intensity around 10,000 lux, which is substantial. For anyone suffering from a seasonal affective disorder, exercising for 30 minutes outdoors is the equivalent of a daily session of light therapy, which is usually obtained from a purchased light box. Exercising outside can also raise the oxygen level of our cells, directly impacting how much physical and mental energy we generate. When we breathe deeply, we expedite the removal of carbon dioxide and other waste products from our systems. It is interesting to know that some experts believe that during states of depression, regional blood flow to brain tissue is usually decreased. Exercising helps to remedy this. In fact, some people believe that it is virtually impossible to sustain a mental state of anger, depression or anxiety during and right after vigorous exercise. Some studies have shown that jogging for 30 minutes three times a week can be even more effective than psychotherapy sessions. For women who suffer through the hormonal upheaval of menopause, regular exercise has literally saved them from an emotional crisis and depression.

Dr. John Greist, the author of a renowned discourse entitled "Running Out of Depression," conducted a study of 28 depressed patients and found that those patients who ran controlled their depression much better than those who were treated with psychotherapy. Even if you can only get out three days a week, the emotional benefits of regular exercise cannot be overstated.

Exercise and Stress Management

Understandably, if you are experiencing high stress levels, exercising is the last thing you feel like doing.

Frequently, when we feel stressed we want to withdraw, not only socially but physically as well.

Did you know that some health care experts believe that becoming too sedentary creates stress itself? Numerous studies have discovered that breaking out of a lethargic lifestyle—forcing yourself to move—results in more positive thoughts. Even seemingly minor, low-impact exercise like walking around the block can release tension and create desirable neurochemical changes in the brain.

The psychological and physical benefits of regular exercise cannot be overemphasized. All kinds of exercise can help alleviate nervous tension. For this reason, you need to select the type of exercise that you will like and will do on a regular basis. Brisk walking is, perhaps, the perfect form of exercise. While you're walking, you can think about methods to unravel the tangled web of stress that dominates your life.

Exercise can be a marvelous release and can promote better relaxation and sleep. In light of its connection to the biochemical makeup of the brain, exercise can be an effective tool for alleviating and managing stress. More than any other factor, though, exercise is very inexpensive and helps to control weight and create fitness.

Exercise Is Vital for Weight Control

Those who have lost weight through exercise (in contrast to those who have lost weight through dietary means) are the people who have the most success at losing and managing their weight. If you fit the profile of a "couch potato," I strongly urge you to change your lifestyle—even just a little bit, and start exercising in some way. Exercise has so many unseen health benefits. Chasing away the goblins of depression is one of the most important benefits, although exercise also helps the lymph system to do its job by stimulating circulation, expediting the removal of toxins and waste material from the body.

An added bonus of exercise is that when we increase our heart rate and energy is expended, more calories are burned, weight is lost and sudden drops in blood sugar are usually prevented. In other words, exercising can help stem sudden carbohydrate cravings due to low blood sugar. If you've felt low for an extended period of time, you know how many aches and pains have accompanied the depression. Regular exercise can help to alleviate stiff muscles and joints and can boost the digestive system so elimination is more efficient. Simply put, when you exercise, you sleep better, breathe easier, and think clearer. Remember, any weight loss program that does not incorporate exercise as a primary component will always fail.

The Body-Mind-Spirit Connection: How It Affects Healing

Today, the therapeutic values of touch, massage, chiropractic manipulation, acupuncture, aroma therapy and even prayer testify to the fact that all of the senses of the human body respond to healing. In addition, we are only now starting to comprehend the magnitude of our body's ability to self-heal. Studies show that 90 percent of patients who seek medical help have self-limiting disorders or disorders that will go away by themselves without treatment. Suppressing symptoms with harsh drugs or invasive techniques can actually compromise the body's ability to heal. Natural therapists believe that when augmented with the proper nutrition, when cleansed of toxins, or when balanced through chiropractic or osteopathy, the body will often heal itself.

Sadly, the notion that the physician is a teacher or an advisor has also been forgotten. People will usually spend more time discussing the pros and cons of a car purchase with a salesman than completely going over their health concerns with a doctor. Eating habits, emotional states, etc. are rarely questioned and diagnosis is based on high-tech machinery and laboratory tests. By contrast, natural health practitioners ask detailed questions concerning every aspect of a person's life, including the spiritual and include the patient in the healing process. In many instances, doctors have forgotten how to truly care for their patients and do little more than scratch out prescriptions. Natural protocols have long recognized the effect of negative attitudes and emotions on the physical body.

STRESS: PUBLIC HEALTH ENEMY NUMBER ONE

The evidence is in and it is overwhelming: stress plays a vital role in the origin and development of a number of diseases. Stress significantly contributes to coronary artery disease. Stress depresses the immune system making us more susceptible to cancer, autoimmune diseases, and infections. Stress makes us age faster. Get the point?

Today, we are just beginning to appreciate the profound effect the mind exerts on the body especially in causing and curing disease. The role that stress plays is stunning. Estimates suggest that as many as 80 percent of all visits to the doctor stem from stress-related problems. As mentioned, stress directly impairs the immune system and can act as the single most damaging factor to our overall health and well being—but only if we let it.

According to a 1996 survey of corporate executives, 44 percent of the employees questioned said their work load is excessive as compared to 37 percent in 1988. A quarter of these people felt stressed at work every day, and another 12 percent felt it almost every day.

When we feel stressed, whether it is conscious or not, the brain instantly stimulates the adrenal glands to produce hormones called cortisosteroids, which enter our circulatory systems and inevitably put strain on our immune responses. Consequently, our body becomes more vulnerable to neoplastic (cancer-causing) processes. These hormones, including cortisol, adrenaline and prolactin, inhibit the activities of white blood cells, inhibit the amount of lymphocytes produced and cause the thymus gland to actually shrink.

Studies have found that the incidence of breast cancer was significantly higher in the women who had experienced a traumatic emotional experience during the six years before they developed the tumor. Many other studies support the very damaging effects of stress on immunity, indicating that that T-cell activity is dramatically impaired in people who lose their spouses, lose their jobs or experience other emotionally upsetting events. When the stress becomes chronic, chemical changes occur in the body, inadvertently creating an environment which predisposes to disease.

STRESS TEST: PERSONALITY AND EVENTS

Scientists have a testing criteria for evaluating individual stress levels to determine whether they are reaching the levels that require additional management.

If you answer yes to two or more of the following questions you may have a stress-prone personality.

- Do you try to do more than one thing at a time?
- Do you rush through your meals?
- Are you compulsive about punctuality?
- Do you find it difficult to relax?
- Do others tell you to take things slower?
- Do you often interrupt others while they are talking?
- Are you accident-prone?
- Do you get impatient or upset if something or someone delays you (traffic jams, appointments, etc.)?

Specific Symptoms of Stress

The following symptons can be be indicators of stress:

- tense muscles
- irritability
- anger outbursts
- racing or irregular heartbeat
- increased use of drugs, alcohol or tobacco

- forgetfulness
- crying
- nail biting
- loss of self-confidence
- teeth grinding
- becoming accident prone
- back or neckaches
- fluttery stomach
- heartburn
- increased perspiration
- cold hands or feet
- lack of concentration
- decline in productivity
- excessive sighing
- twitching

Standard Medical Approaches to Stress

Tranquilizers and antidepressants like Prozac are among the most commonly prescribed drugs to relieve anxiety and tension. Using barbiturate hypnotic drugs or narcotic analgesics is not the ideal way to manage stress. Drugs like Valium and lithium are strong and potentially fatal drugs which must never be casually prescribed or taken. Doctors often sense our impatience and our need for a quick fix, when in reality, we need to focus on our lifestyles, diet and spiritual status. Using meditation, herbs, vitamins, minerals and relaxation techniques are certainly much more desirable to potentially dangerous drugs. Masking the symptoms of stress will never solve the problem. A number of excellent herbs exist which can help to safely calm the nervous system and promote restful sleep without addiction or hangover-type effects.

the power of meditation

Meditation can take all sorts of forms. It can include yoga with deep breathing, biofeedback training or formal training such as transcendental mediation. All of these types of meditation have one thing in common: they achieve a state of "mindfulness," the ability to let the mind go completely blank by not concentrating on one particular thought. (Ironically, while the term "mindlessness" may seem more appropriate, the fullness concept refers to the notion that while the mind is full, it is not focused on any one subject.)

Because I have had considerable experience with acupuncture, I have always leaned towards Eastern medicative techniques. I strongly advise everyone to become involved in some form of meditation on a daily basis.

One of the best meditation programs is found in Dr. Herbert Benson's *Timeless Healing*. The method he uses consists of selecting a word or phrase (a mantra), finding a quiet place to sit in, breathing in and out through the nose and with every exhale, repeating the word once in your mind. Words such as "sky," "peace," "love," and "tranquility" work well. Benson found that using words with a particular positive religious connotation greatly enhance the meditative session. Select a word or phrase that is spiri-tual in nature. His method is simple to learn and to implement.

Whether it be his way or another, we should all practice meditation regularly for 15 to 20 minutes every morning or at least 10 to 15 minutes twice a day. Meditation dissipates the cumulative effects of stress. The health benefits of learning to remain in a quiet state are tremendous. Meditaion can enable us to improve many medical and nonmedical conditions. Don't expect overnight results. Just keep at it and practice regularly. Research has shown the positive effects of meditation will last 2 to 3 weeks after one stops, but if you do stop, the benefits will eventually cease.

Relieving Stress With Recuperative Time

Because our world is full of stressors, both good and bad, our health will be compromised unless we create a "recuperative time" to ease and neutralize that stress.

Many years ago, Dr. Herbert Bensen conducted research that supported the idea that meditation practiced 15-to-20 minutes every morning had a cumulative effect. The longer individuals practiced meditation, the greater their health benefits. People who routinely meditated had lower blood pressure throughout the day, less adrenal response to stress and an overall improved sense of well-being. Interestingly, if the meditation stopped, all of these health benefits disappeared after two to three weeks.

Dr. Steven Covey's best-selling book, *The Seven Habits of Highly Effective People*, states that having a recuperative time every day is essential to improved performance in the work place. It is also crucial to preventing the onset of many degenerative diseases we have come to expect as we grow older. Learning one of the meditative arts and implementing it into our lives as an integral part of our daily routine is one of the best ways to stay healthy.

The real question is why go to all the trouble of trying to prolong life, if you're not enjoying it in the first place? Remember, when you decide to make a change in how you live, you should feel comfortable about it. If you could prove that any one change helped you to live an extra five years, the change would be worthless if you didn't enjoy the extra five years.

Each of us will inevitably suffer from illness, depression, injury, or disappointment as integral parts of our mortal existence. No amount of change will enable us to escape these experiences. What we can do is to live our lives in such a way that we are able to handle whatever forms of stress we may encounter. Learning to control our minds and let go of the countless stressful thoughts that cross through our neural pathways is a wonderful beginning.

VISUALIZATION THERAPY

A colleague of mine has written several articles on the power of healing words. He was trained as an intern in this approach and has extensively studied the effect of prayer and visualization on disease. He is often asked to compare this therapy with other natural protocols like acupuncture and chiropractic and which one he would utilize if he were stranded on desert island. Without hesitation, he says he would choose to take the time to relax while visualizing the body healing itself. This kind of self-treatment can be learned and used by everyone on a regular basis. It is very easy to put into practice and is considered a form of meditation. It can be instantly used to better relationships, attitude, health or even body functions like blood flow or immune function.

SPIRITUAL HEALING: LINKING BACK TO OUR CREATOR

Natural medicine rests on the belief that the body and the mind or spirit are intrinsically connected. Virtually every primitive culture embraced the idea that the mind and spirit must also be treated along with the physical body in order to "get well." Recently, much has been published on the body-mind connection and how it relates to health. The general consensus is that until physical, emotional and spiritual entities are harmoniously integrated, real health will not occur. If we are plagued by depression, fear or anxiety, our physical health will suffer. It's as simple as that.

Unfortunately, spiritual issues as they pertain to physical health have been sorely neglected by modern medical practitioners. Now, however, the idea of "drawing on the powers of heaven" is not the taboo it used to be. As we approach a new millennium, great numbers of people are actively searching for ways to boost their spiritual lives in an effort to find a more lasting kind of happiness and satisfaction.

Once again, we must go back to ancient times and relearn what even the most primitive societies knew: the link between the spirit and the body must be acknowledged, that they have a ongoing and inseparable effect on each other.

Within our academic and intellectual circles, the worth of the soul is usually scoffed at or cast aside as rather inconsequential. Because it is considered a "religious" topic, it has been relegated to some outer realm that in no way pertains to issues of medicine or health. In our efforts to employ the scientific method to validate anything and everything, we have forgotten the ultimate healing power of spiritual medicine.

Trust yourself to become spiritually in tune. Trust that there is a loving God who is aware of your struggles. Ask for his help and expect to receive it. Man was created that he might have joy, not despair.

In *The Efficacy of Prayer*, P.J. Collipp, M.D., suggests that prayer does indeed have value in the treatment of disease. Collipp states, "Among the plethora of modern drugs, and the increasing ingenuity of our surgeons, it seems inappropriate that our medical literature contains so few studies on our oldest and, who knows, perhaps most successful form of therapy [i.e., prayer]."

Carl Jung, in his treatise *Modern Man in Search of a Soul*, wrote of his profound dissatisfaction with conventional therapies for the mentally ill. His interest in the metaphysical or the supernatural grew from his observation that Freud's methods of treating people with psychological disorders did not seem to work if they were over the age of 35. He concluded, "It is safe to say that every one of them fell ill because he had lost that which the living religions of every age have given to their followers, and none of them has been really healed who did not regain his religious outlook."

I believe that if you are lacking spiritual roots, you need to cultivate some. Seek out God and learn to have faith. Never underestimate the power of love which helps us to break out of our sometimes obsessive preoccupation with selfish concerns. Eric Fromm said, "In addition to faith, we must possess courage, the willingness to take a risk, even to experience pain and disappointment." As humans, we can forgo some of the most powerful healing tools at our disposal. One of these tools is faith.

PART 2

Alternative Therapies

"I will follow that system which, according to my ability and judgment, I consider for the benefit of my patients, and abstain from whatever is deleterious . . ."

—FROM THE HIPPOCRATIC OATH

Mainstream Medicine and Alternative Therapies: My Story

It's always intriguing to hear how and why a medical doctor chooses to embrace unorthodox therapies for disease. My story has evolved over a number of years as a practicing physician who routinely delivered 160 babies per year, performed hundreds of surgical procedures and saw virtually every ailment suffered by human beings. I discovered that many of my patients would come to me and essentially say, "fix me."

While many of my patients responded to conventional treatments, a significant group that never seemed to improve grew in number. As I pondered the dilemma of determining what treatments to attempt for these individuals, I discovered a rather interesting fact: conventional medicine is rather rigid in its approach to problematic disease; treatment options must be expanded to fit the specific needs of each patient. It was during this time in my practice that I joined the faculty in the residency program at McKay-Dee Hospital in Ogden, Utah, and subsequently

began to explore various alternative treatments and their applications.

I was surprised to learn that the UCLA Medical School students and physicians were learning to perform acupuncture. I wanted to be among them. Throughout the course, I became acquainted with a number of Chinese herbal formulas that I incorporated into my practice. The word spread quickly throughout my community. Soon, I found myself confronted by many different people curious if their herbal preparations were legitimate. Their inquiries motivated me to learn more. I found that incorporating herbal therapies in conjunction with acupuncture and body/mind interventions seemed to be a surprisingly effective treatment trio.

The patient is always the real beneficiary of doctors investigating alternative medicine. Among the many alternative therapies, patients may find more effective methods for treating various diseases. Just as doctors adopt new ideas and methods, patients must be equally open to adjusting their way of thinking since some alternative therapies like acupuncture may be quite unlike more familiar conventional therapies. Most objections by patients to a new therapy vanish as they increase their understanding. When patients are willing to open a book or ask questions, they better understand a new therapy.

No single philosophy of diagnosis or therapy supplies us with all the answers. Nevertheless, the best treatment strategies hinge on integrating various health care methodologies.

Education in Natural Medicine is Crucial to Effective Healing

Today, the idea that orthodox medicine alone holds all the answers is no longer accepted. While the value of mainstream medicine in certain situations remains undisputed, its practices are often limited to strong drug therapies or radical surgeries. Today, when it comes to health care, consumers want to know all of their options. The key is education.

You can be certain that most physicians are unaware of significant clinical data supporting the efficacy of certain herbs like echinacea, the impressive cardiovascular action of garlic, glucosamine for healing arthritic joints, wild yam as a safe source of progesterone, etc. Does your physician know that marine lipids act as natural blood thinners . . . or that St. John's wort can act as a natural treatment for depression without the toxic side effects of prozac or monoamine inhibitors. . . . Has your doctor ever recommended cascara sagrada for chronic constipation? It is extremely effective, gentle, nonhabit forming and can actually improve the muscle tone of the colon wall.

In my view, physicians fall into three major categories when it comes to natural medicine. A relatively small group of doctors on one end of the spectrum are strongly opposed to any treatment that fall out of the realm of conventional therapies. The largest group consists of doctors who tolerate or ignore their patients use of alternative therapies. And finally, the last is a growing group of doctors who have developed a genuine interest in natural medicine and are making the effort to learn more. This last group will inevitably represent the physician of the future who will have the savvy and know-how to incorporate the best alternative treatments with conventional medical practices.

Why Are More Doctors Exploring Alternative Therapies?

Several reasons exist explaining the growing interest physicians are demonstrating in nonconventional forms of treatment. When I discovered that many of my patients did not respond well to traditional therapies, I began to look elsewhere in an effort to alleviate their suffering. Regardless of what motivates them, physicians cannot ignore the profound interest the public has in safe and natural treatments. There is no question that a great number of people in our communities have become disillusioned with established medical practices.

More doctors would integrate alternative therapies into their practices if it were not for two deterring factors: first

of all, doctors spend eight years or more in school concentrating on their individual specialty; time is extremely tight and the notion of taking additional time to learn about alternative therapies is not particularly appealing. Second, even if a physician wanted to investigate alternative medicine, reliable schools and courses of information are hard to find. It is not easy for a doctor to obtain this kind of information but it is certainly possible for any physician who has enough desire.

Medical practices which have evolved over the last fifty years are not the only therapies available. Medicine has devolved from an art dedicated to the healing and preservation of life, to one guided by the latest, high-priced pharmaceutical drug designed to target disease symptoms. We live in a society that is quick to medicate itself without looking into the processes and intricacies of disease.

Dr. Malcom Todd, a former president of the American Medical Association, put it best when he said, "Thus far, physicians have shown little objective interest in promoting health and preventive care. We actually have a disease oriented cure system, rather than a health oriented care system in this country today."

It is tragic that in our vigorous attempts to treat a number of devastating diseases, many of us have overlooked the profound impact of natural therapies. For centuries, the principles of natural healing have been based on

- The healing power of nature
- Doing no harm to the patient
- Identifying and treating the cause of disease, not just its symptoms
- Promoting the role of physician as teacher as well as healer

Most of us would like to find a doctor that is oriented toward the use of natural therapies and luckily, increasing numbers of medical doctors are becoming intrigued by alternative forms of treatment. More and more publications, authored by medical doctors who have embraced natural health treatments, are appearing on newsstands. Medical journals are full of articles on antioxidants, vitamin and mineral therapies and the profound health implications of diet and exercise.

Medical schools which now offer courses in alternative medicine include Harvard, Columbia, Georgetown and Duke. Today, there are 14 accredited chiropractic colleges in the United States.

The National Cancer Institute is actively researching rainforest plants and some insurance companies are beginning to cover alternative treatment costs. Osteopaths and chiropractitioners recognize that the neuroendocrine system coordinates virtually all body functions and rely on manipulation of the spine to restore the proper energy flow and to promote healing. Naturopaths use herbalism, massage, nutrition and manipulation to diagnose and treat disease. Emphasis on fasting, hydrotherapy, nutrition and the elimination of alcohol, coffee, tobacco, etc. are integral to this holistic approach. Homeopathy is based on the belief that minute amounts of certain substances which actually mimic disease symptoms can cure. Homeopathic remedies are approved as over-the-counter medications by the Food and Drug Administration.

Scientific Documentation of Natural Treatments

To the surprise of many physicians, a great deal of credible scientific data exists explaining how certain natural compounds work in the human body. Knowing the physiological mechanisms behind natural medicines is crucial to its acceptance. Most doctors don't have a clue why or how certain herbs or vitamins can help heal, and unfortunately, many don't care to inform themselves on such things.

When a colleague of mine sent out a questionnaire to physicians regarding the use of cranberry for the treatment of urinary tract infections (UTIs), some fascinating trends surfaced. Surprisingly, 50 percent of the medical doctors who returned the survey said they used cranberry for UTIs and half of this number believed it was effective. Obviously a significant number of physicians were willing to use this particular natural treatment and their use did not always depend on their belief that the herb was actually helpful.

Interestingly, a question the survey did not ask was, "If you believe that cranberry works, how does it work?" You can be certain that the majority of physicians would have no idea how to respond. Moreover, they are probably completely unaware of research studies which explain and support the efficacy of certain bioactive ingredients found in botanical medicines.

CRANBERRY AND URINARY TRACT INFECTIONS: MAGIC OR SCIENCE?

When confronted with explaining the biological action of cranberry, the most likely answer would be that it must alter the pH of the urine, inhibiting the growth of bacteria by making it more acidic. However, when this theory was tested with a group of volunteers who took cranberry, the pH of the urine remained unchanged. Regardless of the quantity of cranberry juice they drank, the pH stayed the same. The question remained: how does cranberry work? To address this perplexing question, a number of simple and elegant experiments were designed.

First, it is important to understand that the 85 percent of urinary tract infections are caused by *E. coli* a bacteria that resides in the large intestine where it contributes to friendly flora action. When it makes its way into the urethra, though, an infection can result. The other 15 percent of infections are caused by other bacteria that also live in the bowel. Bacteria must cling to the walls of the bladder in order to cause an infection. Free-floating bacteria in urine are washed away and do not cause inflammation.

When bacteria colonize in the walls of the bladder, destructive enzymes that destroy the bladder lining are released. As a result, capillary bleeding occurs and blood enters the urine. After experimenting with various theories, it was concluded that cranberry contains a natural substance that keeps the bacteria from adhering to the bladder,

flushing them out in the urine (this active antiadherence ingredient found in cranberry is currently in the process of becoming a patented medicine.)

Consider the implications of the experiment's results: Urinary tract infections are extremely common and while generally not life-threatening, they cost millions of dollars in drug treatments and time lost from work. Moreover, repeated antibiotic therapy results in increased susceptibility. If the majority of these infections could be prevented, enormous amounts of money could be saved and spent on more worthy endeavors. Cranberry is a relatively inexpensive, natural and extremely safe way to prevent and treat urinary tract infections. How many other natural herbal agents exist for diseases we are quick to medicate with potent and risky chemical drugs?

PHYTOMEDICINALS: HERBAL MEDICINE

Linnaeus once said, "Herbs and plants are medical jewels gracing the woods, fields, lanes, which few eyes see, and few minds understand. Through this want of observation and knowledge the world suffers immense loss." The advent of modern medicine prompted what has now become a frenzied competition: drug companies racing to patent new synthetic pharmaceutical compounds for immense profit. In the process, traditional herbal treatments were cast aside as old fashioned and obsolete. Referring to conventional medicine as "traditional" is somewhat of a misnomer in that "traditional" more correctly refers to centuries of historical herbal therapies.

Many of us who call ourselves medical practitioners have forgotten that most of the world's population still successfully relies on herbal medicine. While we have an impressive array of sophisticated, high-tech medical procedures, some of our health statistics are nothing to brag about. For example, the United States ranks behind more than 15 other countries in infant mortality, a dramatic indicator that we need to re-evaluate our health-care system and its relation to nutrition. We live in a nation of plenty that is ironically often malnourished. Herbal therapies are often integrated with certain foods to augment their action.

European and Japanese medical establishments have had the guts (for lack of a better term) to research and apply principles of natural healing without the obstacles of suppressive restraints or patent bureaucracies. Meanwhile, physicians in the United States persistently trudge through mazes, nothing more than lab rats in a massive experiment that has become a monumental failure.

In the beginning, all drugs were natural substances extracted from the environment. Each primitive culture discovered the curative properties of certain local plant parts and the practice of phytomedicine evolved. All kinds of interesting therapeutic applications developed and each was based on understanding the curative properties of individual plant parts and how to use them. For example, boiling the bark of the cinchona tree alleviated symptoms of malaria, and capsicum powder helped to ease the pain of a toothache.

The notion that synthetic chemical compounds are the only effective medicine is no longer accepted. After found-

why do drugs produce side effects?

Most prescription drugs wreak more havoc on our health than the original ailment they were designed to treat. While no one wants to dispute the lifesaving value of antibiotics, steroidal anti-inflammatories, etc., drugs are routinely over-prescribed and pose significant health risks as well. Drugs thought to be safe have killed or maimed thousands of people. For example, thalidomide, once prescribed to pregnant women for morning sickness, caused birth defects in hundreds of cases. Also, sleeping pills like Halcyon can cause serious personality changes, and phen-fen, indiscriminately dispersed by careless physicians, has been linked to potentially fatal heart problems.

Our high-tech, high-priced orthodox medical practices frequently harm rather than heal. Drugs are the cause of more than 100,000 deaths per year, and 30 percent of hospitalized individuals are further damaged by drugs.

The over-prescription of antibiotics is a perfect illustration of a good thing gone bad. Using antibiotic therapy for everything from a virally caused sore throat to a hangnail has resulted in the development of antibiotic-resistant bacteria, which may eventually create a modern day plague for which there is no cure. In other words, antibiotics cannot cure these resistant strains of bacteria. And taking antibiotics continually makes an individual more prone to future infections and weakens the immune system.

ing the Bio-Brain Center in Princeton, New Jersey, Dr. Karl Pfeiffer stated, "For every drug that benefits a patient, there is a natural substance that can achieve the same effect."

It has been estimated that as much as 80 percent of the population of this planet relies on herbal medicine. But unknown to many, this impressive use of herbs is not limited to poor or backward countries. Almost half of all medical doctors in France and Germany used herbal therapies as part of their healing protocols. Unfortunately, medicinal practices in the United States aren't nearly as progressive.

Over the last three decades scientific data has been steadily accruing supporting the notion that herbs can provide safer and in some cases, even more effective treatment than prescription drugs. Ironically, while orthodox medicine claims scientific backing, Dr. David Edd asserts that "very little of medicine has been carefully evaluated in well-designed, well-controlled studies. . . . for a large proportion of practices, we really don't know what the outcomes or what the effects are."

The belief held by many that "a little is good, a lot is better" can be very dangerous with respect to both conventional and herbal medications. Occasionally, you will find herbal preparations that are extremely concentrated, such as some sophisticated European extracts and are much like today's potent prescription medicines. If you are not sure about a particular medication, don't guess. Wisdom and prudence should be used with all medicines whether or not they are in a concentrated form. Also, unless otherwise noted, it is best not to use herbs if you are pregnant or lactating without first consulting a health care professional who has good information on the subject.

Some patients may not find the help they are looking for from alternative therapies. And, as a doctor, I don't rely strictly on alternative therapies. If I feel a patient would be better off with a conventional therapy, that is what I recommend. Sometimes I feel a patient would be better off if they used both conventional and alternative therapies.

HERBS VS. DRUGS: A COMPARISON

Unlike synthetic drugs, herbs provide a synergistic array of compounds designed by nature to enhance individual action against disease, avoiding any detrimental side effects. In an attempt to isolate the active components of medicinal plants, drug researchers have inadvertently created a pharmaceutical monster. By assuming that only one of the primary chemical constituents of plants is therapeutically valuable, they have cast aside the so-called "inactive" compounds which played a profound role in the biochemical acceptance of the whole plant in the human body. Isolated, mimicked or potentiated drug compounds are not equivalent to the whole plant or herb.

By refining or synthesizing various compounds, toxicity is created. In other words, because they are presented to the body stripped of other substances that act as balancing agents, these artificial compounds are not well received by the body.

In most cases, each of a drug's therapeutic effects comes with a negative side effect. Granted, the newly created drug may be more potent, administered with great precision and easier to ingest, but the human body has a tendency to recognize it as a foreign and unnatural substance. As a result, a chain of undesirable physiological reactions occurs. Frequently, the body reacts to synthetic and powerful compounds much as it would to a poison.

The bottom line is that nature usually knows best. It is important, though, to remember that unlike the potent, quick and sometimes dangerous effects of synthetic drugs or analogs, herbs work slowly. Rather than just masking symptoms, herbs intrinsically heal—and their effects are longer lasting.

While plants have provided medicine with some of its best drugs, artificial synthesis of chemical compounds found in specific plants has unfortunately snuffed the search for new and better plant sources. Synthesized compounds can be patented, but often, the enormous amount of money needed to bring that compound into therapeutic dispersion is difficult to recoup.

European and Asian countries have continued to study and value the use of herbal preparations and are far ahead of the United States in regard to herbal medicines and their practical applications. Phytomedicinals are legally sold in these countries where laws requiring their safety and efficacy are more reasonable than in American communities. Herbs like ginkgo biloba, milk thistle (silymarin), echinacea, ginseng, and ephedra are commonly used by reliable medical practitioners who have recognized their therapeutic value for decades.

What is frustrating is that even when pharmaceutical drugs are prescribed by doctors, they rarely contribute valuable information on how to minimize some of their risks. For example, have you ever heard your doctor tell you to take acidophilus supplements after taking a course of antibiotics? The effects of drugs on the absorption of dietary nutrients is rarely addressed by physicians.

ARE HERBS SAFE?

Dr. Andrew Weil, yet another physician who has embraced both orthodox and natural medicine states:

"For every prescription I write for a pharmaceutical drug, I give out 40 or 50 for botanical remedies. In almost 10 years of prescribing in that way, I have not yet seen a serious adverse reaction in any patient taking a medicinal plant."

The statistics verify Weil's statement. From 1983 to 1992 herbs did not contribute in any deaths, while dietary supplements caused three deaths, over-the-counter drugs caused 320, food-borne illnesses resulted in 9000 and—most alarmingly—prescription drugs played a significant role in nearly 100,000 deaths. Herbs can be incredibly safe if used as directed because, in many ways, they act like foods in the human body.

Guidelines for Herb Purchasing and Usage

The following are several suggestions to consider when buying and using herbs:

- Purchase herbs from reliable sources that you know provide pure and potent products. Look for standardized products with guaranteed potency.
- Choose herbal forms that are the most effective. Herbs can come in extracts, tinctures, dry capsulized powders and even in ointments and creams. Always look for the percentage of active ingredient, if possible.
- Take dosages that are recommended and do not assume that more is always better.
- If you are prone to allergies, pregnant, nursing or taking other drugs for any condition, check with your doctor before using herbs.
- Herbs are designed to work with the body and usually require consistent use over a long period of time to achieve the desired results.
- Try to use products which come from companies sympathetic to the environment and to ecological awareness.

- Do your homework on the specific herb you have chosen to take as far as its most effective delivery system. Wild yam, for example is better absorbed through the skin rather than through the mouth.
- Herbs can be taken in dried form and are usually available in capsules, as teas, extracts or tinctures. New delivery systems such as sublingual drops or creams may provide even better assimilation.
- Give children only a fraction of the adult dose depending on their age. Don't give children under the age of two any supplement unless you check with your physician. Children six to twelve can receive one fourth of the adult dose. Children twelve to eighteen can receive three fourths of the adult dose.
- Read the contradictions of certain herbs and make sure you do not have a condition or are taking drugs which may cause an unwanted interaction.
- Keep all herbs out of the reach of children.

Herbal Combinations: Balancing the Yin and the Yang

I have found a way to design herbal formulas for my patients based on combining herbs that satisfy each of the following individual categories:

- active herbs (usually bitter)
- aromatic and carminative herbs
- demulcent herbs
- cleansing herbs

Active herbs provide direct, therapeutic action and can have powerful biological effects often accompanied by gastrointestinal upset. Consequently, aromatic or carminative herbs like ginger, cloves or peppermint settle the stomach and intestines and are added to temper this effect. In addition, aromatic herbs help to stimulate digestion and circulation, boosting the efficacy and the delivery of the active herb. Demulcent herbs also soothe the gastrointestinal tract. Cleansing herbs are an integral part of the formula since many seemingly unrelated disease conditions are actually the direct result of poor bowel elimination and the build-up of intestinal toxins. The cleansing herbs gently stimulate the bowel to more efficiently get rid of accumulated wastes.

For centuries Chinese herbalists understood that prescribing herbs in time-tested formulas was more effective than using single botanical preparations. The widespread use of various herbal formulations resulted in the compilation of several thousand herbal blends. Traditionally, these blends were individually adjusted according to the needs of the patient. The time-honored practice of carefully designing herbal formulations is based on the concept of synergistic enhancement. In other words, there are certain plants that exist in nature which function more efficiently when they merge their medicinal attributes.

Today, scientific research supports the ancient idea of herbal "marriages." The notion that combining certain herbs together creates a better therapeutic effect can be supported by clinical studies. It's important to remember that the interaction between certain botanicals can be even more important than the individual properties of each contributing herb. Well-designed herbal formulas can exert impressive therapeutic effects on a number of maladies.

Another of the advantages of blending herbs is that various symptoms can be treated simultaneously. Most herbal blends are comprised of what might be called dominant plants, (which are usually responsible for primary therapeutic actions), and passive herbs that serve to soothe, support and potentiate.

Stimulatory herbs are usually bitter and are nicely complemented by aromatic, carminative and demulcent herbs. For example, senna is a stimulatory and dynamic bitter herb which initiates colon muscle contraction. Adding a carminative herb, like ginger, to senna serves to soothe the stomach and prevent gripping which may occur if senna was taken alone. The addition of capsicum or ginger to any herb formula acts as a catalyst, increasing the efficiency of each individual herb. Herbs like peppermint are potentiated by capsicum. Moreover, the menthol contained in peppermint helps to balance out the "hot" nature of the capsicum. A good herbal blend will combine stimulant herbs with nourishing, protecting and cleansing varieties.

INCORPORATING HERBS INTO YOUR MEALS

Herbs can naturally complement and augment diet, especially in cases when sickness is present. Many cultures routinely use herbs in preparing food, not necessarily for taste enhancement, but to treat specific symptoms. For example, in Asia, if someone in the family comes down with a cold, an herb such as astragalus may be added to their soup to bolster not only the immune system of the sick one, but to help increase disease resistance in the rest of the family.

Certainly, if we were better at using herbs in our day-to-day meal preparation, we would gain tremendous health benefits. Interestingly, we know now that curcumin, one of the active ingredients in turmeric acts as an antimutagen, meaning that it decreases our risk for the abnormal reproduction of cells. Learning to use turmeric regularly in meal preparation may decrease our chances of getting cancer. Get used to adding a wide variety of herbs and spices in cooking your meals.

CHINESE HERBAL MEDICINE

The Chinese have used botanicals as medicines for over a thousand years and even today, they practice a sophisticated form of herbal medicine that is recognized by their professional organizations. Chinese herbalism was adapted by the Japanese a few centuries after the birth of Christ and is widely practiced today along with disciplines like acupuncture. Oriental herbal medicine offers the western world a veritable treasury of tried and true treatments, which, for the most part we have not used until recent decades.

Traditional Chinese medicine dates back as far as 2,500 B.C. and recorded practices and disciplines are still used by modern practitioners. The Chinese have always viewed disease as an indication that an imbalance or disruption in harmony has occurred within the delicate and interwoven systems of the whole person. Consequently, medicinal therapies are designed to realign and restore this balance, enabling the body's own restorative powers to work more efficiently. Herbs or botanical extracts are the most important external agents and augment other therapies such as acupuncture.

The Chinese medical system is based on the "theory of elements," a system that incorporates five elements that constitute every way in which human beings interact with their environment. The elements—wood, fire, earth, metal, and water—are considered linked together and synergistically related. Each of these are connected with specific emotions and parts of the human body, seasons, tastes, colors and sensations. In order to maintain balance and good, the elements must be harmoniously related with none being too dominant (disease may develop). Chinese practitioners became skilled in looking at various parts of the body in terms of these elements and they distinguished when one needed to be emphasized or tranquilized. The five elements include the following:

Wood

Season: spring
Taste: sour
Emotion: anger
Parts of the body: liver, gallbladder, tendons, eyes

Water

Season: winter
Taste: salty
Emotion: fear
Parts of the body: kidneys, bladder, ears, hair, bones

Metal

Season: fall
Taste: pungent
Emotion: grief
Parts of the body: lungs, large intestine, nose, skin

Earth

Season: Indian summer
Taste: sweet
Emotion: worry
Parts of the body: spleen, stomach, mouth, muscles

Fire

Season: summer
Taste: bitter
Emotion: joy
Parts of the body: heart, small intestine, tongue

THE THEORY OF YIN AND YANG

The philosophy of yin and yang is based on the idea that there must be opposition in all things. According to theories, all things created are kept in balance by an opposite force. Yin refers to the female sex, cold and dark while yang is the male, hot and light. Keeping these opposing entities balanced is what maintains good health and prevents disease. Remember, too little or too much of one can cause illness to occur. Each part of the body falls into either a yin or yang category. Herbal medications are designed to either calm an excess of one of these forces or to enhance one that is lacking. Hot versus cold is the basis of almost all medical diagnosis. Chinese medicine also identifies five tastes that are characterized as hot or cold. For example, a sweet or pungent taste sensation causes heating to occur, while salty, bitter or sour tastes have a cooling effect. Herbal combinations can contain a variety of tastes designed to achieve a particular kind of balance. Schizandra, for example, is a botanical that contains five taste sensations.

The Chinese believe that each type of taste will target a specific area of the body. Sweet or pungent herbs are used for the external areas of the body and upper sections of the torso. The sour, bitter or salty herbs are applied to the lower parts and to internal organs. Because different areas of our bodies can be affected by the same disease, an individual assortment of cooling and heating herbs must be selected depending on whether upper or lower areas are involved. The strong or pungent herbs are also considered stimulants, the sweet ones as tonifying and the salty as softening.

The Chinese like to use herbs in standard formulas which number in the thousands. Herbal blends use synergy to achieve better results. Herbal combinations can include up to twenty herbs which complement each other according to individual need. Chinese practitioners use teas, decoctions, soups and even have their patients add herbs to food. The ability to recognize whether a particular body part needs cooling or heating is essential to Chinese herbal medicine.

Major Herbs and Their Applications

ALFALFA (Medicago sativa)

Definition: A nutritive herb rich in minerals and vitamins, especially iron and vitamin K. Considered an estrogen precursor.

Applications: Allergies, anemia, arthritis, asthma, Bell's palsy, blood disorders, bursitis, cholesterol, diabetes, digestive disorders, fatigue, gout, lactation, kidney disorders, morning sickness, menopause, nausea, Cushing's disease, rheumatism, ulcers and urinary tract infections.

Scientific Updates: Contains eight essential amino acids, is a rich source of vitamin B12, natural fluoride and chlorophyll. Alfalfa has demonstrated an antirheumatic effect, lowers cholesterol and improves overall health and vigor.[1] Recent French studies have found that alfalfa can reduce tissue damage caused by radiation exposure.[2] In addition, it has also shown antibacterial and antitumor properties.[3] Because it can neutralize acidity, it is also beneficial for bladder and urinary tract infections.

Safety: Take as directed. No known toxicity.

Complementary Agents: Uva ursi, juniper, parsley, buchu, cornsilk, marshmallow, cranberry, vitamin C, bioflavonoids, proanthocyanidins, vitamin A, B-complex, calcium/magnesium, marine lipids, acidophilus, and phytonutrients.

ALOE VERA (Aloe barbadensis)

Definition: Natural astringent with healing and laxative properties.

External Applications: External: Burns, wounds and minor skin irritations.

Oral Applications: Acne, AIDS, allergies, bed sores, canker sores, chicken pox lesions, colitis, constipation, herpes, insect bites and stings, psoriasis, scar tissue, sores, sunburn, gastric ulcers, leg ulcers, diabetes and asthma.

Scientific Updates: Recent studies have confirmed that aloe has the ability to fight against a variety of bacteria and fungi.[4] Because it has impressive antimicrobial properties, it makes an excellent preparation for the treatment of burns. Its action has been observed against bacteria which include the staphylococcus and streptococcus types.[5] It has also shown significant antiviral activity against HIV.[6] In addition, aloe vera has exhibited itself as an immune system stimulant, an anti-inflammatory agent, a booster of tissue repair and a compound which can actually lower blood sugar.

Safety: Gel extracted from the leaf is recognized as a safe food. Aloe vera can come in a naturally occurring gel, as a concentrate, in juice form or in capsules. Excessive oral doses of aloe vera may cause gripping pains and diarrhea.

Complementary agents: Vitamin E, tea tree oil and wild yam cream.

ASTRAGALUS (Astragalus membranaceus)

Definition: Rich in polysaccharides, astragalus supports T-cell function and is considered an excellent immune system stimulant.

Applications: AIDS, hepatitis, viral infections, peripheral vascular diseases, immune disorders, influenza, hypertension and myasthenia gravis.

Scientific Updates: Astragalus contains various unique chemical compounds which have made it one of the most impressive Oriental health-promoting botanicals. Asian practitioners have used astragalus for a compromised immune system, viral infections of all kinds and for high blood pressure. Recent studies have found that astragalus may be useful for cases of myasthenia gravis.[7]

Safety: No known toxicity.

Complementary agents: Echinacea, boneset, garlic, essential fatty acids, hawthorn, ginseng and schizandra.

BILBERRY (Vaccinium myrtillus)

Definition: Suited for intestinal upsets such as diarrhea and irritated intestinal mucosa. Over long periods of time, bilberry helps to manage eye disorders caused by weak capillaries due to its anthocyanin content.

Applications: Blood sugar, bruising, diabetes, diarrhea, eyesight, gallstones, hemorrhoids, kidney stones, circulatory insufficiency, hypoglycemia, night blindness, urinary disorders and varicose veins.

Scientific Updates: Bilberry is considered an herbal antioxidant which helps to inhibit free radical damage in human tissue. Studies have found that bilberry extract can kill or inhibit the growth of certain fungi, yeast, and bacteria.[8] Bilberry is also effective in cases of diarrhea and intestinal upset.[9]

Safety: Diabetics should check with their doctor before taking this herb.

Complementary Agents: Goldenseal, fenugreek, bilberry, gymnema, sylvestis, blueberry, vitamin C, bioflavonoids, proanthocyanidins, phytonutrients, vitamin E, vitamin A, B-complex, chromium, bee pollen, and bee propolis.

BLACK COHOSH (Cimicifuga racemosa)

Definition: Its antispasmodic properties have made it a favorite botanical remedy for menstrual cramps, muscle spasms and coughs. It is also believed to stimulate estrogen synthesis, making it a desirable supplement for menopause.

Applications: PMS, hormonal imbalances, stress, nervousness, muscle cramping, menopause, lung congestion, inflammatory conditions and hypertension.

Scientific Updates: Modern research has supported the use of black cohosh for hypertension and cardiovascular disorders.[10] Black cohosh can help to tranquilize an irritable or excited nervous system while stimulating certain CNS functions which promote normalcy. Recently, the value of black cohosh as a uterine tonic has been supported by clinical research.[11] Current experimentation strongly suggests that black cohosh has anti-inflammatory properties.[12] Black cohosh significantly relaxes nerves and smooth muscle and is effective in treating irritated nerves and general restlessness. The Russians have recently approved black cohosh extract for use as a central nervous system tonic and a treatment for high blood pressure.[13]

Safety: Black cohosh is considered safe although pregnant women should consult their physician before using it. Avoid large doses.

Complementary Agents: Valerian root, hops, wood betony, scullcap, chamomile, passionflower, mullein, marshmallow, squaw vine, melatonin, calcium/magnesium and B-complex.

BLACK WALNUT (Juglans nigra)

Definition: Rich in organic tannins, this herb has antifungal and astringent properties which predispose its use for parasitic infections, skin fungi and other skin eruptions.

Applications: Athlete's foot, boils, *Candida albicans* (yeast infections), canker sores, cold sores, eczema, fungus, gum disease, herpes, intestinal parasites, tapeworm and tuberculosis.

Scientific Updates: Recent research strongly suggests that black walnut has antifungal properties as well as an antiseptic action.[14] Clinical studies have found that certain constituents in black walnut have anticancer properties.[15] This particular action may link the connection of viruses and parasites to malignancies.[16] The high tannin content of black walnut is primarily responsible for it ability to expel worms and parasites.[17] "Black walnut has been shown to be specific for treatment of *Candida albicans*."[18]

Safety: Use in appropriate amounts as directed. Pregnant or nursing mothers should check with their physicians.

Complementary Agents: Garlic, cascara sagrada, buckthorn, pumpkin seeds, red clover, culver root, acidophilus, vitamin A, B-complex, pantothenic acid, calcium/magnesium, potassium and marine lipids.

BLESSED THISTLE (Cnicus benedictus)

Definition: Traditionally use to increase lactation, blessed thistle also treats fevers, indigestion and diarrhea.

Applications: Anorexia, lack of appetite, circulatory disorders, blood purification, cancer, constipation, digestive problems, fever, gallbladder disease, gas, headaches, heart problems, hormonal imbalances, lactation, liver ailments, lung diseases and painful menstruation.

Scientific Updates: Blessed thistle is an excellent supporting herb for plant combinations. "It helps activate a sluggish liver and corrects stomach and digestive problems, flatulence and tension headaches. It further supports the body's cleansing and detoxifying systems by promoting perspiration and removing excess fluids."[19] Modern studies have found that blessed thistle contains antibacterial and antiyeast properties.[20] It has demonstrated its ability to strengthen the spleen and liver and helps reduce fevers by promoting perspiration.[21]

Safety: Ingesting excessive amounts of blessed thistle may cause nausea. Contact with the skin should be avoided.

Complementary Agents: Lemon grass, sage, slippery elm, chamomile, catnip, peppermint, milk thistle, vitamin C, bioflavonoids, calcium/magnesium and digestive enzymes.

BUCHU (Barosma betulina)

Definition: Used for chronic kidney and bladder inflammations, buchu, a natural astringent, helps to alleviate high acid urine and is also good for healing the prostate gland.

Applications: Bladder infections, diabetes, kidney disease, prostate disorders and water retention.

Scientific Updates: It is the volatile oil content of buchu which enables it to stimulate urination while acting as a urinary antiseptic.[22] Buchu "acts to eliminate mucus, acid urine and irritation, and is given to combat many forms of inflammation and infection, including cystitis, pyelitis, ureteritis and prostatitis."[23] ". . . Diasophenol, which has antiseptic properties is considered by some to be the most important constituent of buchu."[24]

Safety: Use in appropriate doses as directed.

Complementary agents: Uva ursi, parsley, cornsilk, cranberry, juniper berry, alfalfa, marshmallow, bee pollen, vitamin C, bioflavonoids, proanthocyanidins, vitamin A, zinc and mineral and electrolyte supplements.

BUCKTHORN (Rhamnus frangula)

Definition: Buckthorn is a purgative herb that stimulates bowel evacuation and is a considered a tonic for the liver and gallbladder.

Applications: Bowel cleansing, cancer, constipation, fever, gallbladder disease, gallstones and liver ailments.

Scientific Updates: Buckthorn has shown significant inhibition of leukemia in mice studies.[25] Buckthorn contains anthraquinone glycosides which works like cascara sagrada to promote gentle colon peristalsis.[26] European studies have confirmed the advantage of buckthorn's ability to release its active principles in the small intestine rather than the stomach.[27]

Safety: Take as directed in appropriate doses as an excess may cause intestinal gripping. Pregnant or nursing women should avoid this herb due to its laxative effect.

Complementary agents: Cascara sagrada, red clover, pumpkin seeds, culver root, marshmallow, slippery elm, dandelion, black walnut, quassia, ginger, acidophilus, vitamin A, vitamin E, B-complex, bioflavonoids and marine lipids.

BURDOCK (Arctium lappa)

Definition: The insulin content of burdock gives it the ability to promote the healing of sores. It also has the ability to clear the blood of impurities and toxins.

Applications: Abscesses, acne, boils, carbuncles, blood disorders, cancer, canker sores, chicken pox, colds, constipation, eczema, fever, gout; hemorrhoids, herpes, blood sugar disorders, poison ivy, poison oak, psoriasis, tonsillitis, tumors, gallbladder disease, liver disease and weak immune system.

Scientific Updates: Studies have supported the ability of burdock to help restore liver and gallbladder function.[28] In addition, clinical testing has also established both antifungal and antibiotic properties of burdock. Burdock can lower blood sugar, inhibit certain types of tumors and greatly contribute to the healing of specific skin ailments like leprosy and venereal disease sores.[29]

Safety: Burdock can interfere with iron absorption.

Complementary Agents: Chaparral, alfalfa, dandelion, echinacea, yellow dock, Oregon grape, cascara sagrada, buckthorn, blue-green algae, kelp, licorice, milk thistle, aloe vera, vitamin A, B-complex, essential fatty acids, zinc, potassium and lecithin.

BUTCHER'S BROOM (Ruscus aculeatus)

Definition: A natural vaso-constrictor, butcher's broom strengthens weak blood vessels and discourages the formation of blood clots. It also possesses significant anti-inflammatory properties.

Applications: Arteriosclerosis, capillary weakness, diabetic retinopathy, hemorrhoids, inflammation, jaundice, phlebitis, varicose veins, blood clot (prevention), leg cramps, gout and jaundice.

Scientific Updates: Research has confirmed the ability of butcher's broom to constrict vessels and inhibit inflammation. Both of these properties make the herb ideal for fragile capillaries of swollen veins.[30] European practitioners routinely use butcher's broom for any disorder affecting the veins, especially hemorrhoids.

Safety: Generally considered safe, an allergy to butcher's broom can produce stomach upset.

Complementary Agents: Ginkgo, ginger, bilberry, vitamin C, bioflavonoids, grape seed or pine bark extract.

CASCARA SAGRADA (Rhamnus purshiana)

Definition: One of nature's most gentle and effective laxatives, cascara sagrada stimulates a sluggish colon while exerting a tonifying effect. It is one of the most preferred herbal remedies for chronic constipation and is also good for the liver and gallbladder.

Applications: Congestion (general), constipation, colon disorders (sluggish colon etc), gallbladder disease, gallstones, gas, hemorrhoids, jaundice, kidney stone prevention, liver disorders, parasites and worms.

Scientific Updates: The aloe-emodin content of cascara has shown antileukemic properties.[36] The anthraquinones have exhibited potent antibacterial properties against intestinal bacteria.[37] The rhein content of cascara is used in Africa to expel worms.[38] Cascara increases muscular activity in the large intestine.[39] Cascara can prevent the occurrence of calcium based urinary stones.[40] "Cascara is perhaps the safest and most certain laxative available and can be used to restore tone to the colon and thereby overcome laxative dependency in the elderly. The herb is safe and effective for detoxification and cleansing programs."[41]

Safety: At recommended dosages, no toxicity. Cascara should not be used by nursing mothers as its laxative effect can transfer to the infant. Pregnant women should avoid using cascara unless directed by their doctor to do so. People with ulcers or irritable bowel syndrome should check with their doctor before using cascara sagrada.

Complementary Agents: Dandelion, black walnut, quassia, red clover, garlic, buckthorn, pumpkin seeds, marshmallow, slippery elm, culver root, acidophilus, vitamin A, B-complex, vitamin E and calcium/magnesium.

CATNIP (Nepeta cataria)

Definition: By acting as a natural antispasmodic, **catnip** helps to alleviate gas pains, promotes therapeutic perspiration during fevers and calms the central nervous system.

Applications: Colic, intestinal gas, bloating, diarrhea, stomach cramping, insomnia, colds, flu, fevers and pain.

Scientific Updates: Today, catnip is sometimes called "nature's Alka Seltzer" due to its ability to stimulate digestion.[42] It also has some antibiotic properties which may help to control stomach bacteria.[43] It is used for a wide variety of ailments including insomnia, and anemia and is rich in organic iron, which helps to build the blood.

Safety: Catnip is considered a safe botanical medicine if used appropriately.

Complementary Agents: Ginger, fennel, peppermint, papaya, capsicum, saw palmetto berry, myrrh gum, calcium carbonate, pepsin and acidophilus.

CAT'S CLAW (Uncaria tomentosa)

Definition: Cat's claw is a Peruvian rainforest herb with certain alkaloids capable of anti-inflammatory actions, antitumor activity, antiviral actions and the ability to cleanse the intestinal tract. It is thought to signficantly boost the action of the immune system and has been under study for the treatment of both AIDS and cancer.

Applications: Allergies, arthritis, bowel disorders, bursitis, cancer, candida, chemotherapy, chronic fatigue syndrome, cirrhosis, Crohn's disease, edema, fibromyalgia, hemorrhoids, hormonal imbalances, inflammation, intestinal disorders, immune system dysfunction, lupus, parasites, PMS, radiation treatments or exposure, toxic poisoning, ulcers and viral infections (influenza, respiratory infections, etc.).

Scientific Updates: Krallendon is the commercialized name for one of the constituents of this herb that has been used to treat AIDS patients either alone or in conjunction with AZT therapy. It has the ability to activate the immune system. It antiviralviral properties have been confirmed in clinical laboratory studies.

Safety: European studies confirm very low toxicity even when taken in very large doses. Cat's claw shouldn't be used, however, by pregnant or lactating women or by anyone who has had a transplant. Taking the herb may alter bowel consistency in some individuals.

Complementary Agents: Pau d'arco, garlic, echinacea, goldenseal, vitamin C, grape seed extract, bioflavonoids and antioxidant agents.

CHAMOMILE (Matricaria chamomilla)

Definition: As a natural relaxant, chamomile works to soothe the nerves, promote sleep and induce perspiration during fevers. It is also considered a gastrointestinal tonic.

Applications: Insomnia, anxiety, skin irritations, arthritis, menstrual cramps and gastrointestinal distress.

Scientific Updates: Recent studies have confirmed that chamomile works as a uterine tonic, relaxes the nervous system, and interacts positively with other nervine herbs.[49] It has antibacterial properties, can stimulate the liver, and is currently under study for its anticarcinogenic action.[50]

Safety: No toxicity has been found in chamomile. Avoid extreme doses. Do not take chamomile for long periods of time. Allergic reactions are a possibility, but if you are allergic to ragweed, proceed with caution.

Complementary Agents: Valerian root, skullcap, hops, wood betony, black cohosh, mullein, marshmallow, passionflower, peppermint, vitamin B-complex, vitamin C, vitamin A, calcium/magnesium and melatonin.

COMFREY (Symphytum officinale)

Definition: Any condition that involve excess mucus can respond to the action of comfrey which promotes mucus discharge and tissue regeneration.

Applications: Anemia, asthma, blood cleanser, coughs, lung mucus, ulcers, tuberculosis, burns, emphysema, fractures, sores and swelling and pain.

Scientific Updates: It is the allantoin content of comfrey which gives it the ability to stimulate new cell growth and proliferation making it ideal for any type of healing, especially bone fractures.[51] Comfrey is also recommended for any type of wound healing and can contribute to restoring normal and healthy lung function.

Safety: Comfrey should not be used for prolonged periods of time. Use for over three months may be detrimental to the liver.

Complementary Agents: Fenugreek, garlic, capsicum, mullein, horehound, vitamin A, vitamin E, vitamin C, bioflavonoids, grape seed or pine bark extract and slippery elm.

CORNSILK (Zea mays)

Definition: Cornsilk refers to the soft, hair-like growth which accompanies an ear of corn. This fine delicate silk is usually collected when the corn is in milk and is used when still green. Cornsilk compounds, which include maizenic acid, can act as a cardiac tonic and diuretic. Used by the ancient Incas as a treatment for urogenital infections, cornsilk was marketed by Parke-Davis in Europe in 1880. Cornsilk is considered part of a family of herbs which help soothe and heal the urinary system.

Applications: Albuminuria, bladder infections, edema, heart trouble, hepatitis, kidney disorders, prostatitis, urinary tract infections and water retention.

Scientific Updates: The maizenic acid contained in cornsilk has a stimulating diuretic effect. In addition, this compound also benefits the liver and intestines and is considered a "cardiac solution" for the heart.[52] Clinical studies in China and Japan have demonstrated the remarkable diuretic properties of cornsilk.[53] "Cornsilk directly reduces painful symptoms and swelling due to several inflammatory conditions including cystitis, pyelitis, oliguria, hepatitis and all edematous conditions."[54] In China it is also used for hypertension and diabetes.[55]

Safety: Take in appropriate doses as directed. Any substance that acts as a diuretic may cause a potassium deficiency if used in excess. Use potassium supplementation. Cornsilk is considered a mild, nontoxic herb.

Complementary Agents: Buchu, parsley, uva ursi, cranberry, juniper berries, marshmallow, vitamin C, bioflavonoids, proanthocyanidins, B-complex, vitamin E, magnesium, potassium, copper, and mineral and electrolyte supplements.

COUCH GRASS (Agropyron repens)

Definition: Its natural diuretic action makes couch grass ideal for any type of urinary tract infection. It can stimulate urine discharge and help to pass kidney stones.

Applications: Bladder infections, blood purifier, jaundice, kidney disease, kidney stones and rheumatism.

Scientific Updates: Extracts of couch grass have exhibited antibiotic effects on a variety of bacteria and molds.[56] Couch grass has been known to eliminate kidney stones.[57]

Safety: Take in appropriate doses as recommended. An excess could lead to potassium and other mineral deficiency.

Complementary Agents: Uva ursi, cornsilk, parsley, juniper, cascara sagrada, red clover, garlic, black walnut, vitamin C, bioflavonoids, vitamin A, vitamin E, potassium, magnesium, copper and mineral and electrolyte supplements.

CRAMP BARK (Viburnum opulus)

Definition: Used primarily to relieve any condition caused by a spasm, cramp bark treats menstrual cramps, muscle spasms, and abdominal cramps. It is also good for heart muscle and exerts a calming effect in cases of hysteria or nervousness.

Applications: Asthma, colic, constipation, digestive disorders, edema, menstrual cramps, muscle cramps, heart disorders, hypertension, hysteria, leg cramps, nervousness and uterine cramps.

Scientific Updates: Cramp bark has been referred to as a potent muscle relaxant that has "a very specific action on the uterus and is one of the best remedies for menstrual pain."[58] This herb has been recognized in the *National Formulary* as a specific antispasmodic also useful for attacks of asthma and hysteria.

Safety: Use in appropriate doses as directed.

Complementary Agents: Squaw vine, dong quai, damiana, red raspberry, licorice, sarsaparilla, black cohosh, peppermint, valerian root, vitamin B-complex, vitamin E, vitamin C, bioflavonoids, folic acid, calcium/magnesium, chromium, selenium and potassium.

CRANBERRY (Vaccinium macrocarpon)

Definition: Cranberry has astringent applications for the urinary tract and is a traditional remedy for bladder infections and kidney-related disorders. It is a natural diuretic and urinary antiseptic agent.

Applications: Bladder infections, fever, and urinary tract infections.

Scientific Updates: Recent research suggests that cranberry juice may help fight urinary infections which are caused by certain bacteria.[59]

Safety: No known toxicity.

Complementary Agents: Burdock, parsley, uva ursi, juniper berry, goldenrod, marshmallow, alfalfa, corn silk, vitamin C, bioflavonoids, proanthocyanidins, vitamin A, zinc and bee pollen.

CULVER ROOT (Veronicastrum virgincum)

Definition: Used for generations by Native Americans, this herb helps expel old debris from the bowel, boosts liver function, clears congestion and is considered a natural relaxant.

Applications: Blood purifier, constipation, diarrhea, colon congestion, liver ailments and stomach disorders.

Scientific Updates: Culver root works chiefly on the intestines that are chronically constipated due to poor biliary flow. "It has a mild action without causing the depression of physical strength common with many other purgative medicines."[60] "Leptandrin excites the liver gently and promotes the secretion of bile without irritating the bowels."[61]

Safety: Pregnant or nursing mothers should not take this herb without their doctor's consent. Taking fennel or ginger with this herb helps to prevent the formation of intestinal gas.

Complementary Agents: Buckthorn, cascara sagrada, red raspberry, ginger, fennel, black walnut, quassia, garlic, couch grass, acidophilus, vitamin C, bioflavonoids, vitamin A, B-complex, marine lipids, and blue-green algae.

DAMIANA (Turnera aphrodisiaca)

Definition: Primarily used for treating female disorders, damiana is considered a sexual restorative, a remedy for menopause and a reproductive system tonic. It is also considered a central nervous system stimulant.

Applications: Aphrodisiac, bronchitis, depression, emphysema, fatigue, female problems, hormonal imbalances, infertility, impotence, menopause, mood swings, Parkinson disease, PMS, prostate disorders and sexual dysfunction.

Scientific Updates: Clinical studies have found that damiana benefits sexual ability and nervous tension.[62] Damiana has also been used to treat depression as a "stimulating nervine."[63] It has been applied in cases of chronic fatigue and mental exhaustion.[64] Damiana contains beta-sitosterol, a compound ". . . that could have some stimulant effect on the sexual apparatus or could help build sexual health and reproductivity."[65] "It is excellent when used in formulas with herbs such as ginseng, suma, sarsaparilla and saw palmetto."[66] Damiana is useful for both female and male infertility.[67]

Safety: Use in appropriate doses as directed.

Complementary Agents: Saw palmetto, dong quai, red raspberry, licorice, kelp, sarsaparilla, black cohosh, cramp bark, queen of the meadow, ginseng, squaw vine, gotu kola, vitamin E, bee pollen, bee propolis, B-complex, calcium/magnesium, potassium and marine lipids.

DANDELION (Taraxacum officinale)

Definition: Rich in potassium, dandelion works to detoxify the blood, increase the flow of bile from the liver, builds red blood cells and is considered a highly nutritive food.

Applications: Acne, anemia, arthritis, asthma, blood disorders, eczema, gallbladder disease, hepatitis, hypoglycemia, jaundice, kidney infections, liver disorders, psoriasis, PMS, skin eruptions, and weight loss.

Scientific Updates: Several clinical studies have supported the ability of dandelion to treat chronic liver congestion.[68] Dandelion has an impressive bile-stimulating action which helps promote liver and gallbladder function.[69] The ability of dandelion to clear the gallbladder and treat jaundice has been impressive.[70] Modern research has proven the validity of dandelion. It can stimulate the elimination of uric acid from the body and treat anemic conditions of the blood.[71]

Safety: Use as directed in appropriate doses.

Complementary Agents: Milk thistle, burdock, yellow dock, cascara sagrada, fenugreek, garlic, red sage, red clover, black cohosh, vitamin C, bioflavonoids, proanthocyanidins, vitamin A, B-complex, vitamin E, phytonutrients and blue-green algae.

DEVIL'S CLAW (Harpagophytum procumbens)

Definition: Used for treating rheumatism, arthritis and gout in South Africa, the glycoside content of this herb makes it a natural anti-inflammatory agent. It is also considered an antiaging botanical and a vascular tonic. It is an ideal herb for most geriatric applications.

Applications: Arteriosclerosis, arthritis, blood purifier, cholesterol inflammation, edema, indigestion, liver ailments, neuralgia, rheumatism and stomach ailments.

Scientific Updates: Recent studies have confirmed the anti-inflammatory value of this herb for chronic rheumatism, arthritis, neuralgia and gout, rating it equal to phenylbutazone, a commonly prescribed drug for arthritis.[72] It also helps to regulate cholesterol levels.[73]

Safety: Extensive data supports the safety of this herb, but it should never be used during pregnancy becaues it may stimulate uterine contraction.

Complementary Agents: Celery, wild yam, black cohosh, Oregon grape root, ginger, glucosamine, vitamin C, bioflavonoids, grape seed or pine bark extract.

DONG QUAI (Angelica sinensis)

Definition: Considered one of the best herbal uterine tonics, dong quai is very highly regarded by Asian medical practitioners. Used to correct painful menstruation, hormonal imbalance, postpartum conditions and menopausal symptoms, this herb works well with vitamin E to strengthen the reproductive system.

Applications: Atherosclerosis, anemia, bleeding, fatigue, circulatory insufficiencies, high blood pressure, hormonal imbalance, menstrual disorders (irregular periods, painful periods, PMS), menopause, muscle spasms and poor vitality.

Scientific Updates: The chemical constituents of dong quai have an immediate stimulatory effect on the uterus by strengthening and normalizing uterine contractions.[74] Both animal and human studies have found that dong quai improves peripheral circulation.[75] Research indicates that it is the ferulic acid and lulgustilide content of the herb which prevents spasms and relaxes blood vessels.[76] It also has proven estrogenic activities.[77]

Safety: No reported toxicity. Avoid in cases of severe gastrointestinal disease and check with your physician if pregnant or nursing. This herb should not be used by anyone with hemorrhagic diseases or during the first three months of pregnancy. It should also be avoided during severe cases of the flu or in cases of spontaneous abortion.

Complementary Agents: Kelp, black cohosh, cramp bark, squaw vine, queen of the meadow, sarsaparilla, licorice, damiana, red raspberry, saw palmetto, wild yam, vitamin E, vitamin C, bioflavonoids, B-complex, calcium/magnesium, potassium, marine lipids and primrose oil.

ECHINACEA (Echinacea purpurea)

Definition: Because it has natural antibiotic actions, echinacea is considered an excellent herb for infections of all kinds. In addition, it works to boost lymphatic cleansing of the blood, enhances the immune system and has cortisone-like properties which contribute to its anti-inflammatory action. It is recommended for stubborn viral infections, yeast infections and for arthritic conditions.

Applications: Acne, arthritis, blood cleansing, boils, burns, bronchitis, canker sores, chronic fatigue, colds, congestion, contagious diseases, ear infections, fevers, herpes, glandular disorders, infections (viral and bacterial), influenza, immune system disorders, prostate disease, psoriasis, tonsillitis and wounds.

Scientific Updates: Laboratory tests have found that compounds contained in echinacea have the ability to rearrange and recognize enzyme patterns in the body.[78] The ability of this herb to boost immune function deals with thymus gland stimulation.[79] It can actually stimulate the production and action of interferon.[80] Echinacea may help the body neutralize carcinogenic substances.[81] The chemical content of echinacea promoted improved resistance to all septic or infectious conditions.[82]

Safety: High doses of echinacea may occasionally cause nausea and dizziness. This herb has not exhibited any observed toxicity even in high doses. Anyone suffering from any type of kidney disorder should not take echinacea for longer than one week intervals due to possible excrete mineral imbalance. Heavy or prolonged use of this herb is not recommended.

Complementary Agents: Alfalfa, capsicum, ginger, ginseng, cat's claw, goldenseal, astragalus, garlic, vitamin C, bioflavonoids, vitamin A, blue-green algae, B-complex vitamins, calcium/magnesium and zinc.

EYEBRIGHT (Euphrasia officinalis)

Definition: For generations, this herb has been a favorite choice for the treatment of various eye diseases. It is particularly effective for any inflammation of the mucous membrane of the eye, in addition to light sensitivity, minor irritations, weeping, itching, etc.

Applications: Allergic reactions (eye-related), cataracts, conjunctivitis, diabetic retinopathy, eye inflammations, eye infections, eye strain, glaucoma and vision problems.

Scientific Updates: This herb has natural astringent and anti-inflammatory properties contained in its compounds which have not undgergone scientific study as of yet.

Safety: While its specific biochemical actions have not been delineated, eyebright has been successfully used for generation in hundreds of cases of eye irritations and other eye ailments. Its ability to cleanse the blood supply to the eye is thought to be responsible for its therapeutic effect.[83]

Complementary Agents: Bilberry, red raspberry, goldenseal, grape seed or pine bark extract, vitamin A, beta carotene, vitamin C, bioflavonoids and antioxidant array.

FENNEL (Foeniculum vulgare)

Definition: Used as an effective carminative for digestive problems, fennel relieves intestinal gas and colic, boosts the expulsion of mucus, stimulates lactation and has been used for weight loss. Its licorice-like taste makes it a good flavoring agent which also helps to enhance the digestibility of other herbal medicines.

Applications: Appetite suppressant, colic, gas, indigestion, intestinal disorders, lactation booster, morning sickness, nausea, sedative (juvenile), uric acid (gout) and weight loss

Scientific Updates: Recent studies have looked at the estrogenic action of fennel.[84] The flavonoid content of fennel is thought to be responsible for its ability to stop stomach spasms typically seen in colic.[85]

Safety: Generally recognized as safe.

Complementary Agents: Catnip, chamomile, chickweed, ginger, papaya, peppermint, licorice, dandelion, fenugreek, thyme, digestive enzymes, calcium/magnesium, acidophilus and bioflavonoids.

FENUGREEK (Trigonella foenum-graecum)

Definition: Esteemed by the Greeks and Romans, fenugreek was used as a flavoring agent and aphrodisiac. Today it is commonly used to break up and expel mucus, soothe the gastrointestinal tract and stimulate milk production.

Applications: Allergies, bronchitis, cholesterol levels, coughs, diabetes, digestive ailments, emphysema, intestinal gas, headache, lung infections, mucus congestion and skin eruptions.

Scientific Updates: Fenugreek is currently being used to treat diabetes in Middle East countries.[86] Because it contains up to 30 percent mucilage, fenugreek works as an effective anti-inflammatory agent and can heal abscesses and other skin eruptions. Clinical tests have shown that fenugreek significantly reduced blood glucose and cholesterol levels in test animals.[87] Fenugreek seeds, which contain diosgenin and tigogenin, may also help tone uterine muscle and stimulate lactation in nursing mothers.[88] French scientists have found that fenugreek stimulates pancreatic secretion which enhances digestion.[89]

Safety: Fenugreek should be avoided in pregnancy as it is a uterine stimulant. Diabetics should check with their doctor's before using fenugreek for blood sugar control.

Complementary Agents: Dandelion, myrrh, red clover, lobelia, cornsilk, garlic, yellow dock, goldenseal, vitamin C, bioflavonoids, proanthocyanidins, phytonutrients, blue-green algae, vitamin A, B-complex and chromium.

FEVERFEW (Chrysanthemum parthenium)

Definition: Used to treat many of the same disorders aspirin is used for, this herb is most widely known for its therapeutic application for migraine headaches, fever and for arthritis. Folk literature is full of praise for it ability to calm inflammation and treat pain.

Applications: Asthma, inflammatory conditions, arthritis, menstrual pain, migraine headaches and fever.

Scientific Updates: This herb contains a group of chemicals called sesquiterpene lactones which are bitter compounds which inhibit prostaglandin production in the body and decrease histamine release; two functions which cause the inflammatory response.

Safety: Because it acts similarly to salicylates found in aspirin, it is not recommended for pregnant or lactating women or for children. In addition, anyone taking blood thinners should not use this herb.

Complementary Agents: White willow, vitamin C, proanthocyanidins, bioflavonoids, marine lipids and garlic.

GARLIC (Allium sativum)

Definition: Garlic contains more than 200 chemical compounds. Its sulphur-containing substances, such as allicin and ajoene, are what give garlic its antibiotic properties as well as its pungent smell. Garlic has been used for centuries for everything from protection from infection to increased sexual prowess.

Applications: Arteriosclerosis, arthritis, asthma, blood poisoning, blood pressure (high or low), bronchitis, cancer, candida, circulatory insufficiency, colds, colitis, coughs, digestive disorders, ear infections, fever, flu, fungus, gas, heart disease, infections (viral and bacterial), liver ailments, lung disorders, parasites, pinworm, prostate gland disorders, respiratory congestion and yeast infections.

Scientific Updates: Garlic has been the subject of intense scientific study over the last three decades. Recent research has proven the value of garlic in treating and preventing cardiovascular disease. Controlled studies discovered that it can lower cholesterol and triglyceride levels, reduce the tendency of the blood to clot and decrease blood pressure.[92] Garlic has been scientifically proven to inhibit bacterial growth.[93] One milligram of allicin, garlic's primary constituent, is estimated to equal 15 standard units of penicillin.[94] Dr. Erik Block discovered that garlic also protects the liver from drug, radiation and free radical damage.[95] Garlic can also stimulate immunity and is considered an anticancer agent.[96]

Safety: Garlic is considered safe, however, an excess dose can cause stomach upset. When using garlic directly on the skin, coat the area with olive oil first to avoid skin irritation. Do not use garlic in large amounts if you have anemia or ulcers.

Complementary Agents: Parsley, capsicum, alfalfa, blue-green algae, kelp, black walnut, buckthorn, couch grass, echinacea, goldenseal, red clover, vitamin C, bioflavonoids, proanthocyanidins and phytonutrients .

GINGER (Zingiber officinale)

Definition: Native to coastal regions of India, this herb has a long history of use throughout the world for its ability to treat gastrointestinal upsets. Folk medicine is full of records confirming the use of aromatic ginger for its stimulating and carminative properties. It makes a wonderful tea in times of colds and flu and can quiet nausea and indigestion better than any other modern medicinal agent.

Applications: Nausea, morning sickness, motion sickness, indigestion, diarrhea, colon disorders, gas, loss of appetite, colds and flu, pain and earaches.

Scientific Updates: An article found in the March 2, 1982 edition of *Lancet* showed that ginger can be as effective or better than Dramamine, an over-the-counter drug for treating motion sickness.

Safety: Considered safe and nontoxic if used as directed.

Complementary Agents: Peppermint, fennel, papaya, spearmint, chamomile, cascara sagrada, senna, aloe vera, proteolytic enzymes, vitamin C and bioflavonoids.

GINKGO (Ginkgo biloba)

Definition: The most ancient of all trees, ginkgo is native to areas of the Far East and is a favorite of Chinese practitioners for the treatment of respiratory disorders. Today, ginkgo is the subject of widespread scientific inquiry for its ability to increase circulatory oxygenation to brain cells as well as other body areas.

Applications: Antiaging, Alzheimer's disease, asthma, depression, attention deficit disorder, blood clots, circulatory insufficiency, dementia, kidney disease, memory loss, respiratory disease, senility, stress, stroke, tinnitus and vascular disease.

Scientific Updates: Numerous studies have found that ginkgo can protect the neuronal membranes in the brain and help prevent the decrease in cerebral reception that occurs with aging.[101] During an open trial involving 112 geriatric patients who suffered from inadequate cerebral blood flow, 120 mg of ginkgo extract caused a significant regression of pre-existing symptoms.[102]

Safety: Ginkgo is considered nontoxic with few side effects. It can be safely used with other supplements. In rare cases, some gastric upset or incidence of headache or skin rash has occurred probably indicating an allergic reaction.

Complementary Agents: Ginseng, gotu kola, sage, bee pollen, capsicum, suma, St. John's wort, garlic, vitamin B-complex, folic acid, magnesium, choline, antioxidant array and DHEA.

GINSENG SIBERIAN (Eleutherococcus senticosus)

Definition: Used for generations by the Chinese, ginseng was taken to increase life span as well as wisdom. Considered a tonic herb, ginseng has captured the interest of the scientific community and has been found to lower cholesterol, boost cardiovascular function, prevent blood clots, increase stamina and protect cells from radiation. Continuing research on ginseng is currently underway.

Applications: Aging, drug withdrawal, depression, diabetes, colds, hypertension, radiation protection, impotence, lung disorders, prostate gland disease, compromised immunity and sexual dysfunction.

Scientific Updates: A study published in *The American Journal of Chinese Medicine* reported that ginseng can moderate the effects of a high-cholesterol diet in both rates and humans.[103] Clinical testing has found that ginseng can prevent cellular damage from radiation exposure.[104] Ginseng can increase sperm count, lower blood sugar and help to treat alcoholism.[105]

Safety: Generally recognized as safe, ginseng should be purchased from reliable sources to ensure purity and potency. A study published in a 1979 issue of the *Journal of the American Medical Association* erroneously reported that ginseng causes high blood pressure and irritability. The study was subsequently discredited. If used in reasonable amount, ginseng is considered nontoxic.

Complementary Agents: Gotu kola, ginkgo, St. John's wort, bee pollen, saw palmetto, wild yam, DHEA, vitamin-B complex and antioxidant array.

GLUCOMANNAN (Amorphophallus konjak)

Definition: Glucomannan is a unique herb that provides dietary fiber with no calories. It promotes bowel elimination, absorbs intestinal toxins and can help normalize blood sugar. When taken before meals, this herb can help to produce a feeling of fullness, supressing the appetite. As a dietary aid, it can expand to about 50 times its original volume when combined with water.

Applications: Athersclerosis, high cholesterol, constipation, sluggish colon, hypertension, diabetes, blood sugar disorders and obesity.

Scientific Updates: Glucomannan is currently being used in weight reduction formulas to suppress carbohydrate craving. When combined with lecithin, it is thought to help prevent cardiovascular disease.[106]

Safety: Considered nontoxic, but anyone suffering from any blood sugar-related disease should check with their physician before using glucommanan.

Complementary Agents: Lecithin, chromium, garcinia cambogia, garlic, hawthorn, essential fatty acids, carnatine and fiber sources (psyllium, guar gum, etc.).

GOLDENSEAL (Hydrastis canadensis)

Definition: Used by Native Americans for generations, goldenseal root is a favorite among herbalists for its anti-inflammatory effect and antibiotic-like actions. The bitter nature of this herb has also made it an effective remedy for digestive disorders and as a bitter tonic for gastric ulcers. Strained infusions of goldenseal have traditionally been used as a soothing eye wash.

Applications: Diarrhea, eczema, eye inflammations, flatulence, gallbladder disease, gastritis, giardia, hemorrhoids, impetigo, indigestion, infections (viral and bacterial), liver disease, excessive menstrual flow, mouth sores, rhinitis, ringworm, ulcers and vaginitis.

Scientific Updates: Laboratory tests have proven goldenseal's ability to protect against gram-positive and gram-negative bacteria including tuberculosis bacteria.[107] It helps to reduce vaginal and uterine inflammation.[108] Tests have found that berberine-containing herbs can be more effective in treating gastrointestinal infections than standard antibiotics.[109]

Safety: Prolonged or excessive use may kill bacterial flora and raise white blood cell count. Taking unusually high amounts of goldenseal can lower heartbeat and adversely affect the central nervous system. Pregnant women should not use this herb because its berberine content can stimulate uterine contractions. Continual use can lower vitamin B absorption. Goldenseal is not recommended for anyone with low blood sugar or hypertension.

Complementary Agents: Barberry, Oregon grape, echinacea, garlic, capsicum, myrrh, ginger, eyebright, juniper, dandelion, chamomile, black cohosh, comfrey, cascara, gentian, dong quai, vitamin C, bioflavonoids, vitamin A, digestive enzymes and grape seed or pine bark proanthocyanidins.

GOTU KOLA (Centella asiatica)

Definition: Grown in Java and Ceylon, gotu kola is one of the most popular Ayurvedic herbs utilized as a nerve tonic, a remedy for epilepsy and as a brain normalizer in conditions such as memory loss and schizophrenia. Recently, scientists have discovered its ability to treat inflammation and fever.

Applications: Age-related disorders, arteriosclerosis, circulatory problems, epilepsy, high blood pressure, infections, depression, fatigue, hypoglycemia, learning disorders, memory loss, menopause, nervous conditions, PMS, psoriasis, schizophrenia, senility, ulcerations and wounds.

Scientific Updates: Studies have indicated the gotu kola works as a tonic for fatigue without the side effects of caffeine.[110] It also stimulates and builds the nervous system counteracting the effects of stress. Europeans and Asians use this herb for psoriasis, cervicitis and vaginitis.[111] In India, gotu kola has enjoyed widespread use as a brain food with its therapeutic focus on improving memory and promoting longevity.[112]

Safety: No known toxicity. Take in appropriate doses.

Complementary Agents: Chickweed, cascara, bilberry, dong quai, sarsaparilla, ginseng, ginkgo, capsicum, licorice, vitamin C, bioflavonoids, vitamin E, vitamin D, zinc, bee pollen and bee propolis.

GUARANA (Paullinia cupana)

Definition: Also known as Brazilian cocoa, guarana is a caffeine-containing herb which is used as an energy drink and natural stimulant. Guarana contains chemical compounds called xanthines which include caffeine, theobromine and theophylline.

Applications: Appetite suppressant, aphrodisiac, diarrhea, fatigue, gastrointestinal disorders, headaches, migraines, neuralgia and PMS.

Scientific Updates: Guarana is used for its stimulating properties and for its diuretic action. It is also considered antidiarrheic, and antifatigue. Its potential for treating migraine headaches is under current investigation.

Safety: Guarana is a caffeine-containing herb and should not be overused. Pregnant women or nursing mothers should not use guarana. Overuse can cause a strain on the urinary tract, heart palpitations, or insomnia. Combining guarana with herbs such as ephedra can have harmful side effects.

Complementary Agents: Yerba mate, ginseng, gotu kola, kola nut and chickweed.

GYMNEMA SILVESTIS (Gymnema sylvestre)

Definition: As a native tree of Africa and India, gymnema leaves have the remarkable ability to block out the certain taste sensations, especially sweetness. It is an extremely popular herb in Japan and is included in diabetic, hypoglycemic and weight loss formulas.

Applications: Diabetes, fatigue, hypoglycemia, obesity and sugar cravings.

Scientific Updates: Modern research has found the gymnemic acid, the active ingredient of this herb blocks sugar absorption into the body.[113] A clinical study published in 1986 suggests that extract of gymnema can significantly enhance liver and pancreatic function.[114]

Safety: Diabetics should check with their physician before using this herb.

Complementary Agents: Fenugreek, goldenseal, milk thistle, ginger, bilberry, blueberry, dandelion, vitamin C, vitamin A, B-complex, bioflavonoids, proanthocyanidins, chromium, bee pollen and bee propolis.

HAWTHORN BERRY (Crategus oxyacantha)

Definition: Known as a botanical heart tonic, hawthorn berries were popular with the ancient Greeks and traditionally used to treat high and low blood pressure, irregular heartbeat, heart pain and atherosclerosis. Native Americans look to the berry for its therapeutic effect on rheumatism and digestive difficulties.

Applications: Angina, irregular heartbeat, blood pressure disorders, congestive heart failure, hypertension, coronary artery disease, high cholesterol, nervous disorders, insomnia, Reynaud's syndrome and sore throat.

Scientific Updates: The cardiotonic properties of hawthorn are well documented. The flavonoid content of hawthorn berry has been clinically proven to dilate peripheral and coronary blood vessels, alleviating hypertension and angina.[115] Experimental studies have found that hawthorn works in three important ways: it eases blood flow, lowers blood pressure and strengthens heart muscle.[116] One of the most desirable benefits of hawthorn is that its cardioprotective role may actually escalate when used for a prolonged period of time.[117] In addition, hawthorn has the ability to lower serum cholesterol levels and prevent cholesterol deposits from accumulating in arteries.[118] It is an extremely valuable therapeutic agent for the early stages of congestive heart failure and arrhythmias.[119]

Safety: No known toxicity has been found in hawthorn. It may potentiate the action of digitalis and should only be mixed with pharmaceutical drugs when approved by a physician. The effects of hawthorn can be cumulative.

Complementary Agents: Capsicum, garlic, passionflower, valerian, peppermint, ginkgo, vitamin C, vitamin A, vitamin E, vitamin B-complex, calcium/magnesium, potassium, selenium, coenzyme Q10, marine lipids and phytonutrients.

HORSETAIL (Equisetum arvense)

Definition: Used for centuries to treat internal and external injuries, horsetail helps to facilitate the use of calcium in the body and has a high silica content. It is particularly good for boosting circulation, promoting the healing of broken bones and for kidney and urinary tract diseases. It is considered a natural diuretic and astringent.

Applications: Arthritis, bladder ailments, bedwetting, conjunctivitis, bone injuries, glandular disorders, hair loss, kidney stones, nervous tension, tumors and urinary problems.

Scientific Updates: Research has found that horsetail contains antibiotic and hemolytic (blood-clotting) properties.[120] Its rich array of minerals makes it ideal for the healing of injured tissue and bone. It is especially effective in poultice form.

Safety: No known toxicity.

Complementary Agents: Ginseng, marshmallow, plantain, alfalfa, yucca, dandelion, parsley, saw palmetto, glucosamine, shark cartilage, vitamin C, HCL, phosphorus and calcium/magnesium.

HO-SHOU-WU (Polygonum multiflorum)

Definition: Traditionally used by the Chinese to promote longevity, this herb is rich in flavonoids and is primarily used to restore vigor, strengthen the cardio-vascular system, enhance the endocrine system and tone the liver and kidneys. It is good in applications for chronic fatigue or degenerative conditions.

Applications: Aging, cardiovascular conditions, chronic fatigue, circulatory insufficiency, debilitated conditions, glandular disorders, impotency and infertility.

Scientific Updates: Research on this herb is limited but its long history of use by the Chinese in restorative herbal formulas attests to its tonic action.

Safety: Presumed to be safe.

Complementary Agents: Hawthorn, garlic, coenzyme Q10, marine lipids, essential fatty acids, capsicum and vitamin E.

HOPS (Humulus lupulus)

Definition: Hops is best known for its use in the brewing of beer. It is an extremely useful nervine herb which has been traditionally used to calm the central nervous system and safely induce sleep. During the reign of King George, it was used to fill pillows to help promote relaxation during illness. Native Americans utilized hops for and over acidic stomach and for indigestion.

Applications: Insomnia, headaches, hyperactivity, anxiety, fever, nervousness, pain, stress, stomach spasms, inflammation and colon disorders.

Scientific Updates: Recent in-depth clinical studies reveal that hops works to relax smooth muscle and naturally sedates the nervous system. Lupulone and humulone are the active ingredients of hops.[121] The flavonoid content gives hops its anti-inflammatory action.

Safety: Hops has no known toxicity. It is not recommended for anyone who is suffering from clinical depression. Large quantities can have an aphrodisiac effect.

Complementary Agents: Valerian root, skullcap, chamomile, mullein, marshmallow, wood betony, passionflower, vitamin E, B-complex, folic acid, niacin, vitamin C, inositol, calcium/magnesium and melatonin.

JUNIPER (Juniperus, communis)

Definition: Known for its aromatic blue-green berries, juniper has been used in European circles to treat kidney disorders, urinary tract infections and prostate disease. It has blood purifying and antiseptic properties which make it a natural for any disorders affecting the urinary system.

Applications: Adrenal gland disorders, bedwetting, bladder problems, colds, diabetes, fungal infections, hypo-

glycemia, infections, kidney infections, kidney stones, pancreas deficiencies and water retention.

Scientific Updates: Juniper acts directly on kidney function to stimulate urine flow by increasing the rate of glomerulus filtration (blood purification).[122] Studies have found that after kidney disease, juniper can help restore kidney tissue and normalize blood pressure.[123]

Safety: If pregnant, use juniper only with your physician's permission. Long term or excessive use may cause kidney irritation or inhibit iron absorption. Using juniper in herbal blends helps to avoid this possibility.

Complementary Agents: Cornsilk, uva ursi, cranberry, parsley, alfalfa, marshmallow, kelp, buchu, queen of the meadow, vitamin C, bioflavonoids, proanthocyanidins, B-complex, vitamin E, magnesium, potassium, copper and mineral and electrolyte supplements.

KAVA KAVA (Piper methysticum)

Definition: A root native to the South Pacific, kava kava has been used for centuries as a calmative botanical. Its primary usage is to relax the central nervous system.

Applications: Insomnia, nervousness, stress, headaches and anxiety.

Scientific Updates: Research has found that kava kava has mild psychoactive properties which can contribute to a feeling of contentment and peace while actually sharpening the senses.[124]

Safety: No known toxicity.

Complementary Agents: Hops, valerian root, chamomile and melatonin.

KELP (Fucus vesiculosus)

Definition: Technically speaking, kelp is a group of algae which grows in the parts of the Atlantic and Pacific Oceans. Its high mineral content makes it a desirable nutritive herb. It is one of the best natural sources of iodine, making it a good herbal remedy for the treatment of hypothyroidism and obesity.

Applications: Acne, adrenal insufficiencies, colitis, eczema, endocrine gland disorders, energy, fingernails, hypothyroidism, obesity and uterine disorders.

Scientific Updates: Studies conducted in Japan show a direct correlation between the consumption of algin found in kelp and the prevention of breast cancer.[125] The ability of algin to stimulate the T-cells of the immune system is thought to be responsible for this effect. The micronutrients in kelp also enhance stamina and help to balance hormones.[126] Tests have suggested that it may also have antibiotic properties.[127] By boosting thyroid function, kelp may increase energy by regulating metabolism, which may help boost thermogenesis (fat burning).[128]

Safety: Use as directed in appropriate doses.

Complementary Agents: Alfalfa, dong quai, dandelion, black cohosh, damiana, gotu kola, ginseng, Irish moss, licorice, sarsaparilla, queen of the meadow, vitamin A, vitamin C, bioflavonoids, vitamin E, calcium/magnesium, phosphorus, potassium, zinc, phytonutrients, blue-green algae and bee pollen.

LEMON GRASS (Cymbopogon citracus)

Definition: Chinese medicinal practitioners use lemon grass to treat colds, abdominal distress and headaches. It is also considered a blood cleanser and a good remedy for fevers. Lemon grass helps to expedite the removal of mucus from the body during infections.

Applications: Colds, digestive upsets and fever.

Scientific Updates: "Lemon grass is reputed to slow the discharge of mucus, as well as reduce mucus discharge in respiratory conditions, due in part to its astringent properties."[129]

Safety: Use in appropriate dosages as directed.

Complementary Agents: Sage, blessed thistle, marshmallow, mullein, pleurisy root, catnip, chamomile, slippery elm, vitamin C, bioflavonoids, proanthocyanidins, vitamin A and calcium/magnesium.

LICORICE (Glycyrrhiza glabra)

Definition: Licorice is an extremely sweet herb that possesses significant antiarthritic and anti-inflammatory properties which are linked to the release of corticosteroid from the adrenal glands. Licorice has been used for adrenal insufficiencies and has recently shown its effectiveness in preventing and treating ulcers.

Applications: Addison's disease, adrenal exhaustion, allergies, arthritis, circulatory insufficiency, colds, coughs, ear infections, fatigue, female complaints, hoarseness, hypoglycemia and hyperglycemia, immune weakness, liver disease, lung problems, ulcers, and uterine tonic.

Scientific Updates: Licorice has been the subject of much modern study. It has clearly established its estrogenic activity.[130] The glycyrrhizin content of licorice stimulates the productions of hormones such as hydrocortisone which work as efficient anti-inflammatory agents.[131] "Studies have shown licorice to also posseses the ability to counter the effects of two tumor-producing agents."[132] Licorice has proven anti-inflammatory and antiallergic properties.[133] The properties of glycyrrhizin contained in licorice stimulate the production of interferon which boosts immunity.[134]

Safety: Licorice should be avoided if high blood pressure is present. Avoid licorice if you are taking digoxin-based drugs or have rapid heartbeat. Excessive consumption of licorice can cause symptoms resembling high blood pressure. Taking supplements of potassium are recommended.

Complementary Agents: Wild yam, saw palmetto, dong quai, black cohosh, kelp, gotu kola, milk thistle, dandelion, ginger, ginseng, queen of the meadow, sarsaparilla, cramp bark, squaw vine, vitamin E, B-complex, folic acid, calcium/magnesium, potassium and phytonutrients.

LOBELIA (Lobelia inflata)

Definition: Western herbal practitioners have prescribed lobelia for a wide variety of ailments and prize it as a therapeutic herb. Because it has the ability to induce vomiting, it has been the subject of some controversy. It is an effective and powerful agent for treating bronchitis and asthma and can dilate the bronchiole tubes. It also acts as a potent relaxant for the central nervous system.

Applications: Allergies, asthma, arthritis, bronchitis, colds, coughs, croup, emphysema, epilepsy, fever, insomnia, lung disease, migraine headaches, mumps, pleurisy, pneumonia, toothaches, whooping cough and worms.

Scientific Updates: In the past, lobeline was approved for use by the FDA as a deterrent to smoking in cases of nicotine withdrawal.[135] Lobelia is considered an effective expectorant based on its ability to stimulate the adrenal glands to release corticosteroids that promote the relaxation of bronchial muscles.[136]

Safety: Misuse of lobelia can result in vomiting. Lobelia should be taken in exact prescribed dosages. Overdosing on lobelia can cause serious side effects.

Complementary Agents: Capsicum, garlic, licorice, comfrey, fenugreek and mullein.

MARSHMALLOW (Althaea officinalis)

Definition: Hippocrates advocated the use of this herb for wound healing. It has the capability of healing inflamed or injured tissue and has demulcent properties which soothe irritated mucous membranes. It is calcium-rich and has been used to increase lactation and heal the respiratory and urinary tracts.

Applications: Gastrointestinal upset, lung congestion, abrasions, dry coughs, sore throats, colitis, urinary tract infections and nervous exhaustion or breakdown.

Scientific Updates: Recent laboratory findings disclose that marshmallow contains 286,000 units of vitamin A per pound which helps to boost its healing powers.[137] The ability of marshmallow to soothe and heal irritated respiratory passages is well-documented.[138] It does the same for the gastrointestinal system.[139]

Safety: Marshmallow is considered safe and nontoxic.

Complementary Agents: Black cohosh, burdock, slippery elm, hops, valerian root, skullcap, mullein, wood betony, chamomile, melatonin, vitamin E, schizandra, calcium/magnesium, inositol, vitamin C, vitamin A, and niacin.

MILK THISTLE (Silybum marianum)

Definition: Milk thistle has a long history of use as an extraordinary liver rejuvenant. Ancient dioscorides used it to reverse the poisoning effect of a snakebite. Today, European doctors use intravenous applications of milk thistle for mushroom poisoning, which destroys liver tissue and causes death. It has an impressive track record as a liver tonic and protectant.

Applications: Cirrhosis, hepatitis, diabetes, free radical protection, gallstones, chronic fatigue, jaundice, kidney congestion, liver damage, kidney disease, poisoning and psoriasis.

Scientific Updates: In experiments, silymarin, the primary component of milk thistle, was given to test subjects before a deadly mushroom amanita toxin was ingested. It was 100 percent effective in preventing liver toxicity.[140] Studies have shown that taking milk thistle has resulted in a pronounced reduction of cholesterol in the bile which helps to prevent gallbladder disease.[141] Recent studies point to milk thistle as a possible therapy for psoriasis.[142]

Safety: No known toxicity. Taking silymarin can produce looser stools although the effect is rare. The safety of milk thistle extracts in pregnant or nursing women has not been established.

Complementary Agents: Dandelion, bioflavonoids, grape seed or pine bark proanthocyanidins, turmeric, artichoke, schizandra, vitamin E, selenium, germanium, marine lipids, essential fatty acids and psyllium.

MULLEIN (Verbascum thapsus)

Definition: During the Civil War, mullein was used to treat respiratory infections. It has calming properties and can soothe inflammation. Swollen membranes respond to mullein and it has been used for hay fever, as a sleep aid and has reportedly cured warts.

Applications: Colds, coughs, cramps, ear infections, insomnia, nervousness, respiratory problems, sore joints and pain.

Scientific Updates: Recent laboratory studies have found that the saponins and mucilage contained in mullein enable it to heal and soothe inflammation.[143] In addition, testing concluded that mullein can be used as an herbal pain reliever and sleep aid.[144]

Safety: Mullein is recognized as safe.

Complementary Agents: Marshmallow, slippery elm, horehound, hops, skullcap, valerian root, wood betony, black cohosh, lobelia, melatonin, vitamin C, vitamin E and calcium/magnesium.

MYRRH GUM (Commiphora molmol)

Definition: Myrrh is considered a bitter herb with astringent and antiseptic properties. It has been used to treat mouth disorders and is still prized in certain parts of the world as a precious commodity.

Applications: Congestion, indigestion, gas, ulcers, irritable bowel syndrome, ulcerative colitis, diverticulitis, Crohn's disease, wound healing, sore throats and gingivitis.

Scientific Updates: Myrrh normalizes mucous membrane activity.[145] Because the mucous lining of the stomach is so important for its protection from stomach acids, myrrh is considered a valuable digestive aid. In addition, if too much mucus is secreted in the gastrointestinal tract, digestion in impaired. Myrrh helps to ensure the proper function of mucous secreting glands and exerts an antiseptic and antibacterial action at the same time.[146]

Safety: Myrrh has a mild uterine stimulant action and should be avoided in pregnancy.

Complementary Agents: Ginger, fenugreek, catnip, peppermint, fennel, capsicum, acidophilus, saw palmetto, slippery elm, calcium/magnesium, vitamin A, vitamin B-complex, vitamin E and digestive enzymes.

NETTLE (Urtica dioica)

Definition: Also known as stinging nettle, this herb grows in water patches along river and stream banks and has been used traditionally by the Chinese as well as western cultures. Extracts of nettle which have had their stinging properties greatly reduced have been used in everything from hair tonics for baldness to respiratory disorders.

Applications: Asthma, ulcers, bronchitis, jaundice, nephritis, hemorrhoids, dysmenorrhea, gout, arthritis, allergic rhinitis and low blood sugar.

Scientific Updates: It is the histamine, acetylcholine and serotonin present in the leaf bristles of this plant which give it a catalyst like action much in the same way that capsicum works. Nettle compounds actually irritate mucus membranes which creates the needed formation of additional protective mucus. Recent studies have used nettle to treat allergic hay fever.

Safety: Nettle can be highly allergenic, therefore caution should be used in determining if an allergy to its compounds exists.

Complementary Agents: Mullein, marshmallow, vitamin E, slippery elm, vitamin C, bioflavonoids and lobelia.

NONI (Morinda citrifolia)

Definition: Virtually every part of this Polynesian plant has been used for medicinal purposes in the South Pacific for centuries with special emphasis on its fruit, leaves and bark. Noni juice has recently emerged as a valuable therapeutic agent with significant anticancer and anti-inflammatory properties. Like many other botanical medicines, noni has earned a legitimate place in nature's medicine cabinet.

Applications: Arthritis, atherosclerosis, bladder infections, boils, bowel disorders, burns, cancer, chronic fatigue syndrome, cold sores, constipation, depression, diabetes, diarrhea, drug addiction, eye inflammations, fever, fractures, gastric ulcers, gingivitis, headaches, hypertension, immune weakness, intestinal parasites, kidney disease, menstrual disorders, pain, respiratory disease, tuberculosis, tumors and wounds.

Scientific Updates: Noni has an impressive array of terpene compounds that have exhibited natural antibiotic activity. Compounds in the noni fruit have been linked to the synthesis of xeronine in the body which has significant healing properties. The alkaloid content of noni causes a number of therapeutic actions, particularly against inflammatory ailments. Recent testing has found that certain noni compounds such as damnacanthol have inhibited the growth of precancerous RAS cells.

Safety: Extracts of noni are considered safe if used as directed but pregnant or nursing women should consult their physician before using any noni derivative. High doses of root extracts may cause constipation. Taking noni supplements with coffee, alcohol or nicotine is not recommended. It should be taken on an empty stomach for maximum effectiveness.

Complementary Agents: Cat's claw, *Morinda officinalis*, kava kava, pau d'arco, echinacea, aloe vera, bioflavonoids, selenium, germanium, grape seed extract, proteolytic enzymes, glucosamine and shark cartilage.

OATSTRAW (Avena sativa)

Definition: This herb is known for its rich mineral content and ability to treat osteoporosis, menstrual disorders, urinary tract infections and even hysteria. Tinctures made from oatstraw are used in homeopathic preparations for use in arthritis, liver ailments and skin disorders.

Applications: Contagious diseases, insomnia, menstrual disorders, indigestion, urinary tract infections, osteoporosis, nervous conditions and conditions requiring calcium.

Scientific Updates: Oatstraw is an excellent natural source of calcium and magnesium and is best utilized in tea form. It is considered a superior plant source of magnesium. Oatstraw should be a rich green color and have a characteristic odor to be considered of good quality.

Safety: No known toxicity.

Complementary Agents: Plantain, marshmallow, alfalfa, barley grass and calcium/magnesium.

OREGON GRAPE (Berberis aquifolium)

Definition: Oregon grape is another berberine-containing herb which has been used to treat infection. It has the ability to contribute to blood cleansing which makes it a favorite choice for the treatment of skin disorders. It is also considered a glandular tonic.

Applications: Acne, anemia, blood purification, fever, indigestion, immune system, infections, eczema, jaundice, liver disorders, psoriasis, skin ailments, staph infections and vaginal yeast infections.

Scientific Updates: Laboratory studies have confirmed that Oregon grape has a similar bacteriocidal effect as goldenseal.[147] The berberine and hydrastine herbs have some impressive credentials in their natural antibiotic effect.

Safety: Generally considered safe if taken as directed. Berberine containing herbs should not be used for long periods of time or in large dosages. They are not recommended for pregnant or nursing women.

Complementary Agents: Goldenseal, barberry, garlic, echinacea, myrrh, dandelion, burdock, capsicum, vitamin A, vitamin C, bioflavonoids, acidophilus and blue-green algae.

PARSLEY (Petroselinum sativum)

Definition: Much more than just a garnish, parsley supplies chlorophyll, helps to restore the urinary tract and is recommended to increase lactation. It can also alleviate the bad breath caused by eating garlic.

Applications: Bedwetting, bladder infections, blood disorders, diabetes, edema, gallstones, halitosis, jaundice, kidney disease, kidney stones, prostate disorders and water retention.

Scientific Updates: Studies have shown that in comparison to citrus juices, parsley contains three times more vitamin C.[158] Recent experiments have established that parsley can lower blood pressure, kill microbes and tone the uterus.[159] Clinical physicians have also claimed that parsley is effective as a remedy for liver disease.[160] The flavonoid content of parsley stimulates urination and provides relief.[161]

Safety: Pregnant women should not use excessive amount of parsley.

Complementary Agents: Buchu, cornsilk, alfalfa, uva ursi, juniper berry, cranberry, marshmallow, kelp, saw palmetto, garlic, vitamin C, bioflavonoids, vitamin A, vitamin E, zinc, proanthocyanidins, bee pollen and phytonutrients.

PASSIONFLOWER (Passiflora incarnata)

Definition: Used as an effective nervous system calmant in Europe, passionflower is recommended for anyone trying to get off of pharmaceutical sleeping pills. It is also suggested for eye inflammations and hyperactivity.

Applications: Alcoholism, anxiety, eye inflammations, insomnia, nervousness, headaches, hyperactivity, hypertension, cardiovascular disease, asthma, hormonal imbalances and stress.

Scientific Updates: Relatively unknown is the fact that passionflower contains low levels of serotonin, a neurotransmitter that naturally calms the brain.[162] It is the harmane alkaloids in the herb which have demonstrated their ability to relax smooth muscle and expand the coronary arteries of the heart, decreasing blood pressure.[163] Additional research has also found that passionflower exerts an anti-inflammatory action making it useful for conditions like arthritis.[164]

Safety: No known toxicity.

Complementary Agents: Valerian root, hops, capsicum, peppermint, chamomile, melatonin, GABA and calcium/magnesium.

PAU D'ARCO (TAHEEBO) (Tabebuia avellandedae)

Definition: Pau d'arco or taheebo, as it is also known, is relatively new to Western herbalists and is harvested from the bark of the lapacho tree in South America. It has been linked to cancer cures and at one time was investigated by the National Cancer Institute for its anticancer properties. Today it continues to be used for malignancies, especially leukemia, and is also prescribed for herpes, diabetes, arthritis and hypoglycemia. It is under current study for it possible value in treating AIDS.

Applications: AIDS, blood disorders, candida, infections, liver disease, pain (arthritis), prostate disorders, ringworm, ulcers, anemia, cancer (especially leukemia), diabetes, herpes, hypoglycemia, lupus, parasites, skin diseases (including cancer), tumors, venereal disease and yeast infections.

Scientific Updates: Some of the chemical constituents of Pau d'Arco have shown the ability to suppress tumor formation.[148] Some researchers believe that the lapacho content of pau d'arco is one of the most important antitumor agents in the world.[149] Pau d'arco has also proven its antibacterial and antiviral properties.[150]

Safety: Taking this herb in tea form is recommended and generally considered safe. In unusual cases, mild nausea or a laxative effect has occurred. Rotating pau d'arco therapy with mathake tea is sometimes advised. Do not take lapacho compounds which have been isolated from pau d'arco. Use the whole herb.

Complementary Agents: Licorice, garlic, echinacea, goldenseal, black walnut, alfalfa, burdock, kelp, milk thistle, dandelion, Oregon grape, yellow dock and yerba mate.

PEPPERMINT (Mentha piperita)

Definition: Peppermint is one the most popular herbal teas in America and has a wide array of pleasant and therapeutic properties. Used for flavoring and for its menthol content, it has both stimulant and antispasmodic actions. Pennyroyal and spearmint have similar properties.

Applications: Colds, sinusitis, bronchitis, diarrhea, gastritis, enteritis, indigestion, nausea, intestinal gas, bloating, griping, colic, colitis, heartburn, irritable bowel syndrome, gallstones, stomach spasms, ulcers and vomiting.

Scientific Updates: Today, peppermint is recognized for its soothing action on the stomach and intestines. It works as an antispasmodic, which helps to relieve nausea and other stomach maladies. Peppermint relaxes the muscles of the digestive tract and stimulates bile flow, which facilitates more efficient digestion.[151] Increased bile flow results in less indigestion, flatulence and colic.[152] The menthol constituent of peppermint works as a natural analgesic and antibacterial.[153] Peppermint has also been able to dissolve gallstones and may be a nonsurgical approach to gallstone removal.[154]

Safety: When used in normal and appropriate dosages, peppermint is considered quite safe. Oil of peppermint can be irritating to mucous membranes if used excessively. Use with caution if pregnant or breast-feeding.

Complementary Agents: Catnip, fennel, ginger, myrrh, capsicum, saw palmetto, calcium carbonate and digestive enzymes.

PLEURISY ROOT (Asclepias tuberosa)

Definition: Traditionally used to treat any respiratory disorder, pleurisy root has the ability to expedite the removal of lung mucus. It is one of nature's best expectorants.

Applications: Allergies, asthma, bronchitis, emphysema, pneumonia, tuberculosis, cough, sore throat, colds and tuberculosis.

Scientific Updates: Pleurisy root specifically targets the lungs and stimulates the removal of thick mucus. It helps to mitigate pain and inflammation typical of lung infections. The reputation of pleurisy root as an excellent therapeutic for lung ailments extends back for several centuries. Earlier in the century, it was considered the primary expectorant, "acting on organs of respiration, powerfully promoting . . . expectoration."[165] "Pleurisy root opens up the lung capillaries, which action helps release any thick mucus . . . thinning it for easier discharge."[166]

Safety: Use appropriate dosages as directed.

Complementary Agents: Sassafras, slippery elm, wild cherry bark, sage, thyme, saw palmetto, lemon grass, blessed thistle, mullein, fenugreek, capsicum, marshmallow, vitamin C, bioflavonoids, vitamin A, calcium/magnesium, bee pollen and acidophilus.

PUMPKIN SEED (Cucurbita pepo)

Definition: A symbol of health in China, the pumpkin contains seeds which have significant antiparasitic properties and are routinely used to rejuvenate the prostate gland. As a rich source of zinc, they are highly recommended for the male reproductive system. Pumpkin seeds are highly nutritional.

Applications: Prostate disorders, intestinal parasites.

Scientific Updates: Recent Swedish clinical trials found the that oil constituents of pumpkin seed combined with saw palmetto effectively treated an enlarged prostate gland.[155]

"Pumpkin seed has a reputation of being a non-irritating diuretic."[156] Pumpkin seed contains a rare amino acid called myosin found in the seeds of certain *Cucurbita* species, which is the primary protein constituent of muscles.[157]

Safety: Take as directed.

Complementary Agents: Saw palmetto, kelp, garlic, black walnut, red clover, cascara sagrada, quassia, buckthorn, acidophilus, bee pollen, bee propolis, B-complex, vitamin E, bioflavonoids, phytonutrients, blue-green algae, zinc and electrolyte supplements.

PYGEUM (Prunus africana)

Definition: Native to areas of Africa and Madagascar, this evergreen tree has been traditionally used to make a tea for genitourinary disorders. Today, standardized extracts of pygeum are used for prostatic hyperplasia, or for BPH.

Applications: Prostatitis, benign prostatic hypertrophy, prostate cancer, incontinence, dysuria, polyuria and nycturia.

Scientific Updates: The phytosterols contained in this herb have anti-inflammatory properties which also inhibit the formation of prostaglandins which are responsible for the swelling in the prostate gland. One of these called beta-sitosterol has been shown to be helpful in cases of BPH by helping to reduce elevated prostaglandin production. The pentacyclic triterpenoids also work to block enzymatic activity associated with inflammation and swelling in the prostate gland.

Safety: No toxicity has been reported with this herb.

Complementary Agents: Saw palmetto, grape seed extract, cruciferous vegetables, isoflavones and vitamin C with bioflavonoids.

QUASSIA (Picrasma amara)

Definition: Traditionally called a "healer of the sick" quassia is a potent herb which is recommended for those with debilitating conditions. It must be taken correctly, or unpleasant side effects can occur.

Applications: Anorexia, convalescence, elderly emaciation, indigestion, fever and worms.

Scientific Updates: Quassia lessens putrefaction in the stomach and prevents the formation of acid substances during digestion.[167] It is said to be one of the best remedies of noxious substances in the alimentary canal resulting from inadequate digestion.[168]

Safety: Because of its potency, it is better to take quassia in herbal formulations than alone to avoid stomach irritation and nausea.

Complementary Agents: Black walnut, cascara sagrada, garlic, buckthorn, ginger, pumpkin seed, red clover, peppermint, vitamin E, vitamin C, bioflavonoids, proanthocyanidins, B vitamins, acidophilus, phytonutrients and blue-green algae.

QUEEN OF THE MEADOW (Eupatorium purpureum)

Definition: Particularly good for joint disorders, this herb helps promote the healing of strains and sprains and helps to alleviate the pain of gout caused by uric acid deposits.

Applications: Arthritis, bladder infections, Bright's disease, bursitis, gallstones, gout, joint pain, kidney infections, kidney stones, neuralgia, prostatitis, rheumatism, urinary disorders and water retention.

Scientific Updates: Queen of the meadow simulates the gland and organs that clear the body of toxic waste.[169] It has been clinically established as a good treatment for rheumatic and gouty joints due to uric acid deposits.[170] It is considered a tonic for the genito-urinary system and can promote suppressed urine flow.[171] Queen of the meadow works as a therapeutic agent on the uterus and prostate gland.[172]

Safety: Take in appropriate doses as directed.

Complementary Agents: Kelp, saw palmetto, capsicum, red raspberry, dong quai, black cohosh, gotu kola, damiana, uva ursi, parsley, vitamin C, bioflavonoids, B-complex, vitamin E, potassium, magnesium and copper.

RED CLOVER (Trifolium pratense)

Definition: A sweet herb, red clover is considered an excellent blood purifier with some antibiotic action. It is often suggested in any infectious conditions, especially skin eruptions.

Applications: Acne, bladder infections, blood cleanser, boils, bronchitis, cancer, leukemia, liver disorders, nervous conditions, psoriasis, skin ailments, and tumors.

Scientific Updates: Clinical studies have found that red clover contains antibiotic properties against several bacteria including those that cause tuberculosis.[173] Scientists have discovered that red clover contains molybdenum, a trace element that is now recognized as essential in clearing the body of nitrogenous waste material.[174] "Many naturopathic physicians use the herb as an alterative including it in regular cleansing programs."[175]

Safety: Take as directed. No known toxicity.

Complementary Agents: Licorice, buckthorn, cascara sagrada, sarsaparilla, alfalfa, quassia, black walnut, kelp, blue-green algae, phytonutrients, vitamin C, bioflavonoids and acidophilus.

RED RASPBERRY (Rubus idaeus)

Definition: Known for its soothing properties, red raspberry helps to ease female discomforts while strengthening uterine muscle. It also promote tissue healing and healthy skin, bones and teeth.

Applications: After-birth pains, bowel disorders, childbirth, colds, diarrhea, digestive problems, female complaints, fever, flu, heart disease, lactation, menstrual irregularities, miscarriage, morning sickness, mouth sores and nausea during pregnancy.

Scientific Updates: Research has found that a particular constituent of the raspberry leaf caused either contraction or relaxation of uterine muscles as needed.[176] "Raspberry leaf tempers the effects of hormonal runaway, such as might occur during menstruation, pregnancy and delivery."[177] It is also thought to build the tissue of the cervix to prevent tearing during delivery.[178]

Safety: While mild doses are recommended during pregnancy, excessive amounts should be avoided.

Complementary Agents: Licorice, dong quai, saw palmetto, cramp bark, damiana, queen of the meadow, squaw vine, sarsaparilla, black cohosh, kelp, gotu kola, wild yam, vitamin C, bioflavonoids, B-complex, folic acid, vitamin E, calcium/magnesium and primrose oil.

RED SAGE (Salvia officinalis)

Definition: Associated for millennia with wisdom and longevity red sage has traditionally been used for menstrual disorders, to reduce night sweats and as a natural mouth deodorizer. The volatile oils in red sage have antiseptic and astringent properties and are also used to help dry up milk supplies when breast feeding has ceased.

Applications: Coughs, depression, diabetes, digestive disorders, fever, liver ailments, lactation inhibitor, memory (failing), menstrual pain, mouth sores, nausea, nervous conditions, nigh sweats, sores, sore throat and worms.

Scientific Updates: The volatile oils and tannins in red sage are responsible for its ability to stop excessive perspiration. The oils also have an antiseptic and astringent property which makes them useful in the healing of sores and irritations.[179] Red sage also acts as a powerful antioxidant and boosts circulation. Its estrogenic properties may explain its believed ability to dry up breast milk.

Safety: Avoid medicinal dosages in pregnancy and in cases of epilepsy. Nursing mothers should not take red sage due to its milk drying action.

Complementary Agents: Capsicum, dandelion, garlic, yellow dock, quassia, milk thistle, cascara sagrada, black walnut, acidophilus, blue-green algae, phytonutrients, proanthocyanidins, vitamin C, vitamin A, B-complex and calcium/magnesium.

ROSE HIPS (Rosa species)

Definition: Rose hips is the fruit of a plant blossom that is an unusually rich source of vitamin C. It was used in England during World War II to offset the shortage of citrus fruits and prevent scurvy. It contains 60 times more vitamin C than lemons.

Applications: Arteriosclerosis, bladder infections, blood purifier, cancer, circulatory insufficiencies, colds, contagious diseases, fever, flu, infections, PMS, sore throat and stress.

Scientific Updates: Linus Pauling's research on vitamin C literally put it on the map as a therapeutic agent. His work points to using large, daily doses to prevent all kinds of illness and to promote longevity. Rose hips provide a superior natural source of vitamin C which has been linked to the prevention and cure of certain cancers.

Safety: Vitamin C can be taken in high doses although stomach upset and diarrhea can occur in some cases. People who have trouble with kidney stones should consult their physicians before taking supplemental doses of vitamin C. Taking calcium/magnesium with vitamin C increases its assimilation.

Complementary Agents: Bioflavonoids, grape seed or pine bark proanthocyanidins, calcium/magnesium, capsicum and alfalfa.

SAGE (Salvia officinalis)

Definition: Known for its use in traditional stuffings and meat dishes, sage can significantly reduce excess perspiration and soothe mouth and gum sores. It is an aromatic herb whose fragrance has also been used to promote feelings of well being and relaxation.

Applications: Cankers, coughs, diabetes, digestive disorders, fever, laryngitis, memory, mouth sores, nausea and worms.

Scientific Updates: Sage relaxes peripheral blood vessels, reduces perspiration, salivation and lactation. It is a natural antibiotic and can reduce blood sugar and promote bile flow.[180] The astringent properties of sage make it useful in treating cold symptoms, and relieving the irritation of cankers or mouth sores.[181] Sage is also credited with being a potent antioxidant.[182]

Safety: Pregnant or nursing women should check with their physician before taking sage. Anyone with epilepsy should not use sage for prolonged periods of time.

Complementary Agents: Thyme, peppermint, verbena, ginger, chamomile, lemon grass, blessed thistle, pleurisy root, capsicum, fenugreek, saw palmetto, vitamin C, bioflavonoids, proanthocyanidins, vitamin A and calcium/magnesium.

SARSAPARILLA (Smilax ornata)

Definition: Native to the Pacific coast of Mexico, sarsaparilla was used with sassafras to make root beer. Compounds in this herb promote the production of testosterone and progesterone while cleansing the blood of toxins. This herb is routinely included in formulas designed to balance hormones.

Applications: Blood disorders, male and female hormonal imbalances, infertility, menopausal symptoms, joint aches, psoriasis, sexual dysfunction and skin problems.

Scientific Updates: Clinical tests have discovered antibiotic attributes in sarsaparilla primarily due to its saponin content.[183] Sarsaparilla also has strong diuretic capabilities and dramatically lowers the urea content of the blood.[184] Chinese research has found that as a tonic, sarsaparilla has value in that it can help rejuvenate the nerves, blood and glands.[185] In Mexico, South America and China, the herb is used to treat infertility.[186]

Safety: No known toxicity.

Complementary Agents: Saw palmetto, licorice, damiana, ginseng, kelp, squaw vine, black cohosh, red raspberry, bee pollen, bee propolis, vitamin E, vitamin C, bioflavonoids, folic acid, calcium/magnesium, zinc and marine lipids.

SAW PALMETTO (Serenoa repens)

Definition: The saw palmetto berry was used by ancient Mayans to treat disorders of the genitourinary tract. Interestingly, today's scientists are discovering that compounds in saw palmetto can prevent the conversion for testosterone to dihydortestosterone, which helps to prevent the development of prostate disease. The herb is considered an overall glandular tonic.

Applications: Prostate disease, genitourinary problems, endocrine disorders, infertility, impotence, bronchitis, colds, menstrual disorders, ovarian dysfunction, lactation, thyroid deficiencies, digestive problems and painful menstrual periods.

Scientific Updates: The ability of saw palmetto to treat prostate disease has been the subject of recent clinical studies. The results have been impressive and strongly suggest that saw palmetto may be a viable alternative to the use of Proscar, a pharmaceutical drug used for treating enlarged prostate glands.[187] Its inclusion in digestive formulas is based on its ability to stimulate normal appetite and boost nutrient assimilation.[188] Saw palmetto may also be useful for women who suffer from hormonal imbalances by helping to normalize estrogen levels.

Safety: No toxicity has been reported with saw palmetto.

Complementary Agents: B-complex, calcium/magnesium, calcium carbonate, ginger, proanthocyanidins, phytonutrients, bee pollen, fennel, catnip, peppermint, capsicum, acidophilus, kelp, sarsaparilla, ginseng, digestive enzymes, bee pollen and bee propolis.

SKULLCAP (Scutellaria lateriflora)

Definition: Skullcap, named for its flower formation, acts like a sedative without the deleterious effects of narcotic drugs. It has a relaxing and sleep promoting action which can help to quiet nervousness and treat insomnia. It has also been used in assisting with drug and alcohol withdrawal and has been used for headaches.

Applications: Anxiety, insomnia, muscles spasms, neuralgia, tension, hysteria and pain.

Scientific Updates: Skullcap continues to be used as a mild neural sedative which has the ability to relieve headaches and other related pain. Studies have shown that it can tranquilize a restless and excited nervous system.[189] In addition, nervous twitching and muscle spasms were also calmed by skullcap.[190] An added bonus of skullcap is its ability to lower blood serum cholesterol and prevent high blood pressure.[191]

Safety: Skullcap is considered safe when taken in appropriate dosages. One advantage of using skullcap in an herbal blend is that its dose has been metered out in proportion with other herbs.

Complementary Agents: Valerian root, chamomile, hops, passionflower, wood betony, marshmallow, mullein, black cohosh, B-complex, folic acid, melatonin and calcium/magnesium.

SENNA (Cassia acutofolia)

Definition: Senna is a powerful purgative herb that acts as an intestinal cleanser and strong laxative. It grows in shrub form in regions of the Nile. Today, it is commonly added to colonic formulas to stimulate peristalsis of the large intestine.

Applications: Constipation, jaundice, gallbladder disease, liver disease and worms.

Scientific Updates: Anthrquinone compounds give senna its laxative effect and stimulate the bowel to move within six to eight hours of ingestion. These compounds do not work directly on the bowel but are absorbed through the walls of the small intestine and subsequently stimulate the nerves of the large intestine.[192]

Safety: Because senna is absorbed systemically, it should not be used by pregnant or nursing mothers. Anyone with colon disease should not use this herb unless it is part of a carefully desinged formula. Taking senna can cause significant gripping pains in the abdomen suffesting that it always be taken as part of a combination which helps to neutralize gripping. Senna can become habit forming if it is taken in excess or for long periods of time.

Complementary Agents: Aloe vera, ginger, cloves, peppermint, fennel, cascara sagrada, slippery elm, calcium/magnesium, essential fatty acids, marine lipids, digestive enzymes and acidophilus.

SLIPPERY ELM (Ulmus fulva)

Definition: Slippery elm comes from elm tree bark and is a mucilaginous compound used for generations by Native Americans to soothe irritated mucous membranes. Its protective and healing action make it an excellent herb for treating diarrhea, colon disorders, sore throats or intestinal ulcers.

Applications: Abscesses, asthma, bronchitis, colitis, constipation, coughs, diarrhea, digestive disorders, lung ailments, gastritis, ulcers and heartburn.

Scientific Updates: Clinical studies have proven the value of slippery elm for the treatment of diarrhea, coughs, stomach upsets, colitis and a variety of lung problems.[193] The antitussive action of slippery elm can soothe raw throats and inhibit chronic coughing.[194] In addition, the high mucilage content of this herb helps to heal and restore the mucous membranes of the gastrointestinal tract.[195] The fact that slippery elm is found in over-the-counter medications in the U.S. and Great Britain attests to its versatility.[196]

Safety: No known toxicity.

Complementary Agents: Marshmallow, fenugreek, saw palmetto, mullein, thyme, pumpkin seed, yucca, aloe vera, capsicum, yerba santa, wild cherry, vitamin C, bioflavonoids, vitamin A, B-complex, vitamin E, zinc and acidophilus.

SQUAW VINE (Mitchella repens)

Definition: Also known as "partridge berry," this plant was extensively used by Native Americans as a pregnancy tonic. It was believed to strengthen uterine contractions and ease childbirth. Today it is commonly used in female corrective formulas dealing with menstrual disorders.

Applications: Childbirth, lactation, menstrual disorders, miscarriage, skin problems, tonic (female), uterine disorders and vaginal yeast infections.

Scientific Updates: Squaw vine is a natural for herbal combinations designed to correct female complaints or strengthen the female reproductive system. "Squaw vine is extremely useful for the treatment of water retention."[197] It is accepted as a uterine tonic and a stimulant to the ovaries.[198]

Safety: Use as directed in appropriate doses. If pregnant or nursing, check with your physician before using squaw vine.

Complementary Agents: Kelp, red raspberry, wild yam, black cohosh, dong quai, damiana, cramp bark, licorice, queen of the meadow, saw palmetto, vitamin E, vitamin C, bioflavonoids, B-complex, proanthocyanidins and phytonutrients.

ST. JOHN'S WORT (Hypericum perforatum)

Definition: Used for wound healing during the Crusades, this herb has the ability to cleanse tissue and reduce inflammation, and has recently emerged as an effective antidepressant.

Applications: AIDS, after-birth pains, cancer, menstrual cramps, depression, viral infections, bacterial infections, sleep disorders and wounds.

Scientific Updates: In 1942, a compound called hypericin was isolated from St. John's wort and used as a natural antidepressant. It can also relieve pain and cause a mild sedating effect. It has been shown to be a more powerful antidepressant than placebo and many standard antidepressants.[199]

Safety: This herb can cause photosensitivity, although incidence is rare in humans, with the exception of AIDS patients who have taken large doses. Exposure to strong sunlight for anyone with fair skin is not recommended.

Complementary Agents: Capsicum, thyme, vitamin B-complex, vitamin B6, vitamin B12, (sublingual), folic acid, calcium/magnesium, wild yam, phenylalanine, tyrosine and taurine.

TAHEEBO (see Pau d'Arco)

THYME (Thymus vulgaris)

Definition: Used by the ancient Greeks for its aromatic properties, thyme works to relax stomach spasms and promotes healing. Thymol, or thyme oil, is used in Listerine for its antiseptic action.

Applications: Bronchitis, coughs, digestive ailments, gas, gingivitis, gout, headaches, laryngitis, lung disorders, sciatica pain, sore throats, stomach problems, throat maladies and worms.

Scientific Updates: The thymol content of thyme works as an expectorant and cough suppressant and is frequently used in cough syrups prescribed for lung ailments like bronchitis.[200] When combined with fenugreek, thyme works to relive the pain of migraine headaches.[201] The carminative properties of thyme make it an effective treatment for stomach upsets.[202]

Safety: Use in appropriate dosages. Check with a physician if pregnant or nursing before taking thyme.

Complementary Agents: Fenugreek, capsicum, yerba santa, marshmallow, mullein, saw palmetto, wild cherry, licorice, vitamin C, bioflavonoids, vitamin A and acidophilus.

UVA URSI (Arctostaphylos uva-ursi)

Definition: Uva ursi contains a compound called arbutin,

which has the ability to drain excess water from the cells, promoting an antiseptic effect on the kidneys.

Applications: Bladder infections, Bright's disease, cystitis, diabetes, nephritis, water retention, liver ailments and chronic diarrhea.

Scientific Updates: The primary constituent of uva ursi is a glycoside called arbutin which is responsible for its diuretic action. In addition, when it is excreted from the kidneys, arbutin produces an antiseptic effect on the mucous membranes of the urinary tract.[203] Chemical compounds in uva ursi also help to balance the pH of urine.[204] American research found that uva ursi was effective against nephritis and kidney stones and possessed all-around tonic properties.[205] In addition, tests have found that extracts of uva ursi have shown some anticancer properties and antibiotic action.[206]

Safety: Must be used as directed. Pregnant women should consult their physician before using uva ursi. Prolonged or excessive use may cause gastric irritation.

Complementary Agents: Parsley, buchu, alfalfa, cornsilk, juniper berries, marshmallow, cranberry, lemon grass, vitamin C, bioflavonoids, vitamin B6, proanthocyanidins, B-complex, bee pollen, phytonutrients and mineral and electrolyte supplements.

VALERIAN ROOT (Valeriana officinalis)

Definition: The ester-containing compounds in this herb give it a characteristic odor and help to promote its natural and safe sedating effect.

Applications: Insomnia, headaches, hyperexcitability, hypertension, heart disorders, afterbirth pains, anxiety, tension, high blood pressure, stress, nervous stomach, palpitations, menstrual cramps and muscle spasms.

Scientific Updates: Valerian tranquilizes and regulates the autonomic nervous system, enhances higher brain functions, and eases childhood psychosomatic disturbances and behavioral disorders.[207] Valerian improves sleep quality with none of the drawbacks of barbiturates.[208] Valerian is also recommended for anyone who suffers from cardiovascular disease or hypertension in that it helps to relax smooth muscle and ease tension.

Safety: No known toxicity exists. Extreme doses should be avoided. Pregnant women should consult their physician before taking valerian.

Complementary Agents: Hops, chamomile, passionflower, skullcap, mullein, marshmallow, wood betony, hawthorne berries, black cohosh, niacin, calcium/magnesium, vitamin B6 and melatonin.

WILD CHERRY (Prunus virginiana)

Definition: Found in old fashioned lozenges because of its cough-soothing properties, wild cherry can help calm dry coughs and lubricate irritated mucous membranes.

Applications: Allergies, asthma, congestion, coughs, colds, sore throats, bronchitis fever and tuberculosis.

Scientific Updates: Wild cherry has the ability to calm and soothe irritated mucosal tissue.[209] "Wild cherry bark's use for reducing the symptoms of respiratory distress is without

equal in the herb kingdom."[210] It can benefit asthmatics by relaxing the nerves which feed the lungs.[211]

Safety: No known toxicity.

Complementary Agents: Slippery elm, capsicum, fenugreek, yerba santa, mullein, saw palmetto, marshmallow, thyme, vitamin C, bioflavonoids, proanthocyanidins, phytonutrients, vitamin A, B-complex, vitamin B12, potassium and calcium/magnesium.

WILD YAM (Dioscorea villosa)

Definition: Traditionally used for its hormonal properties, Mexican wild yam root is considered a phytoestrogen (progesterone) with none of the side effects of synthetic hormones. Its use in cream form is emerging as a viable treatment for osteoporosis, menstrual disorders and menopause.

Applications: Hormonal imbalance, PMS, menstrual disorders, infertility, moods swings, fibrocystic breasts, uterine fibroids, ovarian cysts, menopause, osteoporosis, cancer (hormonally related), fibromyalgia and prostate disease.

Scientific Updates: Dr. John Lee's studies impressively delineate the ability of transdermal wild yam to effectively raise progesterone and balance estrogen, which may help to prevent and treat certain cancers and a myriad of hormonally related symptoms.[212]

Safety: Considered safe and nontoxic if used in appropriate amounts. A contraceptive effect only occurs with extremely large doses.

Complementary Agents: Dong quai, black cohosh, damiana, saw palmetto, sarsaparilla, vitamin E, vitamin B complex, folic acid, essential fatty acids, vitamin C, bioflavonoids and grape seed and pine bark proanthocyanidins.

WOOD BETONY (Betonica officinalis)

Definition: As a medieval remedy for head ailments, wood betony's glycoside content can help to alleviate head pain and dilate blood vessels. It is considered a nervine calmant herb.

Applications: Nervous disorders, headaches (especially tension), insomnia, hysteria, facial pain, migraines, liver protectant and Parkinson's disease.

Scientific Updates: Today, scientists have found that wood betony has the ability to dilate blood vessels and promote relaxation.[213] Its vascular effect has been linked to its ability to relieve headache pain, hence causing muscles to relax.[214]

Safety: Wood betony is considered safe when taken in appropriate doses. Because it has the ability to mildly stimulate the uterus, it should be avoided in pregnancy.

Complementary Agents: Valerian, hops, skullcap, marshmallow, mullein, chamomile, black cohosh, melatonin, lavender, vitamin B-complex and calcium/magnesium.

YELLOW DOCK (Rumex crispus)

Definition: As one of the best blood-cleansing herbs, yellow dock helps to rid the body of toxins and purges the lymph glands. It is unusually rich in iron and is an excellent liver tonic.

Applications: Anemia, blood disorders, blood cleanser, boils, cancer, coughs, hives, iron deficiency, liver ailments, psoriasis, rheumatism, skin disorders and sores.

Scientific Updates: Yellow dock enhances the liver's ability to filter the blood.[215] Antibacterial properties have also been observed in yellow dock.[216] "Yellow dock root achieves its tonic properties through astringent purification of the blood supply to the glands . . . It is often used in seasonal cleanses and blood detoxification programs. Among all herbs, it has one of the strongest reputations for clearing up skin problems, liver and gallbladder ailments, and glandular inflammation and swelling."[217]

Safety: Use as directed.

Complementary Agents: Dandelion, capsicum, burdock, garlic, fenugreek, quassia, kelp, black cohosh, red sage, blue-green algae, vitamin C, vitamin A, bioflavonoids, B-complex, proanthocyanidins and phytonutrients.

YERBA SANTA (Eriodictyon spp.)

Definition: Considered a lung tonic, this herb helps to open respiratory passages and stimulates the production of natural cortisone.

Applications: Allergies, asthma, bronchial congestion, colds, flu, laryngitis, hemorrhoids and bladder infections.

Scientific Updates: Yerba santa exerts a strong stimulant action on the lungs enabling them to expel mucus.[218] It also helps to open respiratory passages affected by allergic reactions, and can help decrease nasal discharge.[219] In the past, it has also been recommended for hemorrhoids and bladder infections.[220] In addition, yerba santa increases the therapeutic effectiveness of other herbs.

Safety: Use in the appropriate dosage.

Complementary Agents: Fenugreek, capsicum, mullein, marshmallow, slippery elm, wild cherry, saw palmetto, thyme, comfrey, vitamin C, bioflavonoids, vitamin A, calcium/magnesium, phytonutrients and proanthocyanidins.

Endnotes

1. Daniel B. Mowrey, Ph.D. The Scientific Validation of Herbal Medicine, Keats Publishing, Connecticut, 1986, 2.
2. P. De Froment. "Unsaponifiable substance from alfalfa for pharmaceuticals and cosmetic use." French Patent2, 187,328, 1974.
3. E. Tyihak and B. Szende. "Basic plant proteins with antitumor activity." Hungarian Patent 798, 1970.
4. M.C. Robson, et al., "Myth, Magic, Witchcraft or Fact: Aloe Vera Revisited, Journal of Burn Care and Rehabilitation,(3): 1935: 157-62. See also L.J. Lorenzetti, "Bacteriostatic property of Aloe Vera, Journal of Pharmacological Science, (53): 1964: 1287.
5. R.W. Shelton, "Aloe Vera, its chemical and therapeutic properties," International Journal of Dermatology, (30): 1991: 679-83.
6. J.B. Kahlon, et al., "Inhibition of AIDS virus replication by acemannan in vitro," Mol Biother (3): 1991: 127-35.
7. Rebecca Flynn, M.S., and Mark Roest. Your Guide to Standardized Herbal Products. One World Press, Prescott, Arizona: 1995: 4.
8. Alma E. Guinness, Family guide to Natural Medicine, Reader's Digest Association, New York, 1993, 324.
9. Mowrey, 240.
10. James Duke. Handbook of Medicinal Herbs. CRC Press, Boca Raton: 1985, 120.
11. Michael Murray, N.D., and Joseph Pizzorno, N.D. Encyclopedia of Natural Medicine. Prima Publishing, Rocklin, California: 1991, 462.
12. Guinness, 298. See also J. Young. American Journal of Medical Sciences. 9, 310, 1831, N. R. Farnsworth and A.B. Seligman. "Hypoglycemic plants." Tile and Till. 57(3), 52-56, 1971, and P.S. Benoit, H.H.S. Fong, G.H. Svoboda and N.R. Farnsworth. "Biologic and phytochemical evaluation of plants. XIV. Anti-inflammatory evaluation of 163 species of plant." LLoydia. 39(2-3), 160-61, 1976.
13. A.R. Hutchens. Indian Herbology of North America. Merco, Ontario, Canada: 1973.
14. Penelope Ody, The Complete Medicinal Herbal, Dorling-Kindersley, New York, 1993, 71.
15. U.C. Bhargava AND B.A. Westfall, "Antitumor activity of juglans nigra (black walnut) extractives, Journal of PHarmaceutical Sciences, 57 (10), 1674-1677.
16. Ibid.
17. Mowrey, 230.
18. Jack Ritchason, The Little Herb Encyclopedia, Woodland Publishing, Pleasant Grove, Utah, 1994, 30.
19. Paul Barney M.D., Clinical Applications of Herbal Medicine, Woodland Publishing, Pleasant Grove, Utah, 1996, 66.
20. Michael A. Weiner Ph.D. and Janet A, Weiner. Herbs that Heal. Quantum Books, Mill Valley: California: 1994, 87.
21. Peter Holmes, The Energetics of Western Herbs, Artemis Press, Boulder, 1989, 278.
22. V.E. Tyler, L.R. Brady and J.E. Robbers. Pharmacognosy. 7th ed. Lead and Febiger, Philadelphia: 1976.
23. H.W. Youngken. Textbook of Pharmacognosy. 5th ed. Blakiston, Philadelphia: 1943.
24. M. Grieve, F.R.H.S. A Modern Herbal. Dorset Press, New York: 1994, 134.
25. S.M. Kupchan and A. Karim. "Tumor inhibitors 114: Aloe emodin: antileukemic principle isolated from Rhamnus fangula L." Lloydia, 39, 223-224, 1976.
26. H.W. Youngken; Textbook of Pharmacognosy. 5th ed. Balkiston, Philadelphia, Pennsylvania: 1943.
27. P. Behrns. "Healing remedies in word and illustration." Krankenpflege. 29(3), 101-04, 1975.
28. Mowrey, 68.
29. Ibid., 58 and 249.
30. Flynn, 10.
31. T. Koloata and D. Chungcharcon. "The effect of capsaicin on smooth muscle and blood flow of the stomach and intestine." Siriraj Hospital Gazette. 24, 1405-1418, 1972.
32. Paul Barney, M.D. Clinical Applications of Herbal Medicine. Woodland Publishing, Pleasant Grove, Utah: 1995, 55.
33. Ibid., 20.
34. Peter Holmes. The Energetics of Western Herbs. Artemis Press, Boulder: 1989, 322.
35. Murray and Pizzorno, 419.
36. Mowrey, 58.
37. M. Marchesi, M. Marcato and C. Silvestrini. "A laxative mixture in the therapy of constipation in aged patients." Giornale de Clinica Medica. Bologna: 63, 850-63, 1982.
38. Mowrey, 58.
39. Murray and Pizzorno, 235.
40. Flynn, 12.
41. Ibid.
42. Mowrey, 76.

43. L. D'amico. "Ricerche sulla presenza di sostanze ad azione anatibiotica nelle piante superiori." Fitoterapia. 21(1), 77-79, 1950.

44. "The Cats. Claw," The Energy Times, May-June, 1995: 12.

45. Riccardo Cerri, "New Quinovic Acid Glycosides from Uncaria Tomentosa," Journal of Natural Medicine Vol. 51, No. 2, Mar-Apr, 1988: 257-61.

46. R. Aquino, et al., "Plant Metabolites: structure and in vitro antiviral activity of Quinovic acid glycosides from Uncaria Tomentosa," Journal of Natural Products, Vol, 52, No. 3, may-June, 1990: 559-64.

47. Philip A. Steinberg, "Uncaria Tomentosa (Cat's Claw): A Wondrous Herb From the Peruvian Rainforest," TOWNSEND LETTER, 130, May, 1994: 2.

48. Ibid., New Editions Health World, Feb. 1995: 43.

49. T. Shipochliev. "Extracts from group of medicinal plants enhancing uterine tonus." Veterinary Sciences (SOFIA). 18(4), 94-98, 1981.

50. J. Breinlich and K. Scharnagel. "Pharmacological properties of the ene-yne dicloethers from atricaria chamomilla, anti-inflammatory, anti-anaphylactic, spasmolytic, and bacteriostatic activity." Arzneimittel-Forschungen, 18(4), 429-31, 1968. V. Yakolev and A. Von Schlichtegroll. "Anti-inflammatory activity of alpha-bisabolol, an essential component of chamomile oil." Arzneimittel-Forschungen. 19(4), 615-16, 1969. O. Isaac and G. Kristen. "Old and new methods of chamomile therapy. Chamomile as example for modern research of medicinal plants." Medizinische Welt. 31(31-31), 1145-49, 1980. J.L. Hartwell. "Plants used against cancer: a survey." Lloydia. 31, 71, 1968.

51. Jack Ritchason, The Little Herb Encyclopedia, 3rd ed. Woodland Books, Pleasant Grove, Utah: 1994, 63-64.

52. Ibid., 65.

53. A.Y. Leung. Chinese Herbal Remedies. Universe Books, Now York: 1984, 47-49.

54. Mowrey, 235.

55. Ibid. 82.

56. Louise Tenney. Today's Herbal Health, 3rd ed. Woodland Publishers, Pleasant Grove, Utah: 1992.

57. Ritchason, 66.

58. Ody, 113.

59. Guinness, 302.

60. Ritchson, 68.

61. Grieve, 111.

62. Alma R. Hutchens. Indian Herbology of North America. Merco, Ontario, Canada: 1969, 108.

63. Ody, 164.

64. Holmes, 300.

65. L.S.M. Curtin. Healing Herbs of the Upper Rio Grande. Southwest Museum, Los Angeles: 1965.

66. Tenney, 46.

67. Ibid.

68. Michael Murray, N.D., and Joseph Pizzorno, N.D. Encyclopedia of Natural Medicine Prima Publishing, Rocklin, California: 1991, 462.

69. Guinness, 298.

70. J. Young. American Journal of Medical Sciences. 9, 310, 1831.

71. N. R. Farnsworth and A.B. Seligman. "Hypoglycemic plants." Tile and Till. 57(3), 52-56, 1971,

72. Mowrey, 282.

73. Ibid., 283.

74. Flynn, 18.

75. Ibid.

76. Ibid., 19.

77. Murray and Pizzorno, 462.

78. Gary Gillum, "Echinacea," Today's Herbs, Provo, Utah: Woodland Books, Vol. 1 issue 11, July, 1981: 1.

79. Murray, ENCYCLOPEDIA OF NATURAL MEDICINE, 58.

80. V.H. Wagner and A. Proksch, "Immunostimulatory Drugs of Fungi and higher Plants," Economic Medicinal Plant Research, 1985: (1), 113053.

81. Ibid.

82. Ody, 176.

83. Mowrey, 98.

84. Ibid., 19-20.

85. Ibid., 279.

86. Ritchason, 85.

87. G. Valette, Y Sauvaire, et al. "Hypocholesterolemic effect of fenugreek seed in dogs." Atherosclerosis. 50, 105-111, 1984.

88. W.A. Thompson. Herbs that Heal. Charles Scribner's Sons, New York: 1976, 160-61.

89. G. Ribes, Y. Sauvaire, J.C. Valette, et al. "Effects of fenugreek seeds on endocrine pancreatic secretions in dogs." Annals of Nutrition and Metabolism. 28, 37-43, 1984.

90. Ritchason, 91.

91. Ibid.

92. Guinness, 308.

93. Mowrey, 122-123.

94. C.J. Cavallito and J.H. Bailey. "Allicin, the antibacterial principle of allium sativum. I. Isolation, physical properties and antibacterial action." Journal of the American Chemical Society. 66. 1950-51, 1945.

95. Weiner, 160.

96. Guinness, 308.

97. Mowrey, 104.

98. Flynn, 28.

99. "Ginger." The Lawrence Review of Natural Products: Facts and Comparisons. St. Louis: Nov. 1991.

100. Weiner, 164.

101. F. Juguet, et al., "Deceased cerebral 5-HT1A Receptors during aging: reversal by Ginkgo biloba extract," J. Pharm Pharmacol., April, 1994: 46 (4), 318-28.

102. G. Vorberg, "Ginkgo biloba extract (GBE): A long term study of chronic cerebral insufficiency in geriatric patients," Clinical Trials Journal, (1985) 22, 149-57.

103. Deanne Tenney, Ginseng, Woodland Press, Pleasant Grove, Utah: 1996, 20.

104. Ibid., 21.

105. Ibid., 31.

106. Louise Tenney, 76.

107. Mowrey, 158.

108. Rita Elkins, M.H. Goldenseal, 16.

109. Ibid., 17.

110. List, vol. 2-5.

111. Ibid.

112. R.N. Chopra. Indigenous Herbs of India. 2nd ed. Arts Press, Calcutta: Chopra R.N. et al. 1933.113 Betty Kamen. "Gymnema Extract." Let's Livd. Sept. 1989, 40-41.

114. Journal of Ethmorpharmacology. 1986, 143-46.

115. Flynn, 47.

116. Guinness, 311.

117. "Hawthorn." The Lawrence Review of Natural Products: Facts and Comparisons. St. Louis: May, 1987.

118. Murray and Pizzorno, 383.

119. R. Blesken, "Crataegus in cardiology," Forsch Med, 110, 1992:

290-92

120. Mowrey, 32.

121. Mowrey, 164-65.

122. Ibid., 83.

123. Ibid., 84.

124. Flynn, 52.

125. Ibid., 130.

126. Holmes, 366.

127. Mowrey, 123.

128. Ibid., 268.

129. Ritchason, 133.

130. C.H. Costello and E.V. Lynn. "Estrogenic substances from plants: glycyrrhiza glabra." Journal of the American Pharmaceutical Association. 39, 177-80, 1950.

131. Ody, 65.

132. Guinness, 315.

133. Michael Murray N.D. The Healing Power of Herbs. Prima Publishing, Rocklin, California: 1992, 431.

134. "Licorice." The Lawrence Review of Natural Products: Facts and Comparisons, June, 1989.

135. Murray, Healing Power of Herbs, 241.

136. Ibid.

137. Jack Ritchason, 145.

138. P.H. List and L. Hoerhammer. Hagers Handbuch der Pharmazeutischen Praxis.. Vol. 2-5, Springer-Verlag: Berlin. P. Schauenber and F. Paris. Guide de Plantes Medicinales. Delachaux et Niestle, S.A., Neuchatel, Switzerland: 1969. R.W. Wren. Potter's New Encyclopedia of Botanical Drugs Preparation. 7th ed. Health Science Press, Rustington, England: 1970.

139. "Marshmallow" The Lawrence Review of Natural Products: Facts and Comparisons. St. Louis: Dec. 1991.

140. A. Desplaces, et al., "The effects of silymarin on experimental phalloidin poisoning," Arneimittel-Forsch, 25, 1975: 89-96.

141. Murray, The Healing Power of Herbs, 244.

142. Ibid., 248.

143. "Mullein." The Lawrence Review of Natural Products: Facts and Comparisons, St. Louis: Sept. 1989.

144. James F. Balch M.D. and Phyllis A. Balch, CNC. Prescription for Nutritional Healing. Avery Publishing, Garden City Park, New York: 1990, 56.

145. F. Ellingwood. Therapeutics and Pharmacognosy. Eclectic Medical Pub. Portland, Oregon: 1983.

146. G. Majno. The Healing Hand: Man and Wound in the Ancient World. Harvard University Press, Cambridge: 1975, 217-18.

147. Mowrey, 57.

148. Ibid., 75.

149. Tenney, Encyclopedia of Natural Remedies, 80.

150. H. Gershon and L. Shanks, "Fungitoxicity of 1,4-naphtho-quinones to Candida albicans and Truchophyton mentagrophytes," Canadian Journal of Microbiology, 21, 1975: 1317-21.

151. Penelope Ody. The Complete Medicinal Herbal. Dorling Kindersley, New York: 1993, 79.

152. Murray and Pizzorno, 399.

153. Ody, 79.

154. J.D. Bell and J. Doran, "Gallstone dissolution in man using an essential oil preparation," British Medical Journal, 278, 1979: 24.

155. Barney, 72.

156. Mowrey, 236.

157. Ritchason, 190.

158. Ritchason, 163.

159. A.Y. Leung. Encyclopedia of Common Natural Ingredients. New York: 1980, 257-59.

160. D.M.R. Culbreth. A Manual of Materia Medica and Pharmacology. Philadelphia: 1927.

161. Mowrey, 234.

162. Flynn, 61.

163. Ibid.

164. Guinness, 319.

165. Mowrey, 240.

166. Ritchason, 181.

167. Grieve, 663.

168. Tenney, 114.

169. Mowrey, 4.

170. Ibid.

171. J. King. The American Dispensatory. Cincinnati: 1866.

172. Ritchason, 192.

173. Mowrey, 54.

174. Ritchason, 193.

175. Mowrey, 54.

176. Mowrey, 186, 109.

177. Ibid., 109.

178. Ritchason, 195.

179. Ritchason, 206.

180. Ody, 95.

181. Guinness, 321.

182. Ritchason, 207.

183. Mowrey, 19.

184. Ibid., 19.

185. Ibid., 287.

186. Leung, 152.

187. J. Braeckman. "The extract of Serenoa repens in the treatment of benign prostatic hyperplasia: A multi center open study." Current Therapy Res. 55, 776-85, 1994.

188. Mowrey, 77.

189. B.A. Kurnakov. "Pharmacology of skullcap." Farmakologiia I Toksikologiia. 20(6), 79-80, 1957.

190. S. Shibata, M. Harada, and W. Budidarmo. "Constituents of Japanese and Chinese crude drugs. III. Antispasmodic action of flavonoids and anthraquinones." YAKUGAKU ZASSHI. 80, 620-24, 1960.

V. Usow. Farmakologiia I Toksikologiia. 21(2) 31-34, 1958.

A.F. Gammerman and I.D. Yourkevitch, eds. Wild Medicinal Plants. Bello-Russia Publishers, Academy of Science, Institute of Experimental Botanics and Microbiology, Minsk: 1965.

191. T. Usow. Farmakologiia I Toksikologiia. 21(2), 31-34, 1958.

192. Pederson, 157.

193. Shook, 163.

194. Barney, 98.

195. Ibid., 136.

196. Ibid., 29.

197. Ritchason, 226.

198. Ibid.

199. Murray, 296.

200. Guinness, 324.

201. Velma Keith and Monteen Gordon, The How To Herb Book, Mayfield Publishing, Pleasant Grove, Utah: 1984.

202. Guiness, 324.

203. Ibid., 233.

204. B.S. Barton. Collections for an Essay Toward a Materia Medica of the United States. 3rd ed. Edward Earle and Co., Philadelphia: 1810.

205. J.L. Harwell. "Plant Remedies for Cancer." Cancer Chemotherapy Reports. July, 19-24, 1960. 206 R. Benigni. "The presence of antibiotic substance in the higher plants." FITOERAPIA. 19(3), 1-2, 1948.

207. U. Boeters. "Treatment of autonomic dysregulation with valepotriates (Valmane)." Muenchener Medizinische Wochenschrift. 37, 1873-1876, 1969. V. Kempinskas. "On the action valerian." Farmakologiia I Toksikologiia. 4(3), 305-309, 1964. R. Klich and B. Gladbach. "Childhood behavior disorders and their treatment." Medizinische Welt. 26(25), 1251-1254, 1975.

208. P.D. Leathwood and F. Chauffard. "Aqueous extract of valerian reduces latency to fall asleep in man." Planta Medica. 54, 144-48, 1985.

209. Mowrey, 131.

210. Ibid. 240.

211. Barney, 10.

212. John R. Lee, M.D., Natural Progesterone: The Multiple Roles of a Remarkable Hormone, BLL Publishing, Sebastopol, California: 1993.

213. Daniel P, Mowrey. The Scientific Validation of Herbs. Keats Publishing, New Canaan, Connecticut: 1986, 193. T.V. Zinchenko, and I.M. Fefer. "Investigation of glycosides from betonica officinalis." Farmatsevt Zhurnal. 17(3), 35-38, 1962.

214. Ritchason, 255.

215. Mowrey, 19.

216. List, vol. 2-5.

217. Mowrey, 207.

218. Ritchason, 262.

219. Ibid.

220. Grieve, 865.

An Overview of Other Natural Supplements

ACIDOPHILUS

Definition: Certain substances which sour, such as active cultured yogurt, buttermilk and certain cheeses, contain *Lactobacillus acidophilus* that enhance digestion and elimination by effectively digesting proteins in the bowel. Acidophilus also helps to detoxify harmful bacteria by helping to restore "friendly bacteria" that keep certain microorganisms in check. Non-dairy sources of acidophilus are available. All sources, whether liquid or capsule, should be refrigerated and taken on an empty stomach in the morning. Check expiration dates before purchasing any acidophilus products. Acidophilus supplements should be taken after antibiotic therapy or their effects will be neutralized.

Applications: constipation, yeast infections, mouth sores, colon problems, fungal and bacterial infections, diarrhea, high blood cholesterol, indigestion and malnutrition.

Safety: Acidophilus is considered safe but anyone suffering from an allergy to milk products should use only non-dairy acidophilus products.

Recommendations: Acidophilus can be taken in capsule, tablet, liquid or edible forms such as buttermilk, yogurt, etc. Always check for expiration date and use guaranteed bacterial count products with lacto and bifido bacteria.

ALPHA LIPOIC ACID (ALA)

Definition: ALA is a powerful antioxidant compound which has recently emerged as even more effective than other antioxidants due to its water and fat solubility and its ability to greatly potentiate the action of vitamin E and glutathione. ALA can be defined as an antioxidant compound which is synthesized in the body in extremely small amounts, although it must also be supplied from food or supplement sources to augment intrinsic supplies. It is a vitamin-like substance which contains sulphur and plays a vital role in energy reactions in mitochondrial electron transport. This function is intrinsically related to the metabolism of glucose into energy (ATP).

Applications: Aging, AIDS, alcoholism, atherosclerosis, Bell's palsy, cataracts, cancer prevention, cirrhosis, diabetes, diabetic neuropathy, multiple sclerosis, liver disease, radiation sickness or exposure, memory/Alzheimer's disease, senile dementia, stroke, Huntington's disease, Parkinson's disease and heavy metal poisoning.

Safety: Generally considered safe, ALA has been used for over 20 years in Europe with no reported toxicity or adverse effects. It is well tolerated and assimilated through the stomach. Animal studies have found that doses over 400 to 500 mg per kilogram of body weight can create some toxicity. This amount translates to dosages higher than most people would use as a preventative antioxidant compound. Children and pregnant or lactating women should not take this supplement. Anyone who is under the care of physician or has a serious medical condition should check with their doctor before using ALA. This supplement is considered safe if used as directed. ALA may interfere with vitamin B1 assimilation; anyone suffering from a thiamine deficiency, such as many alcoholics, should take a thiamine supplement in conjunction with ALA.

Recommendations: Generally speaking, taking between 40 to 50 mg of ALA is considered a therapeutic dose for maintaining health, while doses in the 100 mg range are used for chronic conditions. Diabetics can take between 200 and 300 mg per day and even more if their physician feels it is necessary. AIDS patients can exceed this dose but must do so under the supervision of their physician. ALA therapy is a long-term treatment and is usually not associated with short-term results.

BEE POLLEN

Definition: Bee pollen is a fine powdery substance that has been collected from the stamen found within flower blossom and stored by honeybees in honeycomb hives. It is considered a highly nutritious and complete food and contains a rich supply of B-complex vitamins, vitamins C, A, E, carotenoids, folic acid, amino acids, a wide array of minerals and some essential fatty acids.

Applications: Most allergies, anemia, asthma, athletic endurance, chronic fatigue, immune system disorders, impotence, infertility, kidney disorders, menopause, prostate disease and ulcers.

Safety: A very small percentage of the population is allergic to bee pollen. If you suffer from pollen allergies, you should use bee pollen with caution. Start with a very small granule and work up to larger doses. If you experience throat itching or any other allergic symptom, discontinue use immediately. Using pollen that has been harvested from local bees helps to avoid allergic reactions.

Recommendations: Bee pollen can be purchased as a powder, granules, canned, chewable wafers, capsulized or in tablet form. It should be purchased from a reliable source and kept refrigerated. It has been used for centuries to promote stamina and longevity.

BEE PROPOLIS

Definition: Bee propolis is a resinous substance gathered by honeybees from deciduous tree bark and leaves. It is a sticky material that bees use to seal hive holes or cracks. Before it is used in the hive, honeybees take the propolis, combine it with nectar found in their own secretions and eventually end up with a mixture of wax, pollen and bee bread. Propolis has been used for thousands of years as a protection against infection, a promoter of healing and as a superior source of energy and endurance.

Applications: Allergies, bruises, burns, cancer, herpes zoster, fatigue, sore throats, nasal congestion respiratory ailments, acne, sunburn, shingles, flu, colds, coughs, and ulcers.

Safety: Generally considered safe although it should be initially taken in small amounts to check for potential allergic reactions.

Recommendations: With any bee product, potency is vital. Freeze-dried products or vacuum-packed supplements are better than simple capsulized varieties. Bee propolis is very delicate and can break down rapidly.

BENTONITE

Definition: Bentonite is a highly absorbent clay-like substance that helps to lift impacted waste matter which has accumulated on the walls of the gastrointestinal tract. It is usually used in colon cleansing programs and with enema therapy. It should be used under the direction of a health care practitioner.

Applications: Blood and colon purification, constipation, parasitic infections, and food allergies.

Safety: Bentonite therapy should be used under the care of a health care professional. Check with your doctor before using any colonic treatment.

Recommendations: Bentonite is usually sold as a powder and should be used judiciously.

BIOFLAVONOIDS

Definition: Bioflavonoids (also referred to as "flavonoids") comprise a group of plant pigments that provide excellent cellular protection by modifying the action of allergens, carcinogens, and viruses. Bioflavonoids are responsible for giving plants and their blossoms color pigment and are also found in the white material located just beneath the peel of citrus fruits. While they are not technically vitamins, bioflavonoids are sometimes referred to as vitamin P. They are remarkable free radical scavengers and include hesperetin, hesperidin, quercetin, eriodictyon, and rutin. Because the body cannot produce bioflavonoids, they must be supplied through diet or supplementation..

Applications: Bruising, bleeding (including heavy menstrual), high cholesterol, cataracts, oral herpes, allergies, asthma, liver disease and gum disease.

Safety: Excessively high doses may cause diarrhea.

Recommendations: Bioflavonoids are usually combined with other vitamins such as vitamin C and are generally taken in capsule or tablet from. Some citrus derived powders that can be mixed with liquid are also available. When buying any vitamin product, make sure that it contains adequate amounts of bioflavonoids.

BLUE-GREEN ALGAE (see Spirulina and Chlorella)

BOVINE CARTILAGE

Definition: Bovine cartilage helps to promote wound healing and inhibit inflammation. Compounds in bovine cartilage have the ability to block angiogenesis, the process by which tumors are fed by a network of new blood vessels.

Applications: Rheumatoid arthritis, psoriasis, ulcerative colitis, lupus, firm tumors, connective tissue diseases and inflammatory joint conditions.

Safety: Bovine cartilage is considered a nontoxic substance if taken as directed.

Recommendations: Make sure to purchase clean and pure

dried-powder forms that come from cattle which are disease and hormone free. Like shark cartilage, bovine varieties must be taken in rather large doses in order to work. Loose powdered forms are much more practical, although the capsulized product can be used preventatively.

CELL SALTS

Definition: Cell salts are trace minerals that comprise the 12 compounds believed to contain the active ingredients used in the practice of traditional homeopathy. On a cellular level, chelated trace minerals are absorbed up to 80 percent better than unchelated or inorganic minerals. Typical cell salts include magnesium phosphate, calcium sulfate, silica oxide, etc. They are usually taken in tablet form and placed under the tongue to dissolve.

Applications: A vast number of ailments. Every disorder has a particular cell salt formula.

Safety: Mineral overdoses can occur but cell salt therapy is considered safe.

Recommendations: Cell salts are often sold as numbered homeopathic preparations under various label names and should come from reliable sources.

CHITOSAN

Definition: Chitosan is a fiber-like product made from ground shrimp shells that inhibits fat absorption. It is not digestible and has the ability to absorb many times its weight in fats, preventing their absorption through the intestinal wall.

Applications: Obesity, high cholesterol, hypertension, heartburn and gout.

Safety: Considered nontoxic but anyone with a shellfish allergy or who is pregnant or nursing should not use chitosan products. Like fiber supplements, chitosan can inhibit the absorption of lipid-based vitamins and should be taken at a different time. Drink at least eight glasses of water per day when taking chitosan supplements.

Recommendations: Chitosan comes in capsules and powders and should be taken just prior to eating a meal with fat content. Four to eight capsules per meal is the usual amount required to absorb adequate amounts of fat. Using simple chitosan for fat absorption is better than blends which do not contain enough of the compound to be effective.

CHLORELLA

Definition: Chlorella are single-celled green algae, thought to have the richest content of chlorophyll. They are traditionally used as a blood de-toxifier. Chlorella contains an impressive array of vitamins and minerals including 19 amino acids, RNA and DNA. Like other forms of algae, it is recommended for blood building, boosting the immune system and inhibiting both bowel and blood toxicity. Testing is underway to evaluate its phycocyanin content for cancer treatment. Like spirulina, chlorella can help to protect against ultraviolet radiation.

Applications: Blood builder, blood purifier, cataracts, chronic diseases, chronic fatigue, diabetes, food supplement, hepatitis, hypoglycemia, gastritis, glaucoma, obesity and weight loss.

Safety: It is important to obtain any type of blue-green algae from a reliable source to ensure purity. Excess ingestion of chlorella may cause fatigue.

Recommendations: Chlorella is available in capsules, tablets, powder, flakes, freeze-dried crystals, premeasured packets and extracts. It can be a good source of vitamin K. Make sure to look for pure products.

CHLOROPHYLL

Definition: Chlorophyll is the green pigment that plants use to carry out the process of photosynthesis. The greater amount of chlorophyll, the greener the plant. As a food supplement, mineral-rich chlorophyll prompts tissue repair, purifies the blood and the liver and helps to build red blood cells. It also works as a natural deodorizer and tissue healer. In addition, chlorophyll can inhibit the growth of infectious microorganisms, sanitize the colon and treat gum disease. It also promotes the proliferation of friendly intestinal flora. Chlorophyll can also be an excellent source of vitamin K.

Applications: Anemia, blood toxicity, exposure to radiation and ulcers.

Safety: No known toxicity. Use in appropriate doses.

Recommendations: Chlorophyll is available in liquid and capsulized supplements. Look for high quality sources. Fat-soluble chlorophyll is preferable to water-soluble and can be found in fresh juice sources.

CHONDROITIN SULFATE

Definition: Chondroitin sulfate is a promising new supplement. When combined with glucosamines sulfate, it helps to alleviate the painful symptoms of osteoarthritis and can facilitate cartilage healing and regeneration in affected joints. The chemical constituents of chondroitin help to create spaces in the matrix enhancing flexibility and cushioning by enabling it to hold more water. Chondroitin is a naturally occurring compound found in joint tissue. Initial data suggests that both chondroitin sulfate and glucosamine sulfate may be the most valuable and effective natural treatment for arthritis.

Applications: Osteoarthritis, rheumatoid arthritis, gout, lupus, connective tissue diseases, bursitis, joint trauma.

Safety: Considered nontoxic, although side effect studies have not been conducted for longer than a six-year time period.

Recommendations: Look for supplements labeled either chondroitin sulfate or mucopolysaccriarides. These products should be pharmaceutical grade to ensure purity and potency. This compound is usually found in capsule or tablet form. NOTE: Chondroitin sulfate should always be used in combination with glucosamine sulfate.

CITRIN (See HCA)

CONJUGATED LINOLEIC ACID (CLA)

Definition: CLA is a form of linoleic acid, an essential fatty acid that naturally occurs in some vegetable oils and in beef, veal and dairy products. It has impressive antitumor and antioxidant properties. It seems to have the ability to prevent the build-up of cholesterol deposits in the arteries and to promote the burning of fat stores.

Applications: Obesity, atherosclerosis, high cholesterol, cancer deterrent and natural antioxidant.

Safety: CLA is generally considered safe. If you have liver disease, consult your physician. Taking fat absorbing compounds like chitosan can inhibit the absorption of CLA, if taken at the same time. The beneficial effects of CLA take time to occur.

Recommendations: Make sure you are getting pure CLA. Adding vegetable oils to a product technically means it has CLA content but this is not the form of CLA you want. Take in recommended doses only. If you have trouble with fat digestion, taking a lipase supplement may enhance assimilation.

CMO (CETYL MYRISTOLEATE)

Definition: CMO, or cetyl myristoleate, is a fatty acid which is absorbed in the intestines after being orally ingested. It can be extracted from living tissue or synthetically produced. CMO occurs in certain mice species, male beavers and in sperm whale oil. Currently, it is being produced synthetically without using any animal extracts. Simply stated, CMO has the ability to inhibit the symptoms of arthritic disease including pain, and inflammation and is also considered an immunizing agent against the development of rheumatoid arthritis.

Applications: Osteoarthritis, psoriatic arthritis, lupus, back pain, joint injuries, Reiter's Syndrome, autoimmune diseases, ankylosing spondylitis and rheumatoid arthritis (several reports claim that CMO is also effective for rheumatoid arthritis as both a preventative and therapeutic agent).

Safety: Tests which have been run on CMO containing products have found no side effects or toxicity. CMO should not be given to children unless under the supervision of a qualified health care provider. The effects of CMO on pregnant or nursing mothers has not been studied. Anyone suffering from liver disease or asthma should not take CMO without the approval of their health care professional. As is the case with any fatty acid supplement, care should be taken to use the product in recommended doses only.

Recommendations: Generally, a CMO protocol involves a three-to-six week course of treatment. A minimum of thirty days is recommended for maximum efficacy. Therapy typically involves taking a recommended number of capsules or liquid several times a day with a break of several days and eventual resumption of treatment until the entire amount of CMO has been consumed. NOTE: If you have trouble digesting and assimilating fats, taking lipase may help to ensure proper absorption of CMO which is a fat-based compound. Taking fat-absorbing supplements like chitosan may interfere with the proper assimilation of CMO.

COENZYME Q10

Definition: Coenzyme Q10 is a substance which resembles vitamin E and is found in living cells. Natural supplies of this particular compound decrease with age. Recent studies have found that re-supplying the body with coenzyme Q10 may significantly reduce hypertension and heart disease and enhance the immune system. Current studies are underway using coenzyme Q10 as a treatment for AIDS. In addition, this substance has been shown to enhance weight loss, heal periodontal disease, relive angina and inhibit the aging process on a cellular level. It has also demonstrated its ability to reduce the mortality rate of laboratory animals suffering from leukemia and tumors.

Applications: Cardiovascular disease, cancer, high blood pressure, respiratory disease, asthma, mental illness, Alzheimer's disease, candida, obesity, multiple sclerosis, periodontal disease, gastric ulcers, weakened immune systems and AIDS.

Safety: Always look for pure and reliable sources of coenzyme Q10. Supplements should be stored in a dark, cool environment.

Recommendations: The most common form of coenzyme Q10 is in capsulized form. Soft gel caps that are lipid-based are recommended. This compound is also commonly included in antioxidant combinations and cardiovascular formulations.

CREATINE

Definition: Creatine is considered a naturally occurring nutrient found in skeletal muscles that is comprised of arginine, glycine and methionine (three amino acids). Creatine assists in providing muscle fibers with the energy needed to facilitate quick and forceful movements. While most of the body's creatine is obtained from dietary sources, using it in supplement form to enhance muscle building and athletic performance is currently in use. Several clinical studies suggest that creatine supplementation allows for more energy storage, increased stamina, strength and synthesis of protein and lean muscle mass.

Applications: Athletic endurance, muscle building and weight loss.

Safety: No significant long-term studies on the safety of creatine exist. Its usage for several decades is considered relatively safe with an increase in muscle mass. Short-term side effects reported by athletes using large doses of creatine include diarrhea, gas and intestinal upset. Creatine should not be used by anyone suffering from any medical problem without their physician's approval. People suffering from kidney disorders should not take creatine.

Recommendations: Creatine is best utilized in powder form. Exact measurements can be obtained with specific dispensing cups packaged with powdered forms.

DESICCATED LIVER

Definition: When liver is reduced to a concentrated and dry powdered state it is considered desiccated. This particular form of liver is easy to capsulize or add to other health formulations. Desiccated liver is rich in iron and a number of vital vitamins and minerals. Its primary function is to build red blood cells, making it an excellent supplement for any debilitated condition.

Applications: Anemia, chronic fatigue, weakness, stress, liver disease and athletic endurance.

Safety: Desiccated liver that comes from organically raised beef is recommended.

Recommendations: Powder or tablet forms are available. Make sure the product is 100 percent pure.

DHA (DOCOSAHEXAENOIC ACID)

Definition: DHA is an omega-3 fatty acid that is found in coldwater fish lipids and can also be extracted from microalgae. It is considered one of the primary building blocks of the retina and of the brain. It is the most plentiful fatty acid found in human breast milk and serves to ensure the proper function of nerve cell membranes. DHA is also found in eggs, organ meats and red meats—people who have cut down on these foods may be low in the compound.

Applications: Memory disorders, senile dementia, vision problems, nerve disease, brain dysfunction and mental conditions.

Safety: If you are taking DHA that has been isolated from a marine lipid source, you need to rule out fish allergies and check with your physician. DHA obtained from marine lipids should be combined with vitamin E. Long-term studies on taking DHA alone are not yet available.

Recommendations: DHA is now available as an isolated compound which is derived from fish or microalgae sources. Look for pure product from reliable companies. Note: Don't confuse DHA for DHEA, which is a hormone and not a fatty acid compound.

DHEA

Definition: DHEA is the most abundant hormone found in mammals and plays an integral role in a number of vital physiological processes. It significantly contributes to immune function, supplies the biochemical building blocks for the synthesis of other hormones and has recently been linked to many other biological functions. Like coenzyme Q10, it diminishes with age, a fact that has linked DHEA depletion with almost every major degenerative disease. It is considered a significant antiaging compound and its depletion has been linked to stress exposure.

Applications: Lupus, rheumatoid arthritis, psoriasis, diabetes, prostate disease, menopause, high cholesterol and obesity.

Safety: DHEA supplementation should be done with the consent of your physician. While no significant reactions have occurred to supplementation, some minor acne has occurred in some people. DHEA is not recommended for anyone suffering from breast, ovarian, uterine or prostate cancer since these can be hormonally stimulated malignancies. Long-term effects of extended supplementation with DHEA have not been studied.

Recommendations: Tablets or capsules of DHEA are available. Look for standardized potency and pure products with no fillers. NOTE: DHEA levels can be assessed through a blood test.

DMAE (DIMETHYLAMINOETHANOL)

Definition: DMAE is a compound which, among other things, is considered a neurostimulant. It has been used for everything from memory and learning enhancement to increased stamina. It is most commonly used as a mild stimulant that boosts energy without interfering with sleep patterns. DMAE is believed to contribute to increased mental awareness and stamina without the significant side effects of caffeine or amphetamine drugs. In relation to weight loss, DMAE also contributes to heightened metabolism and thermogenesis by boosting energy levels and by helping reduce body fat stores while building muscle. It is thought to work in tandem with herbs like ephedra to help maximize thermogenesis, although no clinical studies supporting this action exist.

Applications: Memory impairment, learning enhancement, stamina, weight loss and thermogenesis.

Safety: DMAE can have significant side effects if taken in large quantities or if overused. Insomnia, headaches, muscle stiffness above the neck or in the legs indicates that DMAE dosages are too high. While there are no adverse reactions to DMAE on record, anyone with manic-depressive illness and epilepsy should not use DMAE without the approval of their physician. The rule with DMAE is to begin with the smallest possible dose. When DMAE is included in formulations, its amount is usually proportionate to its therapeutic purposes.

Recommendations: DMAE can be found in certain seafood and is naturally present in very minute quantities in brain tissue. It is considered a nutritional supplement and is available in capsules, liquids or powdered forms. DMAE may be added to various formulas designed to boost energy, fight fatigue or burn fat. NOTE: If using the liquid form of DMAE, refrigeration is required to preserve potency.

DMSO (DIMETHYLSULFOZIDE)

Definition: This compound is actually a by-product of the paper manufacturing process. It is an oily liquid with a slight garlicky smell and is used as a solvent in commercial products like degreasers. The external application of this compound has proven itself valuable for muscle strains and sprains, joint injuries and even on broken bones. It seems to alleviate pain and promote healing simultaneously. It is absorbed through the skin into the bloodstream and has been used in this way to treat arthritis, muscle problems, headaches, herpes, and even cancer.

Applications: Muscle injuries, joint injuries, bone trauma, strains and sprains, back pain, sciatica, Down's syndrome, acne, sinusitis, skin ulcer, herpes, cataracts, keloids and burns.

Safety: This product should never be taken orally and should be kept out of the reach of children. Long term studies evaluating its safety have not been conducted to date. It should be used judiciously, according to individual instruction.

Recommendations: DMSO usually comes bottled in liquid form and resembles mineral oil.

ENZYMES

Definition: Enzymes are biochemical compounds composed of protein which initiate and regulate virtually every function of the human body. Enzymes are essential for life and cannot be manufactured synthetically. Each and every enzyme has a specific function and recent research strongly suggests that the health ramifications of enzyme therapy is only just now emerging. Our culture's overconsumption of cooked foods has resulted in enzyme depletion, paving the way for a variety of disorders and diseases. Only raw foods contain enzymes which convert stored energy for use, utilize ingested food, detoxify harmful substances, and initiate and govern almost every biochemical reaction needed by all body systems. Cooking destroys most of the enzyme content of foods. Supplemental enzymes can be made from animal enzymes such as pancreatin or pepsin or from plant sources such as aspergillus, papaya or pineapples. Digestive enzymes include amylase, protease and lipase. Proteolytic enzymes include bromelin, papain, pectinase and pancreatin.

Applications: Allergies, digestive disorders, constipation, colon diseases, ulcers, heartburn and autoimmune diseases.

Safety: Use as directed.

Recommendations: Over-the-counter varieties come in tablets, capsules, powders, gums and liquid forms and may be combined in other formulations containing herbs, antioxidants, etc. Take just prior to eating and between meals if you like.

ESSENTIAL FATTY ACIDS

Definition: Also known as vitamin F, these are fatty acids which must be supplied thorough the diet and cannot be produced by the body. These are polyunsaturated acids commonly used to treat high cholesterol, heart disease and to prevent strokes. The most essential of the fatty acids is called linoleic acid. Omega-3 fatty acids include EPA (eicosapentaenioic acid) and DHA (docosahexaenoic acid) from marine lipids. Coldwater fish contain two essential fatty acids referred to as EPA and DHA which have been shown to significantly reduce the risk of cardiovascular disease, contribute to nerve health and act as natural anti-inflammatory agents. Omega-6 fatty acids include GLA (gamma linolenic acid, also referred to as *linoleic acid*) and are usually found in plant sources. These acids can be found in flaxseed oil, a rich plant source of the omega-3 factors, low in saturated fats and cholesterol-free; black current oil, naturally high in GLA (linoleic acid, which must be obtained from dietary sources); and evening primrose oil, the richest source of GLA (linoleic acid) found anywhere. (Borage oil is also rich in omega-6 fatty acids.) Anyone with hormone-related cancers should limit their intake of primrose oil and use black current instead.

Applications: High blood pressure, heart disease, arthritis, breast cancer, psoriasis, eczema, weight loss, multiple sclerosis, brain function, and PMS.

Safety: Diabetics should not take fish oil. Other sources of essential fatty acids are highly recommended, including eating fresh coldwater fish. If you must take fish oil, take a vitamin E supplement also.

Recommendations: Use liquid or capsulized liquid forms. Products that need refrigeration and come in dark or light protected containers are preferable. Combination capsules which contain a variety of essential fatty acids are also good.

FIBER SUPPLEMENTS

Definition: Fiber supplements are products comprised of one or a combination of fiber sources that can be combined with certain herbs and other supplements in order to provide more dietary fiber and colon health. Today, few of us eat the recommended 25 to 45 grams of fiber per day and could benefit from the many health advantages of increased dietary fiber. A number of supplements are available and can be added to liquid. They are also available in bar form or as dry supplements.

Applications: Cardiovascular health, high cholesterol, obesity, cancer preventative, bowel disorders, constipation, varicose veins and hemorrhoids.

Safety: Fiber is considered safe if it is dietary in nature and not taken in such excess that diarrhea of obstruction could occur. Drink plenty of water when taking fiber and if you suffer from any type of colon disorder or digestive system disease, check with your doctor before adding a fiber supplement. Take vitamin and mineral supplements at different times than fiber as absorption may be impaired.

Recommendations: Fiber supplements commonly include herbs such as aloe vera, cascara sagrada, rhubarb, slippery elm or acacia which help to tonify and heal the mucous membranes of the colon. The primary fiber source of most products is psyllium although there are other sources. These include psyllium, which has a colorless transparent mucilage that forms around its insoluble seed; bran, with its low solubility and good water-holding properties; gums, which form a homogenous adhesive gelatinous mass in the lower intestine to expedite waste transit; methyl cellulose, whose slow solubility creates a viscous solution for expulsion; and ispaghula husk, which swells rapidly to form a mucilage.

GLA (Gamma linolenic acid)

Definition: GLA is an essential fatty acid found in plant sources. It belongs to the omega-6 variety and can be obtained from certain oils such as borage, flaxseed, etc. Americans are particularly at risk for GLA depletion in that sources of GLA are not typically consumed in our country.

Applications: Weight loss, high cholesterol, PMS, cardiovascular disease, nerve disease (multiple sclerosis) autoimmune disorders, natural blood thinner, alcoholism, breast cancer, immune dysfunction and arthritis.

Safety: GLA is considered safe if taken as directed. As with any fatty acid compound, check with your doctor before starting supplementation. Make sure not to take this supplement at the same time as a fat blocker like chitosan, or its absorbability will be compromised.

Recommendations: Using GLA as an isolated compound does not have a long track record. If you take a fatty acid supplement that is comprised of certain oils like borage, you will automatically get GLA.

GLUCOSAMINE SULFATE

Definition: Glucosamine sulfate holds some very exciting potential as a safe treatment for osteoarthritis and other inflammatory joint conditions. It is a naturally occurring amino-monosaccharide found in the joints of mammals. When taken as a dietary supplement, glucosamine appears to significantly restore normal biochemistry in supporting the rebuilding and healing of osteoarthritic cartilage. A glucosamine deficiency has been linked to osteoarthritis. Some studies have supported the ability of glucosamine to heal anti-inflammatory disease.

Applications: Arthritis (especially osteoarthritis), cartilage injuries, connective tissue disease, joint pain and TMJ.

Safety: Considered nontoxic, easily tolerated and absorbed. Rare side effects include nausea or stomach upset. Take with meals.

Recommendations: Look for pharmaceutical grade products with strong potency and guaranteed purity. This supplement should always be taken in conjunction with chondroitin sulfate for maximum benefit. Dosages should be higher initially with a tapering off over time. Results will be noticeable within a month to six weeks.

GLUTATHIONE

Definition: This compound is technically a protein which is synthesized in the liver from three amino acids (cysteine, glutaminic acid and glycine). It is a powerful antioxidant agent. It seems to have some remarkable protective properties against radiation, chemotherapy, heavy metals, toxins and other poisons. When combined with selenium, it is particularly helpful; it forms an enzyme galled glutathione peroxidase, which protects the body from harm on a cellular level. It is particularly good as a liver protectant and may play a role in lowering the risk of cancer.

Applications: Relief from the side effects of chemotherapy, exposure to radiation, heavy metal poisoning, liver disease, alcoholism, liver cancer and free radical protectant.

Safety: The effects of long-term usage of this compound have not yet been explored. As with any amino acid compound or derivative, check with your doctor before taking this supplement.

Recommendations: Some controversy exists as to whether glutathione is very effective when taken as an oral supplement. Enhancing its natural production by increasing levels of N-acetyl cysteine or L-cysteine and L-methionine may be preferable. Using alpha lipoic acid has also proven its ability to enhance the action of glutathione.

GRAPE SEED OR PINE BARK EXTRACT
(Proanthocyanidins or OPCs)

Definition: Also commonly referred to as *pycnogenol*, this substance has impressive antioxidant properties and is considered substantially more effective than either vitamin C or E in scavenging free radicals. It also has pronounced anti-inflammatory actions due to a flavonoid called proanthocyanidin. It can be extracted from grape seeds or pine bark and is especially good for vision problems, nerve inflammations, water retention and cardiovascular conditions. It has the ability to stabilize collagen and retard skin aging.

Applications: Free radical protection, Bell's palsy, diabetes, skin aging, bursitis, ulcers, eyesight, cancer, heart disease, arteriosclerosis, multiple sclerosis, colds and flu, prostate disease, lupus, psoriasis, arthritis, senile dementia, stroke and Parkinson's disease.

Safety: When used as recommended, grape seed or pine bark extract is considered a safe supplement with no adverse side effects.

Recommendations: Some controversy exists as to whether pine bark or grape seed is a better source of proanthocyanidins. Both can be good if manufactured by reliable companies that guarantee potency and purity.

HOMEOPATHY

Definition: Homepathy is a system of medicine developed in the 19th century based on the concept of "like cures like." Essentially, substances are used to produce the same symptoms as the troubling disease. These substances, also called cell salts, are heavily diluted and introduced into an infected system. Homeopathic practitioners see symptoms as positive signs that the immune system is in action. More than 2,000 homeopathic remedies exist and are extracted from plant, mineral, animal or chemical sources.

Applications: Allergies, anemia, headaches, arthritis, colitis, peptic ulcers, high blood pressure, obesity, hormonal imbalances, infections or any other chronic diseases.

Safety: Homeopathic remedies may initially worsen symptoms. For dangerous symptoms, care should be taken. Homeopathy is usually reserved for less serious conditions.

Recommendations: Homeopathic remedies are available in tablets, granules, liquids or ointments. Look for established products with a good track record.

HYDROXY CITRIC ACID (HCA or Citrin)

Definition: Found in the herb *Garcinia cambogia*, HCA is a form of citric acid which inhibits the ability of the liver to make fats from carbohydrates. When HCA is present, carbohydrates convert to glycogen rather than fat, ensuring more efficient energy reserves, stamina and weight control. The ability of HCA to augment weight loss without artificial stimulation is impressive.

Applications: Endurance, obesity, appetite suppressant and high cholesterol.

Safety: No known toxicity, but pregnant or lactating women should not use this compound unless advised to do so by their doctors.

Recommendations: HCA is usually sold as citrin or in *Garcinia cambogia* supplements. Look for standardized products with guaranteed potency.

ISOFLAVONES

Definition: A class of phytochemicals found in soybeans that were isolated in the 1970s and have very impressive breast cancer-inhibiting properties. These plant estrogens have the ability to block the negative action of estrogen in breast tissue. One of these isoflavones, "genistein," actually reduces the growth of breast cells and inhibits two key enzyme pathways that contribute to the formation of a tumor.

Applications: Breast cancer, breast cancer risk, hormonal imbalances, PMS, menstrual irregularities and menopause.

Safety: Considered nontoxic if used as directed.

Recommendations: Often these valuable phytochemicals will be combined with cruciferous extracts (indoles) for added protection against the bad effects of estrogen associated with the development of breast tumors. Eating soybean products like tofu is a good source of these compounds.

LECITHIN

Definition: Lecithin is a vital compound necessary to maintain the health of cell membranes which largely regulate life preserving processes on a cellular level. It is comprised of choline, a B vitamin and also contains inositol, choline and linoleic acid. While it is technically a fatty substance, lecithin works to emulsify fats, an important factor in preventing arteriosclerosis and cardiovascular disease. It also contributes to better brain function. Lecithin expedites the removal of fats like cholesterol. Most lecithin is commercially extracted from soybeans or egg sources.

Applications: AIDS, herpes, chronic fatigue, arteriosclerosis, high cholesterol, heart disease, high blood pressure and obesity.

Safety: No known toxicity.

Recommendations: Lecithin is commonly sold in granule form or as a capsulized substance either alone or in combination with other nutrients like glucomannan.

LYCOPENE

Definition: Lycopene is a carotenoid compound found in tomatoes that acts as an impressive antioxidant and can help to prevent the damaging effects of oxidants on DNA, thereby inhibiting the formation of tumors.

Applications: Hormonal imbalances, breast cancer and breast cancer risk.

Safety: Considered safe although long-term studies on using this compound in isolated form have been conducted.

Recommendations: Lycopene may be somewhat difficult to purchase at this time. If you do find it, look for pure varieties with no fillers and add it to your antioxidant and cruciferous extract array.

MELATONIN

Definition: Melatonin is a naturally occurring hormone which is secreted by the pineal gland located in the midbrain. Darkness triggers the production of melatonin which, in turn, brings on sleep. It is believed that melatonin regulates the body's internal clock. The hormone has also been linked to antiaging properties, works as an antioxidant, may inhibit the growth of some types of cancer, may slow the progression of the AIDS virus and may play an integral role in cardiovascular health.

Applications: Aging-related disorders, insomnia, jet lag, weak immune system, high cholesterol, arteriosclerosis, mental illness and cancer prevention.

Safety: Several studies have established the relative safety of taking melatonin supplements, although its long-term effects are yet to be observed. It has no known toxicity, even in relatively high amounts. Some individuals have experienced strange dreams or a feeling of next-day depression following a nighttime dose. It is not recommended for pregnant or nursing mothers or for anyone with severe allergies, leukemia, lymphoma, autoimmune diseases, or severe depression. Anyone who is taking antidepressants or is trying to conceive should not take melatonin. Caution should be used when using the supplement for children.

Recommendations: Melatonin is usually sold in capsulized form and should be taken in very small amounts as directed. You may want to begin with half the dosage and assess the results. Taking too much can result in feelings of lethargy and perhaps even depression.

MUSHROOMS (MEDICINAL)

Definition: These usually refer to shitake and reishi varieties, which are Japanese mushrooms with impressive therapeutic properties. They contain specific polysaccharides which boost T-cell activity in the immune system. Recently, they have been used as a viable cancer and AIDS treatment and may prove to be invaluable for immune deficiency disorders.

Applications: Hypertension, immune dysfunction, infections, chronic fatigue, autoimmune disease, cancer, heart disease, high cholesterol.

Safety: These mushrooms are considered safe if used appropriately. Make sure to look for clean products that have been packaged properly.

Recommendations: Both mushroom types are available in fresh or dried form and can be soaked for twenty minutes before use. They can also be purchased in capsule or extract form.

PHYTOCHEMICALS

Definition: Phytochemicals are non-nutritive compounds found in plants that have potential disease-inhibiting capabilities. Phytochemicals give plants their color and fragrance and may also protect the plant against certain fungal or bacterial infections. Today, phytochemicals are undergoing intensive research as anticarcinogenic compounds. For anyone who has trouble eating ample amounts of vegetables, taking certain phytochemicals in supplement form is highly recommended.

Indoles, a certain phytochemical—found in cabbage, broccoli, and Brussels sprouts—may offer protection against certain types of cancer. Research strongly suggests that these particular phytochemicals may be extremely beneficial. For example, studies have found that indoles have the ability to block estrogen receptor sites in breast tissue. (Estrogen stimulation of the breast has been linked with tumor growth in some women.) In addition, there is some data which suggests that indoles actually inhibit the secretion of estrogen. Indoles may offer significant protection against breast and other types of hormone-linked cancers. They can now be taken in supplement form. Anyone at high risk for breast cancer should take indole supplements.

Allyl sulfides, found in onions, leeks and garlic, have anti-tumor, antibiotic and antitoxin actions.

Flavonoids, found in certain fruits and vegetables, have antioxidant properties and may also inhibit the development of certain cancers. They highly complement vitamin C.

Dithiolthiones, found in cruciferous vegetables (cabbage, Brussels's sprouts, broccoli, cauliflower) may protect cell DNA from carcinogenic threats.

Isoflavones, found in soybeans and soy by-products, may lower the incidence of breast and prostate cancer.

Lignins, found in flaxseed, help to protect the heart and may lower the risk of colon cancer.

Limonene, found in the rind of citrus fruits, stimulates certain enzyme synthesis and has an antitumor effect.

PREGNENOLONE

Definition: Pregnenolone is a naturally occurring hormone that recently proved to have potential health benefits. It is a chemical derivative of cholesterol and is technically considered a steroid like DHEA, cortisol, progesterone, testosterone and estrogen. Pregnenolone is synthesized from cholesterol in several organs. Pregnenolone can be metabolized into progesterone and easily converts into DHEA.

Applications: Pregnenolone is currently in use as a supplement for enhanced brain function, memory deficiencies, Alzheimer's diseases, mood disorders, chronic fatigue, cholesterol levels, lupus, immune weakness, multiple sclerosis, PMS, prostate disease, psoriasis, rheumatoid arthritis, scleroderma, stress and trauma.

Safety: Because pregnenolone is converted to DHEA, androgens and estrogens, it should not be used without your physician's approval. Although studies have found the compound to be nontoxic, pregnenolone has not been subject to intensified long-term investigation. Because it converts to aldosterone, blood pressure could rise when taking Pregnenolone. It is not recommended for anyone suffering from hypertension. High doses of pregnenolone could suppress immune function. The effects of pregnenolone on pregnant or nursing women has not been established.

Recommendations: Pregnenolone is usually sold in capsule form and should be taken as directed.

PYCNOGENOL (see Grape Seed Extract)

PYRUVATE

Definition: Pyruvate is a naturally occuring compound that is the result of carbohydrate metabolism in the body.

Technically, pyruvate is really a combination of highly unstable pyruvic acid and other substances like calcium, sodium or potassium, added to stabilize pyruvic acid. This relatively new compound is thought to enhance fat burning, boost endurance, increase lean muscle mass, decrease blood glucose and lower blood cholesterol. Pyruvate is found in some cheeses and other foods but is normally consumed in very small amounts.

Applications: Weight loss, endurance, muscle building, cardiovascular health, cancer prevention, diabetes and high cholesterol.

Safety: Pyruvate studies have not found serious side effects from usage. But pregnant or lactating women should not use this supplement. Dosages of five grams or more are not recommended, but the efficacy of a dose lower than 5 gram dosages has not been established. Check with your doctor before using pyruvate. Higher dosages have caused some gastrointestinal upset. Long-term studies on the use of this supplement have not been conducted.

Recommendations: Pyruvate can be found in capsule, powder or drink form and is often combined with other compounds that enhance weight loss or build muscle. Calcium, magnesium and zinc pyruvate are the most common types. Sodium pyruvate is not recommended. Pyruvate seems to work synergistically with DHA.

NOTE: The exact amount needed to promote weight loss has not been established. Taking too little of this compound may be ineffective.

ROYAL JELLY

Definition: Royal jelly is a rich, creamy white liquid manufactured by worker honeybees exclusively for the nourishment and cultivation of the queen bee. It literally transforms a common honey bee into a queen bee, extending its longevity from six weeks to five years while greatly boosting its physical prowess. A highly complex compound, royal jelly contains a mixture of protein, lipids and carbohydrates in addition to several vitamins, and an impressive array of 17 amino acids. It has been reputed to stop the aging process and restore vitality and sexual potency. It has also been used as a natural antidepressant, for weight control purposes and to reduce cholesterol.

Applications: Depression, menopause, impotence, infertility, chronic fatigue, weak immune systems, viral and bacterial infections, endocrine system disorders, hormonal imbalances, high cholesterol, weight control, retarded growth, bladder, infections, wounds, anemia, cancer, arthritis, diabetes, athletic endurance, malnutrition, mental exhaustion and ulcers.

Safety: Although royal jelly is generally considered safe, like other bee-related products (bee pollen and propolis) it should initially be taken in small amounts to check for potential allergic reaction.

Recommendations: Royal jelly can be purchased in pure jelly-like material that should be kept refrigerated or frozen. It is also available in capsules, tablets, soft gels and in honey itself. Local products are preferable if possible. Royal jelly is very delicate and can lose its potency rapidly if not processed or packaged correctly.

SEA CUCUMBER

Definition: Sea cucumbers are not vegetables. They are marine-like animals related to starfish. Traditionally used by the Chinese to treat arthritis, the compounds found in these animals are proving themselves scientifically valuable for their anti-inflammatory properties. Some of the compounds found in sea cucumbers include chondoritin, and mucopolysaccharides.

Applications: Arthritis, inflammatory joint conditions, lupus, gout and ankylosing spondylitis.

Safety: Considered safe if used as directed.

Recommendations: Look for a pure product from reliable sources.

SHARK CARTILAGE

Definition: Shark cartilage is a nutritional supplement gleaned from the exoskeleton of the shark. It contains chemical compounds with the impressive ability to inhibit the growth of new blood vessel systems (antiangiogenesis), cutting off the blood supply to some types of tumors, resulting in their shrinkage or disappearance. Cancers characterized by solid tumors seem most susceptible. Continuing research is underway for the use of shark cartilage not only for cancer, but for AIDS, arthritis, diabetic retinopathy, neovascular glaucoma, psoriasis and enteritis as well.

Applications: Acne, asthma, cancer (breast, cervix, Karposi's sarcoma, prostate, pancreatic, ovarian, testicular), colitis, eczema, glaucoma (neovascular), diabetic retinopathy, high blood pressure, poison ivy and oak, pruritus ani (intense anal itching), cataracts, emphysema, gastritis, enteritis, hemorrhoids, joint inflammation, mandibular alveolitis and psoriasis skin disorders.

Safety: Shark cartilage is not considered a toxic substance. Because it inhibits the growth of new blood vessels, it should not be used in under certain conditions. Shark cartilage should not be used by anyone recovering from a heart attack, anyone who has recently had surgery, anyone wishing to conceive or by children who are still in physiological development. Taking shark cartilage for extended periods of time (more than eight weeks) may result in delayed wound healing or in contraception. The long-term side effects of preventing capillary growth in healthy adults are not known.

Recommendations: Obtaining a reliable source of whole shark cartilage that has been properly processed is vital to potency and action. Look for 100 percent pure, powdered forms with no fillers or binders that can be used in appropriate dosages, especially for cancer treatment. Loose powders may be the most practical form and can be mixed with juice. If you have cancer, large dosage of this compound is required. Supplements are also available in gel caps or liquid forms. Topical ointments or creams are also available for skin disorders.

SPIRULINA

Definition: Spirulina is a type of blue-green microalgae, considered to be a rich source of chlorophyll, protein, essential fatty acids and beta carotene. It has an impressive array of vitamins, minerals and amino acids and is generally used as a tonic, nutritive or blood purifier.

Applications: Compromised immune system, liver disease, digestive problems, blood disorders, debilitated conditions, malnutrition, athletic endurance, diabetes and anemia.

Safety: Because spirulina grows in water that may appear to be stagnant, it may be associated with bacterial contamination. If purchased from a reliable source, spirulina should be one of the most sterile foods found in nature. Ingesting very large amounts of spirulina may cause lethargy. When used as directed in a pure form, this supplement can be considered safe.

Recommendations: Spirulina comes in capsules, tablets, powders, flakes, freeze-dried crystals and extracts. Pre-measured packets must be mixed with liquid using a blender.

STEVIA

Definition: Stevia is a South American herb with three hundred times the sweetening power of white sugar without any of white sugar's side effects. It is commonly used to satisfy cravings for sweets and as a sugar substitute. It is non-caloric and can be used in various foods.

Applications: Diabetes, food cravings (especially sweets), hypoglycemia, nicotine cravings, weight loss and sugar substitute.

Safety: Studies have confirmed that stevia is safe to use even in cases of severe sugar imbalance.

Recommendations: Liquid concentrate that is used by the drop.

SUPEROXIDE DISMUTASE (SOD)

Definition: As an enzyme, SOD has particular value as an antioxidant that can help to protect against cell destruction. It has the distinct ability to neutralize superoxide, one of the most damaging free radical substances in nature. Like so many other protective compounds which naturally occur in the body, it decreases with age, making cells much more vulnerable to the oxidants which cause aging and disease. It occurs naturally in broccoli, Brussels's sprouts, wheat grass and in the majority of green plants.

Applications: Antiaging, cancer protectant and overall antioxidant usage.

Safety: The long-term use of this compound as a supplement has not been adequately evaluated. It should be used as directed.

Recommendations: Two varieties of SOD are available. Copper/zinc SOD and manganese SOD both work in different ways to provide two types of cellular protection. SOD is sold in pill form and should be enterically coated so that it does not digest in the stomach, but rather in the intestines for better absorption.

TEA TREE OIL

Definition: Extracted from the leaves of the *Melaleuca alternifolia* tree in Australia, tea tree oil is an essential oil that has impressive antiseptic and healing properties for treating almost every kind of skin affliction. Its antibacterial and antifungal actions make it ideal for wounds, burns, insect bites and yeast infections.

Applications: Abrasions, acne, arthritis, athlete's foot, bites, blisters, boils, burns (minor), canker sores, cold sores, cradle cap, cuts, dandruff, dermatitis, diaper rash, pet shampoo, eczema, fungal nail infections, gingivitis, head lice, hemorrhoids, insect repellant, poison oak and ivy, psoriasis, rashes, ringworm, sunburn, vaginal rinse and warts.

Safety: Tea Tree oil should not be taken internally, although douches using a solution of the oil can be used for vaginal yeast infections. Topical application is considered nontoxic.

Recommendations: Concentrated oil, creams, shampoos, ointments, lotions, and toothpaste are available. Look for 100 percent pure products from reliable sources.

WILD YAM CREAM (Transdermal Applications of Natural Progesterone)

Definition: Wild yam cream is a cream base which contains diosgenin, a plant percussor for the synthesis of progesterone extracted from wild yam. Mexican wild yam is one of the richest phytoestrogen botanicals and provides the human body with a natural and safe source of progesterone. Currently, wild yam is experiencing a resurgence in an attempt to use safe, natural hormonal therapy rather than synthetic varieties. Because the molecule is fat-based, it can be more efficiently absorbed through the skin than when taken orally.

Applications: PMS, menopause, hormonal imbalances, irregular or heavy periods, hormonally induced moods, fibrocystic breasts, uterine fibroid tumors, ovarian cysts, osteoporosis, as a preventative from uterine, ovarian and breast cancer, obesity, fibromyalgia and prostate disease (in proper amounts).

Safety: Although wild yam cream is considered nontoxic and safe, some symptoms may occur when initially taken. Hormonal shifts take place and result in headaches, spotting, and some menstrual irregularities.

Recommendations: Creams, oils and roll-ons are available under different product labels. Make sure you are getting whole wild yam in its natural form without too many other filler compounds which would weaken its potency. The addition of progesterone to wild yam is frequently seen to strengthen its effects, however the desirability of such an addition is debated by some health experts.

Learning About Other Natural Protocols

I want to again reiterate the idea that many ailments can be resolved through self-care. This next section briefly explains a number of other natural therapies that can be applied to various maladies. All of us would do well to acquaint ourselves with these disciplines so we can be aware of all of our health options. The beauty of many of these is that they can be practiced at home once their particular technique is mastered, something that can offer enhanced health care for not only one individual, but their family as well. Different forms of massage, reflexology, acupressure, biofeedback, meditation, relaxation therapy, homeopathy and the use of Bach flower remedies, enemas, fasting, and visualization are all effective self-help techniques. I strongly believe that we need to become much more self-reliant when it comes to health choices and treatments. If we do, we will better the quality of both our mental and physical health. Among other therapies, I would also like to mention NAET, which is a combination of a massage, kinesiology, and acupuncture which is used to eliminate allergic reactions. If a person is interested in using this technique, the following number will provide names of practitioners in their area: Medical Academy of Acupuncture (800) 521-2262.

I would like to discuss in more detail acupressure, acupuncture, aromatherapy and chiropractic, after which a brief description of other therapies will be offered in alphabetical order.

Acupressure

Discipline involving the application of pressure to certain points on the body with the fingertip or fingernail. This therapy is based on the notion that pressure helps to dissipate pain or circulatory blockages by boosting the flow of "chi" or vital energy. It has been used by the Chinese for thousands of years and is a respected medical protocol in China. Like acupuncture, this methodology is based on stimulating certain acupoints in order to balance the flow of internal energy which gets "out of sync" during disease or injury. Using the thumbs, middle or index finger is common and one can learn to apply this discipline to themselves. Pressure is applied to specific points for anywhere from one to several minutes and is repeated throughout the day. Acupressure has been successfully applied to the arm for motion sickness, above the upper lip for nasal congestion and on either side of the lower back for sciatica pain. Ailments which respond well to Acupressure include headaches, fatigue, back pain, constipation, and asthma. Acupressure is sometimes used in combination with acupuncture and is generally not considered as quick, as specific, or as effective as acupuncture. For anyone who suffers from a needle phobia however, it may serve to produce similar results.

NOTE: Consult your doctor before undergoing this therapy. There is some consensus that it may mask the symptoms of serious disease, thereby postponing appropriate treatment.

Acupuncture

Acupuncture involves the stimulation of specific acupoints by the insertion of very fine needles. Like acupressure, it is designed to augment the flow of "chi" thereby restoring the proper balance to affected organs. Determining the right points to target is essential. Careful evaluation of symptoms is necessary and is based on physical parameters as well as a series of questions. While acupuncture needles appear intimidating, their insertion is rapid and is usually painless. Acupuncture needles come in a variety of sizes geared toward their particular insertion point. Blood is usually not drawn if the needles are inserted correctly. Acupuncture has the distinct ability to either stimulate or tranquilize certain nerves. The acupuncturist may use pulse analysis in combination with a visual assessment to arrive at a diagnosis. I believe that it is vital to incorporate herbal medicines and good lifestyle changes with acupuncture to achieve maximum healing. Acupuncture is commonly used to treat headaches, joint disorders, respiratory problems, insomnia, back pain, sinusitis, allergies, anxiety, and some mental illness. This particular healing discipline is not usually employed in cases where a fever or an infection is present.

Aromatherapy

Aromatherapy uses concentrated plant oils to achieve certain desired effects. These essential oils have individual aromatic properties which can prompt a variety of physical and emotional reactions and are generally used to either relax, stimulate or to relieve pain. The term aromatherapy originated with Rene Maurice Gattefosse, a French chemist. Today over 40 essential oils are used for treating ailments. Essential oils also possess other therapeutic properties making them valuable as anti-inflammatory or antiseptic agents. When used topically, a carrier oil is added to the essential oil in order to facilitate its application and avoid irritation. Carrier oils commonly include apricot kernel, avocado, borage, evening primrose, flaxseed, jojoba, olive, sesame, soy, vitamin E and wheat germ. These oils can be used directly on the skin in massage form, can be placed in steam for inhalation, in atomizers, on light bulb rings or in special nasal inhalers. Frequently oil combinations are used for their varied effects. Some common oils and their actions include:

BASIL OIL: Stimulant, nerve tonic, mentally invigorating. *Therapeutic Applications:* depression, fevers, muscle cramps and spasms, nervous tension.

BERGAMOT OIL: Antiseptic, emotional tonic, calming. *Therapeutic Applications:* sitz baths, cold sores, eczema, anxiety or panic attacks, depression.

CHAMOMILE OIL: Anti-inflammatory, analgesic, tonic, calming. *Therapeutic Applications:* PMS, eczema, psoriasis, muscle pain, irritability.

GERANIUM: Astringent. *Therapeutic Applications:* sores, skin disorders, bruises, insect repellent.

NEROLI: Relaxant, sleep promoter. *Therapeutic Applications:* insomnia, anxiety disorders, depression, PMS, tension related syndromes.

EUCALYPTUS: Antiseptic, decongestant. *Therapeutic Applications:* allergies, sinus congestion, coughs, skin irritations.

LAVENDER: Analgesic. *Therapeutic Applications:* headaches, joint pain, pain in general, acne, insomnia, insect bites.

ROSEMARY: Stimulant. *Therapeutic Applications:* chronic fatigue, depression, arthritic pain, asthma.

JASMINE: Antidepressant. *Therapeutic Applications:* depression, hormonally related mood swings, PMS.

Chiropractic (Joint Manipulation Therapy)

Early in my practice, I set up an office and shared a building with a chiropractor. We were treating a young mother who had been in a automobile accident and was suffering from neck and back pain. Her son, who was two years old and had been in a car seat, was checked out in the emergency room and seemed fine. However, for a month after the accident, he was very irritable and would walk around in a state of frustration and was not easily calmed. His appetite was down, and he did not sleep through the night. This chiropractor was treating the family and asked me if I would do some possible pediatric-style acupuncture on the infant in that the child was so irritable and unmanageable, he was not able to apply treatment. A second chiropractor who was working in the same office felt that an adjustment might be very important for this child and with the cooperation of the mother administered one adjustment. Within 5 minutes the child crawled up into the mother's lap and went to sleep, which was the first time he had done so in over a month. Subsequently, he had a second treatment and then returned to his usual self. I later found out that this was the first time these chiropractors had treated such a young patient. I have since come to know that there are many influences on health that we medical professionals don't always associate with a certain set of symptoms. Often, the answer is something as simple as a spinal manipulation. A very simple, quick chiropractic adjustment balanced the child and allowed him to return to normal.

Chiropractic adjustments provide us with one more piece of the puzzle and reinforce the notion that there are many ways of improving a person's health and the more familiar we become with treatment options, the better our chances of success. Find a physician with an open mind who believes in and uses chiropractors or acupuncturists. Chiropractic adjustments are useful for: allergies, asthma, back pain, sciatica, general pain from injury or stress, headaches, joint sprains, muscular pain and stiffness. They can also be useful in helping to treat many different maladies that may not seem to be related to the spine at all.

Alexander Technique

This comprises a balance and movement therapy which is usually used in the treatment of body aches, neck pain, bad posture and headaches.

Art Therapy

Using art to calm the mind or release stress can be very useful in cases where behavioral problems exist. Mental disorders, ADHD and autism may respond to creative art outlet. It can also help to treat digestive disorders, headaches, and stress.

Autogenic Training

This technique involves using relaxation therapy to improve health. It focuses on the mind/body connection. It is good for AIDS, depression, fatigue, stress, headaches, hypertension, indigestion, colon problems, insomnia, migraines, and ulcers.

Ayurveda

This is a traditional Indian discipline which addresses balancing the mind with the body and the spirit to facilitate healing. It can be used in the treatment of arthritis, diabetes, eczema, stress, tuberculosis, ulcers and other diseases.

Bach Flower Remedies

This approach uses flower essences to stimulate both mental and physical responses. It is typically used for the treatment of anxiety, depression, eczema, pain, and shock.

Bates Method

This refers to a particular set of exercises for the eyes which helps to strengthen eye muscles and enhance vision. It is useful in the treatment of eyesight problems, glaucoma and squinting.

Biochemic Tissue Salts

This practice involves using certain salts or minerals to treat disease conditions It is useful for aching feet and legs, brittle nails, colic, coughs, fibromyalgia, hair loss, hay fever, headaches, heartburn, indigestion, teething pain, menstrual pain, migraine, muscular pain, nervous exhaustion, neuralgia, sciatica, sinus disorders, and stomach upsets.

Bioenergetics

Bioenergetics focuses on integrating the body and mind through a series of exercises and has been used for asthma, irritable bowel syndrome, migraines, stress and stress-related disorders.

Biofeedback

Biofeedback teaches the patient to control physical function through mental instruction. It is a technologically supported relaxation therapy and has been used to treat anxiety, headaches, high blood pressure, migraines, stress and epilepsy.

Biorhythms

This refers to the ability to identify individual physical, intellectual, and emotional cycles which we all experience and impact our behavior and health. Understanding biorhythms can help to treat depression and general ill-health.

Bowen technique

This discipline involves using balance and movement therapy and is geared to impact acute or chronic pain of musculoskeletal origin, back pain, muscle problems, joint pain, neck pain, and sprains and strains.

Breathing

Also used in naturopathy, this technique involves controlled inhaling and exhaling to facilitate relaxation and dispel stress. It is good for anxiety, asthma, bronchitis, eczema, hiccups and tension.

Cognitive Therapy

This involves boosting self-confidence in behavior to treat anxiety, behavioral problems, depression and insomnia.

Colonic Irrigation

This process involves sending a water solution throughout the length of the colon to clean it of residue or toxins. It is also called colonic hydrotherapy and is useful in the treatment of candida, circulatory disorders, constipation, diarrhea, and diverticulitis.

Color Therapy

This is using color and light to enhance health and awareness. It is useful in the treatment of arthritis, asthma, blood pressure, circulatory disorders, depression, eczema, insomnia, migraine, rheumatic pain, stress, and tension.

Cranial Osteopathy

This is a treatment that must be administered by a specialist who has the ability to manipulate the bones of the skull. It is useful in the treatment of labor pains, hyperactivity, colic, digestive and gynecological disorders, glue ear, headaches, learning difficulties, meningitis, painful sinusitis, reduced jaw mobility, and tinnitus. It is closely related to craniosacral therapy.

Expression Therapies

These involve using therapeutic activities to express emotion and include dance movement therapy, art therapy, and sound therapy. These are useful in the treatment of anorexia and bulimia, anxiety, behavioral problems, depression, headaches, heart disorders, manic depression, schizophrenia, and stress.

External Visualization

The ability to vividly imagine therapeutic mental pictures can positively impact physiological function and has

been used for anxiety, asthma, cancer, depression, heart disorders, pain, and stress.

Fasting

Abstinence from most or all solid foods and sometimes liquids is the technical definition of fasting (see section on fasting). Fasting can be beneficial for asthma, chronic health conditions, diarrhea, infections, digestive upsets, eczema, fevers, headaches, and skin rashes.

Flotation Therapy

This approach uses floating on water to create true relaxation and is good for anxiety, arthritis, high blood pressure, insomnia, pain and stress.

Gestalt Therapy

Through a series of mental exercises, this discipline involves promoting personal growth through self-awareness. It can be helpful in cases of anxiety, behavioral problems, hyperactivity, insomnia, and tension.

Homeopathy

This discipline uses natural remedies to boost the body's own healing ability. It concentrates on the notion of "like treating like" as far as symptoms are concerned. It has been used for allergies, anxiety, arthritis, asthma, bruising, burns, cold sore, colds, influenza, constipation, cramps, cystitis, deafness, depression, diarrhea, dizziness, earache, eczema, eye conditions, fear, panic, fever, food poisoning, headaches, heat exhaustion, indigestion, insomnia, irritable bowel syndrome, joint problems, low blood pressure, menopausal problems, muscular problems, nausea, rheumatic pain, sciatica, shock, skin problems, stings, swelling, and tinnitus.

Hydrotherapy

This is nothing more than using water therapeutically and usually involves hot and cold temperatures. It is good for anemia, arthritis, asthma, back pain, blood or circulation problems, gallstones, glaucoma, headaches, labor pain and childbirth, menstrual problems, muscle problems, pain, rheumatism, stress and tension.

Hypnotherapy

Using hypnosis to promote healing and well-being is the definition of this approach which focuses on subconscious suggestions. It is useful for addictions, anxiety, asthma, behavioral problems, childbirth and labor pain, insomnia, irritable bowel syndrome, migraines, phobias, stress, and ulcers.

Internal visualization

This approach involves imagining the inner functions of one's body to boost healing and mental well-being. It is good for anxiety, arthritis, headaches, cancer, migraine, pain, rheumatism, stress-related disorder, and tension.

Light Therapy

Using light therapeutically with either sunlight or light boxes has been used for anxiety, depression, hyperactivity in children, overeating, SAD, and fatigue.

Macrobiotic Diet

This nutritional regimen uses certain vegetables and brown rice to balance the body for the elimination of degenerative diseases and the promotion of health. It has been used for arthritis, cancer, depression, digestive disorders, skin problems, and stress.

Magnetic/Electromagnetic Therapy

Using magnets to re-direct energy fields to treat pain and balance the body's energies to encourage healing is what this therapy entails. It is used for the treatment of anxiety, back, neck and shoulder pain, bruising, depression, inflammation, lumbago, rheumatic pain, sciatica, stress, and whiplash.

Massage

Relaxing the body through touch and muscle manipulation is a very effective therapy which can help women with fibromyalgia and even boost the development of premature infants. Using essential oils or other ointments can enhance the positive effects of massage which is used for anxiety, back pain, cancer, circulation problems, colds, depression, headaches, heart disorder, high blood pressure, hyperactivity, insomnia, sinusitis, and tension (all of us could benefit from massage therapy).

Meditation

This involves reaching a state of mental tranquillity which can help to refresh and restore the mind and body and effectively dispel stress. It is useful in the treatment of addictions, anger and aggression, anxiety, chronic pain, circulatory disorders, depression, headaches, hyperactivity, insomnia, nervousness, and physical tension.

Megavitamin Therapy

Also known as orthomolecular therapy, this involves taking large doses of vitamins for disease conditions and is used for acne, addictions, aging, anemia, cancer, common cold, depression, diabetes, hyperactivity, premenstrual syndrome, schizophrenia, and viral infections.

Moxibustion

This involves the application of heat to acupuncture points and is used for arthritis, chronic illnesses like eczema and asthma, fatigue, shoulder problems, pain, stiff neck, and weak back muscles.

Myotherapy

This muscle treatment uses electrical or manual stimulation of certain trigger points in muscles to relieve pain. It is used for addictions, arthritis, backache, chronic recurrent pain of musculoskeletal origin, colic, Epstein-Barr, headaches, migraines, sinusitis, sports injuries, tinnitus, and TMJ.

Naturopathy

This is a broad term referring to a philosophy which utilizes a number of therapies to help the body cure itself from within. It is useful in the treatment of allergies, anxiety, arthritis, asthma, bacterial infections, bronchitis, colds, deafness, depression, diarrhea, digestive disorders, fatigue, heart disorders, influenza, kidney problems, skin problems, ulcers, and viral infections.

Osteopathy

This manipulative therapy is akin to chiropractic and is geared toward treating mechanical problems of the skeletal framework. It is useful in the treatment of aches and pains following childbirth, arthritic pain, back pain, digestive and respiratory difficulties, gynecological problems, headache, joint sprains, muscular pain, osteoarthritis, painful sinuses, recurrent strain injuries, reduced jaw mobility, sciatica, sports injuries, and stress.

Reflexology

This involves massaging reflex points located on the feet and hands to encourage health and well-being and to control pain. It is useful in the treatment of back pain, digestive disorders, heart disease, infertility, insomnia, liver problems, menstrual problems, migraine, multiple sclerosis, pain, sinusitis, and stress.

Relaxation

Many activities can fall under this heading which aims to calm the mind in order to boost the functions of the body and to reduce the deleterious effects of stress. It is useful in the treatment of anxiety, asthma, depression, digestive disorders, eczema, infertility, insomnia, mental tension, pain, physical tension, pins and needles, psoriasis, respiratory disorders, and stress.

Shiatsu

This ancient discipline involves stimulating the vital points along the body's meridians in order to encourage healing, good health, and well-being. It is used for back/neck pain, circulatory disorders, constipation, depression, diarrhea, headaches, immune problems, insomnia, menstrual problems, mental problems, migraines, nervous system problems, osteoporosis, stiff joints, stress, tension, and toothache.

Spiritual Healing

While the traditional definition of this is to use a healer to channel divine healing energies, it can also refer to the establishment of a spiritual link through prayer and mediation for enhanced health. It is good for virtually any condition.

Tai Chi

This ancient Chinese discipline involves the development of the life force of the body through a series of slow-moving, circular movements. It is useful in the treatment of anxiety, blood pressure, chronic health problems, circulatory disorders, insomnia, postural problems, stress and stress-related disorders, and tension.

Therapeutic Touch

Using the hands to touch lightly or even over the body to facilitate enhanced immune response on a cellular level. This therapy has been used for the treatment of chronic health conditions such as AIDS, asthma, cancer, and psoriasis.

Transcutaneous Electrical Nerve Stimulation (TENS/TNS)

This is a non-invasive method using electrical impulses for pain relief that works by stimulating endorphins and blocking nerve response to pain. It is useful in the treatment of arthritis, back pain, circulatory problems, labor pains, lumbago, sciatica, and sports injuries.

Visualization (see External or Internal Visualization)

Yoga

These set of spiritual and physical exercises encourage health and well being and help to diffuse stress. Yoga is excellent for anxiety, arthritis, backache, blood pressure, body tension, diabetes, headaches, migraine, multiple sclerosis, osteoporosis, pain, postnatal illnesses, pregnancy problems, premenstrual syndrome, rheumatism, rheumatoid arthritis, squint, stress, tinnitus, and ulcers.

PART 3

Individual Ailments and Their Recommended Treatments

ACNE

Acne is a frustrating skin condition characterized by blackheads, white heads and red cystules which form when hair follicles in the skin become blocked. It is more common in males and afflicts over half of our adolescent and young adult population. Because we are such an "appearance-sensitive" society, acne can create a great deal of stress and significantly inhibit social confidence. Acne usually appears around the age of fourteen for girls and sixteen for boys. While it typically eases before the age of 21, it can persist into middle age. Three out of four teenagers suffer from some form of acne.

Symptoms

Acne is characterized by pimples, whiteheads and inflamed red areas of swelling generally found on the face but can also appear on the neck, back and chest or buttocks.

Precautions

Severe cases of acne can involve the multiplication of whiteheads under the skin which eventually rupture and lead to serious inflammation and swelling. This condition is called cystic acne and can leave noticeable scarring if not treated properly. If red streaking develops around an inflamed area or a fever is present, contact your physician.

Causes

While the exact cause of this condition is not fully understood, it is known that acne results from the blockage and subsequent infection of a sebaceous gland which produces oil. Apparently, hormonal changes typically seen in puberty, during pregnancy, the menstrual cycle or at menopause affect these glands, causing an overproduction of oil. When the oil becomes trapped, bacteria are allowed to grow, hence an inflammation causes the formation of a pimple.

Other agents which have been linked to the eruption of acne include certain antiepilepsy drugs like dilantin; phenothiazine; iodides; steroids; exposure to petroleum, coal tar or oil; complications as a result of diabetes; birth control pills and pregnancy (called the pregnant mask).

Conventional Therapies

In simple cases of acne most doctors will prescribe ointments or gels designed to peel off the surface layer of the skin to discourage the formation of new blemishes such as Retin-A (retinoic acid). Antibiotics like tetracycline are also used. Acutane (isotreinoin), which inhibits the production of skin oil and shrinks the sebaceous gland has also been used, but is considered a powerful drug which must be taken with the strict supervision of your doctor. Both Retin-A and Acutane have significant side effects and should not be used by pregnant or nursing women

Dietary Guidelines

- Good intestinal function and diet is often overlooked as a contributing factor to acne. Eat a high-fiber diet.
- Increase your consumption of raw fruits and vegetables.
- Eat whole grain, complex carbohydrates.
- Avoid sugary, fatty foods.
- Cut down on dairy products (milk can contain hormones).
- Use olive oil and cut down on saturated and polyunsaturated fats. Food containing trans-fatty acids such as dairy products, margarine, shortening, fried oils or other vegetable oils should also be avoided.
- Drink plenty of water. Keep a pitcher in the fridge and drink throughout the day.
- Fresh cherries or cherry juice helps to clear the blood of toxins.
- Foods high in iodine such as fish and iodized salt should be eliminated.

Recommended Nutritional Supplements

PRIMARY NUTRIENTS

VITAMIN A Boosts the strength of the epithelial layer of the skin and helps to reduce the excess production of sebum (oil).[1] *Suggested Dosage:* 10,000 IU each day. Vitamin A can be taken in beta carotene form or in fish oil combinations. If you are pregnant, you should not take over 5,000 IU per day. Check with your physician when using larger doses of vitamin A.

CHROMIUM Helps to reduce skin inflammation and improve glucose tolerance. Some studies indicate that glucose tolerance can be impaired in some people suffering from acne.[2] *Suggested Dosage:* 400 mcg daily of the GTF or picolinate type. Brewer's yeast is a good source of chromium, although it should not be used with anyone who has a yeast sensitivity or is prone to yeast infections.

VITAMIN B6 Contributes to maintaining good skin tone, boosts peripheral circulation and helps the body fight infection. Extra niacin helps to boost blood circulation to the skin prompting better waste removal and healing to affected areas. Vitamin B6 helps to normalize the metabolism of hormones which can initiate an acne outbreak.[3] *Suggested Dosage:* Take as directed.

VITAMIN E Helps prevent scarring and also contributes to maintaining normal levels of vitamin A. Vitamin E should be taken with selenium. Studies have found that this combination can significantly improve acne conditions. *Suggested Dosage:* Take 400 IU everyday.

SELENIUM A powerful antioxidant which helps to scavenge from free radicals created during periods of inflammation and infection.[4] *Suggested Dosage:* Take as directed with a vitamin E supplement.

ZINC PICOLINATE Vital in treating acne due to its involvement in hormone normalization, tissue regeneration, immune function and vitamin A activity.[5] Studies have shown that zinc levels are notoriously low in adolescents. *Suggested Dosage:* 50 mg to 100 mg everyday for several weeks to a month. Then reduce to 25 to 50 mg per day Do not exceed 80 mg per day. Zinc lozenges are available. The picolinate form is more absorbable.

ESSENTIAL FATTY ACIDS Supplies gamma-linoleic acid which contributes to skin elasticity and repair while helping to breakdown fatty deposits. A deficiency of EFAs has been linked to outbreaks of acne. These acids also help control abnormal fatty secretions in the skin. *Suggested Dosage:* Take as directed in liquid or capsulized form. Supplements can be in the form of evening primrose oil, flaxseed oil or borage oil.

PROTEOLYTIC DIGESTIVE ENZYMES Help to completely digest food macronutrients. Faulty digestion has been linked to the outbreak of blemishes. *Suggested Dosage:* Take as directed just prior to eating.

GARLIC Considered a natural antibiotic that fights bacterial infection and stimulate the immune system. *Suggested Dosage:* One capsule with each meal. Deodorized varieties are available.

ECHINACEA As an herb with antibiotic properties which also stimulates the immune system, echinacea helps to fight infection.[6] *Suggested Dosage:* Take as directed, but do not take for more than three weeks at a time.

BURDOCK Works to detoxify the blood which helps to clear the skin. Burdock root's cleansing power is multifaceted. It has a diaphoretic action (promotes perspiration) which expels toxins from the skin and blood. It promotes liver function and increases bile flow, which in turn cleanses the blood and reduces toxin production in the gastrointestinal tract. In addition, burdock root is a mild laxative and diuretic which action further cleanses toxins from the body and improves general health. *Suggested Dosage:* Take as directed. Can interfere with iron absorbtion.

MILK THISTLE (SILYMARIN) Boosts liver function helping to efficiently detoxify waste from the blood stream. All of us can benefit from the therapeutic properties of milk thistle. This wonderful herb cleanses, strengthens, and protects the liver and its functions. Used extensively throughout Europe, milk thistle is one of the only herbs known to treat some forms of psoriasis. *Suggested Dosage:* 50 mg three times per day.

HERBAL COMBINATION This combination should contain gotu kola, yellow dock, dandelion root, bilberry, red clover blossoms, kelp, and sarsaparilla. *Suggested Dosage:* Two to six capsules daily. For chronic conditions use the maximum dosage of six capsules per day for a prolonged period. For best results, use every day.

GOTU KOLA: Even though this herb has a similar sounding name to a popular soft drink, it is not related to the kola nut nor does it contain any caffeine. Gotu kola is supported by tremendous clinical research performed in Europe. This research demonstrates that gotu kola is effective in the treatment of various skin disorders associated with cellulitis and lupus. It also possesses wound-healing activity and has been shown to decrease scarring. YELLOW DOCK: Yellow dock root is a reputed blood purifier and has been pre-scribed for all types of skin problems including leprosy, boils, and eczema. It has also been reported to clear a con-gested liver. Its laxative effect is well-documented and sup-ports the body's detoxifying ability. DANDELION ROOT: The common yard weed dandelion has a long history of use in herbal medicine. It is part of this formula for its ability to strengthen the liver, improve bile formation, regulate the bowels, purify the blood and tonify the skin. RED CLOVER BLOSSOM: Red clover blossoms are a reputed blood purifier and officially recognized in the United Kingdom for treat-ment of skin conditions such as psoriasis, eczema, and rash-es. KELP: Kelp is thought to be a blood purifier with the ability to alleviate skin problems, burns and insect bites. SARSAPARILLA ROOT: Sarsaparilla root has many benefits including the treatment of acne, psoriasis and eczema. As a result of its diuretic and diaphoretic action sarsaparilla cleanses the body, it is also thought to help balance hor-mones. Because acne can sometimes be due to glandular overstimulation by dihydrotestosterone, using saw palmetto with good diet can help to block this activity.

SECONDARY NUTRIENTS

CALCIUM/MAGNESIUM:Helps to promote tissue healing. *Suggested Dosage:* 1,000 mg calcium and 400 mg of mag-nesium per day.

CHLORELLA: An excellent blood builder and purifier which contributes to clearing the skin. Its astringent properties make it an excellent healing agent. Chlorella also decreases the chance of bacterial growth. *Suggested Dosage:* Take as directed in liquid form.

FIBER SUPPLEMENT: Keeps the bowels working efficiently to remove waste products and prevent the reabsorption of toxins into the blood. *Suggested Dosage:* Take as directed with plenty of water.

VITAMIN C with bioflavonoids: Reduces the inflammatory response and helps to boost immune function to fight infection. *Suggested Dosage:* 3,000 to 5,000 mg everyday in divided doses.

ACIDOPHILUS: Replaces friendly bacteria lost if taking an antibiotic for acne. *Suggested Dosage:* Take as directed. Either the capsulized or liquid form is effective. Look for products with guaranteed bacterial counts.

ALOE GEL: Used to help heal and minimize scarring. *Suggested Dosage:* Use as directed.

MYRRH GUM SPRAY: Works as an astringent and natural anti-septic agent. *Suggested Dosage:* Take as directed.

TEA TREE OIL: Works as a topical antiseptic agent which helps to promote faster healing with less scarring and helps to dry out excess oil. *Suggested Usage:* Apply morning and night. Because tea tree oil is strong, you may want to use it in a carrier substance such as rose water or use a tea tree oil-based lotion or soap. Do not take internally.

SASSAFRAS: May help to adjust hormone levels which are involved in the development of acne. *Suggested Dosage:* Take as directed. Do not use if pregnant or nursing or give to children.

Home Care Suggestions

◆ Keep the skin clean by washing it with a tea tree oil-based soap in the morning and at night.
◆ Shampoo hair frequently to prevent excess oil produc-tion.
◆ Use a warm wash cloth to help remove oil plugs.
◆ Over-the-counter creams which contain benzoyl perox-ide can help to control mild acne but should not be used around the eyes or other delicate areas due to its drying effect.
◆ Girls should avoid foundation makeup that is oil-based. Cosmetics which contain lanolins, isopropyl myristate, sodium lauryl sulfate, laureth-4 and red dyes should also be avoided.
◆ Avoid medications which contain bromides or sulfides.
◆ In the case of pimples with distinct whiteheads, some doctors reccommend gently removing the white core with a special tool (called a "comedo") and applying an antiseptic.
◆ Avoid using topical steroid creams which can prolong infection.

Other Supportive Therapies

ACUPUNCTURE: Acne is a disorder which can respond to proper acupuncture treatment.

HOMEOPATHY: Pulsatilla helps to clear the skin of blemishes, and Lycopodium and Graphites help to breakdown the infected cystules. Kali bichromicum has also been used for chronic acne. Homeopathic preparations of sulfur also work well.

HYDROTHERAPY: Gently rubbing the arms, legs and trunk of the body with cold water and a natural sponge can help to promote healing through enhanced stimulation.

Scientific Facts-at-a-Glance

Interestingly, when dermatologists noticed that insulin was an effective treatment for acne, the link was made between acne and glucose intolerance. It is the skin's glucose—not necessarily the blood's glucose—that is the culprit.[7] For this reason, chromium, which helps to boost the action of insulin, is highly recommended as a treatment for acne.

Spirit/Mind Considerations

The emotional factors which accompany or even may even cause acne should not be overlooked. Acne can cause feelings of withdrawal and can initiate a poor self-esteem. If you have a child who suffers from acne, talking together about treatment options is crucial. Parents who brush off acne as just another side effect of puberty that isn't worth treating need to think again. Find a physician who shows a genuine interest in finding the best treatment combination. Dr. T.G. Olsen, of the Yale University School of Medicine, suggested using oral vitamin A for patients suffering from acne and emphasized the fact that the successful treatment of acne depends to a large extent on the amount of interest the physician is willing to give the patient.[8] The role that sudden stress plays in initiating acne has also been studied. Some people who have suffered an emotional trauma may temporarily break out in acne-like blemishes.

Prevention

♦ While a genetic predisposition to acne has been observed, good facial hygiene coupled with a healthy low-fat diet which emphasizes fresh fruits and vegetables, whole grains and lean sources of protein can help to prevent or lessen the severity of acne.
♦ Keeping the bowels functioning properly by eating high-fiber diets and drinking plenty of water is also thought to be acne-preventative.

Doctor's Notes

I can specifically remember a 15-year-old girl who suffered from a horrible case of acne. She had been advised by her dermatologist to use several different methods of treatment. Her mother did not want her to use systemic antibiotics and so they focused on diet, stress reduction and nutrient supplementation. She was to take 10,000 IU of vitamin A, 50 to 100 mg of zinc (which tapered off with time), a combination of *Centella asiatica* and gotu kola, butcher's broom and billberry. Her dermatologist chose this particular herbal blend because gotu kola is very effective for skin problems, boosts healing and enhances circulation. In addition, butcher's broom has a natural anti-inflammatory effect. She responded well and the number of new lesions decreased over a three to four-week period. Because she continued to suffer from a few lingering spots of deep acne, she occasionally took an injection of diluted cortisone. The

herbal formula listed in this section is designed to cleanse the body by activating all its methods of elimination which include cleansing, strengthening and supporting liver function. Longer-lasting and more wide-ranging results can be achieved by improving the diet and abstaining from chocolate, nuts and stimulants such as caffeine.

Acne runs in families and is often an inevitable problem for certain individuals who have a genetic predisposition. It can, however, through proper diet and good supplementation be successfully treated. Keeping the colon functioning well is rarely addressed for conditions like acne, but can be a significant contributing factor. Incomplete or faulty digestion can also contribute to complexion problems. Fiber supplements and colon cleansing formulas may be of great value to certain individuals who find acne problematic. In addition, adding a good digestive enzyme to your meals may help you to digest more efficiently. Herbs designed to normalize hormones and detoxify the blood are also very good.

Even though the link between diet and acne has not been scientifically documented, certainly eating some foods will aggravate acne in some people, the most common being chocolate. Stop consuming foods you know cause problems.

Additional Resources

American Academy of Dermatology
930 North Meacham Road
P.O. Box 4014
Schaumburg, IL 60168
(708) 330-0230

Endnotes

1. A. Kugman, O. Leyden, et al., "Oral vitamin A in acne vulgaris," International Journal of Dermatology, 20: 1981, 278-85.
2. K.M. Abdel, e. Mofty et al., "Glucose tolerance in blood and skin of patients with acne vulgaris," International Journal of Dermatology, 22: 1977, 139-49.
3. B. Snider and D. Dieteman, "Pyridoxine therapy for premenstrual acne flare," Arch Dermatol., 110: 1974, 103-11.
4. G. Michaelsson and L. Edquist, "Erythrocyte glutathione peroxidase activity in acne vulgaris and the effect of selenium and vitamin E treatment," Acta Derm Venerol, 64:1984, 9-14.
5. G. Michaelson, et al., "A double-blind study of the effect of zinc and oxytetracycline in acne vulgaris," British Journal of Dermatology, 97:1977, 561-65.
6. V. Tyler, et al., Pharmacognosy, 8th ed., (Lew and Febiger, Philadelphia: 1981), 480-81.
7. T.G. Olson, "Therapy of acne," Med Clin North Am, 66 (4): 1982, 851-71.
8. K.M. Abdel, et al., "Glucose tolerance in blood and skin of paitents with acne vulgaris," International Journal of Dermatology, 22: 1977, 139-49.

AIDS/HIV

AIDS is a blood-borne disease which is caused by HIV (human immunodeficiency virus). This virus specifically attacks the body's immune system eventually crippling its defense mechanisms through the inhibition of a lymphocyte called the T-helper cell. Consequently, disease organisms are allowed to flourish with death usually occurring from a secondary infection, such as pneumonia or other opportunistic diseases.

African cases of AIDS afflict homosexuals, although in the United States, male heterosexuals, bisexuals, intravenous drug users and hemophiliacs who need frequent transfusions constitute the primary risk group for AIDS. It is important to understand that AIDS does not effect all individuals who are HIV-positive although symptoms of AIDS will usually appear in between one and five percent of those who have HIV. Many infected individuals can remain symptom-free for years. At this writing, approximately 50 percent of individuals who have been exposed to HIV have come down with AIDS.

Currently, there is no curative treatment or vaccine for AIDS. Symptoms and complication of AIDS can respond to specific antibiotics, antiviral drugs, radiation and anticancer therapies. AIDS is considered a fatal disease.

Symptoms

It can take years (usually between two to five) for the symptoms of AIDS to appear after initially becoming infected with HIV. A person who has been infected with HIV, but does not actually have AIDS, may experience weight loss, fever and enlarged lymph nodes. These symptoms are referred to as ARC (AIDS-related complex). It is possible, however, to be infected with HIV and not know it. After activation of the virus, symptoms can significantly vary for each individual. Possible symptoms include persistent fatigue, weight loss, appetite loss, inflamed gums, mouth sores, swollen glands, unexplained fever, night sweats, chronic diarrhea, dry coughing, short-lived illnesses (sometimes resembling mononucleosis), skin disorders such as dermatitis,(especially in the facial area), oral thrush, yeast infections and an enlarged liver or spleen. Other conditions that can develop in a person with AIDS include shingles, Epstein-Barr, tuberculosis, herpes simplex and salmonellosis. Almost half of AIDS patients will contract Pneumocystis carinini pneumonia, 30 percent will come down with Kaposi's sarcoma, and 12 percent will suffer from other infections. If the brain is involved, dementia can result.

Precautions

If you think you have been exposed to the virus, get tested immediately. Early treatment and the protection of others is vitally important. Getting on an intensified nutritional program using diet and supplements can help to boost the immune system.

Causes

HIV has been isolated from body fluids including blood, tears, semen, saliva, breast milk, nervous system tissue and female genital tract secretions.

The major methods of transmitting the disease are through sexual contact, tainted transfusions or needle sharing, from a pregnant woman to her unborn child or from a nursing mother to her child.

In very rare instances infection can occur through accidental needle injury, kidney or organ transplant or through artificial insemination.

The frequency of sexual contact plays a major role in raising the risk of becoming infected with HIV. There is some speculation that venereal diseases, such as genital herpes may predispose individuals to HIV infection.

The AIDS virus has never been shown to spread from sweat, tears, urine or feces. No evidence exists that AIDS can be spread from casual contact including a dry kiss, a handshake, a telephone receiver, a swimming pool, a toilet seat or through insect bites. However, recent research suggests that the virus can live outside the body for up to ten days, prompting the notion that the virus is more virulent than previously assumed.

Conventional Therapies

Confirming the presence of HIV involves blood testing for the presence of antibodies to HIV. Testing may not always be accurate in that a negative test result may occur in a person carrying the virus if it was contracted recently. A repeated test after six months is recommended for someone who believes they are at risk.

Currently, no known cure for AIDS exists. A number of anti-viral drugs such as AZT (zidovudine) and acyclovir are currently in use. Other drugs employed such as HIVID (zalcitabine) actually try to replace parts of the virus involved in the replication process, thereby halting viral reproduction.

While AZT has serious side effects, it does slow the progression of the disease and can help to prevent the transmission of the virus from a pregnant woman to her unborn child. AZT is often used in combination with other drugs. Other drugs which show some promise in treating AIDS include protease inhibitors which block enzyme reactions necessary for the virus to replicate itself; cyclophilin inhibitors, which keep infected cells from attaching to healthy ones; antisense compounds which interfere with the genetic codes of the virus; glucosidase inhibitors which attack the viral coat and reverse transcriptase inhibitors which keep an enzyme necessary for the virus to duplicate itself dysfunctional.

Supportive therapy for complications resulting from AIDS include using antibiotics such as pentamidine for pneumonia. If Kaposi's sarcoma is present, anticancer drugs and radiation are used but are rarely curative.

Combining AZT with other drugs can cause kidney damage and should be done so only with the supervision of your physician. It is important to know that acetaminophen (Tylenol) and aspirin can increase the toxicity of AZT.

Dietary Guidelines

- Protecting and boosting the immune system with a regimen of diet and supplementation is of utmost importance. Studies confirm that individuals suffering from AIDS experience continual stress on their immune systems resulting in a variety of diseases related to immunodeficiencies. Moreover, anyone who suffers from a compromised immune system needs a rigorous supply of nutrients.

- RDA requirements do not address the nutritional needs of the body when fighting disease. Frequently, people with AIDS suffer from malnutrition and while drugs may help to stem the disease, their side effects often contribute to more weakness and debility. Studies have found that victims of AIDS suffer from low serum zinc levels and intestinal nutrient malabsorption.[1] This fact alone is rarely addressed by orthodox practitioners. The bowel and liver need to be strengthened. Nutritional deficiencies including lack of vitamin A, zinc, and pyridoxine in and of themselves may cause decreased immunity.

- For the immune system to function properly, adequate levels of vitamin A, thiamine, riboflavin, pantothenic acid, pyridoxine, folic acid, vitamin E, vitamin C, magnesium, iron, zinc and several amino acids must be maintained.

- Several herbs and other supplements can contribute to immune defenses. Boosting and augmenting the immune system while addressing individual symptoms with nutritional therapy are the most important physical treatment factors in helping to cope with the disease.

- Adding therapies designed to contribute emotional and spiritual support are also intrinsically important to the success of all treatment strategies.

- Learn to eat a diet high in raw foods. Emphasize fresh fruits and vegetables with particular attention to onions, yellow vegetables, dark green vegetables, seeds, whole grains and alfalfa. Drinking freshly juiced fruits and vegetables with the addition of garlic and onion is recommended.

- Green drinks are excellent and adding liquid chlorophyll makes them even better.

- Foods to emphasize are cruciferous vegetables which include cabbage, broccoli, cauliflower and Brussels sprouts; legumes such as millet, lentils, red beans and brown rice; unsalted nuts and seeds, and low-fat or non-fat active yogurts.

- Use olive oil and eat fish (salmon or other coldwater varieties) for protein.

- Use a good protein supplement to help keep protein consumption adequate without eating red meats or cheese.

- Avoid all processed foods, salt, bacon, hot dogs, pickled products, hydrogenated and polyunsaturated fats, potato chips, soda pop, lunch meats and cheeses, alcohol, caffeine and sugar.

Recommended Nutritional Supplements

PRIMARY NUTRIENTS

ACIDOPHILUS Replenishes friendly bacteria destroyed by antibiotic therapy and helps to prevent yeast infections which commonly occur when the immune system is compromised. *Suggested Dosage:* Take in the morning before breakfast and at night before retiring. Use nondairy sources and keep refrigerated. Look for varieties that guarantee bacterial count.

GARLIC CAPSULES Helps to boost the body's defenses through immuno-stimulation. Garlic is also considered a natural antiviral agent.[2] *Suggested Dosage:* Take double the recommended dosage with each meal. Deodorized products are available.

CAROTENES Taking beta carotene in large doses has been shown to boost the production of T-helper cells, which are directly affected by the AIDS virus.[3] Unlike vitamin A, carotenes can be taken without the risk of toxicity. *Suggested Dosage:* Take as directed.

SELENIUM Studies have shown that people with AIDS may be selenium deficient.[4] Selenium also works to take up free radicals which are produced when disease is present. *Suggested Dosage:* 400 mg each day.

GERMANIUM Helps to oxygenate tissues and is believed to contribute to interferon production. In a recent study, 80 percent of patients with AIDS improved their overall health after 18 months of using germanium.[5] *Suggested Dosage:* 200 mg each day.

ZINC Some studies have shown AIDS patients to be low in zinc which boosts thymus gland activity that supports the immune system.[6] The picolinate form seems to be absorbed most efficiently and should be taken with meals. *Suggested Dosage:* No more than 150 mg per day.

COENZYME Q10 Helps to stimulate immune function and also scavenges for free radicals. Its ability to help counteract cellular immunosuppression is what makes it valuable for HIV patients.[7] *Suggested Dosage:* 100 mg each day.

EGG LIPID EXTRACT Extracted from egg yolks, this substance helps to protect cellular membranes which may slow the spread of HIV.[8] *Suggested Dosage:* 10 g after fasting or on an empty stomach.

FREE FORM AMINO ACIDS (combination including arginine, cysteine, cystine, and methionine) Various studies have found that supplementation with these amino acids works to enhance natural killer cell activity and may also inhibit the reproductive processes of the HIV.[9] *Suggested Dosage:* Take as directed on an empty stomach with fruit juice.

PROTEOLYTIC ENZYMES May help to reduce immune deficiency and also supports immune defense mechanisms.[10] *Suggested Dosage:* Take as directed.

CAT'S CLAW Constituents of this rainforest herb have been used to treat AIDS patients either alone or with AZT. Compounds in cat's claw help to inhibit the reproduction of HIV while simultaneously activating the immune system.[11] *Suggested Dosage:* Take as directed with guaranteed potency products. Do not use if pregnant or nursing or if you have had a transplant.

ST. JOHN'S WORT Very recent studies on hypericin, the main bioactive compound of this herb have found that it can protect T-cells from HIV infection in a cell culture.[12] It is considered a promising herbal treatment for AIDS. *Suggested Dosage:* Take as directed. Look for guaranteed potency products.

GLUTATHIONE Helps prevent cellular damage from free radicals caused by viral invasion and may be deficient in people suffering from HIV.[13] *Suggested Dosage:* Take as directed.

ALPHA LIPOIC ACID Recent studies by Dr. Lester Packer of the University of California-Berkeley show that taking ALA can boost glutathione levels while also inhibiting the replication phase of the HIV virus.[14] *Suggested Dosage:* Take as directed.

SHARK CARTILAGE Helps to treat opportunistic infections which can accompany AIDS such as Kaposi's sarcoma by inhibiting tumor growth.[15] *Suggested Dosage:* Take large therapeutic dosages with pure, dried bulk forms.

ESSENTIAL FATTY ACIDS These fatty acids help to prevent the disruption of prostaglandin E1 which plays a vital role in the regulation of T-lymphocytes.[16] *Suggested Dosage:* Take as directed. Fish oils and evening primrose, borage, flaxseed and soy oil can supply these fatty acids. Capsules are available.

CHONDROITIN SULPHATE This compound currently used with glucosamine for arthritis has some impressive antiviral activity in laboratory tests.[17] *Suggested Dosage:* Take as directed with glucosamine. Look for products which combine both.

VITAMIN B-COMPLEX Studies with vitamin B12 have found that supplementation may help to reverse neurological symptoms associated with AIDS.[18] *Suggested Dosage:* Take as directed using high potency varieties.

VITAMIN C WITH BIOFLAVANOIDS Experimentation with vitamin C administered intravenously for AIDS has shown some positive results.[19] Check with your physician about this option. Vitamin C can help to protect the liver and also has anti-viral and bacterial properties. When combined with bioflavonoids, it acts as an antioxidant as well. *Suggested Dosage:* Up to 20,000 mg per day with meals in divided doses.

VITAMIN E Helps to maintain cell membrane integrity which inhibits the course of T-4 cell derangement usually associated with AIDS.[20] *Suggested Dosage:* Take as directed.

HERBAL COMBINATION This combination should include astragalus, Siberian ginseng, shitake mushroom, reishi mushrooms, St. John's wort, schizandra, ginger root, licorice root and Irish moss. *Suggested Dosage:* Four to eight capsules daily.

ASTRAGALUS: Recent scientific studies have confirmed astragalus benefits the immune function. Astragalus has been shown to increase phagocytosis and interferon production.[21] In another study it was shown to increase the action of interleukin II, a cancer chemotherapeutic agent. Astragalus has also been shown to increase T-lymphocytes of the helper type. Do not use if a fever is present. SIBERIAN GINSENG: Siberian ginseng has a clinically-supported reputation as a stress fighter. It will also improve energy levels and mental function and stamina, which are often lacking in chronically ill people. In the past ten years, research has demonstrated Siberian ginseng's ability to increase important T-lymphocytes of the helper variety. These lymphocytes are significantly reduced in HIV infections. SHITAKE AND REISHI MUSHROOMS: Shitake mushrooms have received considerable attention for their immune system-building abilities. This mushroom has been scientifically studied and shown to stimulate interferon production and increase helper T-lymphocytes. Shitake is very safe and is used in foods around the world. ST. JOHN'S WORT: St. John's wort contributes to this ideal herbal formula in two ways. First, St. John's wort has potent antiviral activity. It has been used to fight the viruses associated with chronic fatigue, herpes simplex, mononucleosis and AIDS. Second, it has clinically proven antidepressive activity which may be of benefit to the chronically ill. St. John's wort may cause a skin reaction when exposed to the sun. GINGER ROOT: Ginger root has a strong carminative (settling to gastrointestinal tract) action. It is also one of the best herbs for stimulating and improving digestion and circulation. These properties will improve the effectiveness of the other herbs in this formula. And for those people who experience nausea with their chronic ailments, ginger root has been clinically proven more effective than prescription medication for nausea. LICORICE ROOT: Licorice root is one of the most used plants in Chinese medicine and is referred to as the "Great Adjunct" because it increases the effectiveness of other herbs. Additionally, studies have shown licorice to enhance the production of interferon and macrophage activity.[22] Do not use for more than a week at a time or if you are pregnant, nursing, have high blood pressure or suffer from diabetes, glaucoma, heart disease, menstrual difficulties or have a history of stroke. IRISH MOSS: Irish moss contains iodine and large amounts of mucilage. A deficiency in iodine has been associated with reduction in the ability of some leukocytes to fight bacterial infections. Mucilage is nutritious and soothing to the gastrointestinal tract.

SECONDARY NUTRIENTS

PROTEIN SUPPLEMENT DRINK: Helps supply easily assimilated forms of protein for cell repair and energy. Look for milk-free varieties. *Suggested Dosage:* Take as directed.

POLYPORUS UMBELLATUS: A Chinese tonic mushroom which increases resistance to infection. *Suggested Dosage:* Take as directed.

MANGANESE: Essential for iron deficient anemics and also acts to boost the immune system. *Suggested Dosage:* Take as directed. Do not take with calcium/magnesium, which would compete with manganese for absorbtion.

SILYMARIN: Expedites liver damage repair which can occur as a complication of AIDS. *Suggested Dosage:* Take as directed. Look for guaranteed potency varieties.

PAU D'ARCO: A rainforest herb which has been used to treat AIDS in South America and has significant anti-viral activity. *Suggested Dosage:* Take as directed. Do not use if pregnant or nursing.

Other Supportive Therapies

HYPNOTHERAPY: Can help to counteract the effects of stress which enables the immune system to function better. Clinical tests support the notion that a positive state of mind and a relaxed body can help to raise T-cell count.

MEDITATION: Disciplines like yoga can help to also facilitate complete stress relief and relaxation.

MASSAGE: Massage techniques designed to expedite the lymphatic flow can help to carry waste away from the body through the blood, helping the body to detoxify.

Scientific Facts-at-a-Glance

Recent research has discovered that individuals infected with HIV often suffer from an imbalance of sulphur-rich antioxidant compounds such as glutathione (GSH) and cysteine.[23] Supplementation with glutathione and cysteine may help to boost immune defenses which become further impaired by the oxidative stress created by the immune response triggered by the virus. Genetic engineers have recently identified a natural molecule that prevents HIV from infecting cells by physically blocking the portal used by the virus to invade lymphocyte cells. This therapy, called chemokine treatment, is under development at the University of Maryland.

Spirit/Mind Considerations

AIDS, more than any other disease in recent history, has caused widespread fear and misunderstanding. Dispelling misconceptions about the way in which AIDS is spread can help to create a more relaxed and compassionate approach to anyone with HIV. Those who have AIDS must cope not only with the sobering prognosis of the disease itself, but with its social stigma as well. Being looked at much in the same way as the lepers of old, AIDS patients often feel as though they have been marked by society. As a result, feelings of alienation, isolation and loneliness frequently develop. Learning to meditate to achieve the type of serenity which undoubtedly augments physical healing is necessary.

Prevention

♦ The only 100 percent safe sexual relationship involves practicing abstinence from sexual contact or faithfully participating in a monogamous relationship with a partner who is free from the virus.

♦ Casual sexual activity of any kind can be risky. While the regular use of condoms can decrease the risk, condoms do not totally protect against infection.

♦ Do not use intravenous drugs. If intravenous drugs are used, never share needles or syringes.

♦ Do not have sexual contact with people who are intravenous drug users.

♦ People who test positive for the HIV virus should not donate blood, plasma, organs, any kind of tissue or sperm.

♦ There should be no exchange of body fluids during any kind of sexual activity, including oral sex.

♦ Use a condom when having sexual intercourse. The effectiveness of condoms in preventing HIV infection has never been conclusively proved, but their consistent use may reduce the incidence of transmission since contact with body fluids is known to increase the risk of contracting AIDS.

♦ Any implement that could become contaminated with blood should not be shared, including razors, toothbrushes, etc.

♦ If in doubt about blood supply for an upcoming surgery, go to the hospital and donate some of your own blood ahead of time. The screening of blood supplies and the use of disposable needles has greatly decreased the incidence of AIDS-contaminated blood.

♦ Keep your immune system strong. Avoid steroids, the indiscriminate use of antibiotics, avoid exposure to radiation or harmful chemicals and eat a healthy diet that is low in fat and protein and high in complex carbohydrates, fresh fruits and vegetables.

Doctor's Notes

Since the discovery of AIDS, many Americans have become more aware of the importance of the body's immune system. AIDS has painfully taught the difficult lesson that life can be short without proper immune function.

Of course, many people have suppressed immune function for various reasons unrelated to HIV. Generally, the degree of suppression influences the degree of disease. Some people are unable to get the upper hand on sickness, experiencing one ailment after another.

The body's defense mechanism is complex. In some cases an organism or virus must penetrate several lines of defense in order to cause a problem. Some defense lines are acquired over time—washing hands to prevent the spread of disease-causing germs is a good example. Properly storing and preparing food to prevent food-borne illness is another line of defense. However, the body has many built-in defense systems which, when functioning properly, can lead to a long, healthy life.

If the body's ability to properly produce interferon or a class or subclass of leukocyte is impaired, the health of the body may be successfully challenged by intruding disease. Therefore, it is easy to understand the critical nature of healthy immune function.

Additional Resources

AIDS Hot Line
(800) 342-AIDS (English)
(800) 344-7432 (Spanish)

National Association of People with AIDS (NAPWA)
1413 K Street NW, Suite 700
Washington, DC 20005
(202) 898-0414

Endnotes

1. M. Moseson, et al., "The potential role of nutritional factors in the induction of immunologic abnormalities in HIV-positive homosexual men," Journal of Acquired Immunodeficiency Syndrome, 1989, 2 (3): 235-47.

2. K. Nagai, "Experimental Studies on the preventative effect of garlic extract against infection with influenza virus," Jpn J Infect Dis, 1973, 47, 321.

3. M. Alexander, et al., "Oral beta-carotene can increase the number of OKT4+ cells in human blood," Immunol Letters, 1985, 9: 221-24.

4. B.M. Dworkin et al., "Selenium deficiency in the acquired immunodeficiency syndrome," J. Parenter Enteral Nutri, 1986, 10 (4): 405-07.

5. "Germanium," Artsenkrant Belgium, 1988, 20: 397. See also, Report from International AIDS Treatment Conference, (Tokyo, Japan: Feb. 13-14, 1987).

6. R.K. Chondra, et al., "Serum thymic factor activity in deviances of calories, zinc, vitamin A and pyridoxine," Clin Exp Immunol, 1980, 42, 332-35.

7. Emile G. Bliznakov, M.D., and Gerlad L. Hunt, The Miracle Nutrient, Coenzyme Q10, (Bantam Books, New York: 1989), 208-09. See also K. Folkers et al., "Biochemical deficiencies of coenzyme Q10 in HIV-infection and exploratory treatment," Biochem Biopys Res Commun, 1988, 153: 888-96.

8. M. Shinitzky, et al., "Lipid regiments for the treatment of AIDS in RR Watson, ed. Cofactors in HIV-1 infection and AIDS, (CRC Press, Boca Raton: 1990).

9. K.M.G. Park, "Stimulation of lymphocyte natural cytotoxicity by L-arginine," Lancet, 1991, 337: 645-46. See also G. Saez et al., "The production of free radicals during the auto-oxidation of cysteine and their effect on isolated rat hepatocytes," Biochem Biophys Acta, 1982, 719: 24.

10. G. Sttauder et al., "The use of hydrolytic enzymes as adjuvant therapy in AIDS/ARC/LAS patients," Biomed Pharmacother, 1988, 42: 31-34.

11. Philip A. Steinberg, "Uncaria tomentosa (Cat's Claw) Wonder Herb from the Amazon," New Editions Health World, February 1995, 41-44.

12. American Journal of Hospital Pharmacy, 1994, 51 (18): 2251-67.

13. R. Buhl et al., "Systemic glutathione deficiency in symptom-free HIV-seropositive individuals," Lancet, 1989, 2: 1294-97.

14. Lester Packer, Ph.D. et al., "Alpha lipoic acid as a biological antioxidant," Free Radical Biology and Medicine, 1995, 19: 227-250, and L. Packer, et al., Free Radical Biology, 1995, 227-50.

15. I. William Lane and Linda Comac, Sharks Don't Get Cancer, (Avery Publishing, Garden City, New Jersey: 1993), 83-84.

16. S.H. Marcus, "Breakdown of PGE1 synthesis is responsible for the acquired immunodeficiency syndrome," Med Hypotheses, 1984, 15: 39-46.

17. E. Jurkiewicz, et al., "In vitro anti-HIV activity of chondroitin polysulphate," AIDS, 1989, 3 (7): 423-27.

18. K. Kieburtz et al., "Abnormal vitamin B12 metabolism in human immunodeficiency virus infection," Arch Neurolm 1991, 48: 312-14.

19. S. Harakeh, R.J. Jariwalla and Linus Pauling, "Suppression of human immunodeficiency virus replication by ascorbate in chronically and acutely infected cells," Proc Natl Acad Sci USA, 1990, 87 (18): 7245-49.

20. T.D. Hollins, "T-4 cell receptor distortion in acquired immune deficiency syndrome," Hypotheses, 1988, 26 (2): 107-11.

21. H. Yunde et al., "Effect of radix astragalus on the interferon system," Chinese Med, 1981, 94: 35-40.

22. R. Pompeii, et al., "Antiviral activity of glycyrrhizic acid," Experientia, 1980, 36: 304.

23. R. Buhl, "Imbalance between oxidants and antioxidants in the lungs of HIV-seropositive individuals," Chem-Biol Interact, 1995, 91: 147-58.

ALLERGIES

Allergies are a disorder caused by the body's hypersensitivity to what can be a variety of substances that can be eaten, inhaled or come into contact with the surface of the skin. This hypersensitivity is actually a malfunction of the immune system, which normally attacks allergic invaders with sticky proteins known as antibodies. It is this malfunction that precipitates the onset of allergic symptoms. When the immune system is triggered by an allergen, antibodies produce histamine and serotonin which cause inflammation.

An allergen is defined as a substance that causes an allergic response. Allergens can be inhaled from the air as dust, dander, pollen, smoke, perfumes, chemicals, etc. They can come from foods such as wheat, corn, chocolate, etc., or drugs like penicillin. They can be acquired through infectious organisms such as bacteria, viruses or parasites. Also, allergens can come from touching things such as plants, animals and chemicals, etc.

Not everyone suffers from allergies. Some people seem to be much more sensitive than others to potential allergens. Some allergies may be genetically passed on. The symptoms of an allergic reaction are often the result of histamine release in the body and usually manifested through the respiratory tract in the form of bronchial asthma, hayfever or allergic rhinitis, etc., and through the skin as eczema or hives. Headaches also often accompany allergic response. The very best way to avoid allergies is to avoid contact with the allergen. For some people it may be impossible to avoid allergen contact especially if the allergen is of the airborne variety such as pollen.

Symptoms

Allergic symptoms are irritating. Some of these include hives, which can cause itchy swollen palms; skin rashes, which almost always itch; sneezing, runny nose, itchy watery eyes; nasal congestion; asthma; swelling of the mouth or throat; diarrhea (which typically affects allergic infants); persistent sinusitis; and irritable bowel syndrome. Arthritic like pains may also be symptoms of a masked allergy.

Precautions

A violent reaction to a bee sting, insect venom, penicillin, aspirin, some vaccines, shellfish or to nuts is probably anaphylaxis. It is a grossly exaggerated immune system reaction which causes the entire respiratory tract to swell, including the bronchial tubes and the larynx, which cuts off breathing. A drastic drop in blood pressure also occurs and the heart and kidneys can cease to function. Symptoms of anaphylactic reaction are flushed face, fear, dizziness, weakness, swelling of the eyes, face or tongue, nausea and vomiting, abdominal cramps or pain, difficulty breathing, wheezing, tightness of the chest, difficulty swallowing and/or unconsciousness. If you have any of the above symptoms, seek out medical care immediately. In the future, wear a medical identification tag and carry an adrenaline kit if appropriate.

Do not take any corticosteroid when pregnant or nursing without your doctor's permission. Do not become vaccinated against any infectious disease when on any corticosteroid due to its interference with physiological reaction to the vaccination. Do not increase, decrease or stop the dosage without specific instructions from your doctor. Corticosteroids may cause a significant loss of potassium and they can interfere with laboratory test results.

Causes

Allergies are caused by a wealth of normal, every-day things including certain types of foods, pollens, pets, dust mites, insect venoms, cow's milk, perfumes, chemical substances and fabrics.

Why a particular individual becomes allergic to certain substance such as cow's milk remains unclear and somewhat controversial. But it has been proven that heredity plays a major determining factor. Other foods typically associated with allergies are wheat, eggs, citrus fruits, beef, veal, shellfish and nuts.

Pollens which come from ragweed and other plants can also cause seasonal allergies. Certain types of grasses are considered common allergens. In addition, contact with dog, cat and horse dander frequently causes allergic reactions. Mold and house dust are also allergic culprits, and insect bites and stings can bring on severe allergic reactions which, in some cases, can be life threatening. Drug sensitivities, such as allergies to penicillin, which is made from a mold, and reactions to bee stings can produce anaphylactic shock in an allergic individual, a condition which can be fatal.

Conventional Therapies

Routine medical treatment involves a combination of avoiding the offending substance and alleviating symptoms. Antihistamines, which block the release of histamine by increasing the number of antibodies, are usually recommended. In more severe cases of allergies or when asthma is involved, corticosteroid drugs such as prednisone may be used to treat asthmatic symptoms and severe nasal congestion.

Nebulizers or spray medicines can also be corticosteroids, such as beconase and vancenase. Cromolyn sodium (nasalcrom, intal, gastrocrom, opticrom), which can come as an inhalant spray or eye drops, is a rather new allergy treatment. Cromolyn does not treat symptoms that are present. Instead it prevents the future onset of allergic reactions by stabilizing mast cells so histamine is not released.

Nasal sprays such as Afrin, Dristan, etc., should be used very sparingly, if at all. They can cause an intensified reverse effect, which only compounds the problem and creates an even greater reliance on the chemical involved.

Dietary Guidelines

- Avoid foods such as wheat, eggs, dairy products, caffeine, chocolate, shellfish, strawberries, nuts, eggs, tomatoes and citrus fruits.
- Avoid consuming FDC yellow no. 5 dyes, along with BHT, BHA, monosodium glutamate and vanillin.
- If taking any corticosteroids, eat high potassium foods, such as bananas or melons.
- Brown rice and stone fruits help with better elimination and are nonallergenic foods.
- Raw honey contains pollen dust and may help to build resistance to certain allergens.
- Brewer's yeast, grapefruit and wheat germ blended together works to strengthen cell walls and provide natural immunity.
- If you suspect you may suffer from uncommon food allergies, you should test yourself by keeping a journal of what you eat and how you feel. Food allergies can manifest themselves a day or two after ingestion and come with a wide variety of seemingly unrelated symptoms.

Recommended Nutritional Supplements

PRIMARY NUTRIENTS

BEE POLLEN Works to establish immunity against flower pollens. Clinical tests have shown that over 17 percent of people with hay fever and 33 percent of asthmatics significantly improved with bee pollen supplementation.[1] *Suggested Dosage:* Start with just a very small amount and work up to 1 to 2 teaspoons per day to check for allergic sensitivity. Capsulized pollen can also be used. Look for local varieties if possible and start taking supplements before the onset of allergy season. Make sure to purchase potent and pure products. Raw types are recommended. Bee pollen can cause an allergic reaction in some individuals and should be initially taken with caution.

VITAMIN C WITH BIOFLAVONOIDS Essential for maintaining cell and tissue integrity which may be compromised when histamine is released. Recent studies confirm the ability of vitamin C to help reduce histamine levels and calm allergic symptoms while mitigating the inflammatory response.[2] *Suggested Dosage:* 5,000 to 10,000 mg per day in divided doses. Ascorbic acid can be purchased in powdered form for larger than normal dosages.

QUERCETIN A flavonoid that can help to stabilize the mast cell, which leaks histamine during an allergic reaction and inhibits enzymes and leukotriene formation.[3] *Suggested Dosage:* 1 to 2 g daily divided into three to six doses.

BROMELAIN Another flavonoid which also works to inhibit histamine response and boosts the action of quercetin. *Suggested Dosage:* 100 to 200 mg per day.

CATECHIN This naturally occurring flavonoid helps to inhibit the enzyme which converts histidine to histamine.[4] *Suggested Dosage:* Take as directed.

NIACIN Helps to inhibit the symptoms of seasonal allergies by slowing histamine release.[5] *Suggested Dosage:* Take as directed. Do not exceed recommended dosages. Some people experience a niacin flush after taking this supplement which causes a nonharmful reddening of the skin.

PANTOTHENIC ACID Combats allergy symptoms by alleviating nasal congestion and excess mucus production.[6] *Suggested Dosage:* Take as directed. Large doses may cause excessive dryness in the nasal passages.

VITAMIN B12 Trials have shown that vitamin B12 significantly improved cases of allergic asthma and contact dermatitis.[7] *Suggested Dosage:* Take 200 to 300 mg with sublingual or lozenge tablets. In addition, you can recieve injections from your physician.

CALCIUM, MAGNESIUM W/ VITAMIN D This particular combination helped to significantly reduce asthmatic allergic responses.[8] The rhinitis that usually accompanies allergies also decreased with calcium supplementation. *Suggested Dosage:* 1,000 to 2,000 mg per day with normal supplementation of vitamin D. Use gluconate or citrate forms and look for chelated varieties for better assimilation.

TYROSINE An amino acid which has been used to treat allergies from hay fever and grass pollens. *Suggested Dosage:* Take as directed on an empty stomach with fruit juice. This amino acid should not be taken by anyone taking beta blocker drugs or suffering from high blood pressure.

ESSENTIAL FATTY ACIDS Several studies suggest that these oils may be depleted in people with allergies. These oils may also inhibit the inflammatory response.[9] *Suggested Dosage:* Take as directed. Fish oils and flaxseed, borage or evening primrose oil supply these essential fatty acids. If using fish oil, take a vitamin E supplement as well.

ZINC Supplementation may help reduce chemical sensitivities and may also inhibit the release of histamine from mast cells.[10] *Suggested Dosage:* Take as directed and do not exceed recommended dosages. Zinc lozenges are available.

ACIDOPHILUS A depletion of intestinal bacteria may predispose an individual to food allergies. Tests support the notion that if we lack friendly bacteria, we may develop a wide range of food sensitivities.[11] *Suggested Dosage:* Take as directed using high bacterial count supplements in either pill or liquid form. Use formulas that are not milk-based.

FEVERFEW Significantly reduces the inflammatory response.[12] *Suggested Dosage:* Take as directed. Do not use if pregnant or nursing.

NETTLE Works in a paradoxical way by actually irritating mucous membranes to increase blood flow, which promotes healing. It is also considered a catalyst herb which helps boost the action of other herbs. *Suggested Dosage:* Take as directed. Nettle can cause an allergic reaction in some individuals and should be used with caution and in initial small amounts.

HERBAL COMBINATION This combination includes montmorillonite clay, horehound, mullein, wild cherry bark, barberry root and peppermint leaves. *Suggested Dosage:* Four capsules daily. Continue using as symptoms persist.

MONTMORILLONITE CLAY: Orally-consumed montmorillonite clay has great applications for reducing symptoms of allergies and the effects of allergens. It absorbs toxins and reduces histamine. Montmorillonite clay also improves gastro-intestinal tract function, which will prevent substances that could cause an allergic response from being absorbed into the blood. Montmorillonite clay also is an antibacterial which may reduce allergic response to toxins produced by bacteria.[13] HOREHOUND: Horehound has a spasmolytic property which means that it can reduce spasms. This is particularly useful for allergen-induced asthma since asthma is caused when bronchial muscles spasm (contract). Horehound will also reduce cough and phlegm produced by the allergen. It further cleanses the body of toxins through its diuretic properties and ability to produce perspiration. Horehound candy has been popular for years in treating these conditions.[14] MULLEIN LEAVES: Mullein, like horehound, has an ability to help control asthma by reducing spasm. This is probably because of its nerve-calming attributes. Mullein leaves are useful in treating bronchitis, sinusitis, and coughs. Many herbalists have found mullein useful in treating headaches and migraines which can result from allergies. Mullein contains high levels of mucilage which can soothe and coat the gastrointestinal tract and improve bowel function. Recent laboratory studies have found that the saponins and mucilage contained in mullein enable it to heal and soothe inflammation.[15] WILD CHERRY BARK: Wild cherry bark has been a favorite in cough and cold medicines, but perhaps its greatest contribution in this formula is found in its ability to relax respiratory nerves that cause asthma. Wild cherry bark also improves stomach function and digestion which may be a great help in reducing the allergic response. BARBERRY ROOT BARK: Barberry root bark's application in this formula is one of general health service. Barberry supports the cleansing of the liver and gall bladder, which will remove toxins and improve digestion. Occasionally, improper digestion is the cause of an allergic response. A partly digested protein is absorbed into the blood and since the body doesn't recognize or know how to utilize this partial protein, antibodies are created to remove it. This unwanted protein may be responsible for initiating a histamine response as well. Do not use if pregnant or nursing. PEPPERMINT LEAVES: Peppermint leaves enhance the effects of the other herbs in this formula. Anyone who has breathed in its pleasant, cooling aroma knows that it has an ability to clear congested nasal passages and improve breathing. Peppermint's volatile oil is described in the *British Herbal Pharmacopeia* as a potent spasmolytic suggesting possible applications with asthma.

SECONDARY NUTRIENTS

MOLYBDENUM: This trace element helps to detoxify sulfite converting it to the sulfate form. Research suggests that people with sulfite allergies may be suffering from a deficiency of molybdenum.[16] *Suggested Dosage:* Take as directed.

BETA CAROTENE: Helps to scavenge for free radicals caused by allergic inflammations and boost the functions of the immune system.[17] *Suggested Dosage:* Take as directed.

VITAMIN E: Thought to possess antihistaminic properties, this vitamin also acts as an antioxidant helping to neutralize the damaging cellular effects of inflammatory oxidant compounds.[18] *Suggested Dosage:* Take as directed, not exceeding 800 IU per day.

ROYAL JELLY: Helps to boost glandular function and cellular regeneration. *Suggested Dosage:* Take as directed. Use small amount initially to check for allergic reactions.

Home Care Suggestions

◆ A nasal wash with warm saline solution can help alleviate soreness and encourage drainage.

◆ Eye drops like Visine can help control redness but are not recommended on a long-term basis. These preparations can have a rebound effect if used longer than three days and actually cause more eye redness.

◆ Installing an industrial strength air purification system may also be beneficial.

◆ Dehumidifiers can bring relief from pollens, molds and pet dander.

◆ For allergies caused by inhalants, air conditioning your house or environment is very effective in controlling molds, pollens and dust mites. The cool temperature along with air filtering devices cuts down on the presence of these allergens.

◆ Use a fungicide like Clorox to keep the growth of mold and mildew in check.

◆ Throw out rugs and carpets that carry pet dander and dust mites.

◆ Replace your furnace filters often. These can become heavily laden with dust and pollen.

◆ Use synthetic pillows which can be washed and keep sheets and pillow cases changed often.

◆ Wear a mask when dusting or mowing the lawn.

◆ Stop smoking.

◆ Avoid using aspirin, which reportedly allows food allergens to be more effectively absorbed by the body.

◆ Ask what's in your food before you eat it.

◆ Look carefully at ingredient lists at the grocery stores and avoid offending substances.

Other Supportive Therapies

ACUPUNCTURE: Treatments can be designed to help balance organ energies that assist in coping with invading allergens. Initially, symptoms will be treated with subsequent treatments focusing on body weaknesses that cause the allergy in the first place.

BACH FLOWER REMEDIES: Clematis is generally used for allergic sensitivities.

HOMEOPATHY: Recent clinical trials have supported the use of Arsenicum, Euphrasia, Nux vomica, Belladonna, Sabadilla and Wyethia for allergic symptoms, although medical acceptance of these treatments has been reluctant, to say the least.[19]

HYPNOTHERAPY: Hypnotic techniques may help to alleviate the physiological stress caused by allergies.

Scientific Facts-at-a-Glance

Recently children in West Germany were found to be more allergic than those in East Germany. The higher rates of allergies among young people in West Germany have been seen as a possible result of the large number of automobiles that produce gas fumes which contain nitrogen dioxide. Doctors in the Netherlands have also recently found that using a goose down comforter or pillow can cause severe allergic reactions. Goose down or goose feathers can contain significant numbers of dust mites, which are considered highly volatile allergens.

Spirit/Mind Considerations

Some physicians have made a connection between emotional stress and the onset of an allergic reaction. This type of allergy must be treated for both it physical and mental ramifications. Allergies have a strong psychological component. Often just the suggestion of a certain weed or even the sight of a silk plant can produce an allergic reaction.

Prevention

◆ Do not introduce cow's milk, citrus juices, eggs, meats, nuts or wheat too early into an infant's diet. Check with your doctor or allergist as to a recommended time table for introducing new foods.

◆ Keep your immune system healthy by avoiding junk foods, empty calories, caffeine, tobacco, alcohol, white sugar and white flour foods and salt.

◆ Taking a vitamin C supplement with bioflavonoids can help boost the immune system.

◆ Keep yourself regular by eating lots of high-fiber foods and drinking plenty of water. There is some discussion that allergies may be caused by an excessive accumulation of waste in the system due to the consumption of an incorrect diet which can promote inappropriate immune responses.

Doctor's Notes

One of my patients, a 45-year-old male who had suffered from hayfever for 10 years, had tried many over-the-counter antihistamines. Although they worked, they made him feel drowsy. Because his allergies occured mostly in the spring, it was obvious they were triggered by pollens. I put him on QVC Plus, a combination of quercetin, bromelain and vitamin C, which reduces the release of histamines, the culprits responsible for allergies. He responded well to the treatment and required no further medication.

Anyone suffering from allergies should make sure that vitamin C, zinc and calcium-magnesium is adequately supplemented. Make sure to use cal-mag supplements that are easily absorbed like calcium citrate or gluconate varieties that are in chelate form. Stinging nettle has been proven to be quite effective in treating people with allergies. Combining nettle with feverfew may also be an effective herbal duo. The trio combination of quercitin, bromelain and vitamin C has also shown good efficacy without the side effects of prescription medications for allergies. It's a good idea to start supplementation with nettle and other supplements at the beginning of the allergy season.

Food sensitivities may play a much more significant role in allergies than most of us may have assumed. In addition, poor protein digestion can result in protein molecules which stay in the body and are recognized by the immune system as foreign invaders, triggering inappropriate immune responses. A predisposition to allergies may be caused by impaired digestion.

Additional Resources

Asthma and Allergy Foundation of America
1717 Massachusetts Avenue, Suite 305
Washington, DC 20036
(202) 265-0265

Endnotes

1. Murray L. Maurer and Margaret Strauss, "A new oral treatment for ragweed fever," Journal of Allergy, 1961, 32: 343.

2. C.A. Clemetson, "Histamine and ascorbic acid in human blood," Journal of Nutrition, 1980, 110 (4): 662-68. See also C. Bucca, et al., "Effect of vitamin C on histamine bronchial responsiveness of patients with allergic rhinitis," Annals Allergy, 1990, 65: 311-14.

3. H. Ogasawara et al., "Effects of selected flavonoids on histamine release and hydrogen peroxide (H2O2) generation by human leukocytes," Journal Allergy Clin Immunology, 1985, 75: 184. See also T. Yoshimoto, et al., "Flavonoids: Potent inhibitors of arachidonate 5-lipoxygenase," Biochem Biophys Res Commun, 1983, 116: 612-18.

4. P. Wendt, et al., "The use of flavonoids as inhibitors of histidine decarboxylase in gastric disease: experimental and clinical studies," Naunyn Schmiedebergs Arch Pharmacol, (suppl), 1980, 313: 238.

5. E. Bekier and C.Z. Maslinski, "Antihistaminic action of nicotinamide," Agents Actions, 1974, 4 (3): 196.

6. W.G. Crook, "Letter," Ann Allergy, 1987, 49: 45-46.

7. S. W. Simon, "Vitamin B 12 therapy in allergy and chronic dermatoses," Jour Allergy, 1951, 2: 183-85.

8. G. Utz, et al., "Oral application of calcium and vitamin D in allergic bronchial asthma," MMW, 1976, 118 (43): 1395-98.

9. L. Gallad, "Increased requirements fro essential fatty acids in atopic individuals: A review with clinical descriptions," Jour Amer Coll Nutri, 1986, 5 (2): 213-28.

10. S.A. Rogers, "Zinc deficiency as model for developing chemical sensitivity," Int Clin Nutri Rev, 1990, 10 (1): 253-59.

11. I. Kuvaeva, et al., "The micro ecology of the gastrointestinal tract and the immunological statis under food allergy," Nahrung, 1984, 28 (6-7): 689-93.

12. S. Heptinstall, et al., "Extracts of feverfew inhibit granule secretion in blood platelets and polymorphonuclear leucocytes," Lancet, 1985, I: 1071-74.

13. B.H. Erschoff et al., "Physiological effects of dietary clay supple-

ments," Final Report on contract # NAS 9-3905, 1965, NASA Manned Spacecraft Center, Houston Texans.

14. M.O. Karryev, et al., "Some therapeutic properties and phytochemistry of common horehound," Izvestiya Akademiya Nauk Turkmenskoi SSR, Seriya Biologicheskekj Nauk, 1976, 3: 86-88.

15. "Mullein." The St. Lawrence Review of Natural Products: Facts and Comparisons, St. Louis: Sept. 1989.

16. R. Papaioannou and C.C. Pfeiffer, "Sulfite sensitivity: unrecognized threat: Is molybdenum the cause?" Journal of Orthomolecular Psychiatry, 1984, 13 (2): 105-10.

17. Journal of Nutrition, 1989, 119: 135-136.

18. M. Kamimura, "Anti-inflammatory activity of vitamin E," Journal Vitaminol, 1972, 18 (4): 204-09.

19. Dana Ullman, "Review of Homeopathy, Allergy/Asthma Research and Science Friction," Quarterly Review of Natural Medicine, Fall, 1995: 241.

ALZHEIMER'S DISEASE

Alzheimer's disease is a progressive, degenerative condition that involves the deterioration of nerve cells in the brain, resulting in memory loss and disorientation. The disease is thought to be responsible for 75 percent of dementia in those 65 years and older. The disease progresses over several years. Unfortunately, the intellectual and personal decline that typically results from Alzheimer's cannot be curtailed as of yet. The disease affects over 4 million Americans and is responsible for 20 percent of patients in nursing homes or chronic care facilities. The disease rarely manifests itself before age 60. Up to 30 percent of people over 85 suffer from Alzheimer's.

Symptoms

There are three general stages to the disease. Initial symptoms include increasing forgetfulness, which may be addressed by the almost obsessive writing of lists.

As the disease progresses, forgetfulness becomes severe memory loss, particularly when dealing with short term events although long-term memory may not be affected. Disorientation may also occur and it is not uncommon for a victim of the disease to lose his way home. Mathematical calculations may also become difficult, indicating a decrease in intellectual ability in addition to becoming unable to find the right words (dysphasia). Anxiety, mood swings and apprehension may become evident and personality changes can also become apparent.

During the final stage of Alzheimer's, severe disorientation and confusion are the rule as are hallucinations and paranoid delusions.

Symptoms of this disease typically intensify at night. In addition, involuntary actions, incontinence of urine and feces, belligerence and violent behavior are not uncommon, although some victims become more docile and withdrawn.

Tendency by Alzheimer's victims to wander and neglect their appearance and hygiene often necessitates confinement to a bed. Once exiled, life expectancy dramatically decreases.

It has been found that many older individuals suffer from malnutrition, which can cause a number of psychological symptoms ranging from depression to a dementia that can be mistaken for Alzheimer's disease. Consequently, it is vital that diet be assessed and that vitamin and mineral supplements be added to determine if nutritional depletion is the cause. The B vitamins are particularly important. In addition, certain drugs can cause memory deficits or altered psychological behavior.

Make sure the cause of what appear to be age-related symptoms are not drug-induced.

Causes

The causes of Alzheimer's remain unknown although several theories exist which range from blaming exposure to aluminum to the existence of prolonged infection. Recently, speculation that Alzheimer's disease may be caused by a specific virus have been proposed.

Other possible causes include reduced levels of acetylcholine, a brain chemical have been found in people suffering from Alzheimer's disease. In addition, nerve fibers in the brain become tangled and certain areas of brain tissue can shrink during the course of the disease.

A genetic factor may also be a determining factor and is currently being investigated. A hereditary connection has been strengthened by the fact that the disease is more prevalent in Down's syndrome cases. In addition, approximately 15 percent of victims of Alzheimer's have a family incidence of the disease.

There has been significant speculation that an intake of aluminum from foods, antacids, cookware or antiperspirants may play a role in contracting Alzheimer's disease. The same speculation exists concerning silicon and mercury. There is no scientific evidence accepted in the medical community which confirms this connection, although autopsies of Alzheimer's victims have shown excessive amounts of aluminum and silicon in the brain. Mercury from dental amalgams may be a contributing factor.

In addition, a deficiency of vitamin B12, zinc, potassium, selenium and boron was also found to exist. Consequently, there is evidence to suggest that increased contact with aluminum in combination with a lack of certain vitamins and minerals may predispose one to the disease. A hair analysis test can determine if aluminum or any other heavy metal toxicity is present. In addition lower levels of vitamin A and E have also been linked to the disease.

Regarding the possibility of a viral component, similarities between Alzheimer's disease and Creutzfeldt-Jakob disease have been noted by some who see a growing viral connection with both disorders.

Another correlation that has been recently investigated regarding possible causes of Alzheimer's disease is the finding that women with Alzheimer's had lower estrogen levels than healthy women of the same age.

Immune system dysfunction and low zinc levels have also been linked to changes in aging brain tissue which may predispose one to Alzheimer's disease.

Higher than normal levels of glutamine synthetase have been found in Alzheimer's patients. Alcohol abuse has also been linked to this disease.

Conventional Therapies

The only way to absolutely diagnose Alzheimer's disease is with a brain biopsy or post mortem examination of brain tissue. As a result, an EEG (which records brain wave patterns) will show slower waves. There are no lab tests that can prove the existence of the disease. Alzheimer's disease is particularly difficult to diagnose. Consequently, some symptoms of dementia can be misdiagnosed as Alzheimer's.

Senile dementia, unlike Alzheimer's disease, can be caused by treatable conditions such as hypothyroidism, vitamin B12 deficiency, alcoholism, pernicious anemia, a series of strokes or a brain tumor. In some cases, the elderly may experience severe depression, which can mimic

Alzheimer's disease in several of its symptoms. Over-medication of the elderly is another factor which should be addressed as a possible cause of Alzheimer's-like symptoms.

No medical treatments, including attempts at restoring acetylcholine nerve cell function have proven successful. The provision of good nursing care is vital, which includes, a good diet, social interaction and using tranquilizers if behavior becomes difficult. Treatment with sandostatin and tetrahydroaminoacridin may prove helpful in treating the symptoms of Alzheimer's and should be discussed with your physician.

Dietary Guidelines

- ◆ Incorporate a good dietary regimen with an emphasis on a high-fiber diet that stresses fresh fruits and vegetables, sprouts, seeds, nuts, pressed oils, millet, brown rice, oat bran, whole grains, fish and low-fat foods.
- ◆ Do not stress the immune system by consuming alcohol, nicotine, caffeine, white sugar, processed foods and red meat.
- ◆ Do not use aluminum pots, pans or other cooking utensils.

Recommended Nutritional Supplements

PRIMARY NUTRIENTS

PHOSPHATIDYL CHOLINE Increases acetylcholine levels in the brain which directly impact memory function. Clinical data suggests that elevating acetylcholine in the brain may improve memory in Alzheimer's patients.[1] *Suggested Dosage:* 10 to 20 g daily. Use high quality preparations.

PHOSPHATIDYL SERINE This compound is one of the primary phospholipids found in brain tissue and plays an important role in brain function. Animal and human studies have found that supplementing this nutrient can improve memory and age-related changes in brain chemistry.[2] *Suggested Dosage:* 300 mg divided out in three doses with meals.

LECITHIN Contains choline which stimulates the production of acetylcholine and may help with memory function. *Suggested Dosage:* 100 mg three times daily with meals. Use granules or capsulized varieties.

COENZYME Q10 Increases brain cell oxygenation and boost circulation. *Suggested Dosage:* 100 mg per day.

ALPHA LIPOIC ACID German animal studies have found that ALA supplementation caused an improvement in the long-term memory of aged mice while younger mice showed no difference. What this finding implies is that ALA must help to reverse age-related memory impairment. It is assumed that the mechanism behind this action involves protecting brain cells from the kind of deterioration brought on by oxidation over time. *Suggested Dosage:* Take as directed.

GINKGO BILOBA Clinical studies are supportive of this herb's ability to reverse the metal deterioration associated with early stages of Alzheimer's disease.[3] It improves brain cell oxygenation and circulation and is highly recommended. Ginkgo is good for treating the early symptoms of Alzheimer's. *Suggested Dosage:* 60 mg of 24 percent extract taken two to three times a day.

VITAMIN B12 AND FOLIC ACID A distinct depletion of these vitamins have been found in Alzheimer's patients suggesting that deficiencies that may not even show in blood serum tests may precipitate the progression of this disease.[4] *Suggested Dosage:* 1,000 to 2,000 mg daily of vitamin B12 which can also be administered in injections. Folic acid supplements should be taken as directed.

VITAMIN B6 A lack of this vitamin has been closely linked with a number of neurological disorders including depression and schizophrenia. Elderly people can easily become deficient in vitamin B6. *Suggested Dosage:* 50 mg per day. Sublingual forms or injections are available.

VITAMIN E Helps transport oxygen to brain cells and scavenges for free radicals which can cause brain tissue damage. Vitamin E has been shown to help stabilize the symptoms of this disease and retard its progression. *Suggested Dosage:* 800 IU to 1,200 IU per day.

VITAMIN C, CALCIUM AND MAGNESIUM This trio may help reduce the presence of aluminum accumulations. Vitamin C is a potent antioxidant; calcium/magnesium work to calm the central nervous system. *Suggested Dosage:* 6,000 mg of vitamin C per day divided in equal doses with meals. Buffered forms are best. Doses of 1,500 mg of calcium and 500 of magnesium are recommended daily.

ZINC Prevents zinc depletion which has been linked to a number of brain disorders. *Suggested Dosage:* No more than 100 mg per day. Take with meals.

GERMANIUM Oxygenates brain cells and acts as an antioxidant agent. *Suggested Dosage:* Take as directed.

HERBAL COMBINATION This combination should include peppermint leaves, Siberian ginseng, gotu kola, kelp, rosemary leaves, damiana leaves and butternut root bark. This herbal formula is designed to improve circulation, and oxygen uptake and transport, and reduce the effects of stress. This mix will improve the ability to concentrate and retain memory, and help arrest the progression of age-related memory dysfunctions. *Suggested Dosage:* Two to four capsules daily. In more severe cases a person may consume up to twelve capsules daily.

PEPPERMINT LEAVES: Peppermint relieves tension and stress which can contribute to more normal breathing. This means that more oxygen will be available for the red blood cells to carry throughout the body including to the brain. The anti-stress factor will assist with concentration as well. SIBERIAN GINSENG: Siberian ginseng is considered to be an adaptogen agent or a substance with the ability to normalize systems of the body, irrespective of the direction, deficiency or excess of the pathologic state. Clinical studies have demonstrated ginseng's ability to improve physical assertion, mental alertness and the body's resistance to the effects of stress. Ginseng can protect the body against the effects of toxic chemicals and radiation, modulate immune system function in fighting disease and is considered an antiaging herb.[5] GOTU KOLA: Gotu kola is a popular herb used throughout the world and is particularly popular in India. Ayurvedic doctors use it as a central nervous system tonic and to improve mental stamina and enhance memory.[6] Clinical studies performed in Europe show gotu kola has the ability to increase circulation. KELP: Kelp's high concentration and broad range of trace elements nourish the central nervous system and boost brain function. The algin in kelp soothes and improves gastrointestinal tract function, and it also binds with cholesterol and toxins to remove them from the body. Kelp improves nutrition and general health. ROSEMARY LEAVES: Rosemary helps maintain a healthy nervous system. It assists in combating stress and improves circulation especially in the elderly who may be experiencing chronic poor circulation. Long-term use improves memory. In addition, this herb acts as a powerful antioxidant which can reduce brain tissue damage caused by free radicals. DAMIANA LEAVES: Germany's drug regulatory board suggests using damiana for the "fortification and stimulation in cases of overwork, mental stress, and nervous debility, and for enhancement and maintenance of mental and physical efficiency." In Britain it is used as an antidepressant. Damiana can interfere with iron absorbtion. BUTTERNUT ROOT BARK: Butternut root bark has been included in this formula as a laxative to cleanse toxins from the body and to improve health.

SECONDARY NUTRIENTS

NADH: May help to improve symptoms. *Suggested Dosage:* Take 5 to 15 mg per day.

SELENIUM: An excellent free radical scavenger which should be taken with vitamin E. *Suggested Dosage:* Take as directed.

ALFALFA AND BURDOCK: Improve cerebral circulation which helps to oxygenate the cells and promote better brain function. *Suggested Dosage:* Take as directed.

CAPSICUM: Helps in supplying nutrients to the brain. *Suggested Dosage:* Take as directed. Capsicum can cause a burning sensation in the stomach.

LADY'S SLIPPER: Supplies nutrients to the nervous system. *Suggested Dosage:* Take as directed.

Doctor's Notes

The cause of this disease is still in question and has been associated with increased amount of aluminum deposits in the brain. However, many researchers have neglected to make the link.

A recent study showed that taking products with Ibuprofen reduced the risk of developing Alzheimer's. Vitamin E, NADH and ginkgo can be helpful, although as the disease progresses, ginkgo is not as effective.

Doctors often hear complaints from patients who are experiencing memory loss, poor memory or an inability to concentrate. Some of these people may also experience other possibly related conditions like poor circulation or tinnitus (ringing in the ear). Memory loss can be caused by many different factors such as head trauma or injury, ischemia or stroke (a condition where blood flow to parts of the brain has been cut off), poor circulation and oxygen flow to the brain and organic brain disease. Alcoholism, smoking and even environmental pollutants may also lead to memory dysfunction. In such cases it is important that the person change environments or habits to stop the progression of the condition. Inability to concentrate may be caused by stress or nervous disorders. Formulas used most commonly for age-releated memory problems include *Ginkgo biloba,* gotu kola and bilberry. These all help boost cerebral circulation, enhance memory and improve mental function.

Home Care Suggestions

◆ Those that suffer from this disease are usually very limited in their ability to be self-sufficient. Consequently, home care falls to the caregiver. Because home care is so intensive, contact should be made with the Alzheimer's Disease Society for specific instructions and support (see address below).

Other Supportive Therapies

ACUPUNCTURE: Certain trigger points can help stimulate certain regions of the brain.

Scientific Facts-at-a-Glance

Recently a team at John Hunter Hospital in Newcastle, Conn., reported that high levels of aluminum exist in some canned soft drinks. Their studies reveal that the aluminum content of noncola drinks in cans was almost six times that found in bottles. For cola drinks, the amount was three times higher. Apparently, the acidity of soft drinks erodes the imperfections in the protective covering which lines the cans. As a result, aluminum dissolves into the beverage.

Spirit/Mind Considerations

In its initial stages, victims of Alzheimer's usually try to compensate for their forgetfulness and will sometimes try to solicit others to help them. Depression and anxiety brought on by memory loss are common and should be addressed. As mentioned earlier, personality changes are common. Those caring for someone suffering from Alzheimer's should definitely take advantage of support groups available. The disease can be devastating to families. Often the care-giver in this situation will need as much psychological support as the patient. Emotional, as well as financial, stress can result as the disease demands more care. Self-help groups should be used. Counseling is recommended to prevent the possibility of abuse due to the stressful nature of this disease. Because the victim of Alzheimer's cannot be reasoned with, the care giver needs external support and advice.

Prevention

◆ Avoid sources of aluminum which are commonly found in food additives (can be found in cake mixes, processed cheese, frozen dough etc.); baking powder, which can have from 5–50 mg of sodium aluminum phosphate per teaspoonful; pickling salts; some salad dressings; table salt; some white flours; some water sources; douches; some feminine hygiene products; some lipsticks; antacids (there are a number available that are aluminum free); some brands of buffered aspirin; antidiarrheal medications; aluminum coated cookware (cooking tomato based ingredients, which are acidic, can cause some leeching into the food from the pot or pan); some antidandruff shampoos; aluminum cans and other containers, especially soda pop cans.

◆ While the origins of the disease remain a mystery, keeping active and staying involved during post-retirement years has been known to prolong life and enhance its quality. Join senior citizen clubs, travel, exercise and keep yourself occupied.

◆ Eat a diet high in antioxidants, such as carotenes, flavonoids, zinc and selenium.

◆ Take a high-potency multiple vitamin daily to prevent nutrient depletions associated with this disease.

◆ Avoid alcoholic beverages.

◆ Only take drugs that are absolutely necessary.

Additional Resources

Alzheimer's Association
919 North Michigan Avenue, Suite 1000
Chicago, IL 60611
(800) 272-3900 or (312) 335-8700

Alzheimer's Disease Society:
2 West 45th Street, Room 1703
New York, NY 10036,
(212) 719-4744.

Association for Alzheimer's and Related Diseases
70 East Lake Street, Suite 600
Chicago, IL 60601-5997
(800) 572-6037
(800) 621-0379

Endnotes

1. D.J. Canty and S.H. Zeisel, "Lecithin, and choline in human health and disease," Nutr Reviews, 1994, 52: 327-339.
2. T. Crook, et al., "Effects of phosphaditylserine in Alzheimer's disease," Psychopharmacol Bull, 1992, 28: 61-66. See also E. W. Funfgeld, et al., "Double-blind study with phosphaditylserine in Parkinsonian patients with senile dementia of Alzheimer's type (SDAT)," Prog Clin Biol Res, 1989, 317: 1235-24.
3. B. Hofferberth, "The efficacy of Egb761 in patients with senile dementia of the Alzheimer type: A double-blind, placebo-controlled study on different levels of investigation," Human Psychopharmacol,

1994, 9: 215-22.

4. M.G. Cole and J.F. Prichal, "Low serum vitamin B 12 in Alzheimer-type dementia," Age Aging, 1984, 13: 101-05. See also G.M. Craig, et al., "Masked vitamin B 12 and folate deficiency in the elderly," British Journal of Nutrition, 1985, 54: 613-19.

5. D. H. Zhou, "Preventative geriatrics: an overview from traditional Chinese medicine," American Journal of Chinese Medicine, 1982, 10, (1-4): 32-39.

6. R. N. Chopra, Indigenous Drugs of India, 2nd ed. (Arts Press, Calcutta: 1933).

ANGINA

Angina is chest pain that occurs when the muscles of the heart wall are temporarily deprived of some of their oxygen supply. Angina is a common condition usually affecting men after the age of 30 and is almost always caused by some stage of coronary artery disease. In women, the occurrence is generally later and has been also linked to anemia. Angina is usually the first symptom of heart disease and should receive prompt medical attention.

The average heart beats over 100,000 times a day and about 38 million times per year. To illustrate, this remarkable organ raises the equivalent of one ton to a height of 41 feet every 24 hours. The heart muscle must beat 24 hours a day to sustain life. Heart defects can be of various origins. Some are inborn errors; others are caused by aging, disease, or illness, such as rheumatic fever and beriberi. Fortunately there are many herbs that support the function of the heart.

Symptoms

Pain which radiates from the center of the chest is the main symptom of angina. This pain can move into the back, upper jaw, throat and arms and, in particular, the left arm.

Angina pain has been described by patients as being more of a squeezing or pressure sensation than a sharp or stabbing pain. While strenuous physical activity usually precedes angina, a spasm of a coronary vessel may trigger the reaction at any time.

In addition to the pain, difficulty in breathing and nausea, sweating and dizziness may also occur. This combination of symptoms can easily mimic a heart attack.

Angina may progressively become worse, with episodes appearing more frequently and lasting longer. As a result, people suffering from angina typically become less and less active to avoid the possibility of triggering an attack.

Precautions

If chest pain does not subside in ten to fifteen minutes, the condition may be a heart attack and emergency medical treatment is required immediately. Prolonged angina may also increase the risk of a heart attack. A change in lifestyle could dramatically enhance your longevity and should be seriously considered.

Causes

Cholesterol sometimes builds up in the smaller arteries of the heart and can narrow the vessels enough to stem the flow of blood. When the blood flow is cut off altogether, a heart attack will usually occur. Under normal sedentary conditions, enough blood may pass through the vessel so that the symptoms of angina are not present. In the case of strenuous activities, such as mowing the lawn or stair climbing or even after a large meal or emotional upset, the oxygen requirements of the heart increase. Consequently, blood flow in these situations is not sufficient to feed the heart muscles and the oxygen deprivation causes the heart to work harder and chest pain to occur. When the oxygen requirement falls, the pain will usually subside.

Conventional Therapies

A class of drugs known as nitrates (nitrostat, nitrolingual) are often prescribed. They are usually dissolved under the tongue when an attack occurs. Nitrates dilate blood vessels and increase the blood flow to the heart muscle. Pain is usually relieved within minutes and relief can last up to 30 minutes. Isosorbide dinitrate (isordil, sorbitrate) takes longer to act by a few minutes, but it remains effective for one or two hours.

Oral nitrates such as isordil, peritrate and nitro-bid are used to increase blood flow to the heart over a 24-hour period. Nitrate patches are also available, although the body will build a tolerance to the patches when used over a longer period of time.

Beta blockers are another class of drugs which are used to keep the heart from overexertion by reducing the amount of oxygen it needs. Beta blockers are also prescribed for high blood pressure. Some of these are known as lopressor, tenormin, corgard and blocadren. Beta blockers inhibit the release of adrenaline (which speeds up the heart under conditions of stress). In other words, beta blockers slow the heartbeat. A complication of this treatment is that a heart rate that is too slow results.

Calcium blockers (isoptin, calan, cardizem) which interfere with tiny amounts of calcium that regulate the contraction of the heart muscle, may also be prescribed. These drugs cause relaxation and increased blood flow to the heart. This therapy also causes the heart to beat with less strength and must be used carefully. Calcium blockers are usually prescribed for angina that is thought to be caused by a spasm of the coronary artery.

Surgical Options

Bypass surgery is an option if angina does not respond to drug therapy. This procedure involves detouring a blood vessel around the blocked section and reattaching it at another location. If the left main coronary artery is blocked, bypass surgery is highly recommended. Bypass surgery is remarkably low risk, with a mortality rate of approximately one percent.

Angioplasty is another surgical procedure sometimes used to alleviate angina. A deflated balloon is attached to a wire and threaded through the vessel. The balloon is then blown up at the point of blockage. This succeeds in eliminating the blockage in most cases, but it can necessitate an emergency bypass. Once removed, the blockage will reappear over time if changes in diet and lifestyle are not implemented.

Dietary Guidelines

- Eliminate stimulants such as coffee, tea and caffeine drinks.
- Avoid alcohol, sugar, soft drinks, salt, red meats, fatty dairy products, margarine, shortening and high-fat, sugary foods. Eat foods that contain cholesterol sparingly. Cholesterol is obtained primarily from animal source foods such as meat, eggs and dairy products.
- Eat plenty of fiber, complex carbohydrates, broiled coldwater fish, chicken and turkey, raw vegetables and fresh fruits, garlic and onion.
- Use olive oil and safflower oil, and eat raw almonds (avoid peanuts). Watch out for hydrogenated and even polyunsaturated oils and fats. Monosaturated oleic fats seem to be the best choice of dietary oil and includes olive oil.
- Avoid deep-fried foods and minimize the heating of fats.
- A low salt diet is recommended and the following substances should be avoided: MSG, baking soda, canned vegetables and soups, diet soft drinks, meat tenderizers and softened water.

Recommended Nutritional Supplements

PRIMARY NUTRIENTS

COENZYME Q10 Acts as a catalyst in certain chemical reactions and is thought to directly benefit heart function by increasing tissue oxygenation and is considered a preventative of recurring heart attacks.[1] *Suggested Dosage:* 50 mg with each of three meals per day.

GARLIC Can help to lower blood pressure and also helps in thinning the blood.[2] In addition, it can significantly lower blood cholesterol levels which can cause arterial blockages linked to angina. *Suggested Dosage:* Take two capsules with each meal. Deodorized products are available.

ALPHA LIPOIC ACID A vitamin-like antioxidant which has recently been recognized for its ability to protect cardiac tissue from damage that normally results when oxygen is deprived.[3] *Suggested Dosage:* 50 mg per day.

L-CARNITINE Helps to decrease the risk of heart disease by reducing triglyceride levels while boosting the oxygenation of heart muscle during times of stress.[4] Tests have supported its ability to reduce anginal episodes.[5] *Suggested Dosage:* 1,000 mg per day in divided doses.

PANTHETHEINE Levels of heart panthethine can decrease during periods of oxygen depletion. In addition, supplementation decreases serum cholesterol and inhibits the formation of clots.[6] *Suggested Dosage:* 300 mg with each of three meals per day.

SELENIUM WITH VITAMIN E Clinical trials have shown that supplementing these two nutrients together can reduce the pain of angina.[7] Vitamin E also helps to prevent heart tissue damage and naturally thins the blood. *Suggested Dosage:* 200 mg of selenium per day with 200 to 400 IU of vitamin E per day. Do not exceed 400 IU without the permission of your physician.

CALCIUM CHELATE AND MAGNESIUM Essential for the maintenance of regular heartbeat and helps to control cholesterol levels.[8] A calcium deficiency has been associated with atherosclerosis, a primary cause of angina.[9] Magnesium should always accompany calcium for absorbability and has been successfully used to treat angina.[10] Magnesium deficiencies have been associated with angina. *Suggested Dosage:* 100 mg of each mineral in divided doses. Look for chelated gluconate or citrate varieties.

LECITHIN Works to emulsify fats and may normalize lipoproteins and inhibit the formation of blood clots.[11] *Suggested Dosage:* Six grams daily with meals. Can be taken in capsule or granule form.

FISH OIL SUPPLEMENTS Eicosapentaenoic acid (EPA) and docosahexaenoic acid (DHA), both found in cold water fish, are considered excellent protectants against heart disease. Studies done in Japan, Sweden and the Netherlands where EPA consumption is high, show a marked lower incidence of heart disease. Fish oil helps to thin the blood, protects against atherosclerosis by reducing plasma lipids even when cholesterol levels are high and reduces the pain of angina.[12] *Suggested Dosage:* Take as directed with a vitamin E supplement. Make sure to take vitamin E when increasing omega-3 oils.

EVENING PRIMROSE OIL Supplies essential fatty acids which help to discourage arterial lipid deposits. *Suggested Dosage:* Take as directed. Capsulized or liquid forms are available.

POTASSIUM Ensures proper electrolyte ratios. In addition, a deficiency of potassium has been related to cardiac disturbances.[13] *Suggested Dosage:* Take as directed.

KHELLA An herb which has been used for the treatment of angina and other cardiovascular diseases since ancient Egyptian times. The primary compound of khella has proven its effectiveness in alleviating angina pain and in improving stress tolerance when exercising.[14] *Suggested Dosage:* Take as directed.

HAWTHORN A superior cardiovascular herb which lowers blood pressure and strengthens heart muscle. In clinical trials this herb has proven its ability to treat heart failure.[15] *Suggested Dosage:* 200 to 500 mg of hawthorn can be taken as a tincture or in capsule form, alone or in an herbal combination.

HERBAL COMBINATION This combination should include hawthorn berries, motherwort, rosemary leaves, cayenne, kelp, wood betony and shepherd's purse. *Suggested Dosage:* Four to six capsules daily. May be used daily.

HAWTHORN BERRY: Next to digitalis, hawthorn is probably the most recognized herb for positively affecting the heart. As demonstrated by scientific studies, hawthorn supports metabolic processes in the heart, dilates coronary vessels, reduces peripheral resistance and lowers blood pressure, reduces tendency for angina attacks and strengthens damaged or weakened heart muscles. *The British Herbal Pharmacopeia* indicates hawthorn is reputed to dissolve deposits in sclerotic arteries. Hawthorn is perhaps the best cardiotonic known today.[16] MOTHERWORT: The use of motherwort as a cardiotonic spans centuries. In fact, its other common names—"heart heal" and "heart wort"—are more indicative of its heart benefits. Nevertheless, it has been proven worthy for official recognition in Britain, Germany, and France. Motherwort is especially beneficial in cases of nervous heart conditions which can cause, among other things, palpitation or abnormally rapid or fluttering heart beats. Motherwort normalizes the heart in at least two ways. It asserts a calming action on the central nervous system which can help to normalize heart rate, and it assists in improving thyroid function in cases of hyperactivity. Hyperthyroidism is often associated with heart palpitation. The British recognize motherwort's ability to reduce blood pressure and like hawthorn, it has a mild sedative action.[17] ROSEMARY LEAVES: Like many spices, rosemary contains powerful antioxidants. Antioxidants have clearly been shown to support the integrity of the veins. Rosemary has also exhibited cardiotonic capacity which helps with normal heart function. Rosemary stimulates bile flow which improves digestion. It also causes mild perspiration, releasing toxins from the body and improving health.[18] CAYENNE: Cayenne supports and improves circulation. Cayenne is considered an herb activator that increases the effectiveness of other herbs. It stimulates digestion and promotes perspiration. Cayenne has been shown to reduce blood pressure, especially in conjunction with garlic.[19] KELP: Kelp is a powerhouse of micronutrients that assist with various metabolic processes. Kelp has been considered a blood vessel cleanser and a treatment for atherosclerosis. Kelp contains algin, a soluble fiber that improves bowel function and soothes the gastro-intestinal tract. Kelp has also been suggested in cases of obesity and digestive problems.[20] WOOD BETONY: Wood betony is carminative, diuretic and nervine. The three benefits support a healthy cardiovascular system. In addition it acts to lower blood pressure.[21] SHEPHERD'S PURSE: Shepherd's purse is a common weed that grows all over the United States. It is a diuretic and has an ability to regulate blood pressure and heart action.[22]

SECONDARY NUTRIENTS

VITAMIN B-COMPLEX: Helps to normalize cholesterol and strengthen heart muscle. A deficiency of the B-vitamins has been linked to heart disease.[23] *Suggested Dosage:* Take as directed making sure to add extra vitamin B1 and vitamin B3.

VITAMIN C WITH BIOFLAVONOIDS: Works to toughen capillaries. A vitamin C deficiency has been strongly linked to the development of heart disease and angina.[24] *Suggested Dosage:* 1,000 mg with each meal.

COPPER AND ZINC: A copper deficiency may be associated with the development of heart disease.[25] Zinc has shown its ability to help normalize blood lipids but can decrease copper levels so the two should be taken together.

Suggested Dosage: Take as directed and do not exceed recommended dosages.

CHROMIUM: Chromium supplementation can help to reduce cholesterol levels helping to prevent the atherosclerosis which can precede angina.[26] *Suggested Dosage:* Take as directed using picolinate or GTF varieties. If you suffer from a blood sugar disorder, check with your physician before using this supplement.

TAURINE: This amino acid can help normalize heart rhythms and also acts as a free radical scavenger. *Suggested Dosage:* Take as directed on an empty stomach with fruit juice.

GINSENG: Helps in normalizing blood pressure and is traditionally used to treat angina in China. *Suggested Dosage:* Take as directed. Panax ginseng is usually recommended.

VALERIAN: Works to calm the central nervous system reducing the stress which sometimes precedes an attack of angina. *Suggested Dosage:* Take as directed. Look for guaranteed potency products. Valerian may cause some drowsiness.

Home Care Suggestions

◆ The first and foremost requirement for treating heart disease is to accept the fact that a change in lifestyle must occur, with a sturdy commitment to maintain the new lifestyle.

◆ If you smoke, stop or cut down as much as possible.

◆ If overweight, go on a sensible diet where fats are reduced, with special attention to cutting saturated fats and cholesterol containing foods such as butter, red meats, fats, fried foods, processed "empty calorie" foods, eggs, dairy products, etc.

◆ Avoid stress and use relaxation tapes, or meditation times to alleviate tension. More emphasis is being placed on the body-mind connection in relation to controlling physiological functions which had been thought to be totally involuntary. Regular, low-impact exercise is very effective in releasing stress.

◆ Under a physician's guidelines, begin an exercise program such as walking three to five times a week.

◆ If you know you will probably experience angina before participating in a certain activity, a nitroglycerine tablet, prescribed by your physician, may be taken beforehand.

Other Supportive Therapies

MASSAGE: Stimulates circulation and prompts relaxation.
MEDITATION AND VISUALIZATION: An excellent way to de-stress helping to reduce the strain that anxiety causes on the cardiovascular system.

Scientific Facts-at-a-Glance

Recent studies support the notion that a lack of certain nutrients can cause the development of diseases like angina. We are quick to blame what we consume rather than what we may be leaving out of our diets. Beta carotene, vitamin A, C and E deficiencies have linked to angina pectoris.[27]

Spirit/Mind Considerations

Learning to relieve stress and effectively relax is essential in controlling conditions like angina. Disciplines designed to evoke complete relaxation are very helpful when dealing with conditions like angina. Light a candle and concentrate on the flame, trying to empty your mind of all conscious thought. Controlled breathing can also help create a relaxed state. The spiritual aspects of stress-related diseases are usually ignored, but getting in touch with a higher power can help you to judge less, become slow to anger, trust in those around you and to feel gratitude. Each one of these feelings can help us dispel the tension and negative behavior, which very often contributes to the development of stress-related diseases.

Prevention

◆ The best approach to angina is to take steps to prevent it from ever occuring. Angina is a disease which indicates the presence of other conditions that could have been prevented through proper diet and exercise.

◆ A diet low in fats and high in fiber is recommended along with a daily exercise routine (brisk walking, bicycling, etc.) for at least 30 minutes a day.

◆ Meditation, yoga, breathing exercise, massage, etc., are proven to relieve high levels of stress.

◆ Take lecithin and essential fatty acid supplements daily. The omega-3 oils found in coldwater fish are highly recommended. These two substances play a very significant role in preventing coronary artery disease by decreasing cholesterol levels and through the proper metabolism of dietary fats.

Doctor's Notes

The highly effective heart medicine digitalis is actually a derivative of a botanical commonly known as "fox glove" or *Digitalis purpurea.* While digitalis is associated with a narrow safety margin and not found in this formula, many other botanicals described hereafter are quite safe and effective. This formula can strengthen a weak heart, restore proper heart rhythm, reduce blood pressure and prevent angina.

Additional Resources

American Heart Association
7320 Greenville Avenue
Dallas, TX 75231
(214) 373-6300

Endnotes

1. T. Kamikawa, et al., "Effects of coenzyme. Q10 on exercise tolerance in chronic stable angina pectoris," American Journal of Cardiology, 1985, 56: 247.

2. A. Bordia, "Effect of garlic on blood lipids in patients with coronary heart disease," American Journal of Clinical Nutrition, 1981, 34 (10): 2100-03.

3. R. Passwater, Lipoic Acid: The Metabolic Oxidant, (Keats

Publishing, New Canaan, CT: 1996).

4. A. Cherchi, et al., "Effects of L-carnitine on exercise tolerance in chronic, stable angina: a multicenter, double-blind, randomized, placebo controlled crossover study," Int Journal of Clinical Pharmacol Ther Toxicol, 1985, 23 (10): 569-72.

5. C.S. Rossi and N. Silliprandi, "Effect of carnitine on blood lipid pattern in diabetic patients," Nutrition Rep Int, 1984, 29: 1071.

6. L. Arsenio, et al., "Effectiveness of long-term treatment with pantetheine in patients with dislipidemia," Clinical Ther, 1986, 8: 537-45. See also D. Prisco, et al., "Effect of pantetheine treatment on platelet aggregation and thromboxane A2 production," Curr Ther Res, 1984, 35: 700.

7. D.V. Frost and P.M. Lish, "Selenium in Biology," Ann Rev Pharm, 1975, 18: 259.

8. N. Karanja, et al., "Plasma lipids and hypertension: response to calcium supplementation," Amer Jour of Clin Nutri, 1987, 45 (1): 60-65.

9. R.D. Phari, "Cellular calcium and atherosclerosis: A brief review," Cell Calcium, 1988, 9 (5-6): 275-84.

10. L. Cohen, and R Kitzes, "Magnesium sulfate in the treatment of variant angina," Magnesium, 1984, 3: 46-49.

11. J.G. Brook, "Dietary soya lecithin decreases plasma triglyceride levels and inhibits collagen and ADP-induced platelet aggregation," Biochem Med Metab Biol, 1986, 35 (1): 31-39.

12. R. Saynor, et al., "The long-term effect of dietary supplementation with fish lipid concentrate on serum lipids, bleeding time, platelets and angina," Atherosclerosis, 1984, 50: 3-10.

13. T. Dychner and P.O. Wester, "Magnesium and potassium in serum and muscle in relation to disturbances of cardiac rhythm," Magnesium in Health and Disease, (Spectrum Publishing, 1980), 551-57.

14. H.L. Osher, K.H. Katz and D.J. Wagner, "Khellin in the treatment of angina pectoris," New England Journal of Medicine, 1951, 244: 315-321.

15. M. Tauchert, et al., "Effectiveness of the hawthorn extract LI 132 compared with the ACE inhibitor Captopril: A multicenter, double-blind study with 132 NYHA stage II," Munch Med, 1994, 136 supple, I: S27-S33.

16. H. Leuchtgens, "Crataegus (Hawthorn) special extract WS 1442 in NYHA II heart failure: A placebo-controlled, randomized, double-blind study," Forschr Med, 1993, 111: 352-54.

17. Y.X. Xia, "The inhibitory effect of motherwort extract on pulsating myocardial cells in vitro," Journal of Traditional Chinese Medicine, 1983 3(3): 185-88.

18. A. Boido et al., "N-substituted derivatives of rosmaricine," Studi Sassaresi, Sezione 2, 1975, 53 (5-6): 383-93.

19. K Sambaiah and N. Satyanatayana, "Hypocholesterolemic effect of red pepper and capsaicin," Indian Journal of Experimental Biology, 1980, 18: 521-29.

20. P.B. Searl, et al., "Study of a cardiotonic fraction from an extract of the seaweed undaria pinnatifida," Proceedings of the Western Pharmacology Society, 1981, 24: 63-65.

21. T.V. Zinchenko, et al., "Investigation of glycosides from betonica officinalis," Farmatsevt Zhurnal, 1962, 17 (3): 35-38.

22. K. Kuroda, and T. Kaku, "Pharmacological and chemical studies on the alcohol extract of capsella bursa pastoris," Life Sciences, 1969, 8 (3): 151-55.

23. H. Povoa, et al., "Folic acid and lipoprotein lipase from aorta and blood plasma of atherosclerotic rats," Biomed Biochem Acta, 1984, 43 (2): 241-44.

24. R.A. Riemersma, et al., "Risk of angina pectoris and plasma concentrations of vitamins A, C, E and carotene," Lancet, 1991, 337: 1-5.

25. J.T. Salonen, et al., "Interactions of serum copper, selenium, and low density lipoprotein cholesterol in atherogenesis," British Medical Journal, 1991, 302: 756-60.

26. M. Simonoff, et al., "Chromium deficiency is a risk factor for ASHD," Nutr Rev, 1983, 41: 307-10.

27. Reimersam, et al., 1-5.

ANXIETY

A panic or anxiety attack can be a profoundly frightening and intense experience. Panic attacks can be so devastating that people who suffer from them will often drastically alter their lifestyles in order to avoid triggering one.

An anxiety or panic attack causes an extremely negative emotional state, which is characterized by feelings of intense fear and apprehension. Anyone suffering from an anxiety attack feels a sense of impending doom, although in most cases, there is no actual physical threat present. While anxiety, if kept within limits, is a normal part of life, when it begins to disrupt one's ability to participate in day-to-day activities, it is considered a psychological illness. Anxiety attacks also cause a variety of physical symptoms that can easily be mistaken for serious disorders like heart attacks.

Normal activities such as driving, finding oneself far from home, stepping into a crowded room or going shopping may trigger a set of physical and emotional symptoms which reinforce the anxiety or panic. Frequently, the person who has suffered a panic attack relates that attack to what they were doing at the time. As a result they may want to avoid shopping, driving etc., for fear that another attack will occur in the future. It is not uncommon however, to have one panic attack and then never experience another.

Anxiety disorders are rather common and affect roughly four percent of the American population. Younger adults are more susceptible and the disorders affect men and women equally. A panic attack can last from five minutes to an hour and usually averages about twenty minutes in length. Anxiety attacks can lead to phobias such as agoraphobia in which the person rarely leaves home for fear of losing control in public.

Symptoms

An anxiety or panic attack can produce tightness in the chest, rapid, pounding heartbeat, throbbing or stabbing pains in the chest, breathlessness, heavy sighing or deep inhaling, headaches, neck and back spasms, inability to relax or restlessness, pallor, sweating or clammy skin, fatigue, nausea or diarrhea, difficulty swallowing, belching or vomiting, the urgent need to urinate or defecate, dizziness, hyperventilation, yawning or a tingling sensation in the limbs.

Precautions

Whenever an anxiety attack of a phobia has progressed to the point where it interferes with everyday functioning, get professional help. If you feel incapacitated, contact local phobia centers who will often send phobia aides to help you within your own home.

Causes

Often, victims of anxiety attacks have a heightened level of arousal in the nervous system so that their reactions to certain stimuli are much more intense and over-exaggerated. One area of the brain, the locus ceruleus, controls emotion and when it is stimulated, creates anxiety. Accordingly, panic attacks may be seen as a form of epilepsy in which the locus ceruleus becomes overstimulated and discharges impulses in excess.

People prone to depression seem to suffer more from panic attacks. This implies that a neurochemical imbalance may be the cause of both disorders. Typically, people who experience panic for no obvious reason find it more difficult to adapt to changing situations and environments.

Heredity is a factor—these attacks seem to run in families. Some psychoanalysts believe that anxiety disorders stem from repressed or unresolved childhood experiences or conflicts.

There is some speculation that inner ear disorders can contribute to feelings of anxiety or phobias.

Foods allergies have also been linked to panic disorders and should be investigated as a possible cause.

A lack of B-complex vitamins or other nutrients can precipitate drastic changes in emotional behavior. Make sure to rule out nutrient depletion in assessing symptoms.

Conventional Therapies

Counseling and psychotherapy are routinely prescribed along with antianxiety drugs such as benzodiazepines.

Beta blockers (inderal, tenormin, etc.) can also help to control the adrenalin surges that accompany anxiety attacks.

Clomipramine is considered one of the best treatments for panic attacks and is a relatively new antidepressant. Alprazolam (Xanax), which is derived from valium, is also routinely used; however it is highly addictive and when it is withdrawn, panic attacks can reoccur.

Drugs which block the action of adrenalin may help to control the physical symptoms of panic attacks but do nothing to remove the fear itself.

Finding a good psychotherapist trained to deal with these kinds of disorders is far preferable than becoming dependent on drugs. Often, physicians will rely on tranquilizing or antidepressant drugs to control these disorders and badly ignore counseling or self help measures.

Dietary Guidelines

◆ Avoid caffeine in any form. People who are prone to panic attacks and anxiety disorders will sometimes be sensitive to caffeine. It also makes good sense to avoid stimulants of any kind.

◆ Do not eat white sugar and highly sweetened foods. Experiencing sporadic fluctuations in blood sugar can create feelings of anxiety and stress the adrenal glands. Eat complex carbohydrates such as whole grains and avoid "empty-calorie" junk foods.

◆ Try to rule out food allergies by keeping a careful record of what you eat and the incidence of attacks.

◆ Do not take any drugs that you absolutely do not need. Look for correlations between any drug you might be taking and anxiety attacks. Some drugs which are considered to have tranquilizing side effects can actually agitate the nervous system of some people. Certain decongestants, codeine preparations, cough medicines, etc., can have this effect.

Recommended Nutritional Supplements

PRIMARY NUTRIENTS

VITAMIN B-COMPLEX All of the B-vitamins are vital to the proper functioning of the nervous system and the maintenance of mental health. Strong supplementation of the B-vitamins can improve brain function and help in reducing anxiety and stress.[1] Take extra vitamin B1, vitamin B6 and vitamin B12. *Suggested Dosage:* Take as directed. Use sublingual forms where possible.

VITAMIN C WITH BIOFLAVONOIDS These are important for healthy adrenal glands, which can become overworked during periods of anxiety. Taking high doses of this vitamin has been linked to increased stress resistance.[2] *Suggested Dosage:* 1,000 mg with each meal.

NADH An organic compound which can help to normalize brain chemistry, promoting a feeling of calmness and well-being. *Suggested Dosage:* Take in a reduced form on an empty stomach with an eight-ounce glass of water at 5 mg per day.

CALCIUM AND MAGNESIUM Has a calming effect and helps to decrease feelings of nervousness. *Suggested Dosage:* Take as directed using chelated gluconate or citrate products.

L-TYROSINE An amino acid which can help alleviate symptoms of stress and promote sleep.[3] *Suggested Dosage:* Take as directed on an empty stomach in the morning with fruit juice. Do not use if you are taking beta blocker drugs or suffer from high blood pressure.

GABA WITH INOSITOL Acts as a natural tranquilizer. *Suggested Dosage:* Take as directed.

MELATONIN Promotes relaxation and sleep and has been used to treat mental disorders such as depression and the type of insomnia that accompanies anxiety.[4] *Suggested Dosage:* Take only a directed, starting with very small amounts. Not recommended for pregnant or nursing mothers.

VALERIAN A safe and nonaddictive tranquilizing herb which has proven its efficacy in treating anxiety disorders.[5] Valerian works especially well in combination with passionflower. *Suggested Dosage:* Take as directed only. (Taking valerian may cause drowsiness.)

KAVA KAVA Kavain, the major bioactive compound found in kava kava, has proven its effectiveness in clinical trials with patients who suffered from anxiety disorders.[6] *Suggested Dosage:* Take as directed.

GINKGO BILOBA Improves brain cell oxygenation and has proven antidepressive effects.[7] *Suggested Dosage:* Take as directed, using guaranteed potency products.

ESSENTIAL FATTY ACIDS Supply the nerve sheathes with essential nutrients. *Suggested Dosage:* Take as directed.

HERBAL COMBINATION This combination should include valerian, passionflower, wood betony, ginger, hops, skullcap, chamomile and blessed thistle. *Suggested Dosage:* Four to eight capsules daily.

VALERIAN: Valerian is probably the most widely used botanical in Europe for nervous tension, anxiety and insomnia. In fact, the herb is found in dozens of drugs and teas. Interestingly, valerian is calming and relaxing in cases of nervous tension and anxiety, while at the same time improving alertness and ability to concentrate.[8] It is important to know that consuming too much valerian when fatigued can actually be stimulating. Valerian seems to be just the prescription for the modern human family. PASSIONFLOWER: Considering its name, it might be misconstrued as the perfect aphrodisiac. Passionflower works well in formulas designed to treat insomnia, but it works even better in formulas designed to combat stress, nervous tension, anxiety, restlessness, hysteria and nervous headaches. It contains small amounts of serotonin, which acts to calm the brain.[9] Do not use if you are pregnant or nursing. WOOD BETONY: Wood betony has been well appreciated and prescribed for hundreds of years by old and new world physicians for treating nervous and sleep disorders, with particular application for tension headaches.[10] It also acts as a cleansing tonic to the blood and certain organs. Along with valerian, wood betony is mildly settling to the gastrointestinal tract. Wood betony is officially recognized in the *British Herbal Pharmacopeia*. GINGER: Eating disorders and digestive disturbances often accompany nervous tension and anxiety. A better herb than ginger cannot be found to treat digestive disorders. Ginger assists almost every aspect of digestion. It stimulates saliva and bile production; prevents nausea, gas and bloating; improves peristalsis by toning the intestinal muscle; and optimizes friendly intestinal flora. Its ability to stimulate circulation makes the other herbs of this formula more effective. Ginger root activates the body's cleansing and detoxifying systems through its diuretic, diaphoretic (promotes perspiration) and digestive properties. Ginger root's therapeutic value is officially recognized in Britain, Belgium, and France. HOPS: Hops is widely cultivated in North and South America, England, Germany and Australia for use in beer production. It has been so used for over a thousand years. Perhaps for just as long, hops has been used medicinally to treat restlessness, anxiety and sleep disorders.[11] Hops is officially recognized in Britain, Belgium, France and Germany. SKULLCAP: Skullcap has proven itself useful for sleep disorders, nervous conditions, tremors, and spasms. It has the ability to calm an excited nervous system.[12] In earlier years it enjoyed official recognition in the *United States Pharmacopeia* and the *National Formulary*. Skullcap is still officially recognized in Europe to treat epilepsy, hysteria, nervous tension and insomnia. CHAMOMILE: While chamomile has been modestly employed in this country as a tea and in other health preparations, it does not even approach the success found in western and eastern Europe, especially Germany, where it is considered to be a panacea. Chamomile has been extensively researched where it has demonstrated usefulness in sleep and digestive disorders. It is carminative or settling to the gastrointestinal tract, but also mildly stimulating to the bowel without being a true laxative. It is officially recognized in Britain, Belgium, France, and Germany. BLESSED THISTLE: Blessed thistle plays a supporting role in this formula. It helps activate a sluggish liver and correct stomach and digestive problems, flatulence and tension headaches. It further supports the body's cleansing and detoxifying systems by promoting perspiration and removing excess fluids. Britain, Germany and Belgium officially recognize its medicinal value.

SECONDARY NUTRIENTS

NEROLI OIL: A natural sedative and antidepressant which has been used traditionally as a remedy for hysteria. It also helps to control heart palpitations. *Suggested Use:* In aromatherapeutic applications or as a massage agent.

VERVAIN: Considered a relaxing nerve tonic. *Suggested Dosage:* Use as directed.

L-GLUTAMINE: Works to gently tranquilize the central nervous system. *Suggested Dosage:* 1,500 mg divided into three doses on an empty stomach with fruit juice.

GABA: Helps to nourish the brain and is essential for brain cell health. *Suggested Dosage:* Take as directed.

Home Care Suggestions

◆ Find support groups that have been organized to provide a forum for sharing feelings and contributing to overcoming phobias through a network of mutual sharing and counseling. Your local mental health organization will have a number of support groups that you can contact.

◆ Learn to control your thoughts by conditioning yourself in moments of oncoming panic to invoke positive reassurances about the situation. A therapist or support group can provide a long list of possible and helpful phrases to use.

◆ When you feel a panic attack coming on, immediately recognize it for what it is and kick in a conditioned response such as singing a particular song, popping in a favorite tape, or counting backwards. Learn to help yourself. If your mind is powerful enough to create feelings of overwhelming panic when there is no real danger, then it is powerful enough to quell those fears.

◆ Exercise daily. Exercise is a wonderful outlet for pent-up tension or anxiety. Choose something you enjoy and learn to release your emotional fears in a constructive physical way such as jogging, swimming, rac-

quetball etc. If you feel you cannot leave your home, get a treadmill or pop in an aerobics tape.

◆ Get a regular massage for its relaxation value and if you feel an attack coming on, have your companion give you a deep shoulder and neck massage.

◆ Investigate therapies such as self-hypnosis, breathing exercises, music therapy, and biofeedback. Any of these may offer valuable advice on how to control the mind and subsequently the body in avoiding feelings of panic or anxiety.

◆ Aromatherapy may have some real benefit for anxiety disorder victims. Sniffing certain aromas can have the immediate affect of calming and relaxing the nerves and creating a feeling of well-being. Some of the smells which typically produce a state of happiness are cookies or bread baking, cinnamon and ginger, baby powder, a freshly cut lawn, etc., You may be able to find an aroma that is bottled and can be taken with you to help you feel calmer during times of stress.

◆ Become involved with community groups, church groups, etc., which give you something constructive to do that you enjoy. Teach adults how to read, visit the bedridden, get on a computer network, learn to serve others and concentrate on spiritual enrichment, and learn to truly love by connecting with a higher power.

Other Supportive Therapies

MEDITATION: Learning to meditate can help to dispel feelings of anxiety or tension while teaching us to focus on only what we want to think about. Mind control is an integral part of learning to deal with feelings of uncontrolled anxiety or panic.

VISUALIZATION: The ability to visualize situations which normally precede an attack and deal with time on a rational basis with alternative behaviors can help control anxiety disorders. In addition, bringing to mind certain images when confronted with feelings of panic can help dispel an attack.

CONTROLLED BREATHING: This discipline in invaluable for achieving relaxation amidst great or overwhelming stress and can be perfected with a little practice.

AROMATHERAPY: Certain fragrances like lavender can help dispel stress and promote a tranquilizing effect. Aromatic oils can be carried in one's purse or pocket for use outside the home.

Scientific Facts-at-a-Glance

While most anxiety disorders are linked to stress or other psychological factors, more evidence is mounting that physical disruptions in neurochemistry may be more responsible for triggering an attack than previously assumed. Norepinephrine is the neurotransmitter involved and may inadvertently initiate a cascade reaction of physiological events that create a feeling of panic. Suffering from deficiency of B-vitamins can clearly cause all sorts of abnormal emotional states, implying that what we eat profoundly affects our brain chemistry.

Spirit/Mind Considerations

Anyone who has trouble with panic or anxiety attacks believes that something terrible is about to happen to them when they have the least ability to control it. For this reason, going out in public is particularly frightening. Sometimes, people who are having a panic attack say or do irrational things and may refer to unseen sources of danger. As a result of their impaired social function, many panic attack victims become irritable, increasingly dependent on others, easily fatigued, withdrawn, frustrated and may suffer from insomnia or bad dreams. In severe cases, a sense of that the person feels cut off from themselves or from the real world may occur. It is vital to be empathetic to anyone who battles this disorder. Trying to diminish the reality of the fear will only serve to make the person feel worse. The power of prayer may also be of great worth here, although it is rarely suggested. Learning to pray in situations where emotions are involved can be very empowering.

Prevention

♦ If anxiety attacks run in your family, recognize them for what they are and if you experience one, be smart enough to educate yourself on anxiety disorders, get counseling if you need it and be determined enough not to let something like panic attacks compromise the quality of your life.

♦ Manage stress and learn to relax by setting aside a certain portion of each day for relaxation techniques.

♦ Eating well, getting exercise and becoming involved in enjoyable activities will go far in preventing the onset of anxiety.

Doctor's Notes

I can remember one of my pateints who was a 30-year-old woman who had a history of anxiety and mild depression. She had tried Ativan and Xanax, both prescription drugs that did help to control her anxiety but clouded her mind and interfered with her coordination. She came to me for some natural alternatives and we decided to use valerian root alone for a trial period. I warned her about the smell (dirty gym socks). She took one at 10 a.m. and one at 2 p.m. and found that her anxiety was cut in half. Subsequently, she tried a combination of valerian, chamomile, passionflower, and skullcap. While this formula is typically used for insomnia this woman took it during the day and experienced a significant calming sensation. She had the option of taking these every day or only the days when she felt particularly anxious.

Another 42-year-old male who was experiencing situational anxiety due to a buisness position found that he could not be effective at work and had difficulty sleeping at night. He didn't want to take anything that would impair his mental faculties, so we tried some kava kava. He was also given the choice to take it daily or as needed. For the first week or two he took one or two in the morning, one or two in the afternoon and then again in the evening if he needed to sleep. Over a period of two to three weeks, he started to take it only as needed. While he acknowledges that people who suffer from anxiety need help, he refutes the inevibility of potent and addicting drug therapy. In addition, I have found that teaching my pateints who suffer from stress-related disorders to do simple meditation exercises combined with herbal therapy can do them a world of good. Combining valerian with other herbs such as chamomile, hops, skullcap, and passionflower can help relieve both anxiety and sleep disorders. Valerian can also be combined with kava kava, which has shown in several studies to be as effective as prescription tranquilizers.

Anxiety disorders are also often linked to depression, which explains why allopathic prescriptions such as Prozac are used to treat both. Often, if depressive disorders improve, anxiety attacks will subside. This does not imply that the two disorders always come hand in hand. Some individuals suffer strictly from panic or anxiety attacks without experiencing any symptoms of depressive illness. I have found that exercising on a regular basis can actually benefit both conditions. In addition, taking up to two to three times the RDA for B-complex vitamins may be very helpful for some individuals. Being trained in a form of meditation such as tai chi or transcendental meditation can also be very useful.

Frequently general fatigue is a symptom of anxiety and stress. The more stressed and anxious we become, the more energy we use, consequently, the more fatigue we feel. In this case, natural nervine herbs with effective relaxation properties can be helpful. Valerian root or kava kava are good choices.

Another new and promising treatment for anxiety or panic attacks is in the form of NADH. Taking it in a reduced form at 5 mg per day on an empty stomach with 8 oz. of water can be very effective for some people who suffer from anxiety-related disorders.

There are many situations, both emotional and physical, which contribute to anxiety. Many people are intimately aware of the things that cause stress and try whenever possible to avoid them. However, when stress becomes chronic, it may ultimately become the cause of many mild to serious physical disorders: difficulty in breathing, headaches, back and neck tension, and muscle spasms. If relief is not found for the aforementioned problems, immune function may become impaired which may eventually lead to greater illness or disease.

Since taking medication will not alleviate the causes of anxiety, the treatment of it must focus on symptom reduction. By treating the symptoms of stress, a person will better be able to relax, be calm, and even sleep well. This will help the individual cope with the underlying causes of the anxiety, while keeping the body in a better, uncompromised state of health. Nature has provided botanicals comprising some of the best nervines, calming agents, and relaxants known to mankind with very little or no side effects. These herbs have expertly been brought together in this formula which will help treat everything from tension and spasms to insomnia and digestive disorders.

Additional Resources

The Phobia Society of America
133 Rollins Avenue, Suite 4B
Rockville, MD 20852-4004

Endnotes

1. L. Christiansen, et al., "Impact of a dietary change on emotional distress," Jour of Abn Psychol, 1985, 94: 565-79.

2. A. Kallner, "The influence of vitamin C status on the urinary excretion of catecholamines in stress," Human Nutr Cllin Nutri, 1983, 37: 447-52.

3. G.E. Abraham, "Nutrition and the premenstrual tension syndromes," Jour App Nutri, 1984, 36: 103-24.

4. S.P. James, et al., "Melatonin administered in insomnia, Neuropsychopharmacology, 1990, 3: 19-23. See also A.B. Dollins, et al., "Effect of pharmacological daytime doses of melatonin on human mood and performance," Psychopharmacol, 1993, 112: 490-96.

5. V. Schellenberg, et al., "Quantitative EEG monitoring in phtyo-and psychopharmacological treatment of psychosomatic and affective disorders," Schizophrenia Res, 1993, 9 (2,3): Abstract.

6. W.E. Scholine and H.D. Clausen, "On the effect of d,l-kavain: experience with neuronika," Med Klin, 1977, 72: 1301-06 and D. Lindenberg and H. Pitule-Scholdel, "D, L-kavin in comparison with oxazepam in anxiety disorders: A double-blind study of clinical effectiveness," Forschr med, 1990, 108: 49-50, 53-54.

7. H. Schubert, and P.Halama, "Depressive episode primarily unresponsive to therapy in elderly patients: efficacy of Ginkgo biloba in combination with antidepressants," Geria Forsch, 1993, 3: 45-53.

8. U. Boeters. "Treatment of autonomic dysregulation with valepotriates (valmane)," Muenchener Medizinische Wochenschrift. 37, 1873-1876, 1969. V. Kempinskas. "On the action valerian." Famakologii I Toksikologiia. 4(3): 305-309, 1964. See also R. Klich and b. Gladbach. "Childhood behavior disorders and their treatment." Medizinishce Welt, 26(25), 1251-1254, 1975.

9. Rebecca Flynn, MS and Mark Roest, Your Guide to Standardized Herbal Products, One World Press, Prescott Arizona: 1995: 61.

10. Daniel P. Mowrey. The Scientific Validation of Herbs. Keats Publishing, New Canaan, Connecticut: 1986, 193. T.V. Zinchenko, and I.M. Fefer. "Investigation of glycosides from betonica officinalis," Farmatsevt A-Zhurnal. 17(3), 35-38, 1962.

11. Mowrey, 164-65.

12. B.A. Kurnakov, "Pharmacology of skullcap," Farmakologiia I Toksikologiia,. 20(6): 79-80, 1957.

ARTERIOSCLEROSIS

SEE "CORONARY HEART DISEASE"

ARTHRITIS

Arthritis is a condition characterized by an inflammation of a joint with accompanying pain, swelling, stiffness and redness. The term does not refer to just one disease, but rather to a number of joint disorders which can develop from a number of different conditions. Osteoarthritis, which is a natural consequence of aging joints, attacks the knees, hips, and fingers. It occurs when the cartilage cushion which lines the joints becomes stiffer and rougher; consequently, bone can actually overgrow the joint area, causing swelling and decreased mobility. In its final stages, the pain may actually subside; however the joint is no longer functional. Rheumatoid arthritis is the most severe type of the disease and is classified as an autoimmune disorder. The body's immune system acts against the joints and surrounding tissue the same way it would attack an unwanted invader. Joints in the hands, feet and arms become extremely painful, stiff and eventually deformed. This type of arthritis can effect the entire body. Gout is a disorder associated with a type of arthritis in which uric acid, a waste product, accumulates as crystals in the joints and causes inflammation.

Arthritis may be limited to only one joint or may affect many. It can range from mild aching to severe, debilitating pain, which can result in eventual joint deformities. It is the leading cause of physical disability in the United States. Approximately 50 million people suffer from the disorder. Types of arthritis include osteoarthritis, rheumatoid, ankylosis spondylitis, psoriatic arthritis, Reiter's syndrome, gout, systemic lupus, juvenile rheumatoid arthritis, infectious arthritis, Kawasaki syndrome and lyme disease.

Symptoms

Those who suffer from arthritis typically encounter symptoms like early morning stiffness, swelling, recurring tenderness in one or more joints, changes in joint mobility, redness or a feeling of warmth in joints, unexplained weight loss, fever or weakness.

In cases of rheumatoid arthritis, symptoms may disappear during periods of remission. Damp weather and emotional stress do not cause arthritis but do seem to worsen its symptoms. Also, lyme disease, which is caused by a tick bite, can be misdiagnosed as arthritis.

Causes

Arthritis may be caused by a number of physiological conditions which include endocrine disorders, a defect in the immune system, genetic predisposition, a complication of other diseases, the result of an infection, injury or surgery, excessive mobility, age-related changes in the joints, altered biochemistry, food sensitivities and a lack of HCL (hydrochloric acid).

Conventional Therapies

Drug therapy, exercise and rest comprise conventional medical treatment for the disease. There is no known cure for arthritis. Frequently, nonsteroidal anti-inflammatory drugs will be prescribed for pain control. Some studies have indicated that the use of nonsteroidal anti-inflammatory drugs successfully suppress the symptoms of arthritis but may actually accelerate the progression of the disease. If you feel you must use prescription or over-the-counter medication, ask your doctor about using the drug carafate, which is commonly prescribed for ulcers. It can give the same relief as aspirin or an anti-inflammatory without stomach lining damage.

Recently, hip and knee replacements used in advanced stages of arthritis have proven to be quite effective and should be discussed with a physician as a last resort measure. Synovectomy involves the removal of diseased synovial membrane which surrounds the joint. Several orthopedic procedures can help to realign deformed fingers or toes.

Dietary Guidelines

◆ Avoid foods such as white potatoes, tomatoes, peppers, eggplant, and milk products.
◆ Avoid red meat, which causes uric acid build up and can cause joint inflammation.
◆ Increase your intake of carrots, celery, cabbage, fresh grapefruit or tomato juice.
◆ Decrease vegetable oils high in omega-6 fatty acids. Olive oil and canola oil may be used in moderation. Lower your intake of dietary fat.
◆ A low-sodium diet helps counteract water retention in tissues which can aggravate the swelling that accompanies arthritic inflammation.
◆ Do not take iron supplements; high iron levels have been associated with joint pain.
◆ Make sure to rule out food allergies as a cause of chronic joint pain.

Recommended Nutritional Supplements

PRIMARY NUTRIENTS

GLUCOSAMINE/CHONDROITIN SULFATE These compounds comprise the building blocks of joint cartilage and have recently accrued some impressive credentials in not only alleviating symptoms, but promoting cartilage repair as well. This duo is quickly replacing the use of NSAIDs among many arthritis sufferers. It is better absorbed than cartilage extracts.[1] *Suggested Dosage:* Take as directed using both compounds together.

MARINE LIPIDS Cod liver oil or salmon oil contain omega-3 fatty acids which provide substantial amounts of vitamin D, important for bone growth, and vitamin A, which act as an anti-inflammatory agent. The EPA (eicosapentaenoic acid) content of coldwater fish can significantly decrease pain and swelling.[2] *Suggested Dosage:* Take as directed and add a vitamin E supplement when taking fish oils.

GAMMA LINOLENIC ACID (GLA) Treatment of arthritic symptoms with GLA has provided impressive results, with as much as a 30-percent improvement in some studies. GLA is derived from borage oil and evening primrose oil and can even reduce synovitis.[3] *Suggested Dosage:* Take as directed. Therapeutic doses may be higher than normal preventative doses.

NADH Compounds containing niacinamide are believed to enhance glucocorticoid secretion which can decrease pain and increase mobility.[4] *Suggested Dosage:* Take only as directed. High doses can cause a number of negative side effects.

GRAPESEED EXTRACT Also known as pcynogenol, this compound contains proanthocyanidins, which scavenge free radicals caused by inflammation. *Suggested Dosage:* Take as directed.

BROMELAIN AND PROTEOLYTIC ENZYMES These compounds help to counteract inflammation and reduce swelling. *Suggested Dosage:* Take as directed before meals.

CARTILAGE EXTRACTS Animal cartilage contains a protein that inhibits the development of blood vessels that nourish tumor growth. This mechanism may help to discourage the inflammatory process that takes place in joints as well.[5] *Suggested Dosage:* Take as directed remembering that this therapy takes time to establish itself. Six to eight weeks is initially recommended.

BORON One's intake of boron may be correlated to developing osteoarthritis. In addition, boron supplementation has proven its effectiveness in producing a remission of arthritic symptoms.[6] *Suggested Dosage:* No more than 3 mg per day.

L-CYSTEINE This particular amino acid may be deficient in people with arthritis.[7] *Suggested Dosage:* Take as directed on an empty stomach with fruit juice.

GLYCOSAMINOGLYCANS This compound, which has been isolated from bovine cartilage, has shown marked therapeutic value in treating arthritis. Controlled studies confirm its ability to actually inhibit joint destruction.[8] *Suggested Dosage:* Take as directed.

SUPEROXIDE DIMUSTASE This compound has been tested in various clinical trials and can help to inhibit joint inflammation, function, range of motion and mobility.[9] *Suggested Dosage:* Take as directed. Sublingual forms or injections may be more effective than capsules.

COPPER AND ZINC A correlation between low copper and zinc levels and arthritis has been established.[10] Moreover, zinc helps with proper bone development. *Suggested Dosage:* Use picolinate products and don't exceed over 50 mg of each mineral per day.

ACIDOPHILUS A 1995 study further supports the notion that intestinal derangements can cause arthritic symptoms. An imbalance in the microflora found in the bowel can cause antigen activity that targets the joints.[11] *Suggested Dosage:* Take as directed on an empty stomach in the morning and at night. Look for products with guaranteed bacterial count.

VITAMIN A AND VITAMIN B6 Necessary for the production of collagen and for the nourishment of bone cartilage tissue. Deficiencies in these vitamins can cause joint deterioration. *Suggested Dosage:* Take no more than 10,000 IU of vitamin A and 50 mg of vitamin B6 per day.

VITAMIN C WITH BIOFLAVONOIDS Some studies have confirmed that people with rheumatoid arthritis are deficient in vitamin C. The toxicity of vitamin C is very low and it is believed to bring about some degree of regression in the disease.[12] Vitamin C also helps to strengthen capillary walls in the joints and to counteract bleeding; consequently, it may be beneficial in conjunction with aspirin therapy. *Suggested Dosage:* 5,000 to 10,000 mg per day in divided doses with meals.

VITAMIN E AND SELENIUM May inhibit prostaglandin production, which causes inflammatory response. Clinical studies with people suffering from osteoarthritis have also proven its analgesic effect.[13] Selenium acts as a free radical scavenger and can help relieve pain and increase blood levels of glutathione.[14] *Suggested Dosage:* Take 200 mg of selenium and up to 1,200 IU of vitamin E per day, using organic varieties.

PANTOTHENIC ACID A deficiency of this acid in rats appeared to cause a failure in the growth of cartilage and initiated arthritis-like symptoms. Supplementation can help alleviate symptoms, especially in cases of rheumatoid arthritis.[15] *Suggested Dosage:* 500 mg per day.

HERBAL COMBINATION This combination should include devil's claw, yucca, alfalfa, wild yam root, sarsaparilla root, kelp, white willow bark, cayenne, and horsetail. *Suggested Dosage:* Four to six capsules daily. For extreme cases it is best to use maximum dosage of six capsules per day for a prolonged period of four to six months.

DEVIL'S CLAW: Don't let the name of this herb scare you off. The secondary roots of this plant have a rich history of use as an anti-inflammatory, analgesic and digestive stimulant. There is probably no other herb with a greater reputation for treating rheumatism than devil's claw. It has gained official recognition as an antirheumatic and digestive agent in many European countries, including France, Germany, Belgium, and Britain.[16] Improper digestion can affect joints in that undigested proteins called peptides can trigger an inappropriate immune response. Sometimes the body considers peptides to be a foreign substance, or antigen, and in response produces antibodies or larger amounts of histamine. Some people have found that when they improve the health of their digestive system, rheumatic symptoms disappear. YUCCA: Yucca has a similar action to that of devil's claw. It improves digestion, thereby reducing histamine production and, as a result, flammation and pain may be alleviated. The constituents of yucca which are bioactive are saponins.[17] ALFALFA LEAVES AND SEEDS: As mentioned in the previous two paragraphs, rheumatism may be a result of poor digestion. An impaired digestive system can cause malnutrition by starving the body of much needed macronutrients and micronutrients. If allowed to become chronic, serious and debilitating diseases can be the consequence. Alfalfa leaves and seeds provide a rich nutrient source to help the body to return to a healthy state.[18] WILD YAM ROOT: Other common names for wild yam root include rheumatism root and colic root, suggesting its use as an antirheumatic and digestive aid. Its antirheumatic property is primarily thought to be attributed to its cortisone precursor diosgenin. As diosgenin is converted to cortisone, anti-inflammatory activity results, and the patient may notice a reduction of pain.[19] SARSAPARILLA ROOT: Sarsaparilla which is used as a food flavoring in the United States, is officially recognized in Germany and the United Kingdom for its antirheumatic, anti-inflammatory, and diuretic properties. Its activity is thought to be due to its saponin content. Historically, this herb has been used to treat gout and rheumatism and is classified as a tonic and blood purifier.[20] KELP: Kelp, like alfalfa, is a dense source of nutrients, particularly trace elements which can improve the body's nutrition. It also provides mucilage in the form of algin, which soothes the gastrointestinal tract. WHITE WILLOW BARK: White willow bark has been used for over a thousand years to relieve pain. Salicin, aspirin's forerunner, was discovered to be white willow's active constituent. Apart from its ability to assist with pain, salicin reduces inflammation, but unlike aspirin it will not thin the blood or irritate the stomach. CAYENNE: Cayenne stimulates circulation and makes the other herbs more effective. Cayenne can help to improve digestion. Cayenne's "hot" principle, capsaicin, is also a noted analgesic and can be applied in topical ointment form. HORSETAIL (SHAVE GRASS): While horsetail contributes to this formula as a mild diuretic, its main action is to strengthen and regenerate connective tissues. Connective tissue (found abundantly in joints) is destroyed by inflammation. Silica is vital in regenerating connective tissue and keeping it strong. Horsetail is one of the richest known sources of silica.

SECONDARY NUTRIENTS

GERMANIUM: An antioxidant which can help scavenge free radicals which are created during the inflammatory process and contribute to joint destruction. *Suggested Dosage:* Take as directed.

FOLIC ACID: Some research has shown that victims of rheumatoid arthritis had lower blood levels of folic acid. *Suggested Dosage:* Take as directed.

CALCIUM PLUS MAGNESIUM: Helps to prevent bone loss and muscle cramping. *Suggested Dosage:* Take as directed using chelated, gluconate, citrate forms.

HISTIDINE: Has anti-inflammatory properties which can reduce pain and swelling. This amino acid is also used to stimulate tissue growth and repair. *Suggested Dosage:* Take as directed on an empty stomach with fruit juice.

METHIONINE: An essential amino acid that is important to the structure of cartilage and can act as a natural anti-inflammatory. *Suggested Dosage:* Take as directed on an empty stomach with fruit juice.

CAT'S CLAW: From the Peruvian rainforest, this herb has impressive anti-inflammatory properties. *Suggested Dosage:* Take as directed, however do not use if you have had an organ transplant, are pregnant or nursing.

CAPSAICIN OINTMENTS: These capsicum-based ointments can help to stimulate circulation and warm affected joints. *Suggested Use:* Begin with a small amount and expect reddening of the area, which will subside with continued use. Keep away from mucus membranes and eyes.

Home Care Suggestions

◆ If you smoke, stop. Smoking is directly related to contracting and aggravating arthritis in males.

◆ A combination of rest and exercise is beneficial; however, long periods of bed rest may increase stiffness and muscle deterioration. At the same time excessive exercise can promote increased joint inflammation. A regimen should be designed with your doctor to suit your needs. Stretching, strengthening and endurance exercises should be incorporated into the program.

◆ If your stomach can tolerate aspirin, it works as an inexpensive anti-inflammatory. Aspirin acts as a blood thinner and should be taken under a doctor's care.

◆ Ibuprofen is also an effective anti-inflammatory but should be used with caution to prevent stomach problems. Acetaminophen (Tylenol) is less effective as an anti-inflammatory.

◆ Heat administered as warm baths, hot tubs or wet compresses, helps relieve chronic pain.

◆ Hot wax treatments, where paraffin wax in melted and applied to painful joints is an old remedy which has proven helpful for some.

◆ Raw lemon rubs and hot castor oil packs are traditional treatments for arthritis.

◆ An ice bag may be used after acute pain or injury to the joint has occurred. Apply for 15 to 20 minutes, remove for 10 minutes.

◆ If you are overweight, stress on weight-bearing joints is a contributing factor to arthritis; therefore weight loss would be beneficial.

◆ Relaxation sessions through books and audio tapes can help alleviate muscle tightening and cramping.

◆ Floatation tanks or relaxed swimming produces pain relief through stress reduction. Pool exercises are also excellent.

◆ Physical therapy through the use of exercise, heat, cold, diathermy, ultrasound, etc., are all beneficial in improving the mobility of the joints and will help to reduce pain to some extent.

◆ Use a good muscle ointment at night before going to bed to help with morning stiffness.

◆ Regular eucalyptus ointment massages can feel wonderful and help to alleviate stiffness and pain.

Other Supportive Therapies

ACUPUNCTURE: There are various trigger points which can be stimulated to help control pain and inflammation.

MASSAGE: Massaging joints with essential oils can help restore mobility and relax tense muscles, which further restrict motion. Care must be taken not to massage too deeply, as joint irritation can be aggravated.

CHIROPRACTIC: For some people, chiropractic adjustments can help alleviate joint pain.

HYDROTHERAPY: Using warm water immersion followed by cold can help control swelling and inflammation. Use cold compresses if the joint is inflamed, followed by alternating hot and cold.

Scientific Facts-at-a-Glance

A team of anesthesiologists at the General Hospital in Denmark have recently discovered that acupuncture can significantly improve joint mobility and reduce pain in patients suffering from arthritis in the knee joint. Classic Chinese acupuncture points were used and the needle method was employed. Unquestionably, skilled acupuncture can reduce pain and improve joint movement in other areas and should be investigated as a treatment option that is preferable to taking pain drugs. Another study conducted by the national public health institute in Finland has found that male smokers have about eight times the risk of developing rheumatoid arthritis as nonsmokers. Exposure to tobacco smoke may trigger the production of rheumatoid factors that, when combined with male hormone, may contribute to the development of arthritis.

Spirit/Mind Considerations

As is the case with most ailments, learning to completely relax the body through meditation can help to relieve pain and stiffness. Arthritis sufferers must learn to deal with pain on a daily basis. Becoming spiritually focused can help the body cope with stress. Pain is an inevitable part of this life. Spritiual direction can help us get past pain and to even glean from it. While none of us want to become incapacitated, turning our focus to the spirit can help us to manage pain. Sometimes we need to surrender our pain or affliction to our God and learn to be more trusting.

Prevention

◆ Risk factors for arthritis include obesity, lack of exercise, or injury to a joint. Keeping fit with a regular exercise program, watching your weight and protecting joints from injury, are all effective preventative measures.

◆ Eat a diet that is low in animal fats and proteins to avoid creating a build up of uric acid, which can cause painful joint conditions.

Doctor's Notes

I feel strongly that improper digestion or food intolerances can significantly contribute to arthritic symptoms. A recent study confirmed this idea by investigating the relationship between fasting and arthritic symptoms. The study suggests that the development of arthritis, autoimmune diseases, celiac disease and inflammatory bowel disorders are due to food sensitivities, which cause certain molecules to permeate through the intestinal wall, triggering unwanted immune reactions.[21] Of even more interest is that NSAIDs can actually increase intestinal permeability to food antigens, making a bad situation even worse.[22] Using the herbal blend listed in this section in combination with glucosamine/chondroitin, marine lipids, NADH and grapeseed extract can help alleviate the symptoms of inflammation and pain and also to provide a rich nutrient base to help the body's healing process. Medical science has only addressed arthritic symptoms and has been remiss in finding compounds that actually help to heal the joint and prompt the regeneration of cartilage. New compounds designed to treat arthritis this way are currently under formulation. Nature has provided us with a number of very healing medicines which target both relieving pain and augmenting tissue regeneration. In addition it is important to reduce stress on the joints. For many people, this means losing weight. I have seen this one change profoundly improve symptoms for overweight people with arthritis. Often it is just a matter of a 10 to 20 pound weight loss. I am also impressed with the action of glucosamine sulfate and chondroitin sulfate.

In cases of rheumatoid arthritis, which is considered both a connective tissue and autoimmune disease, the body is attacking itself. For this type of joint disease, immune function must be normalized. Using astragalus, a Chinese herb, is good in combination with shark and bovine cartilage. Refer to the section of boosting immunity for more information.

Additional Resources

The Arthritis Foundation
1314 Spring St. NW
Atlanta, GA 30309
(800) 283-7800

Endnotes

1. Y. Vidal, et al., "Articular cartilage pharmacology: In vitro studies on glucosamine and nonsteroidal anti-inflammatory drugs," Pharmacol Res Commun, 1978, 10 (6): 557-69. See also J.M. Pujalte, et al., "Double-blind clinical evaluation of oral glucosamine sulfate in the basic treatment of osteoarthritis," Curr, Med Res Opin, 1980, 7 (2): 110-14.

2. T. Stammers, et al., "Fish oil in osteoarthritis," Letter in Lancet, 1989, 2: 503. Fish oils also compete with certain fatty acids that are thought to trigger arthritis inflammation.

3. L.J. Leventhal, E.G. Boyce and R.B. Zurier, "Treatment of arthritis with gamma linolenic acid," Ann Intern Med, 1993, 119: 867-73.

4. W. Kaufman, "The use of vitamin therapy to reverse certain concomitants of aging," Jour Amer Geriatric Soc, 1955, 3: 927. See also A.B. Schneider, "Stereometric evaluation of the myocardial cardiomyocyte-capillary ration of thiamine and nicotinamide," Jour Kardiologiia, 1989, 29 (4): 97-99.

5. J.F. Prudden and L.L Balassa, "The biological activity of bovine cartilage preparations," Semin Arthritis Rheum, 1974, 3 (4): 287-321.

6. R.L. Travers, et al., "Boron and arthritis: The results of a double-blind pilot study," Jour Nutri Med, 1990, 1: 127-32.

7. M.X. Sullivan and W.C. Hess, "Cystine content of finger nails in arthritis," Jour Bone Joint Surg, 1935, 16: 185.

8. V. Rejholec, "Long-term studies of antiosteoarthritic drugs: an assessment," Semin Arth Rheum, 1987, supple 1,17 2: 35-53.

9. L. Flohe, "Superoxide dismustase for therapeutic use: clinical experience, dead ends and hopes," Mol Cell Biochem, 1988, 82 (2): 123-31.

10. D.M. Grennan, et al., "Serum copper and zinc in rheumatoid arthritis and osteoarthritis," N. Z. Med Jour, 1980, 91 (652): 47-50

11. M.P Hazenberg, "Intestinal flora bacteria and arthritis: why the joint?" Scand Jour Rheuma 24 1995, supple 101: 207-11.

12. E.R. Scheartz, "The modulation of osteoarthritic development by vitamins C and E," Int Jour Vita Res Suppl, 1984, 26: 141-46.

13. I. Machtey, and L. Ouaknine, "Tocopherol in osteoarthritis: A controlled pilot study during placebo administration," jour Amer Geriatric Soc, 1978, 26: 328.

14. A. Bruce, et al., "The effect of selenium and vitamin E on glutathione peroxidase levels and subjective symptoms in patients with arthrosis and rheumatoid arthritis," in Proceedings New Zealand Workshop on Trace Elements in New Zealand, 1981, Dunedin, University of Otago, 92.

15. J.C. Annand, "Pantothenic acid and osteoarthritis," Letter, Lancet, 1963, 2: 1168.

16. L.R. Brady, et al., Pharmacognosy, 8th ed. Lea and Gebiger, Philadelphia, 1981: 480.

17. R. Bingham, et al., "Yucca plant saponins in the management of arthritis," Jour Applied Nutrition, 1975, 27: 45-50.

18. M.R. Malinow, et al., "Effect of alfalfa saponins on intestinal cholesterol absorption in rats," Amer Jour Clini Nutri, 1977, 30: 2061-67.

19. H.W. Feller, The Eclectic Materia Medica, Pharmacology and Therapeutics, Eclectic Medical Publications, Portland Oregon: 1983, first published in 1922.

20. Kiangsu Institute of Modern Medicine, Encyclopedia of Chinese Drugs, 2 vols. 1977, Shanghia, People's Republic of China.

21. L. Skoldstam and K.E. Magnusson, "Fasting, intestinal permeability, and rheumatoid arthritis," Rheum Dis Clin N Amer, 1991, 17 (2): 363-71.

22. I. Bjarnason, et al., "Intestinal permeability and inflammation in rheumatoid arthritis: Effects of nonsteroidal anti-inflammatory drugs," Lancet, 1984, 2: 1171-74.

ASTHMA

Asthma is a episodic respiratory disease characterized by recurring attacks of breathlessness, which are usually accompanied by wheezing upon exhaling. Two primary classifications of asthma exist: extrinsic, in which an allergy causes the attack, and intrinsic, when no apparent external cause can be found. During an asthma attack, the bronchiole tubes, found deep within the lungs, constrict as a result of a kind of muscle contraction. In addition, mucus is produced, which can block the smaller tubes and trap in stale air. An asthma attack can vary in its severity, and is typically hard to predict. An attack can last from less than an hour to over a week. Recurrences are inconsistent and, while they can be triggered by certain allergens, sometimes occur for no apparent reason.

More than 10 million Americans suffer from asthma, with 4 million being children. Asthma can occur in toddlers, and in some cases will disappear with time. Over half of children suffering from asthma will outgrow the disease. The incidence of asthma is higher for boys. The disease is rarely fatal; however, a bad attack can be extremely frightening. Asthmatic incidences are responsible for over 8 million lost school days each year. Interestingly, asthma is becoming more prevalent in the US and other developed countries, suggesting a link with environmental pollutants typically found in industrial nations. Asthma is considered an incurable disease; however, attacks can be avoided or relieved with treatment. People who suffer from allergies frequently have asthma also. The type of asthma that only occurs during periods of physical stress belongs in a category all its own.

Symptoms

An asthma attack comes on quickly and is usually unexpected. The most obvious symptoms of asthma are difficult breathing, a feeling of tightness in the chest without actual pain, wheezing which can either be easily heard or only detectable with a stethoscope, more difficulty exhaling than inhaling or increased anxiety.

Coughing can accompany an asthma attack due to the presence of mucus.

Severe attacks can cause sweating, rapid pulse rate, bluishness in the face and lips, hunched-over position in order to facilitate breathing or an inability to speak.

Precautions

During an acute attack try to find any inhalers or drugs the asthmatic usually takes. Help the asthmatic find a comfortable position which is commonly sitting up and leaning slightly forward. Stay calm and be reassuring. Call the appropriate physician, if necessary and in severe cases, drive the person to the hospital or call for an ambulance if transportation is not possible.

Causes

In most cases asthma is caused by allergens such as pollen, cat dander, feathers, cigarette smoke, certain foods, molds, certain drugs (especially aspirin), vigorous exercise typically in cold air, a period of emotional stress or upset, laughing too hard, crying, anger or sadness, psychological anxiety or exertion, changes in temperature, the presence of cold humid air, hair spray, paint thinners, bleach, perfumes, etc.

A strong disposition for asthma can run in families. Frequently, no specific reason for a particular asthma attack can be found, and many asthmatics breathe normally in between attacks. In cases of chronic asthma, emphysema can develop. The whys and wherefores of asthma are not fully understood. Bronchiole tube constriction is controlled by nerves that often constrict for no apparent reason.

Conventional Therapies

Typically your doctor will want to find out if an allergen is causing your asthma. If so, immunotherapy in the form of allergy shots may be recommended; however, this particular treatment remains controversial and often is not successful. The most effective use of allergy shots seems to be for asthmatics who are allergic to pet danders and grasses.

Commonly Prescribed Medications

CORTISONE: Used in liquid, tablet, or aerosol spray and come in the form of: beclomethasone (vanceril, beclovent,), triamcinolone, medrol and decadron. All cortisone derivatives are steroid drug therapies and must be carefully monitored in that they come with significant side effects.

BRONCHODILATOR INHALERS: These drugs are used in aerosol form or in metered dose inhalers. They work like adrenalin and include isoetharine, albuterol, metaporternol, and isoproterenol.

THEOPHYLLINE BRONCHODILATORS: Help to relax and open airways and are fast acting. Most individuals with chronic asthma use this type of sustained-release drug therapy. Most bronchodilating inhalers can become somewhat addictive and the cycle of constricting and dilation can be aggravated as in the case of some nasal sprays designed to shrink swollen sinus passages.

EPINEPHRINE OR ADRENALINE: Given through injection or inhalation, the effect is almost immediate. Because of its side effects, this treatment is usually used only in severe cases and must be overseen by a physician.

If the asthma attack is severe enough to require hospitalization, an intravenous injection of aminophylline may be administered. A fine mist breathing apparatus may also be used to administer drugs. The use of a mechanical respirator in conjunction with muscle relaxants is another option.

Dietary Guidelines

◆ Eliminate milk and milk products from your diet. Dairy products can trigger allergic reactions. In addition milk proteins can increase the production of mucous secretions in the bronchiole passageways. Check ingredient labels for nonfat dry milk.

◆ Diet should be composed mainly of fresh fruits, vegetables, oatmeal, sprouts, onions, garlic and honey, and complex carbohydrates.

◆ Beware of food additives such as MSG and metacisulfite, which can bring on an attack. Sulfites are commonly found in beer, wine, shrimp and dried fruits, potato chips and sausages. Consult the section on food allergies for more on sulfite sensitivities. Also avoid BHA and BHT, food additives, FDC yellow dye no. 5 and tryptophan.

◆ Avoid ice cold beverages and ice cream. Extreme cold can sometimes trigger an asthma attack.

◆ Watch culprit foods such as eggs, wheat, nuts, and seafood.

◆ Decrease your intake of salt, which can promote fluid retention.

Recommended Nutritional Supplements

PRIMARY NUTRIENTS

VITAMIN C WITH BIOFLAVONOIDS Calms inflammation and stabilize histamine release from mast cells. Tests show that asthmatics have lower levels of vitamin C.[1] *Suggested Dosage:* Take bioflavonoids as directed with up to 10,000 mg of vitamin C per day in divided doses with meals.

PANTOTHENIC ACID Helps to mediate allergic histamine responses and combat stress.[2] *Suggested Dosage:* 150 mg per day divided in three doses.

CALCIUM/MAGNESIUM Some research has implied that low magnesium levels may play a role in some types of asthma, and may be linked to mucus production and may help to dilate constricted bronchiole passageways.[3] *Suggested Dosage:* 1,000 mg of calcium and 500 mg of magnesium per day. Use chelated varieties for better absorption.

MARINE LIPIDS (EPA AND DHA) Helps to inhibit prostaglandin production, which aggravates inflammation thought to trigger asthmatic episodes. Tests have shown that taking EPA and DHA capsules significantly decreased shortness of breath.[4] *Suggested Dosage:* Take as directed, making sure to add a vitamin E supplement. Make sure to check with your physician if your suffer from diabetes or high blood pressure before taking fish oil.

L-CYSTEINE Tests have shown that supplementation with this amino acid resulted in a reduction of asthmatic medication.[5] *Suggested Dosage:* Take as directed on an empty stomach with fruit juice.

NICOTINAMIDE This nutrient can help to alleviate asthmatic symptoms with oral supplementation. It is also believed that asthmatics may be niacin deficient.[6] *Suggested Dosage:* Take as directed.

VITAMIN B6 Can be low in asthmatics and supplementation can help to significantly improve symptoms especially in childhood asthma.[7] *Suggested Dosage:* Sublingual or injections are available.

VITAMIN B12 Oral vitamin B12 was used in a clinical trial to combat sulfite reactions and asthmatic symptoms and was concluded to be more effective than pharmaceutical drugs in blocking asthmatic reactions.[8] *Suggested Dosage:* Look for sublingual varieties or ask you doctor about vitamin B12 injections.

VITAMIN A Helps to stimulate tissue regeneration and boost the immune system. *Suggested Dosage:* Do not exceed 10,000 IU per day.

VITAMIN E WITH SELENIUM Works to scavenge free radicals from bronchiole tissue. In addition, asthmatics may be low in selenium.[9] *Suggested Dosage:* Take no more than 600 IU of vitamin E per day. Take selenium as directed.

HERBAL COMBINATION This combination should include pleurisy root, wild cherry bark, slippery elm bark, plantain, mullein leaves, horehound, and licorice root. *Suggested Dosage:* Four to eight capsules daily. For chronic conditions it is best to use maximum dosage of eight capsules per day for a prolonged period of three to six weeks or until symptoms subside.

PLEURISY ROOT: The English word *pleurisy* comes from the French word *pleurisis*, which means, "lung trouble," indicating a primary use for this herb. Technically, pleurisy is an inflammatory condition affecting a thin lining covering the lungs and thorax and is usually a complication of pneumonia, tuberculosis, and other infectious diseases.[12] This root has been used for other respiratory problems including bronchitis and catarrh. WILD CHERRY BARK: Wild cherry bark has always been a favorite in cough and cold medicines.[13] However, its most effective action benefits asthmatics by relaxing or sedating the respiratory nerves. SLIPPERY ELM BARK: Slippery Elm bark has a reputation as a medicine for bronchitis, pleurisy and coughs.[14] It has received official recognition in the *United States Pharmacopeia*. The inner bark is known for its demulcent, diuretic and emollient properties attributable to its high mucilage content. PLANTAIN: Plantain is similar to Slippery Elm bark in that it too contains mucilage. Plantain is used as an expectorant and is especially good for those suffering chronic catarrhal problems.[15] MULLEIN LEAVES: Mullein leaves also contain high amounts of mucilage. While it is considered to be a good remedy for coughs, hoarseness, bronchitis, catarrh and whooping cough it stands out as an antispasmodic in treating asthma.[16] HOREHOUND: Horehound is an excellent remedy for coughs and bronchial problems. Its activity is thought to be attributed to a volatile oil called marubiin.[17]

Horehound helps to cleanse the body of toxins through its diuretic properties and ability to promote perspiration. LICORICE ROOT: Licorice root has received official recognition in Britain, Germany, France, and Belgium for its ability to assist with various respiratory problems which include bronchitis, hoarseness, coughs, sore throats, catarrh, and congestion.[18] It shares some of the same properties as other herbs of this formula in cleansing and healing through its mild diuretic and laxative properties. Do not use if pregnant, nursing, if you have diabetes, high blood pressure, glaucoma, menstrual disorders or history of stroke.

SECONDARY NUTRIENTS

COPPER AND ZINC: Deficiencies in these minerals have been linked to asthmatic episodes. *Suggested Dosage:* Take as directed only. Zinc is available in lozenge form.

GRAPE SEED EXTRACT (PYCNOGENOL): Is considered a powerful antioxidant agent and anti-inflammatory compound. *Suggested Dosage:* Take as directed.

GARLIC: Helps to move mucus congestion out of the lungs and works to fight respiratory infections. *Suggested Dosage:* Take as directed. Deodorized products are available.

ROMAN CHAMOMILE: Anti-inflammatory and antispasmodic which helps control allergic reactions in the respiratory tract. *Suggested Dosage:* Take as directed.

FENUGREEK: Helps to expectorate mucous and contributes to fighting infection. *Suggested Dosage:* Take as directed.

LOBELIA: Helps to relax and clear airways of mucous. Using lobelia extract in drops can help control attacks. Lobelia can cause nausea and should not be taken on an empty stomach. *Suggested Dosage:* Take only as directed never increasing the dosage and only take for a limited period of time. Do not use if pregnant or nursing.

Home Care Suggestions

- Avoid exposure to any offending substances, such as dust, molds, pollens, pet dander, chemicals, etc.
- Protect yourself against sudden blasts of cold air by covering your nose and mouth with a scarf.
- Keep a journal of every attack and the conditions which preceded it to determine if certain carpets, dust, fragrances etc, are responsible.
- Do not smoke and stay out of smoke-filled rooms.
- Stay away from products stuffed with animal hair or pillows stuffed with feathers.
- Be careful if starting a fire. Wood stoves and fireplaces can trigger an asthmatic attack due to smoke particulates which can be released into the room.
- Protect yourself against sudden blasts of cold air by covering your nose and mouth with a scarf.
- If you have exercise-induced asthma, build up slowly to the pace you wish to maintain, breathe through your nose so as not to dry out your throat, and use asthma medication 15 minutes prior to exercising. Swimming is an excellent exercise for asthmatics.
- Use pain relievers that are nonaspirin, preferably acetaminophen.
- Install an air purifier and central air-conditioning in your home.
- When in the car, use the air-conditioner on the recirculation setting, so as to not bring in pollens etc. from the outside.
- Watch the kinds of foods you eat.
- If you find yourself without medication and an attack is coming on, ingest caffeine in the form of strong coffee, etc., which may help to alleviate the intensity of the attack.
- Avoid antihistamines as they tend to dry out secretions, which may perpetrate the production of more mucous.
- Sleep in a propped-up position, which facilitates easier breathing.
- Certain yoga techniques have been found to be beneficial in practicing relaxed inhaling and exhaling.
- Drink plenty of water to keep the respiratory tract secretions as fluid as possible.

Other Supportive Therapies

ACUPUNCTURE: Seek the services of a qualified acupuncturist who can help to stimulate certain points which can calm lung inflammation and expedite the removal of mucus.

Scientific Facts-at-a-Glance

A number of studies usually not cited by traditional medicine indicate that low stomach acid may be linked to asthma in children. In addition food additives, including dyes, tartrazine (ornabe) yellow, amaranth, both reds and blue; preservatives such as sodium benzoate, 4-hydroxybenzoate, esters and sulphur dioxide, have also been linked to asthma attacks.[19]

Spirit/Mind Considerations

Intense negative emotions have been linked to asthma attacks, suggesting that certain types of volatile personalities may be more prone to triggering asthmatic episodes. For this reason, learning to control and dissipate feelings like anger, rage, tension, or hatred is very important. Moreover, all of these emotions contribute to the destruction of not only our physical well being, but our spiritual as well.

Prevention

- Prepare for exercise by easing into it.
- Avoid potential allergens found in food dyes, preservatives, junk foods, dairy products, dusts and pollens.
- Don't smoke.
- Don't expose your lungs to dangerous fumes or toxins.
- Use a humidifier to protect your lungs from hot, dry, irritating air.

Doctor's Notes

The same herbal formulas that are good for allergies are effective for asthma as well; however, these formulas are most efficient when *Ginkgo biloba* is added. Use a guaranteed potency form of 60 mg of 24 percent extract, two or three times a day. This dosage of ginkgo has been shown to reduce the severity of asthma attacks as well as their number. Ephedra, although much maligned, can also be very useful in treating asthma. Side effects associated with this herb have made it somewhat controversial; however, these are a problem only if the herb is misused or taken in large doses. Boswella also has some very beneficial therapeutic properties for asthma.

Respiratory distress can be caused by a wide variety of factors and can exhibit itself with many different symptoms. The herbal combination listed is designed to ameliorate the symptoms and assist in overcoming some of the underlying causes. Herbs have been used for respiratory ailment by various cultures all over the world for thousands of years. There is strong historical documentation for these particular applications.

Additional Resources

Asthma and Allergy Foundation of America
1717 Massachusetts Avenue, NW Suite 305
Washington, DC 20036
(800) 7-ASTHMA

Endnotes

1. S.O. Olusi, et al., "Plasma and white blood cell ascorbic acid concentrations in patients with bronchial asthma," Clinical chimica acta, 1979, 92: 161-66. See also R. Anderson, et al., "Ascorbic acid in bronchial asthma," Jour S A Med, 1983, 63: 649-52 and H. Ogasawara, et al., "Effect of selected flavonoids on histamine release and hydrogen peroxide generation by human leukocytes," Jour Aller Clini Immunol, 1985, 75: 184.

2. W. Martin, "On treating allergic disorders", Letter, Townsend Letter for Doctors, 1991, Aug/Sept, 670: 1.

3. G. Utz et al., "Oral application of calcium and vitamin D in allergic bronchial asthma," MMW, 1976, 118 (43): 1395-98. See also D. Falkner, et al., "Serum magnesium levels in asthmatic patients during acute exacerbations of asthma," A, Jour Emerg Med, 1992, 10 (1): 1-3..

4. J. Arm, et al., "The effects of dietary supplementation with fish oil on asthmatic responses to antigen," Jour Clin Allergy, 1988, 81: 183.

5. E.R. Braverman and C.C. Pfeiffer, The Healing Nutrients Within, Keats Publishing, New Canaan, Conn.: 1987).

6. E.F. Maisel and E. Somkin, "Treatment of asthmatic paroxysm with nicotinic acid," Jour Allergy, 1942, 13: 397-403. See also, J. Schwartz and S.T. Weiss, "Dietary factors and their reaction to respiratory symptoms," The Second national Health and Nutrition Examination Survey, Am Jour Epidemiol, 1990, 132 (1): 67-76.

7. P.J. Collip et al., "Pyridoxine treatment of childhood bronchiole asthma," Ann Allergy, 1975, 35: 93-97.

8. R.A. Simon et al., "Sulfite-sensitive asthma," Res Instit Scripps Clin Sci Rep, 1982-83, 39: 57-58.

9. A. Flatt et al., "Reduced selenium in asthmatic subjects in New Zealand," Thorax, 1990, 45 (2): 95-96.

10. D.J. Tinkelman and S.E. Avner, "Ephedrine therapy in asthmatic children," JAMA, 1977, 237, 553-57.

11. M. Koltai, et al., "Platelet activating factor (PAF) A review of its effects, antagonists and possible future clinical implications," Drugs, 1991, 42 (1): 9-29.

12. F.K. Fitzpatrick, "Plant substances active against mycobacterium tuberculosis," Antibiotics and Chemotherapy, 1954, 4 (5): 528-36.

13. H.H. Smith, Ethnobotany of the Ojibwe Indians, Bulletin of the Public Museum, vol, IV, No. 3 Milwaukee, 1932.

14. Ibid.

15. M. Matev, et al., "Clinical trial of a plantago major preparation in the treatment of chronic bronchitis," Vutreshni Bolesti (Sofia), 1982, 21 (2): 133-37.

16. R.N. Chopra. Et al., A Glossary of Indian Medicinal Plants, Council of Scientific and Industrial Research, 1956, New Delhi, India.

17. M.O. Karryev, et al., "Some therapeutic properties and phytochemistry of common horehound," Izvestiia Akad Nauk Truk SSSR, 1976, 3: 86-88.

18. D.M. Anderson, et al., "The antitussive activity of glycyrrhetinic acid and its derivatives," Jour Phar and Pharmacol, 1961, 13: 396-404.

19. G.W. Bray, "The hypochlorhydria of asthma in childhood," Quar Jour Med, 1931, 24: 181-97.

ATHLETE'S °FOOT

Athelete's foot is a common skin fungus that affects the feet, particularly between the toes, and at times the toenails. It is also referred to as "ringworm of the feet."

This fungus thrives in a warm, moist environments, which explains why it is so fond of shoes. The dark, closed habitat of most shoes provide the perfect location for fungal growth. Athlete's foot is extremely common during and after adolescence, and if left untreated, can attack the nail beds. If athlete's foot becomes severe enough, at least a month's worth of treatment is needed to overcome the fungus.

A condition called "dyshidrosis" may mimic athlete's foot. Eczema may also resemble athlete's foot; however, it will not usually attack the toe web between the fourth and fifth toe. If the nails are affected, obtaining a cure is more difficult and oral therapy may be required. Athlete's foot rarely strikes anyone under ten. If a child has apparent symptoms, consult a physician.

Symptoms

Athlete's foot is characterized by fungus present between the fourth and fifth toes, on the sides of the feet, or on the soles of the feet. It can also manifest itself in red, flaky, cracked, blistery, skin that itches; a burning sensation; and an unpleasant smell.

Exposure to sweat or water will make the top layer of skin appear white and soggy during infection.

Causes

Athelete's foot is caused by a form of ringworm fungus known as "dermatophyte." People who spend long periods of time in sweaty socks and shoes are susceptible, hence the name, athlete's foot. The fungus can also develop and spread in locker rooms and showers.

Using snug, poorly ventilated shoes can provide the ideal environment for the fungus to proliferate.

Athelete's foot is considered slightly contagious and can be contracted from others through the shedding of fragments of skin that have been infected.

It is also believed that the use of antibiotics, radiation or certain drugs which kill beneficial bacteria can facilitate the spread of the fungus. Immunity and susceptibility play a significant role in deterring the growth of the fungus.

Conventional Therapies

Over-the-counter antifungal preparations are usually effective in controlling athelete's foot. There are three general types containing either miconazole nitrate (Micatin products), tolnaftate (Aftate or Tinactin), or fatty acids, (Desenex). Tolnaftate is generally considered better in preventing than curing athlete's foot.

Using a 30 percent aluminum chloride solution is also beneficial for its drying properties and can be made up by your pharmacist. This should be used for two weeks after the infection is gone. Don't use this if the skin is raw or cracked, or intense stinging will occur. If the condition is persistent, a physician may prescribe haloprogin (halotex), ciclopirox (loprox), or ciclopirox (lotrimin) in a cream or ointment form. Creams can trap moisture. Another form of the medication may be preferable.

Dietary Guidelines

- ◆ Avoid a diet high in sugar. Sugar provides the perfect feeding medium for yeasts and fungi.
- ◆ Cut down on fatty foods, caffeine drinks, and empty calorie snack foods.
- ◆ Emphasize raw fruits and vegetables, lean meats, legumes and whole grains, and drink plenty of water.

Recommended Nutritional Supplements

PRIMARY NUTRIENTS

ACIDOPHILUS Replenishes friendly bacteria that can help to inhibit the growth of pathogenic organisms. Clinical studies support the fact that replacing this bacteria through supplementation can kill a number of yeast and other microorganisms.[1] *Suggested Dosage:* Can be found in live active culture yogurt or may be purchased in liquid or tablet form. Look for guaranteed bacterial count with bifidobacteria.

VITAMIN B-COMPLEX Contributes to tissue repair and boost immune defenses. *Suggested Dosage:* Use a high potency yeast-free product and take as directed.

VITAMIN C WITH BIOFLAVONOIDS Helps to strengthen the immune system and is important in connective tissue regeneration and capillary wall strength. *Suggested Dosage:* Take as directed, using up to 10,000 mg per day in divided doses with meals.

PAU D'ARCO A rainforest herb with significant antifungal properties. A study published in the *American Journal of Tropical Medicine and Hygiene* addressed the ability of dietary pau d'arco to protect against *Schistosoma mansoni*, an infection caused by worms which penetrate the skin. The tests found that taking lapachol (found in pau d'arco) orally resulted in its secretion onto the skin where it acted as a surface barrier to worm penetration.[2] The fact that decaying lapacho trees do not become moldy or mildewed also support the notion of its possessing antifungal properties. *Suggested Dosage:* Take as directed. Can be taken in capsulized form or as a strong tea.

TEA TREE OIL A strong antifungal oil for topical use only. This oil has proven its ability to kill athlete's foot in clinical trials as well or better than pharmaceutical drugs.[3] *Suggested Usage:* Use directly on the fungus once or twice a day. Not for oral ingestion.

HERBAL COMBINATION This formula should contain garlic, black walnut hull, and myrrh. *Suggested Dosage:* Four to eight capsules daily. Treatment should stop only after the infection is completely gone.

GARLIC: Garlic has been used for centuries to treat viral, bacterial, and parasitic infections. It has proven its ability to kill the athelete's foot fungus in scientific studies.[4] Garlic possesses the ability to prevent infection especially if it is one that is contracted through insect bites. When garlic is consumed in sufficient quantities (a gram per day), its odor can be detected through the pores of the skin, creating a natural insect repellent. BLACK WALNUT HULL: Black walnut hulls have been nearly as popular as garlic over the years in treating parasitic and fungal infections such as ringworm.[5] It possess some very powerful and interesting compounds and should be the study of more scientific research. MYRRH: A natural antibiotic, astringent and anti-fungal herb. Myrrh helps to further potentiate this formula and can also be made into a foot wash for topical application.

SECONDARY NUTRIENTS

VITAMIN A WITH BETA-CAROTENE: Helps to stimulate the immune system and also helps skin tissue to regenerate and heal. *Suggested Dosage:* Take as directed not exceeding 10,000 IU of vitamin A per day.

ESSENTIAL FATTY ACIDS: Promote skin healing. *Suggested Dosage:* Take as directed using evening primrose, borage, or flaxseed sources. Fish oils can also be used (take with vitamin E).

LIQUID CHLOROPHYLL: Acts as a blood purifier and is an excellent supplement for facilitating the removal of toxins caused by bacteria and fungi. *Suggested Dosage:* Take as directed.

THYME OIL: Helps to fight the infection and soothe inflammation. *Suggested Usage:* Six drops to a cup a water rubbed on the feet at least three times daily.

ALOE VERA GEL: Helps to soothe and heal irritated skin. *Suggested Usage:* Apply liberally, using pure, undiluted preparations.

Home Care Suggestions

◆ Avoid wearing vinyl or plastic shoes which do not allow for moisture evaporation. Leather and cotton are preferable to rubber or wool (which can also promote sweating).

◆ Sandals or canvas shoes are recommended while fighting the infection.

◆ Change your shoes every other day and make sure they air out. Likewise, change socks every day.

◆ Keep your toenails clean by using a wood orange stick rather than a metal nail file.

◆ A baking soda paste can also be beneficial. Make sure to rinse thoroughly and dry completely after an application.

◆ Wash the affected area with soap and water at least twice a day and dry thoroughly, especially between the toes.

◆ Use extra hot water when washing socks to control fungal infection.

◆ Use a powder preparation to help keep feet dry. To avoid the mess of applying powder directly, place it in a plastic bag, then put your foot in the bag and shake it around.

◆ Air your feet as much as possible. A hair blower can be used to dry both your feet and your shoes. Exposure to sunlight is also good.

◆ Foot compresses can be used to soothe the infected areas. Domeboro powder or burrow's solution can be used and are available without a prescription. Soak the area with a cotton cloth for at least 15 minutes.

◆ A saltwater foot soak may also prove beneficial. Use two teaspoons of salt per one pint of warm water. Soak for five to ten minutes, and dry thoroughly.

Other Supportive Therapies

MASSAGE: Foot massage can increase circulation which helps to fight infection.

ACUPUNCTURE: Applying pressure or stimulating certain points on the top of the foot is used to treat this type of infection.

Scientific Facts-at-a-Glance

Taking certain supplements on a daily basis can most definitely boost immune support. Zinc, vitamin B6 and vitamin C are crucial to thymic cell activity and a deficiency of any one of these nutrients can cause a drop in immunity.[6] Our bodies were designed to kill fungal infections; however, we live in a less-than-perfect world where our immune defenses are not continually supported by the level of nutrients we need to counteract the detrimental effects of stress, pollution, poor food choices, etc.

Prevention

◆ Keep your feet clean and dry.

◆ Using disinfectants on shower floors and locker rooms may help to avoid the condition.

◆ If you must walk in public shower areas, wear slippers or shower shoes to avoid coming in contact with the fungus.

◆ Nutritionists wholeheartedly agree that keeping the immune system strong through a healthy diet and lifestyle can provide protection against exposure to infection of any kind.

Doctor's Notes

When we battle a fungal infection, all we want to do is to hurry up and get rid of it. While killing the fungus may be effective, boosting the immune system is even better. In other words, the ideal scenario would be to keep our defenses working at an optimal level so that we are not susceptible to fungal or other types of infections. Many people are exposed to athlete's foot fungus every day and do not develop the disease. What this suggests is that it is possible through herbs, vitamins, diet, etc., to enhance our immune mechanisms so that we don't suffer from recurrent infections. So often pharmaceutical drugs are only temporary fixes for this type of infection and may even predispose us to recurring episodes.

Endnotes

1. E.B. Collins and P. Hardt, "Inhibition of Candida albicans by lactobacillus acidophilus," Jour Dairy Sci, 1980, 63: 830-32.

2. Frederick G. Austin, "Schistosoma Mansoni Chemoprophylaxis with Dietary Lapachol," The American Journal of Tropical Medicine and Hygiene, Vol. 23, no. 3, 1974: 412.

3. D.S. Buck, D.M. Nidorf and J.G. Addino, "Comparison of two topical preparations for the treatment of onychomycosis: Melaleuca alternifolia (Tea Tree) and clotrimazole," Jour Fam Prac, 1994, 38: 601-05.

4. M. Amer, M. Taha and Z. Tossen, "The effect of aqueous garlic extract on the growth of dermatophytes," Int Jour Dermatol, 1980. 19: 285-87.

5. A.Y. Leung, Chinese Herbal Remedies, Universe Books, New York: 1984.

6. W. Beisel, et al., "Single-nutrient effects of immunologic functions," JAMA, 1981, 245: 53-58.

ADD/HYPERACTIVITY

Attention deficit disorder is a condition that affects the central nervous system. Often the condition is referred to as "attention deficit and hyperactivity disorder" (ADHD), or can include hyperkinesis. It is a surprisingly common disorder which primarily affects children but can apply to adults as well. ADD has been diagnosed in 4 to 20 percent of school-age children, or approximately two million children in the United States. Boys are four times more likely to be hyperactive than girls. Today, we understand this disorder better and realize that it has its origin in biochemical imbalances. It is not a disorder which originated from parental shortcomings or because the child is bent on being difficult.

ADD usually becomes apparent by the age of three, although significant symptoms may not surface until child is in school. Frequently, ADD can significantly decrease or even disappear when the child reaches adolescence. Children with this disorder can become moody, depressed and sometimes even antisocial. It is heartening to know that in some cases, children with ADD who subjected their parents to a great deal of grief in their childhood become energetic and creative adults.

Symptoms

Symptoms of ADD or hyperactivity are characterized by a short attention span, impulsive behavior, inappropriate responses, and poor concentration.

ADD may be punctuated by other strange behaviors, including an inability to cope with stress, absentmindedness, temper outburst, sleep disturbances, inability to follow through or complete tasks, forgetfulness, speech or hearing impediments, head knocking, nail biting or other forms of self-injury, difficulty concentrating, inappropriate jumping and running, lack of coordination or neurological abnormalities, including electroencephalogram irregularities.

It is possible for a teacher to assume that a child has ADD when, in fact, the child may be suffering from poor vision, impaired hearing or a language problem.

Causes

The exact mechanisms involved in attention deficit disorder are not understood. There are a number of influences, however. Some of these include a genetic predisposition, drinking alcohol during pregnancy, smoking during pregnancy, drug use during pregnancy, heavy metal poisoning, food allergies, synthetic chemicals, oxygen deprivation, drastic swings in blood sugar based on glucose intolerance, or phosphate additives.

Conventional Therapies

The use of Ritalin (methylphenidate) has been the subject of widespread controversy. It is estimated that this drug is currently being taken by over one million children in the United States. Like too many other medical conditions, most fail to address other possible causes for hyperactive behavior. Unquestionably, in severe cases of ADD, drug therapy may be the only viable alternative, although nutritional avenues can have dramatic results. Behavior therapy and counseling are also useful.

Other accepted medical treatments for ADD or hyperactivity are methylphenidate or dextroamphetamine (dexedrine), which are used in extreme cases. Ironically, stimulant drugs (amphetamines or methylphenidate) are used to treat hyperactivity. It is thought that the midbrain may actually be understimulated in hyperactivity, causing a lack of control.

Dietary Guidelines

◆ The role that food additives play in hyperactivity and attention deficit disorder has been the subject of considerable controversy over the last few years. The Feingold hypothesis proposes that food additives, such as BHT, BHA, artificial colors and flavorings, emulsifiers, nitrates and sulphites, induce hyperactivity in children. Feingold came up with 3,000 different food additives that should be investigated. While the final conclusion of the national advisory committee on hyperkinesis and food additives was that there was no significant connection between the two, ongoing studies suggest that a definite correlation exists. In controlled clinical trials, up to 50 percent of hyperactive children improved when their diets were altered by controlling the ingestion of food additives, sugar and eliminating possible food allergens.[1]

◆ Eliminate white sugar from the diet; several studies suggest that hyperactive children have impaired glucose tolerance.[2] A tendency toward hypoglycemia in hyperactive children also supports the negative emotional effects which sugar could induce. Some university studies have revealed that a carbohydrate- and sugar-rich breakfast can lead to an increase in hyperactive behavior. If protein was eaten at breakfast, hyperactivity was reduced.[3]

◆ Eliminate not only food additives, but possible food allergens such as BHA, BHT, red dye, yellow dye, blue dye, preservatives, cow's milk, chocolate, grape flavoring, orange flavoring, cane sugar, tomatoes, wheat products, eggs, dairy products, nuts, and fish. It is widely accepted that food allergens can cause emotional mood shifts.

◆ Eliminate salt, soda pop (high phosphate levels), catsup, mustard, soy sauce, cider vinegar, colored cheeses, boxed diners, lunch meats, hot dogs, smoked meats, ham, wheat, corn, colored butter, margarine, ice cream, candy, and perfumes.

◆ Do not use foods with salicylates; these include almonds, apples, apricots, cherries, currants, berries, peaches, plums, prunes, tomatoes, cucumbers and oranges.

◆ Emphasize fruits and vegetables that are not on the elimination list; cereals, breads, crackers that only contain rice or oats, or millet. Keep a chart for a week of foods consumed and any emotional reaction that may be linked with those foods.

◆ The phosphates typically found in soda pop have been linked to muscular hyperactivity.

Recommended Nutritional Supplements

Dosages should be adjusted according to the age of the person involved. The following doses are for adults or anyone over the age of eighteen. Check with your doctor if you are treating a child under the age of twelve.

PRIMARY NUTRIENTS

MINERAL SUPPLEMENTS Children with ADD can suffer from a variety of mineral deficiencies. *Suggested Dosage:* Get a good, powerful organic-based supplement with chelated minerals.

CALCIUM/MAGNESIUM Helps to calm the nervous system and is vital for normal brain function. One hundred sixty-five boys who had mental disturbances and learning disabilities were found to be magnesium deficient.[4] *Suggested Dosage:* 1,000 mg of each per day. Use chelated varieties and look for calcium citrate or gluconate.

GABA Some studies have shown that giving GABA (gamma-amino butyric acid) can help to decrease hyperactivity as well as benefit children with learning disorders. *Suggested Dosage:* Take as directed.

VITAMIN B6 An extremely important vitamin for normal mental function. Individuals with learning disabilities, schizophrenia and other mental disorders commonly suffer from vitamin B6 depletion. One study confirms the ability of this vitamin to effectively treat schizophrenic individuals who did not respond to psychotropic drug therapy.[5] *Suggested Dosage:* 50 mg with each meal.

GOTU KOLA Can improve the mental abilities of disabled children due to its antianxiety properties. After using gotu kola therapy, 30 children who were considered disabled were able to stay focused on tasks and experienced improved concentration.[6] *Suggested Dosage:* Take as directed, using standardized guaranteed potency products.

VALERIAN ROOT In Germany, this herb has been used with good success to treat a number of childhood behavioral disorders.[7] *Suggested Dosage:* Take as directed.

OMEGA-3 FATTY ACIDS Although research findings are scant, anecdotal surveys have found that for some children with ADD, marine lipid supplementation seems to initiate some improvement. The exact mechanisms involved remain unknown. *Suggested Dosage:* Take as directed and use a vitamin E supplement with fish oil.

SECONDARY NUTRIENTS

VITAMIN C WITH BIOFLAVONOIDS: Considered a good antioxidant, this vitamin also helps to counteract the effects of stress. *Suggested Dosage:* Take as directed.

TYROSINE: Helps to naturally raise serotonin levels, promoting improved mental outlook.[8] *Suggested Dosage:* Take as directed on an empty stomach with fruit juice.

Home Care Suggestions

♦ A hyperactive child, just like any other, needs a structured and well-disciplined environment. Consistency is of utmost importance and, though difficult to achieve, can help to create a more ordered environment. A hyperactive child, more so than a normal child, must be trained to remember and to complete tasks.

♦ It is essential that parents present a united front to the child and agree on rules, expectations, discipline, etc.

♦ Break up every task the child is asked to do in step-by-step requests. Don't give general instructions—give specific ones designed to bring the child to a conclusion. Use a brightly colored chart to help the child succeed. List tasks one by one such as: get out of bed, brush your teeth, take off your pajamas, make your bed, etc. A reward system can be used. This could include assigning stars to a sheet for accomplished tasks; so many stars would equal going to a movie, a trip to the zoo, etc.

♦ Locate a good counseling service for the entire family. Dealing with a hyperactive child can be extremely stressful; therefore additional outside support may be necessary. Often parents become so callous to the demands of a hyperactive child they have a tendency to ignore the child more, which usually aggravates aggressive behavior. Child abuse may become a factor when the hyperactive child is unusually difficult. Hotlines and preventative measures should be taken to avoid this type of situation.

♦ Choose the right kind of activities for your child. Working on puzzles or long-term visual activities requiring exact hand-eye coordination are not recommended, although some hyperactive children are very adept at putting together mechanical objects. Hyperactive children usually enjoy activities such as swimming or soccer, rather than baseball or football.

♦ Some studies suggest that a regular jogging program is as effective as low dose medication in controlling hyperactivity.

♦ Home environment should not be overstimulating. Avoid blaring TVs, video games, loud stereos, etc.

♦ Give the child simple responsibilities such as sweeping the floor; use a great deal of praise to reinforce good behavior.

Other Supportive Therapies

PARENTAL RESPONSE THERAPY: This entails giving absolutely no attention to negative behavior of any kind and lavish praise for positive behavior. This requires a controlled environment where the child cannot harm other children but themselves, and takes particular dedication to pull off. The results from programs that utilize this form of therapy have been very promising.

ART THERAPY: Creative outlets such as finger painting or sculpture may be helpful to channel energy and to encourage personal accomplishment.

Scientific Facts-at-a-Glance

Children with ADD frequently have heavy metal toxicity. While the reasons for this phenomenon remain fairly unknown, having a hair analysis test to determine if the child has an excess of any heavy metal is recommended.

Spirit/Mind Considerations

It can be extremely difficult to show affection to a child who suffers from ADD. They are often resistant to hugging and can be very difficult to manage. The power of unconditional love cannot be overemphasized. Parents should make sure that these children are well loved. Constant attempts to praise and to show affection are recommended.

Prevention

♦ Keep your child on a nutritious diet that is low in refined sugars and high in natural foods. Use a good multivitamin/mineral supplement.

♦ Establish codes of behavior, household chores, etc. early in the child's life.

♦ Keep noise and distraction to a minimum within the home environment.

♦ Keep your children involved in activities where they can expend energy; these include swimming, jogging, gymnastics, soccer, and any running events.

♦ Make sure your child is not exposed to sources of heavy metals, such as lead pipes or leaded paint.

Doctor's Notes

Before a child is assumed to be hyperactive and subsequently treated with drugs, a careful medical evaluation is mandatory to eliminate other possible conditions. The widespread use of Ritalin is cause for concern. Even the *Journal of the American Medical Association* questioned the extent of the current use of drugs prescribed for hyperactivity. Every four to seven years that number of children receiving medication for hyperactivity is thought to be doubling. While Ritalin may be considered a lifesaver in severe cases of ADD, it should only be used as a last resort.

Additional Resources

(CHADD) Children with Attention Deficit Disorder
499 Northwest 70th Avenue
Suite 101
Plantation, FL 33317
(305) 587-3700

(ADDA) Attention Deficit Disorder Association
PO Box 972
Mentor, OH 44061
(800) 487-2282

Endnotes

1. N. Feingold, Why Your Child is Hyperactive, Random House, New York: 1975. See also, C. Connors, et al., "Food additives and hyperkinesis: a double-blind experiment," Pediatrics, 1976, 58: 154-66.

2. R. Prinz, W. Roberts and E. Hantman, "Dietary correlates of hyperactive behavior in children," Jour of Consult Clinical Psychology, 1989, 48: 760-69.

3. L. Sanders, et al., "Refined carbohydrate as a contributing factor in reactive hypoglycemia," Southern Med Jour, 1982, 75: 1972-75.

4. Biological Psychiatry, June, 1984, 19: 871-76.

5. Biological Psychiatry, 1983, 18:11: 1321-28.

6. MVR Roa Appa, et al., "The effect of Centella asiatica on the general mental ability of mentally retarded children," Indian Journal Psychiatry, 1977, 19: 54-59.

7. R. Klich, "Behavioral disorders of childhood and their treatment," Medizinische Welt, 1975, 26 (25): 1251-54.

8. Oscar Janiger and Philip Goldberg, A Different Kind of Healing, (Putnam Sons, New York: 1993), 72.

AUTISM

Autism is a mysterious disorder that is still easily misdiagnosed and misunderstood. While the symptoms of autism can vary with each child, it is usually discovered before the age of three and is characterized by little or abnormal response to touch, speech and environment. These children are incapable of normal interaction and shy away from close relationships. Obsessive behavior, temper tantrums and withdrawal are all typical of autistic behavior. A pervasive disassociation with reality makes the child unresponsive to stimuli or affection. Speech is sometimes impaired, depending on the severity of the disorder. Over 100,000 people in American suffer from autism. Asperger's syndrome is a much milder form of autism where speech and communication skills are not so seriously impaired, enabling the child to become better educated and independent.

Symptoms

Autism is characterized by marked unresponsiveness, failure to develop attachments, withdrawal, unusual or unpredictable behavior, hyperactivity, temper tantrums and anger outbursts, obsessive use of foul language, slow speech development, aversion to change of environment, exaggerated sensitivity to external stimuli, special talent or skill or compulsion toward repetitive activities.

Causes

The exact cause of autism remains a mystery. Studies suggest that a possible cause may be a genetic factor that causes a malfunction in brain neurochemistry. There is some speculation that exposure to excess lead, copper or mercury may lead to the development of autistic behavior. While nutrient deficiency has not been directly linked to autism, vitamin B6 deprivation can cause serious mental disturbances and bizarre behavior.

Conventional Therapies

A wide range of psychoactive drugs and antidepressants have been used to treat autism and range from lithium to Prozac to Ritalin. These powerful drugs may be useful; however, they come with significant side effects. Their usage should be based on individual need. Ideally, good nutrition and supplementation may replace powerful drug therapy and enable the autistic individual to function more efficiently.

Dietary Guidelines

◆ There is some evidence to support a link between food additives and preservatives and mental function. Any food sensitivities should be investigated. Avoiding culprit foods like dairy products, nuts, wheat, eggs, etc., is recommended.

- High-fiber diets with plenty of raw fruits, vegetable, whole grains and legumes are recommended.
- Keep white sugar intake low and use lean meats.
- Make sure that there is no caffeine or alcohol consumption and stay away from processed foods that are high in nitrates, sodium and other preservatives.
- It is wise to keep blood sugar levels up by providing more small meals a day than one or two larger ones.

Recommended Nutritional Supplements

PRIMARY NUTRIENTS

VITAMIN/MINERAL SUPPLEMENT A potent and organically based vitamin/mineral supplement is recommended. *Suggested Dosage:* Take as directed.

VITAMIN B6 WITH MAGNESIUM Essential for emotional and mental stability. Studies confirm the use of this duo for autistic behavior. Vitamin B6 depletion has been linked to a number of mental disturbances.[1] Using vitamin B6 in conjunction with magnesium resulted in the marked improvement of sixty autistic children in a double-blind trial. Vitamin B6 must be taken with magnesium and not alone.[2] *Suggested Dosage:* 150 mg of vitamin B6 in three equal divided doses. Use sublingual varieties. Take 1,000 mg of magnesium per day. Make sure to take these two supplements at the same time.

CALCIUM/MAGNESIUM Helps to calm the nervous system and is vital for normal brain function. One hundred sixty-five boys who had mental disturbances and learning disabilities were found to be magnesium deficient.[3] *Suggested Dosage:* 1,000 mg of each per day. Use chelated varieties and look for calcium citrate or gluconate.

VITAMIN B-COMPLEX A profoundly important vitamin mix for normal mental function. Individuals with learning disabilities, schizophrenia and other mental disorders commonly suffer from B-vitamin depletion. One study confirms the ability of this vitamin to effectively treat schizophrenic individuals who did not respond to psychotropic drug therapy.[4] *Suggested Dosage:* 50 mg with each meal.

GABA Some studies have shown that giving GABA (gamma-amino butyric acid) can help to decrease hyperactivity as well as benefit children with learning disorders. *Suggested Dosage:* Take as directed.

GOTU KOLA Can improve the mental abilities of disabled children. After using gotu kola therapy, 30 children who were considered disabled were able to stay focused and concentrated.[5] *Suggested Dosage:* Take as directed, using standardized guaranteed potency products.

VALERIAN ROOT In Germany, this herb has been used with good success to treat a number of childhood behavioral disorders.[6] *Suggested Dosage:* Take as directed.

SECONDARY NUTRIENTS

VITAMIN C WITH BIOFLAVONOIDS: Considered a good antioxidant, this vitamin also helps to counteract the effects of stress. *Suggested Dosage:* Take as directed.

TYROSINE: Helps to naturally raise serotonin levels promoting improved mental outlook.[7] *Suggested Dosage:* Take as directed on an empty stomach with fruit juice.

GINKGO BILOBA: More and more research supports the use of ginkgo for brain-related disorders. It has the distinct ability to scavenge free radicals and boost brain tissue oxygenation.[8] *Suggested Dosage:* Take as directed using guaranteed potency products.

ST. JOHN'S WORT: This herb has recently come to the forefront as a viable natural treatment for depression. Due to its antidepressant properties and its ability to help normalize sleep disorders, it is recommended for autism.[9] *Suggested Dosage:* Take as directed with meals.

CHOLINE: Works to nourish nerve endings and boosts brain circulation. *Suggested Dosage:* 1,000 mg per day. Check with your physician before using this supplement.

COENZYME Q10: Enhances circulation and is currently under research for brain disorders. *Suggested Dosage:* Take as directed. NOTE: Dosages should be adjusted according to the age of the person involved. The following doses are for adults or anyone over the age of 18. Check with your doctor if you are treating a child under the age of 12.

Home Care Suggestions

- Make sure regular exercise is as a part of daily activities, not only for physical stamina, but also to release stress and to boost brain cell oxygenation.
- Try to provide small meals throughout the day to keep blood sugar levels steady.
- Creating and maintaining a standardized schedule of daily activities helps to create a sense of security and calmness.
- Find something that interests this individual and try to develop it as much as possible. Puzzles, mechanical put-togethers, or activities with repetitive tasks may be helpful.
- Computers can be lifesavers for autistic children. Various programs can help to channel energy and teach focusing skills.
- If capable, giving the child an animal to care for can teach responsibility, increased affection and expand the ability to focus.

Other Supportive Therapies

MASSAGE: If the child will allow it, foot and hand massage with aromatic oils such as peppermint can help encourage touch and also stimulate sensory perception.

MUSIC THERAPY: Music can provide an auditory stimulus which can help to soothe or intrigue the child. Some autistic children have exceptional musical talent, which should be fostered.

Scientific Facts-at-a-Glance

New technologies in software programs have been especially developed for children with autism, and can be found by contacting Angela Patterson at (408) 727-5775, ext. 106.

Spirit/Mind Considerations

Autism can be one of the most heartbreaking conditions a parent may have to face. All of the natural parental instincts which center on physical touch, expression of affection, communication, teaching etc. must be modified with an autistic child. Moreover, the unique way that your child relates to you as a parent cannot be taken as a personal rejection. One must understand that many autistic children feel trapped inside a world where what they perceive and what they wish to communicate become garbled. The power of love and prayer should not be minimized when it comes to disorders like autism. Continual expressions of love, coupled with gentle persuasion and even strong discipline at times, can help autistic children to cope and even progress. Support groups can be very helpful and enrolling your child in the right school is crucial. Having a positive attitude around the child is also very beneficial.

Prevention

◆ While there is no real way to prevent this particular condition, making sure that your baby has an adequate supply of nutrients is vital.

◆ Use organic vitamin drops to augment diet after solid foods are introduced.

◆ Make sure that there is no possibility that your child can be exposed to heavy metals such as lead, copper, cadmium, etc. Check for paint chips or lead pipes if you live in an older home.

Doctor's Notes

Making sure that an autistic individual is receiving even more than RDA levels of vitamins and minerals is vital. Because the disease is relatively misunderstood, the nutritional component must not be minimized.[10] Both the primary and secondary nutrients listed are all important to brain function and emotional stability. The possibility of food allergies must also be considered as a factor.

Additional Resources

Society for the Treatment of Autism
Agnes O'Neill (Program Director)
PO Box 392
Sydney, Australia
BIP 6H2
(902) 567-6441

Autism Research Institute
4182 Adams Ave.
San Diego, CA 92116

Endnotes

1. H. Classen, "Stress and magnesium," Artery, 1981, 9: 182-189.
2. Biological Psychiatry, May, 1985, 20: 467-78. See also Orthomolecular Psychiatry, April-June, 1984, 13: 117-22.
3. Biological Psychiatry, June, 1984, 19: 871-76.
4. Biological Psychiatry, 1983, 18:11, 1321-28.
5. MVR Roa Appa, et al., "The effect of Centella asiatica on the general mental ability of mentally retarded children," Indian Journal Psychiatry, 1977, 19: 54-59.
6. R. Klich, "Behavioral disorders of childhood and their treatment," Medizinische Welt, 1975, 26 (25): 1251-54.
7. Oscar Janiger and Philip Goldberg, as a Different Kind of Healing, (Putnam Sons, New York: 1993), 72.
8. B. Gessner, et al., "Study of the long-term action of ginkgo biloba extract on vigilance and mental performance as determined by means of quantitative pharmaco-EEG and psychometric measurements," Arzneimittel-Forsch, 1985, 35: 1459-65.
9. K.D. Hansgen, J. Vesper and M. Ploch, "Multicenter double-blind study examining the antidepressant effectiveness of the hypericum extract LI 160," Journal of Geriatric Psychiatry and Neurology, Oct. 1994, vol.7
10. L. Christiansen, et al., "Impact of as a dietary change on emotional distress," Journal of Abnormal Psychology, 1985, 94: 565-79.

BACK PAIN

Back pain is one of life's maladies that affects all of us at one time or another. More people are hospitalized for back problems than any other single cause. Lower back pain is the most common kind and can result from a variety of causes. While slipped or herniated discs are responsible for many back problems, muscles that have lost their ability to support vertebrae or that become strained account for the majority of backaches. Muscles can go into a spasm when triggered and in so doing produce lactic acid, which causes them to feel sore. Consequently, chronic pain can result. Resolving a backache can be frustrating and relief can be slow. Unfortunately, most backaches are recurring.

Symptoms

Back pain is a wide-ranging ailment. Some of the more common symptoms are a persistent, dull pain, usually located in the small of the back, shooting pains which radiate from the small of the back down the left leg, limited mobility and stiffness characterized by unnatural positions, and an inability to completely straighten the spine.

See your doctor immediately if you have back pain accompanied by fever, vomiting, chest pain or difficult breathing. In addition, you should see your doctor for back pain that radiates down one leg to the knee or foot region, back pain that appears for no apparent reason, or chronic back pain that persists for longer than a week without relief.

Causes

Most back pain is the result of a spasm of the large supportive muscles found on either side of the spine. This type of backache usually heals naturally and is commonly linked to overexertion of some type.

Back pain that radiates into the legs may indicate a ruptured or crushed disc.

Other possible causes of back pain include using an overly hard or soft mattress, improper lifting, a slipped or herniated disc, muscle spasms, a blow or fall, arthritis, bone disease, curvature of the spine, menstrual cramps, pelvic disorders and disease, kidney problems, a duodenal ulcer, gout, prostate disorders, constipation, the presence of a tumor, poor posture, faulty shoes, calcium depletion, inadequate seating in the workplace or dehydration.

Conventional Therapies

Muscle relaxants and/or anti-inflammatory drugs such as naprosyn and ibuprofen comprise the most common medical treatment for a backache. Over-the-counter analgesics are also prescribed in combination with hot/cold therapy and bed rest. A new consensus regarding complete immobility for backaches suggests that staying off your feet for over two days may actually instigate a backache. New dramatic therapies involve accelerated exercise, which must be done under the supervision of a trained specialist. Avoid using steroids like prednisone because bone loss can occur as a side effect.

Dietary Guidelines

- ◆ Avoid meats and animal protein products if gout is suspected, due to the high uric acid content of these foods.
- ◆ Eat a diet which emphasizes whole grains, fresh fruits and vegetables, and foods rich in protein which are not milk-based; these include kelp, collard greens, kale, turnips, almonds, watercress, chickpeas, beans, sunflower seeds, and endive.
- ◆ Drink at least six to eight glasses of pure water each day to expedite the removal of muscle acids like lactic and pyruvate. Dehydration can cause muscle spasms and pain.

Recommended Nutritional Supplements

PRIMARY NUTRIENTS

GLUCOSAMINE SULFATE/CHONDROITIN SUFLAFE A very effective duo of compounds which relive pain and inflammation while encouraging the regeneration of joint cartilage. Double-blind studies confirm that these two supplements are actually more effective than ibuprofen if taken long term.[1] *Suggested Dosage:* Take both supplements as directed over a four- to six-week period.

CALCIUM/MAGNESIUM Both of these minerals are essential for bone strength and inhibit muscle spasms. Calcium can help prevent bone loss, which can result in increased stress on the spinal column.[2] Suggested Dosage: 1,000 mg of each per day. Use chelated forms for maximum absorbability. Calcium citrate, gluconate and aspartate are recommended.

SILICON Improves the assimilation of calcium and is needed for the proper function of an enzyme which participates in the synthesis of collagen in bone and cartilage tissue.[3] *Suggested Dosage:* Take as directed. Horsetail, an herb, is naturally rich in silicon.

VITAMIN B12 Increases the absorption of calcium and is vital to the production of healthy muscle fiber. *Suggested Dosage:* Take as directed.

MARINE LIPIDS Marine Lipids: The compounds contained in fish oils (omega-3 fatty acids) have potent anti-inflammatory properties.[4] *Suggested Dosage:* Take as directed. Using vitamin E along with fish oils is also recommended.

DL-PHENYLALANINE This amino acid form helps with pain relief. Studies have shown that it can be effective for chronic pain even when standard medications have failed.[5] *Suggested Dosage:* Take as directed on an empty stomach with fruit juice. Do not use if pregnant, nursing, have diabetes, anxiety disorders, high blood pressure or PKU. If your back pain is associated with sciatica, use St. John's wort and ginkgo as herbal supplements. These botanicals target disorders of the nerves rather than muscle spasms. Devil's claw, tumeric, boswella, ginger, and St. John's wort are all good for sciatic symptoms. Use guaranteed potency products as directed.

HERBAL COMBINATION This combination should include white willow bark, blue vervain, feverfew leaves, rosemary leaves, skullcap, and kelp. *Suggested Dosage:* Three to five capsules daily. Do not use this formula if pregnant or nursing.

WHITE WILLOW: The bark contains a substance called salicin which is believed by some to convert to salicylic acid, or aspirin in the body. Unlike aspirin, salicin does not thin the blood or irritate the stomach. BLUE VERVAIN: Blue vervain is recognized in Europe and elsewhere for its ability to reduce inflammation and muscle spasms.[6] FEVERFEW: Used originally to treat fevers, this herb also has pain-reducing capabilities. ROSEMARY LEAVES: Rosemary performs two major functions in this formula: it relieves painful spasms and assists in reducing pain associated with rheumatism. SKULLCAP: This herb helps to alleviate nervous tension and acts as a natural sedative as well.[7] KELP: Kelp provides electrolytes that can help prevent edema, which discourages inflammation and pain.

SECONDARY NUTRIENTS

HORSETAIL: A good herbal source of silicon, calcium and minerals. *Suggested Dosage:* Take as directed.
VALERIAN ROOT AND HOPS: Two nervine herbs which act as natural muscle relaxants to help in easing the muscle spasms that accompany back pain. *Suggested Dosage:* Take as directed.

Home Care Suggestions

♦ A program of exercising designed to strengthen certain back muscles is very beneficial. It is known that improving your fitness and aerobic capacity enhances your recovery. One of the most effective for lower back pain is to bend over gently from the waist and to bow up and down with your arms extended down to your knees. Make sure to warm up and gently stretch your muscles before beginning exercises. Check with your doctor before starting such a program.
♦ Using an ice pack may also help in alleviating pain and should be applied to the area in short intervals. Using ice therapy is good for the first couple of days followed by the application of heat. Moist heat is preferable. Ice and heat treatments can be alternated with 30 minute intervals for each. You can use a conventional ice bag or make your own. Blue ice packs, (soft ones) used for coolers also work well.
♦ Placing a rolled up towel or pillow in the small of the back may increase comfort.
♦ Resting the affected muscles for at least 24 hours by lying flat on the back is very important.

♦ After bed rest, gradually increase physical activity.
♦ Swimming is especially beneficial for backaches. Stretching the back while in the water is easier and less risky.
♦ Sleeping without a pillow on a very firm mattress is recommended. A bed board can be placed under any mattress. Waterbeds are also beneficial in supporting back muscle if the water pressure is not too low.
♦ Keep your bowel movements regular by following nutritional guidelines.
♦ Many people have found relief through chiropractic adjustments. Before you go to a chiropractor, check with your physician and get recommendations.
♦ Jacuzzi or hot tub therapy can alleviate discomfort.
♦ If you sleep on your side, place a pillow between your legs. Don't sleep on your stomach, which exerts stress on back muscles.
♦ Chinese medicine, in addition to the benefits of acupuncture, offers tai chi which is comprised of a series of slow and fluid movements. This could benefit anyone with back troubles.
♦ Yoga is also a good way to strengthen back muscles and promote flexibility.
♦ Hot oil message (eucalyptus, peppermint or wintergreen oil) can be very beneficial. You can massage yourself with electric back massagers or even wood balls designed to roll over the spine. Several message therapists have advocated using a hard rubber ball and placing it under the back in the tender area while lying on the floor. Rolling on the ball gently can produce the same beneficial results of message therapy.

Other Supportive Therapies

CHIROPRACTIC: Chiropractic adjustments can be of great value for certain back conditions and usually need to be repeated over a period of time.
ACUPUNCTURE: For both pain relief and flexibility, acupuncture can be a very helpful therapy in controlling back pain and discouraging future back episodes.
HOMEOPATHY: Homeopathic creams containing Arnica are good for topical application.

Scientific Facts-at-a Glance

There is a new consensus out that bed rest and immobility may not always be the best thing for back problems. New therapeutic approaches encourage exercise which stretches the muscles and movement to warm them up. This kind of therapy needs the supervision of a professional or muscle damage could occur. In addition, while heat has always been accepted as a good idea, for some people, it seems to aggravate inflammation and pain. Using cold and hot applications may be preferable. One of the most interesting theories concerning chronic back pain is that it is a manifestation of food and chemical allergies. One study found that by placing two individuals with chronic back pain on a controlled fast and by regulating their diet, all back pain disappeared and only recurred when offending foods were eaten.[8]

Spirit/Mind Considerations

Relaxation techniques are invaluable as deterrents to stress-induced back pain. So much of the back pain we experience can be traced to stress reflexes which cause us to tighten up. For many of us, stress targets a specific bundle of muscles usually found at the base of the neck, between the shoulder blades or in the lower back region. We very unconsciously cause these areas to respond to our inability to dispel tension or anxiety. Using meditation, breathing exercises or just learning to recognize the warning signs for stress enables us to ward off some of these muscle spasms.

Prevention

- ◆ If you sit in a chair for long periods of time, make sure that the chair has proper back support. Lumbar supports can be placed in car seats.
- ◆ Avoid heavy shoulder bags, or book bags which can throw back alignment.
- ◆ Wearing shoes that have the proper support and have a comfortable heel height can directly affect the incidence of back pain, especially if long periods of time are spent on foot. Check the height of your heels and purchase quality footwear.
- ◆ Don't slouch; also, walk with good posture so as to not put unnecessary strain on back muscles.
- ◆ Learning to lift correctly is of utmost value. Squatting down and lifting, using the legs to bear the weight, can avoid potential back injury. Never lean forward without first bending the knees.
- ◆ Keep yourself physically fit through a regular program of exercise.
- ◆ Use a vacuum with care. Movements associated with vacuuming can trigger a muscle spasm in the back.

Doctor's Notes

Any condition that persists after attempted treatment should be evaluated by a health care professional. There are several levels of treatment for backache, first being pain control and relaxation of muscle spasm. This can be treated with an application of ice. One way of doing this is to get an ice cube or freeze ice in a styrofoam cup and then peel away the top of the cup so that you can hold the ice in your hand. Use a wash cloth to hold the ice and have someone rub it directly over the area of pain back and forth or in circles for a total of ten to fifteen minutes. At first the area will obviously feel cold, then it will burn and eventually it will become numb. It is important to get to this stage to achieve relief.

Herbs used to help relieve anxiety can be helpful as well. Valerian and kava in combination with skullcap, hops, passionflower and chamomile are excellent natural tranquilizers. If your backache is the result of inflamed muscles or discs, herbs that reduce inflammation include devils claw, tumeric, boswella, and bromelain. Gentian is also good. If sciatic pain is a problem, using St. John's wort and *Gingko biloba* are recommended.

Homeopathic creams which contain Arnica are also good for topical application. It is also important to make sure that your mineral supplementation is adequate. Calcium and magnesium are especially helpful. White willow bark, capsicum, (cayenne), feverfew, peppermint and wintergreen offer good pain relief. Sciatica problems are more complex. This is pain which results from the compression of the sciatic nerve caused by a ruptured or bulging disc in the lumbar spine. I have found that many people have been treated for sciatica when in fact they may suffer from muscle spasms in the gluteus minimus or other muscles located in the posterior buttocks and the lateral hip area.

Lesions or inflammatory conditions affecting the joint where the hip bone meets the back bone can cause symptoms which mimic sciatica. Sciatic pain needs to be treated correctly with acupuncture, trigger point injections, and proper manipulation or it can persist for years with no improvement.

Acupuncture works very well when combined with chiropractic manipulation. Remember that sciatic pain may give you a rest for a time, but usually returns. Don't get discouraged if you need occasional recurring treatment to keep it under control.

Endnotes

1. A.L. Vaz, "Double-blind clinical evaluation of the relative efficacy of ibuprofen and glucosamine sulfate in the management of osteoarthritis of the knee in out-patients," Current Med Res Opinion, 1982, 8: 145-49.
2. J.F. Aloia, et al., "Calcium supplementation with and without hormone replacement therapy to prevent postmenopausal bone loss," Annal Intern Med, 1994, 120: 97-103.
3. Robert Garrison and Elizabeth Somer, The Nutrition Desk Reference, (Keats Publishing, New Canaan, Connecticut: 1990), 82.
4. Biochemical Pharmacology, 1986, 35 (5): 779-85.
5. N.E. Walsh, et al., "Analgesic effectiveness of D-phenylalanine in chronic pain patients," Arch Phys Med Rehabil, 1986, 67 (7): 436-39.
6. S. Sakai, "Pharmacological actions of verben officinalis," Gitu Ika Daigaku Kiyo, 1963, 11 (1): 6-17.
7. B.A. Kurnakov, "Pharmacology of skullcap," Farmakologiia I Toksikologiia, 1957, 20(6): 79-80.
8. D.J. Mayberly, and M.A. Honor, "A reversible back pain syndrome: report of two cases," Jour of Nutri Med, 1991, 2: 83-87.

BAD BREATH

Bad breath, or halitosis, refers to a mouth condition we all have to deal with from time to time. Halitosis consists of an unpleasant smell which can originate from the mouth, throat or digestive system. It is a common disorder and can range from mild, stale smelling breath to foul, fetid breath which usually accompanies some type of mouth and gum diseases. Acidy breath may indicate a diabetic condition.

Causes

Bad breath can be caused by a number of factors, including poor dental hygiene, food lodged between the teeth, dentures, gum disease, tooth decay, smoking, chewing tobacco, drinking alcohol or drinking coffee (acidic). And obviously, bad breath can be the result of eating certain foods like onions, garlic, beer, fish, pastrami, sharp cheeses or anchovies.

Other causes of bad breath are fasting, untreated diabetes (acidosis), the presence of sinusitis, (mouth breathing), sore throats or other conditions that cause the tongue to become coated can cause offensive breath.

More uncommon causes of bad breath include certain lung disorders such as bronchiectasis, some gastrointestinal disorders, tuberculosis, and syphilis.

There is also some speculation that intestinal gases from improper elimination can also cause bad breath. Taking certain drugs, such as some antihistamines, some hormonal therapies, lithium and penicillamine may create some degree of halitosis. Being very hungry or going without foods for a long period of time can induce a dry mouth and ultimately cause stale breath.

In children, bad breath can be the result of diseases such as trench mouth, or throat infections, especially chronically infected tonsils. Occasionally, a small child may insert a foreign object in the nose (such as a tissue, cotton ball, etc.) which remains lodged there. A white, or yellow discharge from the nose usually accompanies the bad breath in these situations.

Persistent, unexplained bad breath may be a symptom of a more serious condition and should be checked by your physician. In addition a badly coated tongue that does not improve after brushing or using mouthwash can indicate a disease condition.

Conventional Therapies

Your doctor will want to rule out disease conditions that may cause bad breath. Your mouth, throat and nose will be carefully inspected. A culture may be needed if a sore throat or mouth sores are present. Most people live with common bad breath and rarely make a special trip to the doctor for treatment. Over-the-counter mints, sprays, and mouthwashes offer only temporary relief.

Dietary Guidelines

◆ Some health care professionals believe that impaired digestion and faulty elimination can contribute to bad breath. This notion is based on the idea that undigested food particles give off toxic gases, which can come back up into the mouth area.

◆ It has also been speculated that eating a diet high in fats can contribute to halitosis. Avoid fatty dairy products and cured meats. Naturally, eating sharp pungent cheeses may cause problems.

◆ Drinking fresh lemon water every day helps to chase away stale breath and chewing on whole cloves or fresh parsley supplies the mouth with natural deodorizers.

◆ Eating raw vegetables or fruits such as apples or carrots also helps to keep the mouth clean in between brushings. Oranges and other citrus fruits also help combat a dry mouth.

◆ Some medication can make your mouth extremely dry. Sucking on candy can help to stimulate saliva flow.

Recommended Nutritional Supplements

Something as simple as brushing after every meal can help eliminate most of our bad breath problems. Foods that coat our mouths like whole milk, cream, cheeses etc. can predispose us to bad breath, along with spices like garlic or onions. Again, the value of eating fresh, raw foods emerges for this ailment. Raw, crunchy fruits and vegetables help to keep the mouth clean and the gums healthy.

PRIMARY NUTRIENTS

ACIDOPHILUS Helps keep the lower bowels functioning well and can reduce the formation of gases.[1] *Suggested Dosage:* Take as directed using guaranteed bacterial count products with bifidobacteria.

LIQUID CHLOROPHYLL Natural chlorophyll is an excellent mouth freshener and odor absorbent.[2] *Suggested Usage:* Use both a drink and a mouthwash according to specified instructions. Taking two tablespoons of liquid chlorophyll with water or juice between meals can help prevent bad breath.

VITAMINS A, C, E, AND B-COMPLEX Help the body to eliminate toxins. The ascorbic acid of vitamin C and the properties of bioflavonoids help to reduce the risk of bleeding gums. *Suggested Dosage:* 5,000 mg per day.

ZINC Some cases of bad breath are caused by a zinc deficiency. *Suggested Dosage:* Take as directed. Use picolinate products.

SECONDARY NUTRIENTS

ALOE VERA GEL: Helps clean the digestive tract and contributes to the healing of any mouth sore that may be present. *Suggested Dosage:* Take internally only as directed as aloe has a laxative effect and can cause gripping.

CLOVES, FENNEL OR ANISE: Sweetens the breath and helps with digestion. *Suggested Dosage:* Use as directed.

PARSLEY: Destroys odor. Chewing on fresh parsley can help to eliminate garlic and onion breath. *Suggested Dosage:* Take as directed.

PEPPERMINT: Sweetens the breath and also promotes good digestion. *Suggested Dosage:* Can be taken in tea form or in more concentrated oils or extracts. Homemade gargles can be made with rosemary or peppermint oil. Use two drops to one cup of warm water.

MYRRH: Can be used as an effective mouthwash that helps heal mouth sores and sore throats. *Suggested Dosage:* Take as directed.

Home Care Suggestions

- Stop smoking.
- Use a mouthwash that contains zinc, which combats certain odors more efficiently. Usually these are red in color.
- Use baking soda-based toothpastes or make your own paste with baking soda and water. There are toothpastes out now which have also added peroxide to their baking soda formulas.
- Chew on fresh parsley after eating strong spices or foods with garlic or onions.

Scientific Facts-at-a-Glance

New breath fresheners that work from the stomach have recently become available; the reviews are mixed. If you are keeping your teeth and gums clean, most bad breath problems will not be serious.

Prevention

- Get regular dental checkups to avoid gum disease and tooth decay.
- Carry a toothbrush with you and brush after each meal.
- Replace your toothbrush often.
- Drink water after you are done eating to remove the presence of food particles and rinse your mouth out if you can.
- Keep yourself regular by eating a high-fiber diet.
- Don't smoke or chew tobacco.
- Eat fresh parsley sprigs after a spicy meal.
- Eat plenty of fresh crunchy vegetables to clean the teeth and stimulate the gums.
- Brush after drinking coffee.

Doctor's Notes

Good dental hygiene, including flossing, is the best way to prevent bad breath. If you wear dentures, soak them nightly. A well-designed toothbrush or water pic can also get to hard-to-reach areas of the mouth. Brushing the tongue is also recommended (the tongue has hair like projections which can catch plaque).

Endnotes

1. G.R. Gibson, et al., "Selective stimulation of bifidobacteria in the human colon by ologfructose and inulin," 1995, 108: Gastroenterology, 975-82.
2. M.C. Nahata, et al., "Effect of chlorophyllin on urinary odor in incontinent geriatric patients," Drug Intel Clin Pharm, 1983, 17: 732-34.

BEDWETTING

It is common for a child to wet the bed until four or even five years old. As many as 7 million children suffer from this problem of involuntary voiding of urine. In fact, the problem is so prevalent that it is not considered a disorder unless it persists into puberty and beyond.

Statistically, bedwetting is considered problematic in a small number of adults. It is important to realize that if a variety of treatments fail, most children outgrow the problem naturally, and they should be made aware of this fact.

Bedwetting is considered an involuntary disorder, and is usually hereditary. Approximately one in every seven children experiences bedwetting. Boys are slightly more prone to bedwetting than girls.

Symptoms

Bedwetting can occur once or several times during the night. Patterns are common and can predict to some extent, how long a child will sleep during the night before wetting. Bedwetting can begin shortly after potty training or several months later.

Precautions

If bedwetting persists after the age of six or occurs during the day, check with your physician to eliminate the possibility of a urinary disorder, or a serious psychological problem.

Causes

- It is sometimes difficult to determine whether bedwetting is a physical or psychological problem. In children under the age of six, though, it is a relatively common occurrence.
- Recent investigations have pointed to the fact that a neurophysical component may be responsible in most cases of bedwetting. Most cases are probably due to immature nervous system development which controls bladder function and is not usually connected to any other physical or emotional condition.
- Very heavy sleepers appear prone to bedwetting, although some studies have refuted this.
- Emotional upsets and extreme fatigue have also been linked to the disorder.
- Heredity, weak or small bladders, nutritional deficiencies and urinary tract infections all have a relationship to bedwetting.
- Allergies can affect deep sleep cycles, which is when bedwetting usually occurs. Foods containing salicylates can cause bedwetting in some children.
- Consuming too much liquid after 6 p.m. can lead to bedwetting.
- Structural abnormalities of the urinary system can be a major factor.
- ADD and ADHD have also been linked to bedwetting.
- In a small number of cases, involuntary urination is present during the day and is usually linked to the presence of a physical abnormality or illness such as the presence of diabetes mellitus or spina bifida.

Conventional Therapies

If the problem persists past five or six years of age, a physician will want to determine if there is a specific physical cause for the problem. In older children, a cystometry (which requires catheterization) may be ordered to assess bladder function. If bedwetting continues, imipramine (tofranil, janimine) may be prescribed which helps to contract the sphincter muscle of the urethra. Imipramine is also an anti-depressant and should only be used if you and your doctor feel it is necessary. The benefits of this treatment are are questionable. In cases where it has been used, it has rarely provided permanent relief.

Dietary Guidelines

- If food allergies are present, avoid cow's milk, chocolate and soda pop.
- Protein supplements can contribute to strengthening of bladder muscles of your child (supplements are recommended because children don't usually like protein-rich foods). Supplements are available at health food shops and can significantly improve physiological performance if the child is a poor eater.
- Don't let the child have any liquids after 6 p.m. Cherry juice has been used to help with urinary and bladder problems.

Recommended Nutritional Supplements

PRIMARY NUTRIENTS

ST. JOHN'S WORT The exact mechanisms of this herb for bedwetting is not totally understood although its effect on slow wave sleep may be a factor.[1] *Suggested Dosage:* This herb should be taken in a guaranteed potency form that is 250 mg. Start by taking one a day for several weeks and if no improvement is evident, take one in the morning and the evening. If the child is in their early teens, you can use the St. Johns wort in the guaranteed potency form of 300 mg. Again, take one in the evening up and do not exceed three dosages in one day.

MAGNESIUM Helps to strengthen bladder muscle and to inhibit premature spasm due to its effect on muscle tissue.[2] *Suggested Dosage:* Take as directed in an age-appropriate dose.

VITAMIN A Helps to facilitate normal bladder muscle function. *Suggested Dosage:* Take as directed. Do not exceed 3,000 IU for a child under six.

UVA URSI Helps to keep the urinary tract clear.[3] *Suggested Dosage:* Take as directed.

SECONDARY NUTRIENTS

HORSETAIL: Works to strengthen the bladder. *Suggested Dosage:* Take as directed in appropriate dosages for a child.

SWEET SUMACH: A traditional herbal treatment for bedwetting, considered a tonic for the urinary system. *Suggested Dosage:* Take as directed.

Most herbs are bitter and children do not respond favorably to them. Try making herb tea solutions of any of the suggested herbs and mixing them in fruit juices. Making frozen fruit bars with herbal teas and fruit juices is also recommended. Most herbal preparations come in capsules, and many children can be taught to swallow them.

Home Care Suggestions

◆ Encourage the child to drink during the day and hold off urination as long as possible to condition the bladder.
◆ Bedwetting alarms can be effective and function by sounding off when the child is wet. A moisture sensor is placed on the child's underclothing. They condition the child to eventually awake when the bladder becomes distended. The method is slow and requires a great deal of patience. Allow at least two to four months for this type of approach. This is a negative feedback approach and conditions the child to associate urination with an unpleasant sensation. If your child is a heavy sleeper (and many bedwetters are), the alarm may wake up everyone but the child, defeating its intended purpose.
◆ Use a felt-covered rubber pad under the sheeting.
◆ If the child is old enough, encourage him or her to change into clean clothes. If you have to do it, calmly go about it without any negative comments.
◆ Give the child as much privacy and respect as possible, without referring to the problem as something to be ashamed of.
◆ Some success has been found with setting an alarm at two different times during the night and waking the child to go to the bathroom. This takes a great deal of patience, though, and can be stressful for all involved.
◆ Encourage the child not to drink any fluids after dinner, or at least for two hours before bedtime. (Some experts dispute the benefit of this practice and claim that the amount of liquid consumed has no bearing on the problem). Common sense dictates that drinking less prior to bedtime could only help.
◆ A lack of sleep can actually worsen bedwetting. Consequently, children should retire early rather than be kept up late.
◆ Learning about chronic bedwetting for a parent is invaluable. Knowledge can help alleviate potentially embarrassing situations for the child. There are several good books available at local libraries on the subject.

Other Supportive Therapies

ACUPUNCTURE: Acupuncture has been very useful in treating this condition.

MASSAGE: Some parents have had success alleviating a bedwetting problem by giving their child an intensive foot massage before bedtime.

Scientific Facts-at-a-Glance

Constipation has been associated with bedwetting. If you suspect this is a problem, treat the child with mild laxative herbs. Some professionals are using an antidiuretic hormone (DDAVP), which comes in the form of a nasal spray to treat bedwetting. However, unless your child is over the age of six or seven and still has chronic problems with bedwetting, this medication is discouraged.

Spirit/Mind Considerations

Bedwetting may cause a child to feel ashamed or even afraid if reprisals are harsh and accusatory. Older children, in particular, may equate it with being a baby. Children that are bedwetters over the age of three may fear of sleeping in beds other than their own and may experience a high degree of guilt. The way a parent reacts to chronic bedwetting is crucial to the child's perception of himself and the problem.

Bedwetting should be carefully explained so it does not create extra anxiety. There should be no scolding or reprimanding of any kind. Some psychotherapists have suggested that bedwetting is the result of repressed hostility or sexuality, but the general consensus is that this does not appear to be the case in the majority of bedwetting situations.

The arrival of a new baby or some other threatening situation may also cause bedwetting to commence. As the parent of a child who suffers through a bedwetting problem, the most important thing to remember is to avoid any kind of negative response, which can actually aggravate the problem by causing more stress and by damaging their self-esteem. Bedwetting is not a result of laziness or a desire to get attention. It is simply an involuntary physiological occurance over which the child has no control.

Prevention

◆ Common sense measures like not giving any fluids after 6 p.m. may help, although for some children, bedwetting seems like an inevitable part of their growing-up process.

Doctor's Notes

Children under the age of five or six should not be treated at all for bedwetting. Their situation really doesn't need to be investigated at that point, unless they are complaining about difficult and/or painful urination, in which case you will want to check for the presence of a urinary tract infection. Bedwetting is often an inherited trait and will resolve itself as the child's nervous system matures.

Attempting to treat bedwetting too early can be very frustrating for both parents and children. Decreasing the amount of fluids taken after 6 p.m. may help some children. There is a form of bladder training that can be done during the day. The child, upon feeling the urge to urinate, tells the parents, who then challenge them to wait a certain amount of time before going into the bathroom. This may start out as a 30-second delay which becomes three minutes, and then may extend to 20 minutes. This allows the child to recognize what a full bladder feels like so they can identify the sensation at night and wake up.

Another possible treatment approach is to challenge the child fill up a quart jar or some other kind of container as high as they can with one urination. This encourages the child to learn how to hold their urine until their bladder is full, training both the child and the nervous system to recognize a full bladder.

There have been successful studies showing that children who are allergic to additives such as dyes, and who have milk sensitivities, stop wetting the bed when these substances are removed from their diets. Screening a child's diet is quite an undertaking but can certainly be worth it in cases where allergies exist.

Children who have a daytime loss of urine as well as night-time loss may be suffering from a more serious problem and need to be seen by a professional as soon as possible.

Additional Resources

The International Enuresis Research Center
Institute of Experimental Clinical Research
University of Aarhus, Denmark
Brendstrupgardsveg DK-8200 Aarhus N

Endnotes

1. H. Schulz and M. Jobert, "Effects of hypericum extract on the sleep EEG in older volunteers," Journal of Geriatric Psychiatry, Oct. 1994, vol. 7.
2. Michael T. Murray, Encyclopedia of Natural Supplements, (Prima Publsihing, Rocklin, Ca: 1996), 170-71.
3. A. Leung, Encylopedia of Common Natural Ingredients, New York: 1980.

BEE STINGS

SEE "INSECT BITES"

BLADDER INFECTIONS

Bladder infections typically afflict women because of the structural makeup of the female urinary tract (the anus, vagina and urethra are relatively close, increasing the risk of bacterial infection.)

A bladder infection, also known as a UTI (urinary tract infection) or cystitis, is one of the most common infections treated by physicians. Medically speaking, a bladder infection consists of an inflammation of the urinary bladder. Fifty percent of all women will experience a bladder infection at some time in their life and twenty percent will recur. Men over fifty with enlarged prostate glands are also susceptible to bladder infections. Bladder infections can be miserable but are usually not considered dangerous. Getting prompt treatment is recommended to avoid any complications.

Symptoms

Bladder and urinary tract infections are punctuated with symptoms like an urgent desire to urinate even after bladder has been emptied, pus or blood in the urine, cloudy urine with unpleasant odor, frequent urination, painful, burning sensation when urinating, lower abdominal pain (especially in children) and chills. Fever and nausea may also be present.

Precautions

Painful urination may signal the presence of a vaginal infection or other potentially dangerous condition. In and of itself, this symptom does not necessarily indicate that a bladder infection is present. Blood in the urine is another symptom which should be called to the attention of your physician.

Causes

- ◆ Over 80 percent of all bladder infections are caused by *E. coli* bacterium which normally reside in the large intestine. In rare circumstances, a virus or fungus may be responsible. Bacteria can travel through the urethra and adhere to the walls of the bladder causing an inflammation.
- ◆ Venereal diseases like gonorrhea and chlamydia may also trigger a bladder infection.
- ◆ Honeymoon cystitis, refers to an inflammation of the bladder brought on by frequent sexual intercourse.
- ◆ Childbirth can also increase your chances of getting cystitis as can some drugs or chemicals.

◆ Consuming an excess of caffeine-containing beverages, alcohol and cigarette smoking have also been linked to bladder infections.

◆ Using a diaphragm for contraception can sometimes block the complete emptying of the bladder which may trigger an infection.

◆ Overusing douches may also cause inflammation.

◆ Estrogen level drops associated with menopause can cause increased susceptibility to bladder infections.

Conventional Therapies

If your doctor determines that you are suffering from a bladder infection, an antibiotic will be prescribed. Bactrin, septra gantrisin, ampicillin or amoxicillin may be used. Some doctors prescribe tetracycline as well. If you continually battle recurring bladder infections, your doctor may recommend that you take an antibiotic every day as a preventative measure. Nitrofurantoin is the most common one used for this purpose. I feel that the use of antibiotics as a preventative therapy should be discouraged unless absolutely necessary. If infections continually recur, your doctor may order a cystoscopy, a procedure that allows the bladder to be visually evaluated.

Dietary Guidelines

◆ Put a big pitcher of water in the fridge and drink, drink, drink. One large glass of water every other hour is recommended or several gallons over the first 24-hour period.

◆ Drinking pure cranberry juice is also recommended; however, sweetened fruit juices are not. Pure cherry juice is also good. Stay away from citrus and other acidic juices.

◆ Cut down on white sugar products or rich, refined foods. Bacteria thrive in high-sugar environments.

◆ Eat plenty of watermelon, which acts as a natural diuretic.

◆ Avoid dairy products.

◆ Do not use alcohol, caffeine or sugary beverages.

◆ Drinking barley water made by steeping barley in a small amount of water can help to soothe the urinary tract.

Recommended Nutritional Supplements

PRIMARY NUTRIENTS

CRANBERRY Considered a superior herb for the treatment and prevention of bladder infections. Compounds in cranberry have the ability to inhibit *E. coli* bacteria from sticking to the walls of the bladder.[1] Taking concentrated cranberry capsules seems to work better than juice forms. If you prefer juice, make sure it is pure, 100 percent unsweetened cranberry. This type of juice may not be found in grocery stores. Check your local health food store. *Suggested Dosage:* If taking a pure juice form, drink at least one quart daily.

Cranberry capsules are more efficient taken in stronger concentrations than juice. Start with four capsules per day for the first three to five days and, then dropping off to two.

GARLIC Acts as a natural antibiotic and has proven antibacterial properties. The allium content of garlic has demonstrated its ability to act as a broad spectrum antibacterial and antifungal agent.[2] *Suggested Dosage:* Two capsules at least three times a day. Take with meals. Garlic can be purchased in deodorized forms.

VITAMIN C WITH BIOFLAVONOIDS Helps to make the urine more acidic which inhibits bacterial growth while boosting immune function. Clincal tests have shown that any infection increases our requirement for this vitamin in that it actually localizes itself at the site of an infection.[3] *Suggested Dosage:* 3,000 to 5,000 mg taken throughout the day. Chewable supplements may be taken continually, however, make sure to drink lots of water when taking therapeutic doses of vitamin C. Esterized products may be useful if you have a sensitivity to acidic supplements. Powders are practical and can be mixed with liquids.

ACIDOPHILUS Replaces friendly flora killed by antibiotics which helps to boost immunity and proper food assimilation. Moreover, boosting lactobacilli helps to fight invading microorganisms that cause urinary tract infections. Acidophilus is particularly helpful for bladder infections in that it can correct the growth of gram-negative bacteria which occurs after antibiotic therapy.[4] *Suggested Dosage:* Both quality capsulized or liquid forms of acidophilus should be taken as recommended on the product label first thing in the morning and right before bedtime. Look for varieties that guarantee bacterial count and check the expiration date. The friendly bacteria found in acidophilus supplements will also be killed by antibiotic therapy. Take the supplements following your course of therapy. Women with recurrent infections may want to try acidophilus vaginal suppositories which has been proven to reduce subsequent infections.[5]

HERBAL COMBINATION This combination should include cornsilk, uva ursi, parsley, juniper berries and buchu. *Suggested Dosage:* Take six to eight capsules a day with a large glass of pure water.

CORNSILK: Used for centuries by Europeans as a urinary diuretic and demulcent and has gained official recognition in France, Britain and Belgium. Clinical studies in both Japan and China have supported its remarkable diuretic properties.[6] UVA URSI: As one of the best researched diuretics, it has excellent antiseptic and antibacterial actions due to its arbutin content which is converted to hydroquinone in the body.[7] PARSLEY: The diuretic action of this herb is due to compounds called myristicin and apiole.[8] Parsley is used in Britain and Germany to provide irrigation when treating kidney stones. JUNIPER BERRIES: Juniper effectively expels uric acid from the body which helps to prevent the development of kidney stones.[9] BUCHU: This herb acts to soothe irritated membranes. Diasophenol, which has antiseptic properties, is considered to be the most important chemical constituent found in buchu.[10]

SECONDARY NUTRIENTS

VITAMIN B-COMPLEX: Helps to ensure proper assimilation of other nutrients and strengthens the body during periods of stress. *Suggested Dosage:* Take as directed, although higher doses are recommended if you are taking antibiotics.

VITAMIN E: Helps to fight infection and promote tissue repair by boosting the action of phagocytes and stimulating cellular defense mechanisms.[11] *Suggested Dosage:* One 600 IU capsule daily. Look for organic sources.

VITAMIN A WITH BETA-CAROTENE: Boosts the functions of the immune system, promotes tissue repair and acts as a free radical scavenger. Supplementing this vitamin has been shown to enhance lymphocyte response to infections and may actually raise our resistence to them.[12] *Suggested Dosage:* Take as directed however do not exceed 25,000 IU daily during the infection period. Drop to 10,000 IU when the infection is over. Pregnant women should not take over 10,000 IU per day.

LIQUID CHLOROPHYLL: Helps to purify the blood and eliminate toxins thrown off by bacteria. (Chlorella, a blue-green algae is high in natural chlorophyll and has shown its ability to protect against infection.)[13] *Suggested Dosage:* Take as directed on product label and use fat-soluble varieties.

ECHINACEA: An herb with proven antibiotic action. This botanical has potent immunostimulatory properties which help to boost white blood cell count and has shown good results in treating a variety of infections, including urogenital varieties.[14] *Suggested Dosage:* Take as directed in either capsule or tincture form. Do not use for over three weeks at a time. Look for standardized or guaranteed potency products.

POTASSIUM: An electrolyte which can be lost in the urine if diuretics are used. *Suggested Dosage:* Take as directed only.

KELP: Replaces trace elements lost through urination and contains algin which helps to soothe inflamed tissue. *Suggested Dosage:* Take one capsule daily with meals.

Home Care Suggestions

- Do not hold urine for long periods of time. Try to empty your bladder every two to three hours.
- Hot sitz bathes can help alleviate pain and discomfort.
- Hot water bottles or heating pads can help ease abdominal pain.

Other Supportive Therapies

ACUPUNCTURE: Proper treatments involves points on the kidney, liver, bladder meridians and the spleen.

HOMEOPATHY: Use Staphysagria 6C for infection and Cantharis 6C for burning pains when urinating.

HYDROTHERAPY: Use a hand sprayer to first direct hot water to the pelvic area, then repeat cold water.

REFLEXOLOGY: Massaging the lower pelvic area can ease symptoms and stimulate circulation to promote better healing and recovery.

AROMATHERAPY: Juniper and sandalwood combined with lavender can be used in oil form as an abdominal massage agent.

Scientific Facts-at-a-Glance

In one study, both women and men who drank 16 ounces of cranberry juice per day eliminated bladder infections by 73 percent.[16] An additional trial published in the *Journal of the American Medical Association* reported that consuming eight ounces of cranberry juice resulted significantly inhibiting the proliferation of bacteria in the urine.[17]

Spirit/Mind Considerations

Bladder infections can be increased by high levels of stress, eating on the run or forgetting to drink adequate amounts of water. Essentially, high anxiety states or emotional fatigue can heighten the risk for a bladder infection. In the case of "honeymoon cystitis" make sure that no misunderstandings arise between you and your spouse concerning the cause of this condition. In other words, knowing that bladder infections in newlywed women are commonplace can help to dispel fears or remove any possible guilt experienced by the new husband.

Prevention

- Use good feminine hygiene practices to keep fecal matter from the urethra.
- Wearing cotton underwear is recommended for women with recurring infections.
- Tampon use may predispose some women to bladder infections.
- Drink a lot of water every day, at least six to eight glasses.
- Empty the bladder before and after sexual intercourse.
- Do not use douches or soaps which can alter pH or irritate membranes thereby increasing susceptibility to infection.

Doctor's Notes

My experience with bladder infections is that women typically suffer from recurring infections because the lining of their bladders have not totally healed from a previous infection, making it prone to re-inoculation with *E. coli* bacteria. I tell my patients who get frequent UTIs to take cranberry for three to four months and then assess the results. Cranberry therapy for this time period allows the bladder to heal. Consequently many women can stop taking the supplement and are much less likely to contract another infection.

If the infection recurs, I recommend an taking cranberry for an indefinite period of time. The alternative to this natural and safe therapy is a protocol of life-long antibiotic treatment. Unlike antibiotics, there is no evidence that bacteria become resistant to cranberry. This is probably due to the fact that cranberry does not kill bacteria like antibiotics do. Instead, it very nicely prevents the bacterial attachment that causes an infection to develop in the first place.[15]

Dried and concentrated cranberry is superior to sweetened and diluted juices and should be taken initially in larger doses with a tapering off. If you take antibiotics for this infection, make sure to use a good acidophilus supplement to replace friendly bacteria that are also killed by the drug.

There is some controversy about taking acidophilus simultaneously with an antibiotic or after treatment has stopped. While it is true that some of the replaced bacteria will also be killed, acidophilus can be taken during and after a course of antibiotic therapy.

One of the more serious forms of bladder infection is called interstitual cystitis, an autoimmune disease or a bladder irritation that is an extension of infections elsewhere in the body. People who suffer with intersititual cystitis experince painful urination, bleeding in the urine and lower abdominal pain, even though there may be no infection present in the urine.

I remember a 58-year-old woman with interstitual cystitis who had a cyctoscopy which revealed areas of ulceration inside the bladder, some of which were caused by diagnostic probing. She had been through the standard regimen of uncomfortable and costly treatments. I started her on a cranberry product called supercranactin that contains a concentrated amount of cranberry plus lesion-healing herbs such as uva ursi and nettle. I also put her on some Chinese herbs designed to clear heat out of the body. In addition she also recieved acupuncture treatments. After her fourth acupuncture treatment, she experienced substantial improvement and by the eigth week, had minimal pain. Now, after 20 treatments, she feels little pain for more than two weeks before needing another treatment. She has replaced her costly surgical procedures with natural, more benign treatments and is very happy with the results.

Additional Resources

Home testing kits can be purchased which can help you find out if your are suffering from a urinary tract infection through color changes when placed in the urine. Ask your pharmacist to direct you to the appropriate products.

Endnotes

1. J. Avorn, M. Monane et al., "Reduction of bacteriuria and pyuria after ingestion of cranberry juice," JAMA, 1994, 271: 751-54.
2. M.A. Adetumbi and B.H. Lau, "Allium sativum (garlic): A natural antibiotic," Med Hypoth, 1983, 12(3): 227-37.
3. P.W. Stacpoole, "Role of vitamin C in infectious diseases and allergic reactions," Med Hypoth, 1975, 1: 42-46.
4. Michael D. Murray, Encyclopedia of Nutritional Supplements, Prima Publishing, Rocklin, CA: 1996, 362-63.
5. G. Reid, A.W. Bruce and M. Taylor, "Influence of three day antimicrobial therapy and lactobacillus vaginal suppositories on recurrence of urinary tract infections," Clin Ther, 1992, 14: 11-16.
6. A.L. Leung, Chinese Herbal Remedies, (Universe Books, New York: 1984), 47-49.
7. A.L. Leung, Encyclopedia of Common Natural Ingredients Used in Food, Drugs and Cosmetics, (John Wiley and Sons, New York: 1980), 316-17.
8. Daniel B. Mowrey, That Scientific Validation of Herbal Medicine, (Keats Publishing, Connecticut: 1986), 234.
9. Ibid., 83-84.
10. V.E. Tyler, L.R. Brady and J.E. Robbers, Pharmacognosy, 7th ed., (Lead and Febiger, Philadelphia: 1976). See also H.W. Youngken, Textbook of Pharmacognosy, 5th ed., (Blakiston, Philadelphia: 1943) and M. Grieve, A Modern Herbal, (Dorset Press, New York: 1994), 134.
11. R.P. Tengerdy, "Vitamin E, immune reponse and disease resistance," Ann NY Acad Sci, 1989, 570: 335-44.
12. W.R. Beisel, "Single nutrients and immunity," Amer Jour Clin Nutri, 1982, 35: 417-68.
13. R.E. Merchant, et al., "Dietary chlorella pyrenoidosa for pateints with malignant glioma: Effects on immunocompetence, quality of life and survivial," Phyto Res, 1991, 4(6): 220-31.
14. R. Bauer and H. Wagner, "Echinacea species as potential immunostimulatory drugs," Econ Med Plant Res, 1991, 5: 253-321.
15. A.E. Sabota, "Inhibition of bacterial adherence by cranberry juice: potential use for the treatment of urinary tract infections," Journal of Urology, 131: 1984, 1013-16.
16. P.N. Prodromos, et al., "Cranberry juice in the treatment of urinary tract infections," Southwestern Med., 47:17, 1968.
17. J. Avorn, et al., "Reduction of bacteriuria and pyuria after ingestion of cranberry juice," JAMA, 271: 1994, 751-54.

BOILS

A boil is a localized infection that is the result of a bacteria that inhabits the skin through the hair follicle. A boil is referred to by the medical profession as a "furuncle." Boils are tender, pus-filled areas of the skin and are usually round in shape. Boils may reoccur and persist for years and will often run in families. They may erupt in any part of the body appearing as a single infection or in multiple groups. The *Staphylococcus aureus* bacteria can usually be cultured from a boil or abscess. Boils are painful and unsightly and can leave scars. Unfortunately, they are also extremely common and should never be confused with acne.

Children and adolescents are particularly prone to boils. Boils are considered contagious and if pus comes in contact with other skin surfaces, new boils can develop. If pus enters the blood stream, boils can erupt in other parts of the body as well. Boils will eventually come to a head, burst and heal within two to three weeks.

Symptoms

Boils generally appear on the buttocks, face, underarms, or upper thighs. They are usually red, raised areas that are extremely tender to the touch. Itching, pain, throbbing and swelling around the boil region is common. Fever or swollen glands may or may not be present. In time, a yellowish tip may appear on the boil.

Precautions

If a fever accompanies a boil, it appears on the face or has red streaking or is fluid filled, see your doctor as soon as possible. It can be dangerous to squeeze a boil, especially around the lips and nose region as the bacteria can invade the bloodstream and cause blood poisoning.

Causes

Boils are usually caused by the bacterium staphylococcus aureus (staph) which invades a hair follicle. Other possible causes of boils include diabetes mellitus (which reduces resistance to bacterial infection), poor hygiene, a weakened immune system, poor nutrition, immunosuppressive drugs, exposure to industrial chemicals, obesity, and nephritis.

Conventional Therapies

Treating a boil usually involves making a small incision in the center of the boil (lancing), to allow the pus to drain off. In addition, an antibiotic may be prescribed to fight the infection and a topical ointment may be used. Like many stubborn types of recurring infections, boils can be difficult to cure. Often antibiotic therapy is temporary and can increase susceptibility to subsequent exposures to infections. Using antiseptic soaps like Betadine on the skin are also usually recommended to keep the number of staph bacteria down. However there is some speculation that these chemicals may upset the natural balance of skin chemistry and increase susceptibility.

Dietary Guidelines

- Avoid a diet high in sugars and fat which can increase susceptibility to infection.
- Eat plenty of raw fruits and vegetables.
- A juice fast may help to reduce toxins in the system.
- Drink eight to ten glasses of pure water daily.

Recommended Nutritional Supplements

PRIMARY NUTRIENTS

GARLIC Acts as a natural antibiotic which boosts the immune system and fights infection. *Suggested Dosage:* Two capsules with each meal. Garlic oil can be applied externally. If the skin is broken, irritation and pain can result from garlic application.

COLLOIDAL SILVER Can be used as a topical application to fight infection. *Suggested Dosage:* Use as directed.

VITAMIN A AND ZINC Work together to boost the immune system. Zinc has been successfully used to treat recurring boils.[1] *Suggested Dosage:* 25,000 IU of vitamin A and 50 mg of zinc per day.

VITAMIN C Fights infection and inflammation and assists with tissue repair. *Suggested Dosage:* 10,000 mg per day divided in three equal doses.

HERBAL COMBINATION This combination should include echinacea, goldenseal root, myrrh gum, garlic, licorice root, blue vervain, butternut root bark and kelp. *Suggested Dosage:* Six to twelve capsules daily. This formula should not be used for more than three weeks at a time.

ECHINACEA: In Britain, this herb used to fight chronic, viral and bacterial infections, pathogenic organisms in the blood, boils, various skin complaints, colds and influenza. Immune stimulation is a well known and documented property of echinacea, making it the herb of choice for boils. Echinacea also improves the mobility of infection-combating leukocytes (white blood cells).[2] Echinacea should not be used for longer than two weeks at a time. GOLDENSEAL ROOT: Two of goldenseal's more active compounds, hydrastine and berberine, have demonstrated effectiveness in treating ulcers and various bacterial and viral infections. It also stimulates immune function and acts as an anti-inflammatory agent.[3] MYRRH GUM: Myrrh gum stimulates phagocyte activity and reduces inflammation of the mucus-secreting mucosa. Myrrh gum also helps with skin problems, ulcers and acts as an antiseptic and anti-inflammatory.[4] GARLIC: Garlic is another herb that can be considered a tonic. It is a powerful warrior against infections of various types and origins. Garlic can increase the number of leukocytes, which help fight infections. In addition, garlic increases perspiration which further cleanses the body.[5] LICORICE ROOT: Licorice root boosts adrenal function which augments immune defenses and also exerts anti-inflammatory and antibacterial actions.[6] Long-term use of licorice is not recommended. It may cause weakness, electrolyte imbalances, water retention and hypertension. BLUE VERVAIN: Blue vervain has the ability to break the cycle of chronically occurring infections and helps to reduce fever. BUTTERNUT ROOT BARK: Butternut improves liver function and stimulates bile production and flow. It also acts as a laxative without gripping, helping the body rid itself of toxins. KELP: Kelp's function in this formula is to provide needed trace elements important in many metabolic processes in the body. These nutrients may further support the healing process and return the body to normal function.

SECONDARY NUTRIENTS

PAU D'ARCO: A natural immuno-stimulant with antiviral and antibacterial properties. *Suggested Dosage:* Take as directed.[7]

ALOE VERA GEL: Helps to heal scar tissue when applied externally. *Suggested Usage:* Use as directed.

TEA TREE OIL: Topical applications of tea tree oil can fight against both bacterial and viral invaders. *Suggested Usage:* Apply as directed.

Home Care Suggestions

◆ Use warm compresses on the boil until it comes to a head and breaks on its own.
◆ Take showers instead of baths to reduce the chance of the infection spreading to another part of the body.
◆ After touching a boil, wash your hands thoroughly to prevent staph contamination of food.
◆ Soaking the boil in an Epsom salt solution is also beneficial in bringing the abscesses to a head.
◆ An onion poultice placed between two pieces of cloth and applied directly to the boil may help in expediting healing.
◆ Fresh hot figs applied directly to the boil also helps bring them to a head.
◆ A bag of black tea used as a compress is an old folk remedy for boils.
◆ Steep one tablespoon of goldenseal and one-half teaspoon of myrrh in pint of boiling water and use to wash the infected area.
◆ It's best not to cover a boil with a bandage and to keep the area clean.

Other Supportive Therapies

HYDROTHERAPY: Going from a hot to a cold bath can help to stimulate circulation which enables white blood cells to more efficiently tackle local infections.

Spirit/Mind Considerations

If you are suffering from recurring boils due to immune system weakness, you need to consider physical and emotional causes. Are you eating a healthy diet? Ask yourself if you are coping with stressors in a way that protects your immune system from impairment. Learn to relax, use controlled breathing exercises or mediation everyday. Make use of a daily recuperative time to relieve stress.

Prevention

◆ Keep the immune system healthy by avoiding prolonged use of antibiotics. If they are necessary, use acidophilus to replace friendly bacteria.
◆ Take essential fatty acids found in salmon and evening primrose oil to protect the immune system.
◆ Take a potent multivitamin and mineral formula every day.
◆ Make sure to keep your vitamin C levels up.

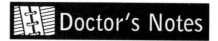 **Doctor's Notes**

Boils are a sign that the immune system has been compromised in some way. Various factors such as poor diet and food allergies may contribute to depressed immunity. Zinc and vitamin A are of particular importance in the treatment of boils. Herbal formulas containing echinacea can also be very good treatments for boils. As a point of caution, some herbs like *Parthenium integrifolium* are labeled as echinacea. Don't accept substitutes. Insist on the real plant and look for standardized or guaranteed potency products.

Other herbs that improve immunity include goldenseal and shitake and rieshi mushrooms (these contain a substance called betaglucan, which improves immune system function). Gotu kola can stimulate immune system function and protect the skin against the spread of infection.

Poultices of goldenseal, oil of bergamot, chamomile and lavender can help to bring the infection to the surface.

Endnotes

1. A. Sanchez, et al., "Role of sugars on human neutrophilic phagocytosis," Amer Jour Clinical Nutri, 1973, 26: 1180-84.
2. B. Luettig, et al., "Macrophage activation by the polysaccharide arabinogalactan isolated from plant cell cultures of Echinacea purpurea, Journal of the National Cancer Institute, 1989, 81: 669-75.
3. Kumazawa, et al., "Activation of peritoneal macrophages by berberine alkaloids in terms of induction of cytostatic activity," Int Jour Immunopharmacol, 1984, 6: 587-92.
4. F. Ellingwood, American Materia Medica, Therapeutics and Pharmacognosy, Eclectic Medical Publication, Portland, Oregon: 1983.
5. B.G. Hughes and L. Lawson, "Antimicrobial effects of Allivum sativum (Garlic)," Phototherapy Res, 1991, 5: 154-58.
6. E. Okimasa, et al., "Inhibition of phospholipase A2 by glycyrrhizin, an anti-inflammatory drug," Acta Med Okayama, 1983, 37: 385-91.
7. A.R. Burnett and R.H. Thompson, "Naturally occurring quionones: The quinone constituents of Tabebuia avellanedae (Bignoniaceae)," Jour Chem Soc, 1967, C: 2100-04.

BPH (Benign Prostatic Hypertrophy)

SEE "PROSTATE DISEASE"

BRONCHITIS

Bronchitis is an inflammation of the mucous membranes that line the bronchi, which comprise the primary airways of the lungs. Bronchitis will usually clear up within a few days if the heart and lungs are healthy.

This disorder commonly occurs during winter months. Chronic bronchitis is a different, more serious disorder usually resulting from prolonged smoking. Continual attacks of chronic bronchitis will cause the lungs to deteriorate.

Symptoms

Bronchitis is a serious infectious disease that is characterized by breathlessness, tightness in the chest, fever, chills, fatigue, wheezing, a very deep cough that can produce grayish or yellow phlegm or sputum, and a cough that may initially be dry.

Bronchitis is also punctuated by a sensation that phlegm needs to be coughed up when in fact, there is nothing there. In addition, pain in the upper chest (which usually worsens upon coughing) may be felt.

Precautions

Contact a physician immediately if you are breathless, cough up blood, have a temperature above 101° F or do not experience improvement within 48 hours.

Causes

◆ Bronchitis can develop as a secondary infection after any respiratory disorder such as a cold, flu or even a sore throat. It is caused by a viral infection and does not respond to antibiotics.
◆ Some forms of bronchitis can also be caused by inhaling dust, pollution or chemical fumes.
◆ Allergies and asthma can predispose one to bronchitis.
◆ While the lungs are particularly resistant to bacterial invaders, they seem more susceptible to the viral infections which cause bronchitis.

Conventional Therapies

Because bronchitis is usually caused by a virus, antibiotics will not be effective unless a secondary infection is present. Addressing the symptoms of the disease will be the primary concern of your doctor. He may prescribe a bronchodilator inhaler and cough suppressants. Cough preparations containing codeine or hydrocodone are routinely used, although these should be used with caution. If the cough produces yellow or greenish mucous, a secondary infection is usually present. In these cases an antibiotic will be prescribed. Nutritional supplements in the form of herbs, vitamins etc. can be of great value in treating viral infections like bronchitis.

Dietary Guidelines

◆ Citrus juices are recommended, though if their sugar content is too high, dilute them with pure water.
◆ Emphasize plenty of fresh fruits and vegetables and stay away from rich, fatty sugary foods.
◆ Hot lemon juice with ginger helps to relieve throat tickling which can provoke coughing and also works to expedite the movement of mucus.
◆ Drink at least eight to ten glasses of pure water daily.
◆ Avoid mucus-forming foods like dairy products.

Recommended Nutritional Supplements

PRIMARY NUTRIENTS

VITAMIN A WITH BETA CAROTENE Essential for lung tissue regeneration and to stimulate immune function. Laboratory tests have proven that vitamin A can help restore immune function even when health has been compromised.[1] *Suggested Dosage:* 25,000 IU during the infection then reduce to 10,000 when better. Do not exceed 10,000 IU if you are pregnant.

VITAMIN C WITH BIOFLAVONOIDS Vitamin C is an antiviral compound which has wonderful anti-inflammatory properties. It also boosts immunity and acts to scavenge dangerous free radicals caused by infection or pollutant exposure.[3] In addition, a recent study of elderly patients hospitalized for bronchitis and pneumonia found that even modest doses of vitamin C were beneficial.[4] *Suggested Dosage:* 10,000 mg daily in three divided doses with meals.

QUERCETIN A bioflavonoid which is capable of antioxidant activity and has the ability to fight against respiratory viruses.[5] *Suggested Dosage:* Take as directed. May be part of a flavonoid blend.

GARLIC A powerful infection fighter against both viral and bacterial infections. When mice were infected with influenza virus, garlic supplementation protected against the development of the disease.[6] *Suggested Dosage:* Take two capsules with each of three meals.

ZINC LOZENGES Helps to stimulate immunity and fights viral infections that cause bronchitis, colds and flu.[7] *Suggested Dosage:* Do not take more than 100 mg of zinc per day. Use zinc gluconate products.

GOLDENSEAL Has natural antiviral and antibiotic properties from its berberine content which can augment immune function.[8] *Suggested Dosage:* Take as directed using guaranteed potency products. Do not take goldenseal for more than two weeks at a time. If you are pregnant, nursing or allergic to ragweed pollen, do not use this herb.

ST. JOHN'S WORT Recent studies have demonstrated the impressive antiviral properties of the hypericin content of this herb.[9] *Suggested Dosage:* Take as directed using guaranteed potency products if possible.

ECHINACEA Considered an immunostimulant, echinacea has the ability to help fight viral infections by potentiating the action of white blood cells. *Suggested Dosage:* Take as directed but do not use for longer than two weeks at a time.

LOBELIA A very effective and natural expectorant, obelia helps to liquefy and move out stubborn lung mucus. It also contains a compound which stimulates the adrenal glands to release certain hormones than can cause the bronchiole tubes to relax.[10] *Suggested Dosage:* Take only as directed with meals. If taken on an empty stomach, lobelia may cause nausea. Do not use on children unless approved by your doctor.

HERBAL COMBINATION This combination should include pleurisy root, wild cherry bark, slippery elm bark, plantain, mullein leaves, chickweed, horehound, licorice root, kelp, ginger root and saw palmetto berries. *Suggested Dosage:* Four to eight capsules daily. For chronic conditions it is best to use maximum dosage of eight capsules per day for a prolonged period of three to six weeks or until symptoms subside.

PLEURISY ROOT: Technically, pleurisy is an inflammatory condition affecting a thin lining covering the lungs and thorax and is usually a complication of pneumonia, tuberculosis and other infectious diseases.[11] This root has been used for other respiratory problems including bronchitis and catarrh. WILD CHERRY BARK: Wild cherry bark has always been a favorite in cough and cold medicines. However, its most effective action for bronchiole spasms or coughs relates to its ability to relax or sedate the respiratory nerves. SLIPPERY ELM BARK: Slippery elm bark has a reputation as a medicine for bronchitis, pleurisy and coughs. It has received official recognition in the United States Pharmacopeia and its inner bark is known for its demulcent, diuretic and emollient properties. PLANTAIN: Used as an expectorant and is especially good for those suffering chronic catarrhal problems such as bronchitis.[12] It is also beneficial for hoarseness and sore throats. It is applicable for virtually all respiratory problems. MULLEIN LEAVES: While considered a good remedy for coughs, hoarseness, bronchitis, catarrh and whooping cough it stands out as an antispasmodic in treating asthma as well. Mullein leaves were officially recognized as an asthma treatment in the *National Formulary* until 1936. CHICKWEED: Chickweed is a folk remedy for asthma, but is also recognized as an expectorant. It has mild laxative effects which will contribute to the cleansing and healing process. HOREHOUND: Horehound is an excellent remedy for coughs and bronchial problems. Its activity is thought to be attributed to a volatile oil found in the herb called marubiin. LICORICE ROOT: Licorice root has received official recognition in Britain, Germany, France and Belgium for its ability to assist with various respiratory problems which include bronchitis, hoarseness, coughs, sore throats, catarrh and congestion.[13] KELP: Kelp's direct application in this formula is in assisting with bronchitis, emphysema and asthma. However, indirectly, kelp provides a very rich storehouse of nutrients which can assist with the healing process. GINGER ROOT: Ginger root makes the other herbs more effective with its catalyst action. Ginger is also an antispasmodic which can quiet coughs. SAW PALMETTO BERRIES: Saw palmetto berries are useful in the treatment of colds, asthma, bronchitis and catarrhal problems. The berries are recognized for their diuretic properties, contributing to overall cleansing.

SECONDARY NUTRIENTS

VITAMIN E: Needed to heal lung tissue and to also increase disease resistance.[14] In addition, if you smoke or are exposed to cigarette smoke, vitamin E supplementation can help to protects against oxidative lung damage.[15] *Suggested Dosage:* Take 400 IU every day.

CYSTEINE: An amino acid which helps build resistance to chronic bronchitis and other respiratory diseases. It also contributes to the thinning of mucus. *Suggested Dosage:* Take as directed on an empty stomach with fruit juice.

WHITE HOREHOUND: Can help relax the bronchiole tubes and ease congestion. Horehound candy is an excellent lozenge. *Suggested Dosage:* Take as directed.

COMFREY AND FENUGREEK: An herbal duo which helps strengthen lungs and facilitates the movement of mucus. *Suggested Dosage:* Take as directed.

Home Care Suggestions

◆ Hang the upper half of your body over the bed, placing your hands on the floor. Stay this way for ten minutes. This position encourages expectorating and is good to initiate mucus drainage.

◆ Over-the-counter cough medicines can be recommended by a physician. Those containing dextromethorphan are preferable if the cough is dry and unproductive. Frequently, if a cough is suppressed, bringing up mucus is also inhibited. Cough medicines should be used sparingly.

◆ Cough drops can help alleviate the tickly feeling that can prompt coughing. Some wonderful herbal lozenges are available in health food shops.

◆ Inhaling vapors made form eucalyptus leaves helps to relieve congestion. Oil-based solutions should be avoided, though, because they may cause irritation.

◆ Mustard poultices have been used for generations as a treatment for lung disorders. Mix one part dry mustard with three parts flour and add water to make a paste. Spread the paste on a cotton pillow case or cheesecloth, flood it and place on the chest for up to twenty minutes. Check to make sure the skin is not becoming overly irritated

◆ Stay in a warm environment and get plenty of rest.

◆ Do not smoke or be around anyone that does. Tobacco smoke can irritate the bronchiole tubes.

◆ A vaporizer or humidifier is recommended. Staying in a closed shower stall with hot water running can substitute for a vaporizer of one is not available. A tent can be fashioned over a simmering pot of water also and steam can be inhaled for at least three to five minutes.

◆ Use a heating pad or hot water bottle applied to the chest for thirty minutes.

◆ Drink plenty of fluids to help facilitate the removal of excess mucous and hydrate the system.

◆ Avoid caffeine due to its diuretic properties. Gaining fluid, rather than losing it, is desirable.

◆ Avoid alcoholic beverages; these can cause dehydration.

◆ Eat hot, spicy foods such as red peppers. In addition to causing a runny nose, the entire respiratory system secretes more fluid, which is beneficial in thinning out mucous.

Other Supportive Therapies

AROMATHERAPY: Inhaling eucalyptus or thyme aromatics can help ease coughing and congestion.

HOMEOPATHY: Aconite, Kali bich. and Pulsatilla are often used for bronchial congestion and coughs.

Scientific Facts-at-a-Glance

Allergies can significantly predispose us to developing bronchitis. If you are continually exposed to lung irritants or allergens like cigarette smoke or other toxic fumes, you can suffer from recurring bouts of bronchitis which, if not resolved early enough, can damage the heart and lungs.

Spirit/Mind Considerations

Bronchitis often occurs when the body is run down from prior infection or perhaps, after a period of high stress. Again, in many cases of bronchitis, the immune system has been compromised, which explains why this ailment is so prevalent among elderly people. Using mediation and relaxation techniques helps to enhance the ability of the body to heal. Coughing spells can be triggered by anxiety or anger, therefore, learning to channel negative emotions is important.

Prevention

◆ Do not smoke or be around anyone that does. Tobacco smoke can irritate the bronchiole tubes.

◆ Protect yourself from environmental hazards in the workplace or home which can continually irritate the lungs.

◆ Keep your immune function strong with good vitamin and mineral supplementation.

◆ Use mega-doses of vitamin C at the first indication of a cold, sore throat or flu to keep secondary infections like bronchitis from developing.

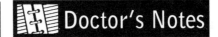 **Doctor's Notes**

Bronchitis is usually treated with antibiotics, which have no effect. A much better approach would be to use a combination of herbs which have known antiviral properties. Using combinations which include echinacea, goldenseal, lobelia and pleurisy root are effective.

Bronchitis can take several forms. Chronic bronchitis is often associated with obstructive pulmonary disease which usually results from smoking or harmful environmental exposure. The more common form of bronchitis is acute bronchitis which is part of an infectious process. By far, the majority of these infections are viral in nature. They should be treated with herbs that have proven antiviral properties, such as echinacea, goldenseal or St. John's wort.

Antibiotics will be of no value for simple virally caused bronchitis. Herbal blends with horehound, cherry bark and pleurisy root are also very helpful. Boiling water on the stove and breathing in the steam can help to break up mucus.

Respiratory distress can be caused by a wide variety of factors and can exhibit itself with many different symptoms. The herbal formula suggested in this section is designed to ameliorate the symptoms and assist in overcoming some of the underlying causes. Herbs have been used for respiratory ailment by various cultures all over the world for thousands of years. There is strong historical documentation for these particular applications. Herbs are very effective and are extremely safe and relatively free from side effects. Conventional drugs used to treat respiratory ailments are often riddled with side effects, making the natural approach the best alternative.

Additional Resources

Lung Line Information Service
(800) 222-5864
(303) 355-5864

National Heart, Lung and Blood Institute
PO Box 30105
Bethesda, MD 20824-0105
(301) 251-1222

Endnotes

1. Pharmacology, April, 1985, 30: 181-87.
2. N.I. Krinksy, "Antioxidant function of carotenoids," 1989, Free Rad Biol Med, 7: 627-35.
3. Annals of Nutrition and Metabolism, May-June, 1984, 28: 186-91.
4. C. Hunt, et al., "The clinical effects of vitamin C supplementation in elderly hospitalized patients with acute respiratory infections," Inter Jour of Vit Nutri Res, 1994, 64: 212-19.
5. I. Musci and B.M. Pragai, "Inhibition of virus multiplication and alteration of cyclic AMP levels in cell cultures by flavonoids," Experientia, 1985, 41: 930-31.
6. K. Nagai, "Experimental studies on the preventative effect of garlic extract against infection with influenza virus," Jpn Jour Infect Dis, 1973, 47: 321. See also N.D. Weber, et al., "In vitro virucidal effects of Allivum sativum (garlic) extract and compounds," Planta Medica, 1992, 58: 417-23.

7. G.A. Eby and G.R. Davis, "Reduction in duration of common colds by zinc gluconate lozenges in a double-blind study," Anti Microb Agents Chemo, 1984, 25: 20-24.

8. Y. Kumazawa, et al., "Activation of peritoneal macrophages by berberine alkaloids in terms of induction of cytostatic activity," Int Jour Immunpharmacol, 1984, 6: 587-92.

9. H. Someya, "Effect of a constituent of Hypericum erectum on infection and multiplication of Epstein-Barr virus," Jour Tokyo Med Coll, 1985, 43: 815-26.

10. D. Halmagyi, et al., "Adrenocortical pathway of lobeline protection in some forms of experimental lung edema of the rat," Dis Chest, 1958, 33: 285-96.

11. F.K. Fitzpatrick, "Plant substances active against mycobacterium tuberculosis," Antibiotics and Chemotherapy, 1954, 4(5): 528-36.

12. M. Matev, et al., "Clinical trial of a plantago major preparation in the treatment of chronic bronchitis," Vutreshni Bolest (Sofia), 1982, 21(2): 133-37.

13. K.M. Nasyrov, et al., "Anti-inflammatory activity of glycyrrhizic acid derivatives," Farmakologiia e Toksikologiia, 1980, 43(4): 399-404.

14. American Journal of Clinical Nutrition, (supplement), 35: 431-33.

15. Journal of Clinical Investigation, March, 1986, 77: 789-96.

BULIMIA

Bulimia literally means "an oxlike appetite" and is characterized by abnormal episodes of excessive eating followed by forced vomiting or purging. It is considered a major eating disorder and often accompanies anorexia. Episodes of vomiting can occur as rarely as once a month or several times a day. Bulimics may also use large amounts of laxatives or diuretics to expel food as quickly as possible.

This disorder is on the increase and usually affects the adolescent or college-aged women. Most victims of this disorder are between the ages of fifteen and thirty. It has been estimated that up to 20 percent of college-age women suffer from bulimia to some extent. Bulimia has become so common among young women, it is considered normal behavior in some circles. Bulimia commonly affects young women who are well educated and come from high-income families.

Bulimia is sometimes considered a variant of anorexia nervosa, a psychiatric disorder, but this is not always the case. Both conditions are motivated by a morbid and profound fear of becoming fat or an obsession to control eating and restrict calorie consumption. Some anorexics may eventually become bulimic. The two disorders can exist simultaneously.

Symptoms

Bulimia is a tragic disorder that can result in erosion of tooth enamel from acid exposure due to repeated vomiting, swelling in the neck region, broken blood vessels in the face, sore throats, weakness, cramps, dizziness, electrolyte imbalance, lack of menstrual periods, low pulse rate and blood pressure, hair loss, jaundice, bad breath, premature wrinkling, fatigue, muscle weakness, underweight or overweight condition, over-exercising, secretive behavior, consumption of large amounts of food at once, frequent illness and infection (sore throats, bladder infections, etc), lack of focus or withdrawal.

In addition to the above physical symptoms, bulimics may leave the house directly after a meal to facilitate vomiting, avoid social situations where food is served, make excuses for not eating such as "I already ate" or "I'm not hungry," or withdraw from the social mainstream. Trips to the bathroom immediately following a meal are also typical. Bulimics also tend to hoard food and impulsively cook and bake.

Precautions

Bulimia can become life-threatening if electrolyte balance is sufficiently impaired. Left untreated, bulimia can cause serious metabolic problems. In addition prolonged bulimic behavior can cause stomach lining ruptures, kidney damage, irregular heartbeat and infertility. If you have induced vomiting in yourself, see a doctor immediately.

Causes

Bulimia can be caused by sexual or physical abuse, neglect, addictive behaviors, unreasonable demands, highly competitive family members, genetic predisposition, biochemical imbalances or societal pressure.

Some bulimics eat to alleviate feelings of depression and then induce vomiting to reduce their feelings of guilt. Athletes, dancers, models and other performers who have to be extremely weight- and appearance-conscious may develop bulimia in order to stay on the team, win the contest, photograph well, etc.

Conventional Therapies

Individual psychotherapy in conjunction with family counseling can successfully treat bulimia. This therapy is usually designed to improve emotional maturity.

Self-help groups and medical supervision are also commonly employed to treat the disorder. Antidepressant drugs such as Prozac or drugs used to treat obsessive-compulsive behaviors are sometimes recommended. Their success rate is questionable, though.

In severe cases, hospitalization may be necessary and supervised treatment is administered over several weeks. Unfortunately, even after exhaustive psychiatric treatments, some bulimics and anorexics may never return to normal eating patterns. In many victims, the risk of a relapse can exist weeks or even months after treatment is complete.

Dietary Guidelines

◆ Keep foods readily available that are visually appealing and healthy. Cut up fresh fruits and vegetables, almonds and dried fruits and eat active-culture yogurt, etc.

◆ Keep healthy low-fat foods around the house. If you crave a certain food eat a very small amount. If you deny yourself, it may precipitate binging later.

◆ Eat three square meals per day. Skipping meals can promote binge eating.

◆ Avoid eating a high-salt, high-sugar or high-fat diet as these foods can induce further food cravings.

◆ Keep hunger in control by nibbling on foods that will keep you from binging later on. Drinking liquid meal replacements can supply much needed nutrients and take the edge off hunger as well. High-fiber foods are also filling and nutritious.

Recommended Nutritional Supplements

PRIMARY NUTRIENTS

VITAMIN SUPPLEMENTS Take a strong multivitamin/mineral supplement. Because extreme vitamin and mineral depletion is common with bulimics, a potent, organically-based vitamin and mineral supplement is recommended. Liquid mineral formulas are quickly assimilated. Take these with some food to avoid nausea. *Suggested Dosage:* Take as directed and look for capsulized or gel-cap products rather than tightly compressed tablets which may not adequately dissolve.

PROTEIN SUPPLEMENTS Liquid drink mixes are available and can be used as sources of calories and protein. These are usually low in fat and calories and high in nutrients and can make all the difference in managing eating habits, hunger and maintaining health. *Suggested Dosage:* Take as directed. Look for soy, vegetable or spirulina sources of protein.

ACIDOPHILUS Helps to stabilize intestinal bacteria and fights fungal and bacterial infections that can frequently occur in people with bulimia due to immune system impairment.[1] *Suggested Dosage:* Take as directed using guaranteed bacterial count products that are not milk-based. Check for expiration date and keep refrigerated.

VITAMIN B12 INJECTIONS May be required to help promote cellular function and treat depression. The B-vitamins are vital to a healthy mental outlook and if they are lacking, which is likely in anyone suffering from an eating disorder, further mental and physical deterioration can occur. Clinical studies have shown that replacing vitamin B12 stores can dramatically elevate mood.[2] *Suggested Dosage:* If you choose to go with oral sources, purchase sublingual products.

ESSENTIAL FATTY ACIDS More than likely, anyone with bulimia is suffering from a serious lack of fatty acids which can predispose them to a number of disorders. More and more research findings point to EFA deficiencies as the causal factor of many diseases including behavioral disorders.[3] *Suggested Dosage:* Take as directed. Look for products that use a variety of oils, such as fish oil, evening primrose, flaxseed, etc.

PROTEOLYTIC ENZYMES Essential for the proper breakdown of food macronutrients and their assimilation into the bloodstream. *Suggested Dosage:* Take as directed just prior to a meal.

ZINC Essential for the metabolism of protein and is quickly lost during periods of starvation. Zinc is involved is every physiological mechanism of immunity as well, which is almost always compromised with eating disorders.[4] *Suggested Dosage:* No more than 100 mg per day. Use picolinate varieties.

POTASSIUM May need to be replaced. Potassium is an electrolyte which can be seriously lost if vomiting is frequent. In addition, the overuse of diuretics can also cause a potassium deficiency. Potassium depletion can cause heart muscle dysfunction. *Suggested Dosage:* Use as directed.

IRON Bulimics frequently become anemic and may need to build up their hemoglobin count. *Suggested Dosage:* Take as directed using organic iron sources.

CALCIUM/MAGNESIUM Calcium deficiencies are very common in bulimics contributing to nervous system anxiety and muscle cramping. Over half of bulimic young women tested were seriously lacking in calcium.[5] *Suggested Dosage:* Take as directed using organic iron sources.

ST. JOHN'S WORT Works to alleviate depression without the side effects of antidepressant drugs.[6] *Suggested Dosage:* Take as directed using guaranteed potency products if possible.

SECONDARY NUTRIENTS

KELP: A good source of essential minerals including iodine which helps to regulate metabolism and hunger.[7] VALERIAN ROOT: Has a tranquilizing effect on the nervous system with none of the side effects of prescription sedatives or barbiturates. It has the ability to relax the intestinal muscles.[8] ECHINACEA AND GINGER: Both of these herbs calm the gastrointestinal tract and can quiet stomach spasms that accompany vomiting. GINSENG: Strengthens the body and improves immunity.

Home Care Suggestions

◆ Often, bulimics are encouraged to record their feelings of anger or depression, releasing negative emotions that sometimes precipitate binge eating.
◆ Use hotline numbers when tempted to binge or purge (see numbers below). If you aren't involved with a self-help group, form your own group hotline and call someone when you're tempted.
◆ If you crave a particular food, wait at least twenty minutes before eating it. Often, if the craving does not result from real hunger, it will pass.
◆ Take a walk or arrange for another activity that is incompatible with eating.
◆ Go to counseling.

Other Supportive Therapies

COUNSELING AND GROUP THERAPY: Very helpful in sharing and strengthening through common experience. Getting to the root of the behavior is easier to accomplish with group input and counselor mediation.
MASSAGE: This therapy can help to create a feeling of well-being and elevate the mood.
ACUPUNCTURE: Can help to restore system energy balances that become so disrupted with any eating-disorder behavior.

Scientific Facts-at-a-Glance

The primary cause of bulimic behavior may, in fact, be related to brain chemistry. Because depression so often accompanies bulimia, compulsive eating may be sparked by a biological need to raise serotonin levels in the brain. Intense cravings for carbohydrate foods typically occur when brain serotonin dips. Interestingly, serotonin manipulation is also intrinsically involved in mood control.

In addition, the nutrient depletion readily apparent in people with eating disorders can disrupt the brain's appestat, making hunger even more unmanageable as the body tries to prompt the eating of certain foods required for survival.

Spirit/Mind Considerations

Bulimia is a disorder that is shrouded by feelings of shame and guilt. Consequently, the bulimic may become preoccupied with becoming withdrawn and isolated in order to ensure the privacy needed to binge and purge. Lying about activities, weight, etc., is also common.

Bulimics are usually distressed about their compulsive behavior and may become depressed, withdrawn or even suicidal. In addition, bulimics may suffer from low self-esteem, emotional stress, frustration, or obsessive perfectionism.

The ability to control weight, as in the case of the anorexic, may be indicative of a deep-seated need for approval or control. In some cases, just the sight of food can induce symptoms of physical stress for the bulimic and can cause a racing heart or sweaty palms.

Other indications of bulimia or a pre-bulimic condition can be eating very fast, eating until the sensation of fullness is very uncomfortable, eating large amounts of food when hunger is really not present and eating alone and feeling disgust or guilt while eating. For these reasons, unconditional support and love are essential. Forcing a bulimic or anorexic to eat is not productive and can be harmful. Supplying a selection of low calorie foods can be helpful. Getting to the root of the problem is also crucial. Often bulimia and anorexia develop from other deep-seated emotional problems that must be addressed. In the case of bulimia and anorexia, the caregiver may have to be the one to take the initiative in helping the bulimic control behavior.

On-going professional counseling is highly recommended for both the victim and the caregiver. It is vitally important that the bulimic feels total support from family and friends and that affection, encouragement and understanding are readily available. The power of love cannot be overstated. The continual outpouring of supportive statements, expressions of love and affection can help to motivate change in a bulimic who may feel unloved or unattractive.

Prevention

◆ Never start to experiment with vomiting, overusing laxatives, diet pills or diuretics.
◆ If you are tempted to resort to drastic eating patterns, read a book, visit a friend or call a helpline.
◆ Accept yourself for who you are and don't become obsessed with thinness.
◆ Eat three good meals a day with plenty of whole grains and raw foods.
◆ Stay away from addictive foods which put on weight and cause drastic blood sugar swings, resulting in abnormal hunger. These include high-fat and high-sugar junk foods.
◆ Exercise moderately every day.
◆ Find out what your talents are and develop them. Join a club, try to excel in school, take music lessons, etc.
◆ Take a strong multivitamin supplement every day.

Doctor's Notes

Clinical studies of bulimic women found that binges often concentrated on high carbohydrate foods and saturated fats and not on protein foods. In addition, calcium, iron and zinc levels were considerably lower than the RDA in over half of these young women. Bulimics often initiate a vicious cycle of eating which emphasized foods that disrupt normal blood sugar patterns and do not supply vital nutrients which help to normalize hunger and appetite signals. As a result, they end up perpetrating a very unhealthy pattern which could be broken if adequate nutrients were supplied and more high protein foods were consumed.

Additional Resources

National Eating Disorders Organization
445 East Granville Rd.
Worthington, OH 43085-3195
(614) 436-1112

American Anorexia/Bulimia Association (AABA)
293 Central Park West, Suite 1R
New York, NY 10024
(212) 501-8351

Institute for the Study of Anorexia and Bulimia
1 West 91st St.
New York, NY 10024
(212) 595-3449

Endnotes

1. G. Perdigon, et al., "Systemic augmentation of the immune response in mice by feeding fermented milks with Lactobacillus casei and Lactobacillus acidophilus," Immunol, 1988, 63: 17-23.
2. H. Curtius, et al., "Tetrahydrobiopterin: Efficacy in endogenous depression and Parkinson's disease," Jour Neural Trans, 1982, 55: 301-08.
3. Michael T. Murray, ND, Encyclopedia of Nutritional Supplements, Prima Publishing, Rocklin, CA:), 255.
4. M. Dardenne, et al., "Contribution of zinc and other metals to the biological activity of the serum-thymic factor," Proc Natl Acad Sci, 1982, 79: 5370-73.
5. K.A. Kendall, et al., "The nutrient intake of women with bulimia nervosa," Inter Jour Eating Disor, March, 1997, 21(2): 115-27.
6. E. Vorbach, et al., "Effectiveness of tolerance of the hypericum extract LI 160 in comparison with imipramine: randomized double-blind study with 135 outpatients," Jour of Geri Psy Neur, October, 1994, 7.
7. G.L. Binding and A. Moyle, About Kelp, Thorson's Publishers LTD, Northamptomshire, England, 1974.
8. B. Hazelhoff, et al., "Antispasmodic effects of Valeriana compounds: An in vivo and in vitro study on the guinea pig ilium," Arch Int Pharmacodyn, 1982, 257: 274-87.

BURNS

Approximately two million people are burned badly enough to require medical attention every year in our country. Burns are categorized according to their severity. A first degree burn is more superficial and is characterized by redness (most sunburns fit this type of burn category). A second degree burn is deeper and results is blistering and splitting of skin layers (scalding and severe sunburn usually belong to this type). Third degree burns, in which the skin and underlying tissue and muscle are destroyed, are usually painless because nerve endings have been destroyed. In addition, skin may be charred. These are the most serious types of burns and can cause significant fluid loss.

Burns are more common in children and the elderly and are usually the result of home accidents, which can be almost always be prevented.

Symptoms

First degree burns cause a great deal of pain and result in skin redness but nothing more. They usually do not require medical treatment and will heal on their own. Pain, restlessness, fever and headache may conicide with a first degree burn.

Second degree burns are deeper and form blisters. Not all of the dermis is damaged and healing usually results without scarring unless the burn is extensive.

In third degree burns, pain is usually absent. In addition, skin tissue and even muscle can be destroyed with bones being visible in some cases. The area will look white or charred red. Loss of body fluids, pulmonary complications and infection are the primary dangers of third degree burns. Scarring is common and skin grafting may be necessary.

In second or third degree burns that affect more than ten percent of the body, shock may occur which is characterized by low blood pressure and rapid pulse caused by the loss of fluids and electrolytes from the burned area. Intravenous fluid must be administered in these cases.

Precautions

Any burn that is extensive or involves the face, hands, feet, eyes or pelvic area requires immediate medical attention. Third degree burns must be treated by a physician immediately. Any burn that shows evidence of infection or doesn't heal within two weeks should be looked at by your doctor.

Causes

Burns are commonplace and can be caused by contact with hot water, radiation, sunlight, chemicals, electricity, fire or any heat source (stove top, curling iron, radiator, etc.)

First Aid for Burns

◆ Apply cold water—not ice water—to the skin for at least five minutes.
◆ If the burn is chemical in nature, continue flushing the area with water.
◆ A cold-water compress can also be used. Remove any watches, jewelry, rings and constricting clothing from the area before swelling occurs.
◆ Dress the area with a clean, nonfluffy material. In the case of severe burns, do not remove clothing that is stuck to the wound. Cover any exposed areas with a clean, dry nonfluffy cloth and secure it until professional treatment is available.

Conventional Therapies

Your doctor will want to determine the severity of the burn and will recommend the following treatments accordingly: antibiotic therapy, skin grafting, antibacterial ointments and dressing and hospitalization if the burn is extensive enough (for the administration of IV fluids to prevent dehydration and shock and to guard against infection).

Dietary Guidelines

◆ In the case of second and third degree burns the diet should be high in both protein and calories for tissue regeneration.
◆ Plenty of fluids should be consumed. Protein drinks can supplement a diet high in raw vegetables, fruits, cereal and nuts.
◆ Citrus fruits, potatoes and broccoli are good sources of vitamin C, which aids the healing process.
◆ In order to heal properly from a serious burn, caloric intake should be higher than normal and should be obtained from good, nutritious sources rather than empty calorie junk foods.

Recommended Nutritional Supplements

PRIMARY NUTRIENTS

POTASSIUM Potassium can be lost from burns and should be replaced as soon as possible. *Suggested Dosage:* Take as directed using chelated products that are food-based. Eating more potassium-rich foods like bananas is also recommended.

VITAMIN A WITH BETA-CAROTENE Contributes greatly to the regeneration of epithelial and mucosal surfaces of the skin.[1] In addition, both of these compounds act as powerful free radical scavengers, especially useful in the case of tissue destruction caused by burns.[2] *Suggested Dosage:* 50,000 IU of vitamin A and 25,000 IU of beta-carotene until healing is sufficient, then drop to 25,000 IU of vitamin A and 10,000 IU of beta carotene.

ZINC Promotes tissue healing by stimulating immune function and by also acting as an antioxidant to inhibit inflammation.[3] *Suggested Dosage:* 75 to 100 mg per day in divided doses. Do not exceed 100 mg per day. Use picolinate varieties.

SELENIUM AND GERMANIUM Two excellent antioxidants which help to minimize tissue oxidants which can result from injuries such as burns. Selenium helps to boost the level of glutathione peroxidase. These help to inhibit the production of prostaglandins and leukotrienes which cause inflammation and pain.[4] *Suggested Dosage:* Take as directed.

VITAMIN E Minimizes scarring if the burn is first or second degree in its severity. Clinical studies have found that vitamin E supplementation enhances tissue regeneration.[5] *Suggested Dosage:* Take as directed.

VITAMIN C WITH BIOFLAVONOIDS Helps in healing processes and can reduce inflammation. A wash made with powdered vitamin C and water can be applied externally. Laboratory tests on mice with burns found that ascorbic acid supplementation retarded the transformation of tissue from second to third degree burns.[6] *Suggested Dosage:* Take as directed.

ESSENTIAL FATTY ACIDS These vital acids contain compounds which profoundly effect prostaglandin synthesis which combined with arachidonic acid, cause swelling, pain and inflammation.[7] *Suggested Dosage:* Take as directed.

GOTU KOLA Extracts of this herb have had remarkable results treating burns cause by scalding, explosions or electrical shock. Taking the herb internally and applying it topically resulted in less skin shrinkage and swelling.[8] *Suggested Dosage:* Take as directed and make poultices out of teas or extract and apply externally.

ST. JOHN'S WORT OIL Helps to heal first or second degree burns due to its ability to speed tissue healing and prevent infection.[9] *Suggested Dosage:* Use as directed on burn. Oil based products are preferable.

GLYCOSAMINOGLYCANS A natural anti-inflammatory agent that contributes to the regeneration of connective tissue.[10] *Suggested Dosage:* Take as directed. (You may need to take this for at least six weeks if your burn is severe enough).

PABA Clinical tests have found that PABA (para-amino benzoic acid) can help to boost skin healing and inflammation.[11] *Suggested Dosage:* Take as directed.

HERBAL COMBINATION This combination contains burdock root, gotu kola, yellow dock, dandelion root and butcher's broom. *Suggested Dosage:* Two to six capsules daily. This formula is designed to cleanse the body by activating all its methods of elimination which include cleansing, strengthening and supporting liver function. This formula will assist with a wide range of skin disorders including eczema, cellulitis, acne, psoriasis, burns and insect bites.

BURDOCK ROOT: If there was ever an herb to promote healthy skin through internal cleansing, burdock is it. Burdock root's cleansing power is multifaceted. It has a diaphoretic action (promotes perspiration) which expels toxins from the skin and blood. GOTU KOLA: Even though this herb has a similar sounding name to a popular soft drink, it is not related to the kola nut nor does it contain any caffeine. Gotu kola is supported by tremendous clinical research performed in Europe. It possesses wound healing activity and has been shown to decrease scarring.[12] YELLOW DOCK: Yellow dock root is a reputed blood purifier and has been prescribed for all types of skin problems including burns. Its laxative effect is well documented and supports the body's detoxifying ability. DANDELION ROOT: The common yard weed dandelion has a long history of use in herbal medicine. It is part of this formula for its ability to strengthen the liver, improve bile formation, regulate the bowels, purify the blood, and tonify the skin. In the case of serious burns, the body must get rid of toxins and metabolites.[13] BUTCHER'S BROOM: This herb helps to facilitate tissue healing, works to detoxify the blood and is a natural astringent.

SECONDARY NUTRIENTS

TEA TREE OIL: Used externally for milder burns, this preparation helps to control pain and expedite healing. It can mix with sebaceous gland secretions and actually penetrate the epidermis and has antiseptic properties as well.[14]

COLLOIDAL SILVER: Use directly on the burn to prevent infection and speed healing.

MYRRH OR GOLDENSEAL POWDER: Can be used to dust a first or second degree burn. It is also available in spray form.

LAVENDER OIL: Diluted in an olive oil base and applied externally, it can help with pain and healing.

WHITE OAK BARK: Contains tannic acid which helps promote healing of skin. Can be used as a compress made from tea.[15]

ALOE VERA: Has healing properties and can reduce scarring with topical application.[16]

MARSHMALLOW: Good for acid or fire burns. Apply directly to the burn in a wet compress and also take internally in capsule form.

Ointments or lotions made from the following combination of herbs can be used for minor burns: malva, chickweed, marigold, plantain, comfrey, marshmallow and mullein.

Home Care Suggestions

- Apply cold water—not ice water—to the burn site. Continue this treatment for at least five minutes.
- Using aloe vera gel after cold water treatment has been administered is considered beneficial by some experts. Keeping a live plant nearby provides fresh juice which can be continually applied for days after the burn has occurred.
- Over-the-counter analgesics, including aspirin and acetaminophen, may help with pain.

- Do not break open blisters that may appear with a second degree burn.
- Elevate the burned area to help prevent swelling and pain.
- Anesthetic creams or sprays are not recommended for burns because they inhibit healing.
- The use of butter, Vaseline or other cream ointments is generally discouraged.
- In the case of minor burns, creams such as neosporin or bacitracin are not helpful.
- Avoid cortisone-based creams or ointments. These can actually increase the risk of infection.
- For minor burns, a compress made from a milk-soaked cloth can promote healing.
- Keep the burn dry, clean and covered with a thick gauze pad that is frequently changed.
- The use of Preparation H for first or second degree burns is advocated by some for its healing properties. It contains yeast, which apparently speeds up the healing process.
- Using raw, peeled potatoes on a minor burn is a traditional home remedy and has been used for generations.

Other Supportive Therapies

HOMEOPATHY: Hypericum can be mixed with pure water and used as a topical application on a burn.

Scientific Facts-at-a-Glance

New skin substitutes and synthetic wound coverings have made it possible to speed healing and avoid surgery in many cases. Dr. George L. Peltier, M.D., and chief of plastic surgery at Hennepin County Medical Center in Minneapolis, has stated, "We don't know all the advantages of substitute skin yet. We're still learning. They're very costly, but they do result in fewer surgical procedures, which means reduced pain for the patient and a shortened hospital stay."

Spirit/Mind Considerations

Anytime our bodies are traumatized by injury, we can slip into a state of emotional shock or depression. For this reason, if someone is seriously burned and disfigured, focus on spiritual and emotional issues. Support systems should be used and honest yet encouraging comments should be elicited by family members and friends. Denying the damage or disfigurement a burn can cause does not really help the victim. Humor, support, and taking time to talk and listen can help overcome the post-traumatic stress of experiencing any kind of an accident.

Prevention

- If you have young children in the house make sure stove controls cannot be reached.
- Turn pot and pan handles away from the edge of the stove so they cannot be grabbed by a child.

- Do not leave plugged-in curling irons, hot curlers, etc., where a child can reach up and grab them.
- Make sure a child is never left alone in the bathtub where scalding can occur. Always check the temperature of the bathwater yourself by immersing your wrist in the water before placing a child in the tub.
- Never leave a child unattended by a campfire or fireplace and make sure to use fireplace screens to prevent sparks from flying.
- Keep electrical outlets covered and cords tucked away.
- Never leave matches or cigarette lighters within the reach of a child.
- Teach your child to stop, drop and roll if their clothes or hair is ever on fire. Practice this exercise regularly.
- Have regular fire drills in the home and use fire safety guidelines provided by the fire department to design your own emergency fire strategy.
- Have a smoke alarm on each floor of your house.

Doctor's Notes

Any burn that causes significant damage needs to be evaluated by someone that is familiar with treating burns. First and second degree burns that are associated with simple redness of the skin or mild blistering, can easily be treated at home. In burns where the skin is intact or has superficial blisters, applications of colloidal silver can be used for pain and healing. Poultices can be made from gotu kola decoctions or extract and placed directly over burn. Taking gotu kola and butcher's broom by mouth can also speed healing.

Applying lavender oil diluted in olive oil can help decrease pain and speed healing. Often we only think to treat a burn externally. There is much nutrient support needed to augment the healing process, to ward off infection, replace fluids and electrolytes and promote new tissue regeneration.

When the body is injured, the immune system is also shocked. Therefore, care should be taken to rest adequately, eat well and take the appropriate supplements.

Botanical salves, gels, sprays, etc., can be invaluable for minor burns and have wonderful healing properties not found in prescription or over-the-counter preparations which usually target pain or inflammation.

Additional Resources

National Burn Victim Foundation
32-34 Scotland Road
Orange, NJ 07050
(201) 676-7700

Endnotes

1. R.D. Semba, "Vitamin A, immunity and infection," Clin Info Dis, 1994, 19: 489-99.
2. N.I. Krinsky, "Antioxidant function of carotenoids," Free Rad Biol Med, 1989, 7: 637-35.
3. J.V. haley, "Zinc sulfate and wound healing," Jour Surg Res, 1979, 27(3): 168-74.
4. L.J. Hinks, et al., "Trace element status in eczema and psoriasis," Clin Exp Derm, 1987, 12: 93-97.
5. G.W. Burton and M.G. Traber, "Antioxidant activity, biokinetics, and bioavailability," Annu Rev Nutr, 1992, 10: 357-82.
6. C.R. Spillant, "The beneficial effects of ascorbic acid in murine burns," Clin Res, 1983, 31:A690.
7. Michael T. Murray, N.D., Encyclopedia of Nutritional Supplements, (Prima Publishing, Rocklin CA, 1996): 252-53.
8. J.A. Gravel, "Oxygen dressings and asiaticosides in the treatment of burns," Laval Med, 1965, 36: 413-15.
9. C. Hobbs, "St. John's Wort, Hypericum perforatum, Herbalgram, 1989, 18-19: 24-33.
10. Y. Vidal, et al., "Articular cartilage pharmacology: in vitro studies on glucosamine and nonsteroidal anti-inflammatory drugs," Pharmacol Res, Comm, 1978, 10(6): 557-69.
11. C.J.D. Zarafonetis, et al., "Paraaminobenzoic acid in dermatitis herpetiformis," Arch Dermatol Syphiolo, 1951, 63: 115-32.
12. T. Kartnig, "Clinical applications of centella asiatica (L), URB Herbs Spices Med Plants, 1988, 3: 146-73.
13. F. Susnik, "Present state and knowledge of the medicinal plant Taxicum officinale," Med Razgledi, 1982, 21: 323-28.
14. P.M. Altman, "Australian tea tree oil," Aust Jour Pharm, 1988, 69: 276-78.
15. Mark Pedersen, Nutritional Herbology, Wendell W. Whitman Co., Warsaw, IN, 1994, 169.
16. D. Grindlay and T. Reynolds, "The aloe vera leaf phenomenon: A review of the properties and modern use of the leaf parenchyma gel," Jour Ethnopharmacol, 1986, 16: 117-51.

BURSITIS

Technically speaking, bursitis is an inflammation of the bursa, a membrane or sac which is found close to a joint, and between tendons and bones. These sacs are actually two layers of tissue that allow motion to take place with decreased friction. Bursa sacs which not longer function are like balloons that have been deflated, causing the two opposing sides of the balloon to rub against each other with increased friction. The result is joint pain and inflammation.

Bursitis usually clears up but typically recurs. It commonly affects the hip, lower knee or shoulder areas. When the shoulder is affected with bursitis, it's referred to as tennis elbow. While bursitis may be miserable, the condition is not considered a serious one. New research and therapeutic approaches to disorders like bursitis are beginning to concentrate on healing and regeneration rather than solely on pain relief.

Symptoms

Swollen, painful and tender joints are common in bursitis. The presence of pain will cause the joint to become immobile, greatly limiting motion. People who suffer form bursitis are commonly seen trying to manually massage the painful area.

Precautions

Symptoms of bursitis may be caused by gout or the presence of infection. Bursitis that persists should always be examined by a physician.

Causes

- Bursitis can result from friction, pressure or injury to the bursa membrane.
- Prepatellar bursitis—"housemaid's knee"—is caused by prolonged kneeling on a hard surface.
- Tibial tubercle bursitis—"clergyman's knee"—can result from long periods of kneeling. A type of bursitis called "student's elbow" is a result of periods of pressure exerted from a desk or table.
- Shoulder bursitis, referred to as subdeltoid bursitis, may eventually cause the joint to become immobile. This type of bursitis is especially problematic for baseball pitchers.
- Bursitis has also been linked to calcium deposits and some experts have associated the disorder to food or airborne allergies. Gluten sensitivity must be ruled out.

Conventional Therapies

Rest is the primary treatment your physician will probably recommend. Ice packs may also be applied, especially if infection is present. Antibiotics and drainage of fluid are also sometimes used. A pressure bandage may also be recommended to stop fluid from re-accumulating. Anti-inflammatory drugs are also routinely prescribed. Injections of corticosteroids are used for severe cases. In unusually persistent cases, a bursectomy may be recommended. This operation is minor and involves making a small incision in the skin where the contents of the bursal sac are permanently removed. Medical practitioners will usually use anti-inflammatory drugs or steroid injections to treat stubborn bursitis which does provide some measure of relief; however, it is usually temporary, rarely curative and comes with substantial side effects.

Dietary Guidelines

- Going on a fast for 24 hours can help you determine if your bursitis could be related to a food allergy.
- In general, staying away from rich, fatty foods or red meats is recommended along with gluten-containing foods.
- High-fat dairy products can also contribute to inflammation.
- Taking green drinks made with chlorophyll and other green vegetables can also help to calm down inflammation and soreness.
- Gluten sensitivity can cause joint and muscle pain which can be mistaken for bursitis, tendinitis, arthritis or fibromyalgia. Make sure you are not allergic to wheat products.

Recommended Nutritional Supplements

PRIMARY NUTRIENTS

GLUCOSAMINE AND CHONDROITIN This powerful duo of compounds helps to protect joint cartilage and is also capable of considerable pain relief.[1] While we know that bursitis affects the sac between joint cartilage, protecting the cartilage from deterioration is important or the bursa sac will be placed under stress. *Suggested Dosage:* Take as directed for at least four to six weeks.

CALCIUM AND MAGNESIUM Essential for bone and muscle function and collagen repair. A deficiency of magnesium can cause joint and muscle pain.[2] *Suggested Dosage:* Take 1,000 mg of calcium and 500 mg of magnesium per day. Use chelated varieties.

PROTEOLYTIC ENZYMES Help to boost efficient metabolic breakdown of food particles and have anti-inflammatory properties as well. Very interesting studies have found that these enzymes can significantly speed the healing of soft tissue.[3] *Suggested Dosage:* Take as directed just prior to eating.

ESSENTIAL FATTY ACIDS Fish oil, evening primrose, flaxseed, borage oils and CLA all contain important Omega compounds. These mediate prostaglandin response, helping to control pain, swelling and the inflammatory response so typical of bursitis.[4] *Suggested Dosage:* Take as directed. Look for products with a variety of oil sources. Always take with a vitamin E supplement if using fish oil sources.

VITAMIN A WITH BETA-CAROTENE Promotes tissue repair and acts as a free radical scavenger to protect inflamed tissue. *Suggested Dosage:* 15,000 IU of vitamin A and 25,000 of beta-carotene every day. Warning: Do not exceed 10,000 IU of vitamin A if you are pregnant.

VITAMIN C WITH BIOFLAVONOIDS Promotes tissue healing and the regeneration of connective tissue and collagen while acting as natural anti-inflammatory agents.[5] *Suggested Dosage:* 5,000 mg daily in divided doses with meals.

QUERCETIN A powerful and very valuable bioflavonoid which inhibits the release of histamine which creates inflammation in bursitis. Quercetin can stabilize cell membranes helping to reduce the breakdown of collagen.[6] *Suggested Dosage:* Take as directed with vitamin C.

BROMELAIN An enzyme compound of pineapple which helps reduce swelling and inflammation. Bromelain is invaluable for its marvelous anti-inflammatory properties. *Suggested Dosage:* Take as directed. Chewable varieties are available.

VITAMIN B12 Some studies indicate that injections of vitamin B12 can help control the pain of bursitis. Sublingual supplements can also be very effective.[7] *Suggested Dosage:* Take as directed.

SUPEROXIDE-DIMUSTASE Clinical tests have shown that this compound has the ability to reduce joint swelling and pain and to inhibit synovial thickening which may be helping in preventing or treating bursitis.[8] *Suggested Dosage:* Take only as directed.

DL-PHENYLALANINE Helps to control pain and, in some studies, was able to work when standard medications failed.[9] *Suggested Dosage:* Take as directed on an empty stomach with fruit juice. Do not use if you have high blood pressure, are taking MOA inhibitors or have kidney disease.

HERBAL COMBINATION Also recommended is an herbal combination that includes devil's claw, yucca, sarsaparilla, white willow bark, cayenne and horsetail. *Suggested Dosage:* Four to six capsules daily. For extreme cases, it is best to use maximum dosage of six capsules per day for a prolonged period of four to six months.

DEVIL'S CLAW: Don't let the name of this herb scare you off. It is so named because the plant's barbed hooks (claw), when stepped on with bare feet, "hurt like the devil." The secondary roots of this plant have a rich history of use as an anti-inflammatory, analgesic and digestive stimulant. YUCCA: Yucca has a similar action to that of devil's claw. It improves digestion and reduces histamine production. As a result, inflammation and pain may be alleviated. The constituents of yucca commonly considered to be its actives are

called saponins. SARSAPARILLA ROOT: Sarsaparilla, used as a food flavoring in the United States, is officially recognized in Germany and the United Kingdom for its antirheumatic, anti-inflammatory, and diuretic properties. Its activity is thought to be due to its saponin content and its ability to bind to endotoxins.[10] Historically, this herb has been used to treat gout and rheumatism and is classified as a tonic and blood purifier. WHITE WILLOW BARK: This herb has been used for over a thousand years to relieve pain. Salicin, aspirin's forerunner, was discovered to be white willow's active constituent. Apart from its ability to assist with pain, salicin reduces inflammation. Unlike aspirin it will not thin the blood or irritate the stomach.[11] CAYENNE: Cayenne stimulates circulation and makes the other herbs more effective. Cayenne can help to improve digestion. Cayenne's hot element, capsaicin, is also a noted analgesic. It is available in ointment form but should not be used around the eyes or other mucus membranes. HORSETAIL (SHAVE GRASS): While horsetail is a mild diuretic, its main action is to strengthen and regenerate connective tissues. Connective tissue (found abundantly in joints) is destroyed by inflammation. Silica is vital in regenerating connective tissue and keeping it strong. Horsetail is one of the richest known sources of silica.

SECONDARY NUTRIENTS

GERMANIUM: Reduces pain and inflammation and scavenges free radicals which are always produced in any inflammatory condition. *Suggested Dosage:* Take as directed.

VITAMIN E: Reduces inflammation by protecting membranes from excess histamine release and its serotonin-promoting action.[12] *Suggested Dosage:* 800 IU daily.

HERBAL OINTMENT: Apply an ointment containing white oak bark, queen of the meadow, skullcap, lobelia capsicum and mullein.

Home Care Suggestions

- ◆ Rest the joint until symptoms improve. Immobilizing it helps facilitate healing.
- ◆ Use ice therapy by applying a soft ice bag to the joint and then removing it for five to ten minutes. Do not use heat if the joint feels hot or is swollen. Alternating heat with ice can also be beneficial and experimenting with hot and cold temperatures is encouraged to see what works best for you.
- ◆ Wrap the area (not too tightly) and elevate it.
- ◆ Use a hot castor oil pack. Soak several layers of flannel in castor oil, place it over the affected area and cover the layers with a sheet of plastic. Then apply a water bottle or heating pad to the layers.
- ◆ Gentle exercise with your doctor's permission may help relieve pain in some cases. Stretching exercises are especially recommended.
- ◆ Physical therapy involving TENS (transcutaneous electrical nerve stimulation) may help with pain control.
- ◆ Ultrasound therapy: Helps control the formation of adhesions and scar tissue in joint injuries.
- ◆ DMSO (dimethyl sulfoxide) solution, applied directly to the joint, penetrates the skin and can help reduce inflammation. It is usually available in health food

stores and should be diluted with water to 70 percent strength. When you dilute this chemical, it will heat up and should be used after it has cooled.

- Wrapping the joint with an elastic bandage may help alleviate discomfort.
- Time spent in a jacuzzi bath may also help with pain control.
- Over-the-counter anti-inflammatory drugs such as aspirin and ibuprofen may be used for pain but do not expedite the healing process.
- A chamomile poultice applied directly to the inflamed area can help reduce pain and swelling in the joints.
- Thyme oil used as a hot compress or in a hot bath stimulates blood flow to damaged tissue and promotes healing.
- Turmeric has been used for centuries in Indian and Chinese traditional medicine for the treatment of inflammation. Make a paste of tumeric and water and apply to inflamed area.

Other Supportive Therapies

ACUPUNCTURE: Can provide some relief from pain and is considered much safer than anti-inflammatory drugs and steroids.

HYDROTHERAPY: Cold compresses can help during an acute bout of bursitis.

MASSAGE: Limbering and warming up muscles with essential oils can be helpful but must be done in a way not to aggravate inflammation.

Scientific Facts-at-a-Glance

Using ultrasound therapy (which employs sound vibrations to boost circulation and create heat in a specific area) helps to eliminate adhesions and scar tissue after an injury.[13]

Spirit/Mind Considerations

Any disorder which causes chronic pain will have a tendency to increase anxiety and stress levels and promote tense muscles. It is vitally important to learn how to relax and relieve stress when dealing with joint or back pains. Stress reaction plays such an integral role in how our muscles and joints function. Tension can be just as damaging to joints and tendons as an athletic injury.

Prevention

- Staying limber seems to protect the joints from bursitis.
- Overuse of certain joints is usually the primary cause of the disorder so "taking it easy" when playing tennis, pitching, etc., is recommended.
- Poor technique in playing racquetball, golfing, bowling, etc., may also predispose one to bursitis and some professional coaching on proper form may prevent the disorder.
- After an injury or a sprain, proper first aid is very important in preventing future bursitis. Rest the injured part, apply ice, use an elastic bandage to limit swelling and elevate the inured area above heart level.
- Use knee pads or protective foam mats if you kneel for extended periods of time.

Doctor's Notes

Bursitis is often treated with injections of cortisone. This helps, but several natural treatments can be more effective. Icing the area followed by a heat press improves circulation, allowing more white blood cells to flood the inflamed area. Anti-inflammatory herbs such as devil's claw, turmeric, bromelain and boswella are also effective. Healing botanicals include gotu kola and bilberry.

The distinction between bursitis and tendinitis is sometimes difficult to diagnose. Often, those diagnosed with one may, in fact, have the other. The treatment with herbal medicine for both would be almost the same. The herbs and herbal blends listed in this section are designed to alleviate the symptoms of inflammation and pain and to also provide a rich nutrient base to help the body's healing process and return the body to normal function.

It is vitally important in any condition involving chronic joint or muscle pain to rule out the possibility of food allergies. A gluten intolerance (often seen in people with celiac disease) can cause all sorts of painful, achy joint disorders which can be mistaken for arthritis or bursitis. In addition, faulty digestion or elimination can promote continual joint or muscle pain which mimics disorders like tendinitis, arthritis, etc.

Additional References

American Pain Society
5700 Old Orchard Rd..
Skokie, IL 60077
1-708-966-5595

Endnotes

1. E.M. Kerzberg, et al., "Combination of glycosaminoglycans and acetylsalicylic acid in knee osteoarthritis," Scand Jour Rheum, 1987, 16: 377-80.

2. J. Eisinger, et al., "Donnees actuelles sur les fibromyalgies: magnesium et transaminases," Lyon Mediterranee Med, 1988, 24: 11585-86.

3. A.J. Cichoke, and L. Narty, "The use of proteolytic enzymes with soft tissue athletic injuries," Amer Chiro, 1981, October, 32.

4. T. Terano, et al., Eicosapentaenoic acid as a modulator of inflammation," Biochem Pharmacol, 1986, 35(5): 779-85.

5. P. Roberts, et al., "Vitamin C and inflammation," Med Biol, 1984, 62: 88.

6. W.W. Busse, et al., "Flavonoid modulation of human neutrophil function," Jour Aller Clin Immunol, 1984, 73: 801-09.

7. A. Hanck and H. Weiser, "Analgesic and anti-inflammatory properties of vitamins," Int Jour Nutr Res, 1985, 27: 189-206.

8. L. Flohe, "Superoxide Dimustase for therapeutic use: clinical experience, dead ends and hopes," Mol Cell Biochem, 1988, 84(2): 123-31.

9. T. Nurmikko, et al., "Attenuation of tourniquet-induced pain in man by D-phenylalanine, a putative inhibitor of enkephalin degradation,"

Acupunc Electro Res, 1987, 12(3-4): 185-91.

10. J.E. Pizzorno and M.T. Murray, A Textbook of Natural Medicine, JBC Publications, Seattle, Washington: 1987.

11. W.H. Lewis, Medical Botany, John Wiley and Sons, Inc., New York: 1977.

12. M. Kamimura, "Anti-inflammatory effect of vitamin E," Jour Vitaminol, 1972, 18-204-09.

13. F.H. Krusen, F.J. Kottke, and P.M. Ellwood, Handbook of Physical Medicine and Rehabilitation, W.B. Saunders, Philadelphia: 1971, 297-321.

CANCER

Cancer is one of the worst of our modern-day plagues, and in spite of the enormous energy and resources that have gone into finding a cure for the disease, it continues to take thousands of lives annually.

Cancer ranks as the second most common cause of death in the United States (heart disease is the first). The term cancer refers to over 100 different diseases in which there is an unrestrained proliferation of cells, either within an organ or body tissue. Benign tumors, unlike malignant ones, do not spread and infiltrate the surrounding tissue, thus causing cell death. Cells from a malignant tumor may proliferate through blood vessels and the lymph system to other areas of the body where new tumors will begin to grow. This process is referred to as metastasis.

Areas in the body where malignant tumors most commonly develop are the lungs, breasts, stomach, colon, skin, pancreas, liver, prostrate, uterus, ovaries, bone marrow, bones, muscles, and the lymphatic system. The term carcinoma refers to cancers of the skin, mucous membranes, glands and organs. Leukemia refers to blood cancer. Sarcoma refers to cancer of the muscles, connective tissues, and the bones. Lymphoma refers to cancer of the lymphatic system.

Symptoms

Cancer can be responsible for a whole host of symptoms. Some of the more common include a sore that does not heal, nagging cough or chronic hoarseness, coughing up bloody sputum, a change in a wart or mole, difficulty swallowing, chronic indigestion, a thickening or lump in the breast or other area of the body, unusual bleeding or discharge, bleeding between periods, obvious changes in bowel or bladder habits, blood in the stool, a persistent low-grade fever, headaches accompanied by visual disturbances, unusual fatigue, excessive bruising, repeated nosebleeds, loss of appetite and weight loss, persistent abdominal pain, blood in the urine with no pain during urination, change in size or shape of the testes, or continuous unexplained back pain.

If any of the above symptoms are present, see your doctor immediately. Often the diagnosis is not cancer, but if it is, early detection is crucial.

Causes

The exact cause of cancer remains a mystery. Over 20 percent of those with cancer never find out why. The primary agents that are involved with cancer are natural parts of food (35 percent of all cases), tobacco (30 percent), sexual history (7 percent), occupational hazards (4 percent), alcohol (3 percent) and food additives (1 percent.)

Other agents that have been linked with uncontrollable cell growth are ionizing radiation, chemicals in the air and diet, vitamin deficiencies, high-fat diets, stress and environmental conditions. The consumption of chlorinated tap water has also been associated with bladder cancer.

The growth of cancer is initiated when oncogenes (genes which control cell growth) are transformed by an agent known as a carcinogen. Once this occurs, the change is transferred to the next generation of cells. Reproduction of these cells is more rapid than normal cells and original function is lost. The clump of cells, known as a tumor, contributes nothing to the function of the body, rather it depletes the body of nutrients. The rate of growth in a cancerous tumor usually depends on its tissue of origin. Tumors located in the lungs and breasts may be present for years before any symptoms appear. Several types of cancers are considered hereditary.

Conventional Therapies

The success rate of standard medical treatment for cancer varies greatly according to the type of cancer involved.

The treatment of cancer can be divided into three categories: radiation, surgery and chemotherapy. Surgical removal of a malignant tumor and the surrounding tissue is the most common form of cancer treatment. A combination of treatments is used to improve the rate of curability. It is common to use radiation therapy prior to surgery to shrink the size of the operable tumor. Unfortunately, orthodox medicine uses therapies that are considered quite toxic and come with a host of negative side effects. Chemotherapy and radiation treatments damage normal tissue while attempting to destroy cancerous tissue. As a result, hair loss can occur, but it is often temporary and sometimes the hair grows back even thicker and more healthy looking than before.

New drugs have been developed to help minimize the nausea and vomiting associated with chemotherapy and should be suggested by your doctor. Corticosteroids, tranquilizers, and the tetrahydrocannabinol (THC) found in marijuana have all been used to control nausea and vomiting.

Other symptoms of chemotherapy may include fatigue, weakness, sterility, kidney and heart damage.

Experimental cancer treatments include the use of interleukin-2, a hormone that stimulates lymphocytes or immune cells in hopes of destroying the tumors through the immune system. Another experimental treatment uses interferon, a body chemical that fights malignancies. Genetic engineering is also being researched because it can produce nonclonal antibodies to attack certain types of cancer.

Medical Diagnostic Tools

BIOPSY: Used to diagnose tumors, a biopsy tests cells removed surgically or through aspiration for microscopic examination.

CYTOLOGY TEST: A test that shows the shedding of abnormal cells. A good example of a cytology test is a pap smear. A urine cytology test is usually given to those who work in industries where bladder cancer is a known risk.

IMAGING TECHNIQUES: Low-dose x-rays such as those used in a mammogram can detect early breast cancer.

Ultrasound scanners can also produce images of organs and may screen for ovarian cancer.

CHEMICAL TESTING: Detects the presence of blood in the feces or elevated levels of enzyme acid phosphates in the blood.

DIRECT EXAMINATION: An endoscope, a tube with a lens, is passed into the area in question and viewed. Cystoscopy, laparoscopy, colonoscopy and gastroscopy are of this type.

ULTRASOUND: A new ultrasound technique used after a mammogram can help reduce uncertainty about whether a breast mass is cancerous or not. The technique uses high-definition, digital ultrasound imaging and reduces the number of biopsies performed.

Dietary Guidelines

The National Academy of Sciences has recently validated what several nutritionally oriented practitioners have said for years: there is a link between diet and cancer. A high-fiber, low-fat diet is now accepted as a valid deterrent to some types of cancer. In addition, animal fats and high-sugar diets that include caffeine and alcohol may increase the risk of several forms of cancer.

Some studies also suggest that if cells are deprived of oxygen, they may become prone to malignant growth. Consequently, because the blood provides all cells with oxygen, the condition of the bloodstream is important in the treatment and prevention of cancer. Vitamins, minerals and herbs that facilitate circulation and the detoxification of blood are valueable.

- ◆ Avoid saturated fats, salt, sugar, alcohols, coffee, caffeine and animal proteins, and restrict dairy foods.
- ◆ Eat a diet high in fiber, raw fruits and vegetables, raw seeds and nuts, and drink plenty of freshly squeezed juices such as carrot, apple, spinach and kale.
- ◆ Keep the bowels active by eating soaked figs, prunes or raisins. A macrobiotic diet is used by some cancer patients who claim good results; this diet includes brown rice and certain vegetables and is worth investigating.
- ◆ Cruciferous vegetables containing indoles should be eaten regularly. These include cabbage, broccoli, Brussels sprouts, cauliflower, turnips, kale and watercress.
- ◆ Soy foods are excellent sources of protein and contain cancer-fighting compounds.
- ◆ A "one-size-fits-all" approach to cancer is not necessarily effective. While certain foods, herbs and vitamins are certainly of value to everyone, your metabolic type and the kind of cancer you have must be considered in designing the right nutritional and supplement protocol for you.

Recommended Nutritional Supplements

PRIMARY NUTRIENTS

VITAMIN/MINERAL SUPPLEMENT With each meal take a strong vitamin and mineral supplement and an array of antioxidants. Use vitamin injections when advised by your doctor. (Taking iron is not advised. Some research suggests that excess iron levels may increase the risk of cancer and may also interfere with normal immune system functions.)

BETA CAROTENE Beta carotene can transform malignant cells, enhance the immune system and retard tumors.[1] *Suggested Dosage:* Take as directed.

COENZYME Q10 May help to reduce toxicity which results from chemotherapy. In addition, this nutrient helps to better oxygenate cells.[2] *Suggested Dosage:* 25,000 IU per day.

PROTEOLYTIC ENZYMES These enzymes help boost the immune system's ability to destroy malignant cells. It is believed by some health-care experts that a lack of digestive enzymes suggests the inability to break down cancer cells. Bromelain is one of these enzymes. Studies prove that bromelain can inhibit the proliferation of lung cancer cells and actually slow the prevention of skin cancer.[3] *Suggested Dosage:* Take five with each meal and take three enteric-coated enzymes in between meals.

ISOFLAVONES The compounds found in soy beans actually resemble tamoxifen, a potent drug used to fight breast cancer. These phytoestrogens have the ability to block the carcinogenic effects of estrogen in breast tissue. They serve to inhibit enzymes that promote cancer cell growth and also interfere with the blood vessel network necessary for a tumor to survive.[4] *Suggested Dosage:* Take three with every meal. Look for supplements that contain genistein.

INDOLE-3-CARBINOL These compounds, extracted from cruciferous vegetables such as cabbage, kale, turnips, broccoli, radishes, cauliflower and watercress, are considered anticarcinogenic phytochemicals and are especially important for the prevention of breast and prostate cancer.[5] *Suggested Dosage:* Take three with every meal. Make sure to watch for products that have no filler ingredients and that have indole-3-carbinol as their primary ingredient.

OMEGA-3 FATTY ACIDS Several studies have shown that fish oil consumption strongly correlates with lower incidences of certain cancers such as breast and colon, and that existing cancers can be inhibited by fish oil supplementation.[6] *Suggested Dosage:* Take as directed and with vitamin E.

ESSENTIAL FATTY ACIDS Although the research is mixed, animal studies have found that linoleic acid suppresses the growth of malignant cells.[7] *Suggested Dosage:* Take as directed. Try to find blends that use a combination of evening primrose, CLA, flaxseed or borage oils.

ACIDOPHILUS Studies have shown that lactobacillus acidophilus may help to prevent colon cancer. Moreover, it may also reduce the diarrhea that accompanies radiation therapy.[8] *Suggested Dosage:* Take two capsules with each meal. Look for guaranteed bacterial count and check the expiration date.

N-CYSTEINE AND ARGININE This duo of amino acids effects the immune system to inhibit the growth of cancer cells.[9] *Suggested Dosage:* Take as directed on an empty stomach with fruit juice.

SHARK CARTILAGE Contains a compound that inhibits the growth of blood vessels that nourish a tumor. Several clinical studies have found that shark cartilage can shrink certain types of tumors, especially those that are hard to the touch.[10] *Suggested Dosage:* Twelve to twenty grams a day of powdered pure product on an empty stomach in noncitrus fruit juice. Bovine cartilage can also be used and requires smaller dosages, although it is considered by some experts to be less effective than shark cartilage.

GERMANIUM Can help to enhance cellular oxygenation and relieve pain. Oral administration of germanium can boost immune function to fight cancer and may also retard the growth of cancerous tumors.[11] *Suggested Dosage:* Take as directed.

SELENIUM Selenium deficiencies have been linked with the development of cancer. In addition, selenium can reduce the effects of chemotherapy and inhibit the growth of malignant tumors. Data supports the fact that soils depleted in selenium can affect cancer rates through the consumption of selenium-poor foods. Adding vitamin E to selenium significantly boosts its anticarcinogenic effect.[12] *Suggested Dosage:* 250 mg per day.

VITAMIN A AND E Important for proper immune function which can be affected by radiation or chemotherapy. Both of these vitamins also participate in damaged tissue repair and regeneration. Supplementing our diets with vitamin A has been shown to improve the course of certain cancers and to act as a protectant to future cancers. A vast amount of clinical data exists concerning vitamin A. It has been used in cases of bladder, cervical, melanoma, and leukemia.[13] Several studies support the use of vitamin E to reduce cancers, enhance the effect of therapeutic drugs, and to slow or inhibit the growth of tumors. Using vitamin E in combination with beta carotene is especially effective.[14] *Suggested Dosage:* Take 50,000 IU of vitamin A for two weeks, dropping to 25,000 IU per day. If you are pregnant, do not take over 10,000 IU per day. Take 1,000 IU of vitamin E daily and be sure to look for organic sources.

VITAMIN B6 A deficiency of vitamin B6 has been directly linked to the creation of some malignant tumors. Mice studies show that a vitamin B6 depletion also increases the size of the tumor and accelerates the disease.[15] *Suggested Dosage:* Take 100 to 150 mg per day in divided doses. Be sure to add in the vitamin B6 content of your B-complex vitamin as part of the total.

VITAMIN B12 Deficiencies of this vitamin can increase your risk of cancer and create a blood condition that is sometimes mistaken for leukemia. Even with heavy cigarette smokers, vitamin B12 supplements improved lung tissue that was already in a pre-cancerous state.[16] *Suggested Dosage:*

Take as directed. Good oral, sublingual varieties are thought to be as effective as injections.

VITAMIN C WITH BIOFLAVONOIDS Considered an anticarcinogen and a powerful antioxidant compound. Over 100 epidemiological studies have investigated the role of vitamin C in cancer prevention and treatment. These clinical trials support the fact that vitamin C can protect against cancer of the stomach, breast, pancreas, rectum, cervix, esophagus and lungs.[17] If you have to have radiation or chemotherapy treatments for cancer, using megadoses of vitamin C may actually enhance the effect of the treatment and protect against certain side effects.[18] *Suggested Dosage:* Take from 10,000 to 15,000 mg per day in divided doses with meals. If you have bowel problems such as diarrhea, cut the dosage.

VITAMIN D Studies with vitamin D have found that it can inhibit the growth of cancer cells in breast and skin cancer. In addition, low serum levels of vitamin D may substantially increase of the risk of developing colon cancer.[19] *Suggested Dosage:* Take as directed.

CALCIUM AND MAGNESIUM Calcium supplementation is extremely important in preventing and treating colon cancer. It can neutralize the negative effects of bile acids and ionized fatty acids in the colon.[20] *Suggested Dosage:* Take 1,000 to 2,000 mg of calcium and 1,000 mg of magnesium per day.

CHLORELLA This freshwater algae actually helped patients with brain tumors to strengthen their immune response. Almost one quarter of 21 patients who received chlorella were alive two years after treatment with no reappearance of the tumor.[21] Chlorophyll, found in blue-green algae, can also be obtained through wheat grass juice and help boost red blood cell development, serving to oxygenate tissue. *Suggested Dosage:* Take as directed.

PANAX GINSENG Can help to boost immune function while providing nourishment as well. *Suggested Dosage:* Take as directed, using only Panax varieties with guaranteed potency.

HERBAL COMBINATION In the early part of the 1900s, a man named Hoxsey had an herbal formula he claimed cured cancer. Many people that were cured of cancer while under his care wholeheartedly agreed with him. Whether it was his formula that cured them or they were cured by unrelated factors is still disputed to this day. Eight of the ten major herbs found in the Hoxsey formula are contained in this primary herbal combination. These herbs may provide needed support to overcome cancer or other serious degenerative diseases. This herbal formula also contains three botanicals not found in the Hoxsey formula. A person with cancer can use this formula as an adjunct to other therapies. Because of the serious nature of cancer, it is important that an individual explore all potential treatments available and consult with a health care professional.

One of the best guides to successful alternative treatments for cancer by physicians is Burton Goldberg's *Alternative Medicine, A Definitive Guide to Cancer.* It relates the personal experiences of over 20 medical doctors who have successfully reversed all kinds of cancer using clinically sound alternative therapies.

This combination should contain red clover blossoms, licorice root, pau d'arco, barberry root bark, stillingia, sarsaparilla root, prickly ash bark, cascara sagrada, burdock root, buckthorn bark, dandelion, echinacea, suma, valerian and kelp. *Suggested Dosage:* Six to eight capsules daily. May be used every day for treatment and during convalescence.

RED CLOVER BLOSSOMS: The use of red clover in treating cancer is not supported by scientific research, but it has long been used as an alterative. In fact, early naturopathic doctors found that it gradually restored overall health. Skin cancers may be prevented if the skin is maintained with red clover blossoms. This herb contains estrogenic isoflavones which may explain some of its benefits.[22] LICORICE ROOT: Licorice root is one of the herbs that is found in the Hoxsey formula. Its main purpose was to make the formula more palatable. However, Hoxsey may or may not have known that licorice also helps to modulate and strengthen the activity of the other herbs. Licorice increases adrenal gland function to stimulate energy. People with degenerative diseases are usually fighting stress which is another condition helped by licorice. In addition, studies suggest that the herb inhibits the growth of certain tumors.[23] PAU D'ARCO (TAHEEBO): Pau d'arco is a popular modern herbal cancer treatment. Its therapeutic constituent, lapachol, has been shown in animal studies to be very effective in treating various types of cancers and tumors. In particular, it has the ability to shrink certain tumors.[24] Like certain saw palmetto supplements, various pau d'arco products lack the very active ingredient that makes them therapeutically active. It is vital to purchase guaranteed potency products with standard percentages of the active ingredient. BARBERRY ROOT BARK: Barberry is used to treat general debilities. It has also been specifically employed to treat tumors of the liver and stomach. In addition, barberry provides a cleansing action through its mild laxative effect. It contains a compounds called berberine which has been used by the Chinese since 1972 to treat leukopenia due to chemotherapy or radiation treatments. Berberine has potent anti-tumor properties.[25] STILLINGIA: Stillingia is an alterative which gradually restores good health. It promotes a healthy liver and treats various skin problems. It is a mild laxative and diuretic further supporting the cleansing action of this formula. In the nineteenth and early twentieth centuries, this herb was used to treat tuberculosis and cancer.[26] SARSAPARILLA: Sarsaparilla root has been used as a blood purifier for centuries. It has been proven to be an excellent treatment for psoriasis, eczema, and other skin disorders because it has the ability to rid the body of endotoxins and counteract the effect of certain deadly poisons.[27] It also protects the liver, a crucial action in fighting any type of cancer. PRICKLY ASH BARK: Prickly ash promotes cleansing by stimulating perspiration. It is part of this formula for its detoxification properties. It has the ability to stimulate the glandular system while helping to rid the body of toxins.[28] CASCARA SAGRADA: Cascara sagrada is included in the formula to help promote proper bowel elimination which substantially contributes to detoxification and healing. This wonderful natural laxative also has antileukemic properties in it anthraquinone compounds.[29] BURDOCK ROOT: Burdock root is also considered an alterative herb with significant cleansing properties. It has demonstrated some interesting antitumor activity as well.[30] It is believed to neutralize and eliminate poisons in the body and has been used in many countries around the world to treat cancers of various types. BUCKTHORN BARK: Included in the Hoxey cancer cure formula, buckthorn bark is a member of the same plant family as cascara sagrada. Besides its laxative effect, it has been used to treat inflammatory tumors and has inhibited lymphocytic leukemia in mice.[31] It also improves digestion and is believed to be able to remove obstructions from the liver and gallbladder. KELP: Kelp contains many trace elements that assist in recovery from almost any degenerative disease. It cleanses the bloodstream and improves resistance against disease. Epidemiological studies demonstrate a strong link between kelp consumption and reduced incidence of breast cancer. The herb has many therapeutic properties linked to cancer prevention.[32] Kelp can protect body tissues against radiation exposure and algin, found in kelp, is very soothing to the gastrointestinal tract. It is needed in this formula since many of the herbs have a modest laxative effect. DANDELION: Helps to clear the blood of toxins and is an excellent liver stimulant. The liver is responsible for detoxifying the system of drugs, radiation effects, etc. and must be kept as healthy as possible. In addition, some chemical constituents of dandelion have exhibited antitumor properties.[33] ECHINACEA: This herb boosts blood purification and boosts the immune response to fight malignancies. Several studies indicate that this herb can improve survival time and inhibit the growth of malignant tumors.[34] Much of the success of herbal therapy depends on its delivery system. European doctors typically use injectable forms of herbal extracts, which can be much more potent and direct. SUMA: Works to help strengthen the entire system and helps to promote stamina. VALERIAN: For external tumors, a valerian tincture applied topically may be beneficial.

SECONDARY NUTRIENTS

SHARK LIVER OIL (ALKOXYGLYCEROLS): This particular compound found in shark liver can help to reduce the growth of tumors and so reduce the cancer mortality rate.[35] *Suggested Dosage:* Take as directed.

GRAPESEED EXTRACT (PROANTHOCYANIDINS): With an antioxidant capability fifty times greater than vitamin C, these compounds can help prevent cancer and treat it by effectively scavenging for free radicals.[36] *Suggested Dosage:* Take as directed.

ESSIAC TEA: Boosts immune function and can actually destroy cancer cells. Essiac tea acts directly on cancer cells and in clinical studies has actually dissolved cancer cells on the skin.[37] *Suggested Dosage:* Take as directed.

CAT'S CLAW: European health practitioners are currently testing and using cat's claw as a potential treatment for various cancers. Cat's claw may work to lower the risk of cancer in two ways: first, it has the ability to act as an antioxidant and may scavenge for carcinogenic substances which can cause the formation of cancerous cells.

Second, scientific studies have shown that it can specifically target cellular mutations such as leukemic cells and inhibits their development. Cat's claw supports the body during chemotherapy and radiation treatments, working as an antioxidant to help remove toxic metabolites and provide support to an already weakened immune system.[38] *Suggested Dosage:* Take as directed.

MAITAKE, REISHI AND SHIITAKE MUSHROOM: The polysaccharide content of these mushrooms gives them immune-boosting properties as well as certain anticancer effects. Lentian, a compound isolated from the shitake mushroom, is used in Japan in an injectable form to treat cancer.[39] *Suggested Dosage:* Take as directed.

D-GLUCARIC ACID: This compound is a phytonutrient found in cruciferous vegetable, citrus fruits and sweet cherries. Using it in supplement form has been shown to inhibit carcinogenesis.[40] *Suggested Dosage:* Take as directed.

GARLIC: Studies have found that taking garlic may increase natural killer cell activity which can help to fight malignancies and inhibit carcinogenesis. New studies now suggest that taking garlic may also help to prevent stomach and colon cancer.[41] *Suggested Dosage:* Take two to three capsules with each meal.

Home Care Suggestions

◆ Use relaxation and self-hypnosis techniques to ease tension and enable you to practice visualization therapy.
◆ Maintain a positive attitude.
◆ Share your feelings with family, friends and self-help groups.
◆ To minimize hair loss apply cold packs to the scalp while taking radiation or chemotherapy.
◆ Keep yourself occupied with things you love to do.
◆ Keep yourself looking attractive.
◆ Engage in mild exercise such as walking and make it a part of your daily routine.

Scientific Facts-at-a-Glance

Isoflavones found in soy products may be the dietary component that explains why Asian women have less breast cancer than Western women. Researchers now believe that isoflavone compounds are able to block the negative effect that estrogen can have on breast tissue. One of these isoflavones—genistein—can actually inhibit tumor growth. Michael Schachter, M.D., is a great advocate of genistein and explains how it can induce apoptosis, which describes the programming of a cancer cell's death. In addition, it has the ability to inhibit clot formation, slow down cell division, move mutated cells back into a normal state, inhibit the availability of sex hormones linked to breast and prostate cancer, and produce angiogenesis, thus discouraging the formation of blood vessels necessary to nourish the tumor (much in the same way as shark cartilage).[42] Such results and their implications are impressive, to say the least. For this reason, it is highly recommended to eat more soy bean products such as tofu. In addition, supplementation with isoflavone compounds is also strongly encouraged.

Spirit/Mind Considerations

There is a great deal of data which shows that our mental attitude and the way we respond to stress can greatly increase our risk of developing a disease like cancer. While stress and attitude are not always involved, they may play a much greater role than we previously assumed. Dr. Douglas Brodie, a physician who regularly treats cancer patients, has concluded that "emotional stress, certain personality traits, and other psychological factors can deeply influence the origin, development, and outcome of almost every disease, including cancer." In his practice he has found that often an event of profound sorrow precipitates the development of cancer. Many theories exist concerning the whys and wherefores of this link, but it is accepted that unresolved grief or anger is often at the root of physiological changes. Personality types that are prone to perfectionism, have a great sense of responsibility, or exhibit a strong work ethic also seem to be more susceptible to developing cancer. It is the inability of these individuals to "de-stress" that is thought to compromise their immune systems, thereby predisposing them to illnesses like cancer. Clearly, being an optimistic and hopeful person has much more to do with physical health than any of us probably realize.

If you ever receive a serious diagnosis of any kind, one of the most important things you can do is to free your mind of daily concerns. Try to resolve anything that is weighing on your mind so you can concentrate on healing. Make amends with friends or family members and avoid negative emotions. Take time each day to meditate and enjoy your surroundings. If necessary, take a leave of absence from work or a relaxing vacation. Most importantly, cultivate a positive mental attitude. Those who have received a diagnosis of cancer will frequently assume the worst, in spite of the fact that the outlook for people with cancer has been steadily improving over the last twenty years. Nearly half of all cancer patients can expect to be free of the disease within five years.

Prevention

- Eat a low-fat diet high in fiber and complex carbohydrates.
- Food such as cabbage, broccoli, Brussels sprouts, and cauliflower are thought by some to protect against cancer.
- Foods rich in potassium such as beans, sprouts, whole grains, almonds, sunflower seeds, sesame seeds, lentils, parsley, blueberries, coconut, endive, leaf lettuce, oats, potatoes with skin, carrots, and peaches are also suggested when designing an anticancer diet.
- Avoid eating fried foods, animal proteins, coffee, tea, caffeine, and salt cured or smoked foods such as bacon, sausage, lunch meats, hot dogs, ham.
- Some professionals recommend avoiding fluoride in the water or toothpaste. Use an air purifier in your home. Do not use artificial sweeteners.
- Do not eat charred or burned foods. Never eat moldy or rancid foods.

- Don't smoke. Smoking is one of the primary causes of lung cancer that can be controlled. Smoking during pregnancy can also increase the risk of cancer to the offspring. Avoid breathing second-hand smoke also.
- Do not drink alcohol heavily. Heavy drinkers are at greater risk for mouth, throat, esophagus and stomach and liver cancer.
- Some studies have showed that germanium may be a factor in the prevention of cancer. A germanium supplement to the diet is recommended.
- Take a good strong antioxidant supplement every day.
- Women need to take cruciferous indole supplements and isoflavones.
- Beta carotene has been recently considered an anticarcinogen, although research is ongoing. The presence of vitamin A may help to protect against several chemically induced types of cancer.
- If cancer runs in your family, get an annual checkup and watch for any warning signs of the disease.
- Take regular doses of vitamin C with bioflavonoids. They may inhibit the formation of carcinogens in the body, thereby lowering the risk of certain kinds of cancer, especially stomach cancer.
- In some countries where breast cancer is low, iodine content in soils is particularly high; therefore, an iodine deficiency may be linked to the incidence of breast cancer. Likewise, areas low in selenium have also been linked to a higher rate of cancer.
- Obesity has been linked to certain types of cancer, such as uterine or breast cancer. Stay at an optimum weight for your height and frame.
- Some studies have linked a higher incidence of prostrate cancer for males who have had a vasectomy.
- Men should take saw palmetto and pygeum supplements after the age of forty to prevent prostate cancer.
- Avoid unnecessary x-rays.
- Avoid exposure to chemicals such as paint, garden pesticides, (considered high-risk carcinogens), hair sprays, and sunlight. Get in the habit of using a strong sunscreen. Avoid exposure to asbestos, vinyl chloride, industrial dyes, and soot.
- Have your home checked for radon gas levels.
- Take screening tests for early detection of breast, cervical, colon and intestinal cancer.
- Exercise regularly. Exercise increases the efficiency of the immune system.
- Practice safe sex. Venereal disease has been linked to the development of cervical cancer. AIDS can also lead to the contraction of cancer.

Cancer Self-Testing Techniques

Self-Testing for Colon Cancer

Chemically treated strips of paper can be used after a bowel movement to detect the presence of blood. If the strip turns blue, retake the test in three days. If the result is positive, see a doctor immediately. The presence of blood in the feces does not always signal cancer and could be the result of a number of conditions.

Self-Testing for Testicular Cancer

Check for a lump after a shower or bath when detection is easier. With the fingers of both hands, roll the testicles between the thumb and the fingers watching for a hard nodule or lump. If one is present, see your doctor right away.

Self-Testing for Breast Cancer

Stand in front of a mirror and raise your hands high over your head, pressing them together. Observe the shape of the breasts. Next, place your hands on your hips and press, watching for any dimpling of the skin on the breast or nipples that appear out of their normal positioning. Also look for any thickening of the skin or nipples or redness. Raise one arm over your head and with the other free hand manually feel the breast, beginning at the outer edge, using a circular motion. Gradually move in toward the nipple. Make sure to completely feel the arm pit area as well. Lymph nodes are found in this area and will move freely and feel soft. Lumps that are hard and not mobile are to be specifically looked for. Repeat this process for the other side. Then lie on your back and perform the same self-exam. Gently squeeze each nipple, checking for a yellow or pink discharge. Doing a breast exam while in the shower is also suggested as lumps are easier to detect on a wet, soapy surface.

Doctor's Notes

Cancer is a degenerative condition that is an unfortunate fact of life for too many people. Arguably, much of the cancer that plagues society could be prevented with the proper lifestyle, diet, occupation, and environment.

Even though cancer often seems to come on suddenly, the body may have long been subjected to stressors leading to the development of cancer. While it is true that 100 percent of people with malignancy will not recover and that many will die of complications attributed to the cancer, others will completely recover with no apparent explanation. Perhaps people who would otherwise die recover when their bodies are given the right nutrient support.

When it comes to nutrients, balanced nutrition is best, focusing on vegetables and fruits in their natural state. Reducing the consumption of refined foods and red meats is always a good idea. Taking megadoses of vitamins, particularly vitamin C (up to 15,000 mg a day as long as it doesn't cause any bowel problems) is warranted. I believe that adding a very good and strong antioxidant is also crucial. I like to suggest herbs that have been shown to improve immune system function to fight cancer; for example, shitake mushrooms contain various types of betaglucan compounds that fight cancerous cells.

More traditional herbs like astragalus and echinacea are also good and should be used in a cycle of two weeks on and two weeks off. Increasing the amount of soy consumption while taking a supplement of genistein (soy isoflavone) is also very important. Look for *Panax ginseng* (Korean or Chinese ginseng), which has the ability to help maintain

immune system function while improving overall nutritional state. Chinese herbs like dong quai can also help the body to fight various cancers. I am also a very strong advocate of joining a support group which afford the opportunity to talk through issues with others who can empathize.

Additional Resources

AMC Cancer Information and Counseling Line
(800) 525-3777

American Institute for Cancer Research
(800) 843-8114

Candlelighters Childhood Cancer Foundation
(800) 366-2333

Endnotes

1. N.I. Krinsky "Effects of carotenoids in cellular and animal systems," Amer Jour Clin Nutr, 1991, 53:238S-46S.
2. K. Okuma, et al., "Protective effect of coenzyme Q-10 in cardiotoxicity induced by adriamycin," Gan To Kagaku Ryoho, 1984, 11(3): 502-08.
3. S. Batkin, et al., Antimetastatic effects of bromelain with or without its proteolytic and anticoagulant activity," Jour Cancer Res Clin Oncol, 1988, 144(5): 507-08.
4. Jon J. Michnovicz, How to Reduce Your Risk of Breast Cancer, Warner Books, New York: 1995, 106-110.
5. Ibid, 17-18.
6. R. Rich et al., "EPA reduces the invasive and metastatic activities of malignant tumor cells," Biochem, Biophys, Commun, 1989, 160:555-64.
7. J. Booyems et al., "Dietary fats and cancer," Med Hypothesis, 1985 17(4):351-62.
8. B.R. Goldin, and S.L. Gorvack, "The effect of milk and lactobacillus feeding on human intestinal bacterial enzyme activity," Amer Jour Clin Nutr, 1984, 39: 756-61. See also S.L. Gorback "The intestinal microflora and its colon cancer connection," Infection, 1982 10(6): 379-84.
9. J. Reynolds et al., "Arginine as an amino modulator" Abstract, Surg Forum, 1987 415-18.
10. R. Langer and A. Lee "Shark cartilage contains inhibitors of tumor angiogenesis." Science, 1983, 221:1185-87.
11. M. Mizushima et al., "Some pharmacological and clinical aspects of a novel organic germanium compound G.E. -132," First International Conference on Germanium, 1984, Hanover Germany.
12. L.C. Clark, "The epidemiology of selenium in cancer," Fed Proc,1985, 44:2584. P.M. Horvoth et al., "Synergistic effect of Vitamin E and selenium in the chemoprevention of mammary carcinogenesis in rats" Cancer Res, 1983, 43(11): 5335-41.
13. S.M. Lippman and ML Meyskens, "Vitamin A derivative in the prevention and treatment of human cancer," Jour Amer Coll Nutr, 1988: 74.
14. E.P. Ripoll et al., "Vitamin E enhances the chemotherapeutic effect of adriomicine of human prostatic carcinoma cells in vitro," Jour Urol, 1986, 136:529-31. See also G. Shaklar et al., "Regression of experimental cancer by oral administration of combined alpha-tocopherol and beta carotene," Nutr Cancer, 1989, 12:321-25.
15. B.M. Chrismey, et al., "Vitamin B6 status of a group of cancer patients, "Nutr Res, 1986, 6(9): 1023-30. C. Ha et al. "The effect of vitamin B6 on host susceptibility to maloney sarcoma virus-induced

tumor growth in mice," Jour Nutr, 1984, 114:938-45.

16. D.C. Heimburger, et al., "Improvement in bronchial squamous metaplasia in smokers treated in folate and vitamin B12: Report of a preliminary randomized double blind intervention trial," JAMA, 1988, 259(10): 1525-30.

17. G. Block, "Epidemiologic evidence regarding vitamin C and cancer," Amer Jour Clin Nutr, 1991, 54:1310S-14S.

18. S. Gupta, "Effect of radiotherapy on plasma ascorbic acid concentration in cancer patients," unpublished thesis found in Prog Clin Biol Res, 1988, 259:307-20.

19. K.W. Colston et al., "Possible role for vitamin D in controlling breast cancer cell proliferaiton," Lancet, 1989, 1:188-91. C.F. Garland et al., "Can colon cancer incidence and death rates be reduced with calcium and vitamin D?" Amer Jour Clin Nutr, 1991, 54:193S-201S.

20. M.J. Worgavitch et al., "Modulating effects of calcium in animal modals of colon carcinogenesis and short-term studies in subjects in increased risk for colon cancer," Am Jour Clin Nutr, 1991, 54:202S-5S.

21. R.E. Merchant, et al., "Dietary chlorella pyrenoidosa for patients with malignant glioma: Effects on immunocompetence, quality of life and survival," Phytother Res, 1991, 4(6): 220-31.

22. G. Schultz, "Content of estrogenic isoflavones in red clover (trifolium pratense) cultivated in sand with different mineral supplies," Deutsche Tiera Wochen, 1967, 74(5): 118-20.

23. I.F. Shvarev, et al., "Effect of triterpenoid compounds from glycyrrhiza glabra on experimental tumors," Vop Izu Ispol Sol v SSSR Akad Nauk SSSR, 1966, 167-70.

24. C.F. Santana, et al., "Preliminary observations with the use of lapachol in human patients bearing malignant neoplasms," Revists do Instituto de Antibioticos, 1980/81, 20: 61-68.

25. H. Nnishino, et al., "Berberine sulfate inhibits tumor-promoting activity of teleocidin in tow-stage carcinogenesis on mouse skin," Oncology, 1986, 43: 131-34.

26. F. Ellingwood, American Materia Medica, Therapeutics and Pharmacognosy, Eclectic Medical Publications, Portland, Oregon: 1983.

27. L. Juhlin and C. Valquist, "The influence of treatment and fibrin microcolt generation in psoriasis," Briti Jour Dermatol, 1983, 108: 33-37.

28. C.F. Millspaugh, "American Medicinal Plants, Dover Publications, New York: 1974.

29. C.H. Chen, et al., "Studies on the Chinese rhubarb: Preliminary study on the antibacterial activity of anthraquinone derivatives of Chinese rhubarb," Acta Pharm Sinica, 1962, 9: 757-62.

30. S. Foldeak, et al., "Tumor growth inhibiting substances of plant origin: Isolation of active principle: artium lappa," Acta Phisolo Chem, 1964, 10: 91-93.

31. S.M. Kupchan, and A. Karim, "Tumor inhibitors, 114: Aloe emodin antileukemic principle isolated from Rhamnus frangula L," Lloydia, 1976, 39: 223-24.

32. Daniel P. Mowrey, The Scientific Validation of Herbal Medicine, (Keats Publishing, New Canaan, Connecticut, 1986): 88.

33. K. Baba, et al., "Anti-tumor activity of hot water extract of dandelion, Taraxacum officinale: correlation between antitumor activity and timing of administration," Yakugaku Zasshi, 1981, 10(6): 538-43.

34. C. Lersch, et al., "Stimulation of immunocompetent cells in patients with gastrointestinal tumors during an experimental therapy with low dos cyclophosphamide, thymostimulin and Echinacea purpurea extract," Tumordiagen Ther, 1992, 13: 115-20.

35. Brohult et al., "Biochemical effects of alkoxyglycerols and their use in cancer therapy," Acta Chem Scand, 1970, 24:30.

36. B. Schwitters and J. Masquelier, OPC In Practice: Bioflavonols and Their Application, Alfa Omega, Rome, Italy: 1993.

37. Burton Goldberg, Alternative Medicine Definitive Guide to Cancer, Future Medicine Publishing, 1997, 270-71.

38. Philip A. Steinberg, "Uncaria tomentosa (Cat's Claw) Wonder Herb from the Amazon," New Editions Health World, February, 1995, 41.

39. T. Taguchi, "Clinical efficacy of leninan on patients with stomach cancer: End point results of a four-year follow-up survey," Cancer Detect Prey (Suppl), 1987, 1: 333-49.

40. Z. Walaszek, "Potential use of D-glucaric acid derivatives and cancer prevention," Cancer Letter, 1990, 54:1-8.

41. O.M. Kandil, et al., "Garlic and the immune system in humans: Its effect of natural killer cells," Fed Proc, 1987, 46(3): 441. See also B. Lau, et al., "Allivum stativum (garlic) and cancer prevention," Nutri Res, 1990, 10: 937-48.

42. H. Wei, "Antioxidant and antipromotional effects of the soybean isoflavone genistein," Proceedings of the Society for Experimental Biology and Medicine, 1995, 208: 124.

CANKER SORES

Canker sores have always pestered human beings. These sores are small painful lesions that commonly erupt on the inside of the cheek, tongue, inner lips and gums. There may be only one or several sores present in an outbreak. The overall consensus is that these sores are virally caused, but this has never been conclusively proven.

Canker sores are painful and annoying and usually heal within a week with or without any specific treatment. Girls are more prone to them than boys, and they occur most frequently in school-aged children. Fortunately, the incidence of canker sores decreases with age, but this is small comfort to any adult who continues to have to cope with them.

Symptoms

Canker sores look like oval, white ulcers that are surrounded by redness. They can range in size from 1/8 inch to more than one inch in diameter. These sores can appear suddenly and disappear just as quickly. Prior to the outbreak of a canker sore, there may be a sensation of tingling or roughness. Depending on their location, canker sores can impede talking or eating. Canker sores may recur two to three times per year and in some cases may be continuously present to some degree.

Precautions

Any lesion or sore that does not heal within two weeks should be examined by a physician. If the sore becomes infected (grayish yellow color with a red ring around the base) see your doctor.

Causes

- While the cause of these sores remains a mystery, in some people physical or emotional stress seems to bring them on. Heredity may also play a role.
- For some women, canker sores occur more frequently during menstrual periods.
- Food sensitivities to walnuts, citrus fruits, chocolate and shellfish have been linked to the outbreak of canker sores.
- Mouth injuries, such as pricks or punctures can lay the groundwork for canker sore development.
- In some people, canker sores have been linked with nutritional deficiencies of iron, folic acid, vitamin B12, or just a poor diet in general. Victims of Crohn's disease have a higher incidence of canker sores.
- Poor dental hygiene may also cause cankers.
- The presence of a fever or a sunburn commonly triggers the formation of canker sores.
- The ulcers may also be a hypersensitive reaction to the hemolytic streptococcus bacteria. These particular organisms have been isolated from canker sores.
- The occurrence of canker sores has also been associated with an abnormal immune response to the presence of normal mouth bacteria.

Conventional Therapies

Unfortunately, medical science offers no cure for canker sores. Treatment is purely symptomatic. Topical pain killers may be recommended. A waterproof ointment, such as Zilactin, may be prescribed to protect the lesion. If the sores become infected, an antibiotic, such as tetracycline may be prescribed. In very severe cases, steroid drugs may be used to reduce inflammation.

Dietary Guidelines

- Allergic reactions to certain foods like pineapple, tomatoes, lemons and walnuts can initiate the creation of canker sores. Identifying these foods and removing them from the diet can lead to marked improvement.[1]
- Eat plenty of salads and raw onions. Onions contain sulfur and promote healing. Try to eat foods with active bacteria cultures such as yogurt or buttermilk.
- Avoid eating sugar, citrus fruits, coffee, nuts, fish or meat. Animal protein produces body acid which can aggravate the ulcers.
- Get vitamin C from foods such as broccoli, cantaloupe, bell peppers, cabbage and cranberry juice.

Recommended Nutritional Supplements

PRIMARY NUTRIENTS

ZINC Zinc supplementation produced good results in 81 percent of a test group who suffered from canker sores. Zinc sulfate paste was also used externally on the sores.[2] *Suggested Dosage:* Use zinc picolinate lozenges as directed but do not exceed more than 100 mg of zinc per day.

ACIDOPHILUS A study showed that breaking open an acidophilus caplet and applying the powder directly on the sore cleared the lesions completely in a few days.[3] *Suggested Dosage:* Take internally using liquid, nonmilk based emulsions. Check expiration date. Use capsules to break open and apply directly to the ulcer.

FOLIC ACID, VITAMIN B12 AND IRON A vitamin B12 deficiency coupled with folic acid and iron depletion can cause recurring canker sores in some people. Supplementing these three nutrients can help to prevent new sores from forming.[4] *Suggested Dosage:* Folic acid can be taken in lozenge form. Take 300 to 400 mg per day.

L-LYSINE A deficiency in this particular amino acid can cause mouth ulcers. In addition, using it therapeutically has resulted in a decreased recurrence rate and in milder symptoms.[5] *Suggested Dosage:* Take as directed with fruit juice on an empty stomach. Do not exceed 1,500 mg per day and do not use longer than three months consecutively.

GARLIC In vitro tests have conclusively shown that the allicin content of garlic combined with its sulfuric compounds killed both herpes simplex viruses 1 and 2 among a whole host of others.[6] *Suggested Dosage:* One capsule with each meal. Garlic extracts can also be applied locally.

ST. JOHN'S WORT This herb has impressive antiviral properties and is even under investigation for its effect on HIV. Its primary bioactive compound, called hypericin, keeps viruses from replicating.[7] *Suggested Dosage:* Take as directed using guaranteed potency products.

ECHINACEA This herb is well known for it antibacterial and antiviral properties. Various clinical studies have demonstrated that it can inhibit the herpes virus in cell cultures.[8] *Suggested Dosage:* Take as directed using guaranteed potency products.

GOTU KOLA This herb contains triterpenes which contribute tremendously to wound or ulcer healing.[9] *Suggested Dosage:* Take as directed using guaranteed potency products.

SECONDARY NUTRIENTS

VITAMIN C WITH BIOFLAVONOIDS: Can help to heal mouth ulcers and promotes tissue regeneration, however an excess of vitamin C has been linked with the development of mouth sores. Some people have found great success in using 1,000 mg of vitamin C every day as a way to prevent canker sores.[10] *Suggested Dosage:* 1,000 to 3,000 mg per day using nonacidic esterized products.

VITAMIN E OIL: Can be applied directly to the sores to promote healing and relieve pain. One study found that topical vitamin E applications resulted in marked pain relief and mouth sores and gum inflammation.[11] *Suggested Dosage:* Buy capsules of organic vitamin E to break open for topical application.

VITAMIN A EMULSION: Use directly on the sores to help promote healing of mucus membranes of the mouth. *Suggested Dosage:* 25,000 IU everyday. Do not exceed 10,000 IU if pregnant. Capsules can also be broken and applied directly to the ulcer.

LEMON BALM: A very recent study of 115 subjects found that if applied early enough, lemon balm extracts in the form of a cream significantly boosted healing.[12] *Suggested Dosage:* Take as directed.

PROTEOLYTIC ENZYMES: Because outbreaks of canker sores have been linked to bowel disorders like Crohn's disease, it is safe to assume that impaired digestion and elimination may be causal factors. *Suggested Dosage:* Take as directed before meals.

Home Care Suggestions

◆ Zinc oxide can be directly applied to the sore as a protectant.
◆ Orabase-B and Zilactin, both over-the-counter preparations, can be applied directly to the ulcers to stop pain and promote healing.
◆ Check ingredients of over-the-counter canker sore

preparations, and use ones with benzocaine, menthol, eucalyptol or camphor.
◆ Sores can be painted with a lobelia tincture several times a day.
◆ Drinking fluids from a straw can be less painful, especially for children suffering from canker sores.
◆ Dab the sores with hydrogen peroxide or make a mouthwash of 1/2 teaspoon of hydrogen peroxide to eight ounces of water. This can be used several times a day.
◆ Sucking on ice can help decrease pain.
◆ Use one teaspoon of potassium chlorate in a cup of water as a mouth rinse.
◆ Raw potatoes contain vitamin P, which helps to heal mouth sores. Place a raw potato directly on the lesion.
◆ A dab of alum on the sore can help prevent infection.
◆ Rinsing the mouth with an antacid like milk of magnesia can coat the ulcers and provide some relief from pain. Do not use this solution if sores are infected.
◆ Placing a wet tea bag, which contains tannin (an astringent and pain killer) directly on the sore can provide some relief.
◆ Making a paste of ground aspirin and water can serve to create a covering on the canker sore and promote healing.

Other Supportive Therapies

AROMATHERAPY: Essential oils such as geranium, myrrh and thyme can be applied directly to the sore.
HOMEOPATHY: Hepar sulfur and Rhus tox. have traditionally been used to treat canker sores.

Scientific Facts-at-a-Glance

Disrupting the acid/alkaline balance of the blood (pH) can result in an outbreak of mouth sores. For this reason, you may want to test your pH with special strips you can buy at your local pharmacy. If you find you lean a bit toward the acid side, you can emphasize alkaline-forming foods and learn to stay away from those that create acid.

Spirit/Mind Considerations

Recurring canker sores can certainly signal a depressed immune system. By now, we are all too aware of how stress can precipitate illness. The bottom line is that all of us need to pay attention to the signals our bodies transmit in the guise of various symptoms or illnesses. We must come to grips with the fact that we cannot continually ignore the metabolic and spiritual needs of our bodies and our minds.

Prevention

◆ Stay away from anything than can irritate or injure the lining of the mouth, such as hard bristled toothbrushes. This also includes sharp foods such as potato chips, nuts, and all salty or very spicy foods.
◆ In some cases, if the sore is caught early enough, drinking water every ten minutes for an hour can inhibit further development.

- Body chemistry must remain in an acid/alkaline balance, which is maintained by a healthy diet high in raw foods and low in meat and fat.
- Taking vitamin C seems to prevent the onset of canker sores. 500 mg a day is recommended. Always check with your physician first before using vitamin C as a remedy for canker sores.
- Eat a diet high in peas, lentils and beans to prevent a deficiency in iron, folic acid and vitamin B, which has been linked to canker sores.
- Keep your life as stress free as possible. Get plenty of rest and exercise and use music, meditation or message therapy to reduce stress.

Endnotes

1. K.D. Hay and P.C. Reade, "The use of an elimination diet in the treatment of recurrent aphthous ulceration of the oral cavity," Oral Surgery, Oral Medicine, Oral Pathology, 1984, 57(5): 504-07.
2. S.W. Wang, et al., "The trace element zinc and aphthosis: The determination of plasma zinc and the treatment of aphthosis with zinc," Rev Stomatol Chir Maxillofac, 1986, 87 (5): 339-43.
3. A. James, "Common dermatologic disorders," CIBA Clinical Symposia 1967, 19(2): 38-64.
4. J. Palopoli and J. Waxman, "Recurrent aphthous stomatitis and vitamin B12 deficiency," Southern Medical Journal, 1990, 83: 475-77.
5. R.S. Griffith, et al., "Success of L-lysine therapy in frequently recurrent herpes simplex infection," Dermatologica, 1987, 175:183-90.
6. N.D. Weber, et al., "In vitro virucidal effects of Allivum sativum (garlic) extract and compounds," Planta Medica, 1992, 58: 417-23.
7. G. Lavie, et al., "Hypericin as an inactivator of infectious viruses in blood components," Transfusion, 1995, 35: 392-400.
8. A. Wacker and W. Hilbig, "Virus inhibition by Echinacea purpurea," Planta Medica, 1978, 33: 89-102.
9. L.M. Balina, et al., "Clinical results of an asiaticoside in cutaneous ulcerous lesions," Diabetes Med, 1961, 33: 1693-96. See also H. Thiers, et al., "Asiaticoside, the active principle of Centella asiatica in the treatment of cutaneous ulcers," Lyon Med, 1957, 197: 385-89.
10. S. Lewis, Vitamin C: Its Molecular Biology and Medical Potential, Van Nostrand Reinhold Co., New York: 1973.
11. S. Starasoler and G. Haber, "Use of vitamin E oil in primary herpes gingivostomatitis in an adult," NY Sate Dent Jour, 1978, 44(9): 382-83.
12. R.H. Wobling and K. Leonhardt, "Local therapy of herpes simplex with dried extract from Melissa officinalis," Phytomedicine, 1994, 1(1): 25-31.

CARPAL TUNNEL SYNDROME

A relatively new disorder, carpal tunnel syndrome (CTS) has become an occupational hazard for many people who spend most of their working time at a computer keyboard. CTS is a disorder which develops over a period of time due to the repetition of stressful movements of the hands or wrists. It involves damage to the nerve that carries brain signals between the brain and the hands. This median nerve passes through the carpal tunnel that is created by the wrist bones and can become constrained if the tissues in the tunnel become swollen or inflamed.

Carpal tunnel syndrome is a fairly common disorder, particularly for middle aged women whose tendons can thicken, causing stress on the median nerve. In carpal tunnel syndrome, one or both hands may be affected.

Symptoms

Carpal tunnel syndrome can cause a tingling feeling in the thumb or other fingers; numbness of the thumb; middle or index finger; an inability to perform tasks requiring dexterity; shooting pains that go into the fingers or up into the forearm; carpal tunnel syndrome numbness will not effect the little finger; a sensation of tingling when wrist is tapped; increased pain at night, especially if wrists are bent; constantly shaking out wrists or pulling them back; swelling; dropping objects; weak grip; morning stiffness of fingers; or shoulder or elbow pain.

Any chronic pain located in any joint could be a symptom of arthritis and should be examined by your doctor.

Causes

Carpal tunnel syndrome occurs when the median nerve is trapped and squeezed in a fibrous passage called the carpal tunnel. An excess of tissue can build up as a result of repeated inflammation and compound the problem. Common activities that can cause carpal tunnel to develop are tennis, canoe paddling, typing, knitting or crocheting, extensive writing, small parts assembly, repeated blows to the front of the wrist, bone fracture or dislocation, meat cutting, hairstyling, playing certain musical instruments, extensive flexing or bending of the wrist commonly seen in gymnastics, using a tool that requires the bending of the wrist over long periods of time or decreased circulation during pregnancy.

There is some evidence to support the fact that a change in female sex hormone during menopause may cause an accumulation of fluid, leading to swelling in the wrists. Women who have just started using birth control pills may also experience symptoms of this disorder. Raynaud's disease, menopause, hypothyroidism and diabetes are thought to increase the risk of developing CTS.

Conventional Therapies

Some cases of carpal tunnel syndrome clear up without medical intervention. Some physicians will prescribe a diuretic to reduce the amount of tissue fluid in the body. If the condition is severe enough, a steroid injection can be administered at the wrist to alleviate inflammation, although this is only a symptomatic approach and is not curative.

If the condition persists and the pain is not manageable, surgery is recommended. A neurologist or plastic surgeon will free the constricted nerve by cutting through the tough membrane of the carpal tunnel, thereby creating more space for the nerve passage. The success rate with this type of surgery is high. The operation requires a brief hospital stay, usually in a same day surgery unit, and the procedure leaves a very tiny scar. If both hands are affected, it is usually recommended that each hand be done at separate times so that the ability to dress, bathe, etc. will not be too difficult during the recovery period. If you are contemplating the procedure, make sure you enlist the services of a neurologist or certified plastic surgeon who has expertise in this area.

Dietary Guidelines

- A diet low in hydrogenated fats is recommended to avoid the accumulation of fatty deposits. It is also beneficial to use monounsaturated oils like olive oil and eat plenty of coldwater fish.
- Foods that promote the production of certain acids are discouraged and include red meats, wines, cheeses, and fatty dairy products.
- Foods to emphasize are brown rice, whole grains, lentils, sunflower seeds, salmon, tuna, avocados, turkey and fresh fruits and vegetables.
- Eating fresh pineapple can provide an excellent source of bromelain, an enzyme that inhibits inflammation.
- Avoid a high-fat diet, smoking, stress, excess salt and caffeine.

Recommended Nutritional Supplements

PRIMARY NUTRIENTS

VITAMIN B6 Recently there has been more emphasis placed on the use of vitamin B6 to help relieve nerve-related disorders. Clinical data strongly suggests that a vitamin B6 deficiency may contribute to carpal tunnel syndrome. Supplementation has been shown to help with symptoms.[1] *Suggested Dosage:* Dosages should be discussed with your doctor because vitamin B6 can be toxic at high levels. Improvement is usually not seen for at least a month to six weeks. Take this supplement with vitamin B2 also.

VITAMIN C WITH BIOFLAVONOIDS Vital to tissue repair and healing and can contribute to reducing inflammation.[2] Vitamin C also plays a significant role in connective tissue regeneration. *Suggested Dosage:* 1,000 mg with each of three meals

BROMELAIN Anyone who requires surgical intervention for carpal tunnel syndrome should take this enzyme for its ability to lessen swelling and inflammation. In addition, if you choose not to opt for surgery, bromelain's ability to inhibit the inflammatory response is well documented.[3] *Suggested Dosage:* Take as directed.

COENZYME Q10 This compound can enhance oxygenation of tissue and also has the ability to protect muscles from exercise induced injury.[4] While CTS is a disorder of nerve conduits, weak wrist muscles subject to constant repetitive motion may also contribute to the development of CTS. *Suggested Dosage:* Take as directed.

GRAPE SEED EXTRACT Also known as pycnogenol, this compound contains powerful oligomeric proanthocyanidins that inhibit swelling and inflammation.[5] *Suggested Dosage:* Take as directed.

HERBAL COMBINATION This combination should include turmeric, devil's claw, capsicum (capsaicin cream), ginkgo, hawthorn and boswella. *Suggested Dosage:* Take as directed.

TUMERIC: A natural botanical anti-inflammatory that can be applied as a paste to the affected area to help control pain and swelling. This herb contains a compound called curcumin which has demonstrated the impressive ability to inhibit pain, swelling and inflammation.[6] DEVIL'S CLAW: The secondary roots of this plant have a rich history of use as an anti-inflammatory and analgesic. Recent studies have confirmed the anti-inflammatory value of this herb for chronic rheumatism, arthritis, neuralgia and gout rating it equal to phenylbutazone, a commonly prescribed drug for arthritis.[7] CAPSICUM: When taken internally, this herb can help to stimulate circulation and blood flow. It can also be used as capsaicin in ointment form and has proven its ability to relieve nerve pain. Various clinical studies on people with neuralgia found that capsaicin cream was a very good analgesic.[8] If you do use capsaicin topically, you can expect an initial reddening of the skin which will subside with time. Keep the ointment away from your eyes and mucus membranes. GINKGO BILOBA: Has the distinct ability to enhance blood flow and oxygenation to nervous tissue. In addition, it acts as a membrane-stabilizing antioxidant with significant free radical scavenging properties.[9] Because deposits in blood vessels can contribute to CTS, this herb may be very helpful. HAWTHORN: Contains natural proanthocyanidins which help to boost the strength of the collagen matrix of arteries and actually lessen the blockage of existing arterial deposits.[10] This herb works well with vitamin C and can help to control cholesterol levels. BOSWELLA: Acts to quell inflammation and works well with other natural anti-inflammatory compounds.

SECONDARY NUTRIENTS

LECITHIN: Helps to supply the body with choline which nourishes nerves. It also contributes to the emulsification of fat which can help discourage arterial plaque deposits in the wrist. *Suggested Dosage:* One tablespoon with each of three meals daily. Use granules if possible.

MANGANESE: Considered a nerve tonic and effective natural anti-inflammatory, this mineral can exert a therapeutic effect of CTS. *Suggested Dosage:* Take as directed. Antacids may inhibit the absorption of manganese.

ANTIOXIDANTS: Purchase a product with a variety of antioxidants, including vitamin A, beta carotene, vitamin E, vitamin C, selenium, germanium and alpha-lipoic acid if possible. These compounds scavenge for free radicals which can cause further nerve tissue damage in CTS. *Suggested Dosage:* Take as directed.

Home Care Suggestions

◆ Over-the-counter medications such as aspirin and ibuprofen are nonsteroidal anti-inflammatory medications and can help to reduce pain. Acetaminophen is not effective in treating inflammation. The continual use of these medicines brings with it significant health risks.

◆ Very mild hand exercises such as rotating the wrists in circles helps to increase circulation and may alleviate some of the tingling. Exercise should be used with caution as resting the wrists is sometimes more effective to control symptoms.

◆ Using a cold pack may also help to relieve swelling if present.

◆ It is not uncommon for people to sleep with their wrists bent against the mattress, which can aggravate symptoms of carpal tunnel syndrome. Before going to bed, use a wrist splint to keep your wrist straight and take stress off of the nerves. These splints are usually made of metal with velcro fasteners and can be purchased at medical supply sources, or can be made to fit your hand by a physical therapist.

◆ Change the position of your hands when crocheting, knitting, typing, holding tools, etc. to facilitate better circulation.

◆ Use handles, pencils, pens, curling irons, scissors, etc. that are substantial in size and easy to operate.

◆ Rotate repetitive tasks and rest from them from time to time.

Other Supportive Therapies

HOMEOPATHY: Rhus toxicodendron is typically used for any condition which causes joint pain or swelling.

PHYSICAL THERAPY: Exercises suggested by the American Physical Therapy Association can help to prevent and to treat CTS. One of the best is to rest your forearm on a table and using your other hand, grab the fingertips of the hand on the table and pull back gently for approximately three to five seconds. Repeat for the other hand.

HYDROTHERAPY: Alternating between cold and hot packs may bring some pain relief, although the effect is usually only temporary.

ACUPUNCTURE OR ACUPRESSURE: Can help to stimulate circulation and alleviate pain.

OSTEOPATHY: Manipulating the bones of the wrist and arm may help to facilitate relief for CTS.

Scientific Facts-at-a-Glance

While carpal tunnel surgery is usually successful, simpler and less invasive techniques are currently under development, including the use of a cold laser to stimulate nerve response and capillary circulation to affected areas.

Spirit/Mind Considerations

This particular disorder typically affects women because women commonly do keyboarding work and other repetitive wrist motions. Moreover, pregnancy and hormonal changes that occur with age can aggravate the problem. Learning to rest and relax during repetitive movements is crucial. Getting in tune with what our bodies need to be protected from injury or stress-related damage is important to our health and well-being. We need to stop and assess our activities and determine how they are impacting our health. Taking some of the precautions mentioned in this section can help prevent or minimize CTS.

Prevention

◆ Learn to stretch your wrist muscles by pressing your hand back. Repeat this action as many times as you can remember to do so.

◆ Use a handrest specifically designed for your typewriter or computer keyboard. This device keeps the hands level while typing rather than bent at the wrist.

◆ Use your whole hand when holding onto an object

◆ If doing a manual job that involves a repetitive movement, take a break from the activity every thirty minutes

◆ Avoid the excessive consumption of protein. In some studies it has been linked to a predisposition to carpal tunnel syndrome.

◆ Avoid taking iron supplements. They contribute to joint problems.

◆ Resistance exercises using stretch bands can help to build wrist and hand strength.

Doctor's Notes

Caused by the compression of the medial nerve as it travels through wrist, CTS can be dealt with through surgery or acupuncture. While most of us who experience a pinched nerve in the neck or back go to a chiropractor for some adjustments, people with carpal tunnel often feel that they have no recourse. Wearing a wrist splint through the night or during work can help tremendously. In addition, taking ten-minute breaks every hour and stretching neck and wrist muscles is also beneficial.

I advise some of my patients to consult a physical therapist for exercises that best suit them individually. It is also effective to take vitamin B6 in higher doses—200 mg for two to three weeks, and then 100 mg for one or two weeks, and then down to 50 mg. Just remember that very high doses of this vitamin should only be taken temporarily. Twenty-five mg of vitamin B6 per day is considered adequate under normal circumstances.

Endnotes

1. J.E. Fuhr, et al., "Vitamin B6 levels in patients with carpal tunnel syndrome, "Arch Surge, 1989 124: 1329-30.

2. C. Spillart, et al., "Inhibitory effect of high dose ascorbic acid on inflammatory edema," Agents Actions, 1989, 27: 401-02.

3. G. Tassman, J. Zafran and G. Zayon, "Evaluation of a plant proteolytic enzyme for the control of inflammation and pain," Jour Dent Med, 1964, 19: 73-77.

4. Y. Shimomura, et al., "Protective effect of coenzyme Q-10 on exercise-induced muscular injury," Biochem Biophys Res Commun, 1991, 176: 349-55.

5. Richard Passwater Ph.D. and Chithan Kandaswami, Ph.D., Pycnogenol the Super Protector Nutrient, Keats Publishing, Connecticut: 1994.

6. A, Mukhopadhyay, et al., "Anti-inflammatory and irritant activities of curcumin analogues in rats," Agent's Action, 1982, 12: 508-15.

7. Daniel B. Mowrey, Ph.D., The Scientific Validation of Herbal Medicine, Keats Publishing, Connecticut: 1986, 282.

8. A. Peikert, et al., "Topical 0.024% capsaicin in chronic post-herpetic neuralgia: Efficacy, predictors of response and long-term use," Jour Neurol, 1991, 238: 452-56.

9. S.S. Chatterjee and B. Gabard, "Studies on the mechanism of action of an extract of Ginkgo biloba, a drug for the treatment of ischemic vascular disease," Naunyn-Schmiedeberg's Arch Pharmacol, 1982, 320: R52.

10. J. Wegrowski, et al., "The effect of procyanidolic oligomers on the composition of normal and hypercholesteremic rabbit aortas," Biochem Pharm, 1984, 33: 3491-97.

CATARACTS

Cataracts occur when proteins in the eye lens change. These alterations cause a thickening, resulting in clouded and distorted vision. In medieval times, people assumed that the milky whiteness associated with this condition was a type of waterfall which sprouted from the brain. Cataracts cause more blindness than any other single cause. Senile cataracts, or those that develop as a result of the aging process, are the most prevalent kind of cataracts and usually affect people over the age of sixty. Free radical damage to lens tissue is what causes a cataract to form. These cellular culprits attack the structural proteins that comprise the lens along with enzymes and cellular membranes. Approximately four million people in this country suffer to some degree from vision impairment caused by cataracts. Cataract surgery is the most common surgery performed in the United States.

Symptoms

Cataracts are characterized by slow and gradual loss of vision with no pain, loss of detail and clarity, pronounced nearsightedness, one eye is usually more affected than the other, disturbed perception of colors or blurred vision.

Causes

Cataracts form when chemical changes take place in the lens of the eye similar to the effect achieved when boiling the whites of an egg. Cataracts can be caused by aging processes, diabetes, eye injury, exposure to radiation, heavy metal poisoning, certain drugs (steroids), nutritional deficiencies, exposure to certain oxidants (ultraviolet light), exposure to low level radiation (x-rays), free radical damage from environmental sources and smoking.

A congenital cataract may result from a rubella infection of the mother during pregnancy or due to drug addiction

Precautions

The sun can cause extensive damage to our eyes and symptoms may not show up for years. UV light exposure is very much linked to the formation of cataracts. Make sure to protect your eyes from these rays.

Conventional Therapies

Once the lens has become clouded, reversing the change is not considered medically possible. For this reason, orthodox medical practitioners assume the lens must be surgically removed and replaced with an implant lens or special kind of contact lens. Cataract surgery is considered simple and very effective and is considered highly successful in at least 90 percent of patients. Surgery is never without its health risks, however. Ideally, if cataracts are treated early enough, surgery can be avoided.

Dietary Guidelines

◆ Eating foods that are rich in natural antioxidants is recommended. Spinach seems especially beneficial as a cataract protectant.

◆ Drink plenty of pure water and avoid drinking water that has been heavily chlorinated.

◆ Foods to avoid include fatty dairy products, saturated fats and hydrogenated oils and fats.

◆ Foods high in refined sugars should also be avoided. Some theories suggest that having to process white sugar or milk sugar causes cataracts to form.

Recommended Nutritional Supplements

PRIMARY NUTRIENTS

BILBERRY This herb contains anthocyanosides which may be able to offer impressive protection against the development of cataracts. One very interesting study found that when combined with vitamin E, bilberry supplementation halted the progression of cataracts in over 95 percent of fifty patients who were suffering from cataracts.[1] *Suggested Dosage:* Take as directed. Look for standardized, guaranteed potency products.

VITAMIN C WITH BIOFLAVONOIDS Helps to scavenge for damaging free radicals and contributes to lower intraocular pressure. Laboratory studies have found that low levels of vitamin C correlate with an increased risk of developing cataracts. Patients who took 350 mg of ascorbic acid experienced significant improvement in their cataracts. Their vision improved by 60 percent.[2] *Suggested Dosage:* 1,000 mg with each of three meals per day.

VITAMIN E WITH SELENIUM This antioxidant duo works together to protect the eye from oxidant damage. Adding vitamin E to you diet may help to restore the corneas of the eyes—even after they have experienced damage.[3] Selenium is required for the proper functioning of an antioxidant called glutathione in the lens of the eye.[4] *Suggested Dosage:* Take 400 IU daily of vitamin E with 400 mg of selenium.

GLUTATHIONE A powerful antioxidant agent which slows cataract progression and protects tissue from oxidant poisons. The lower amounts of glutathione that exist in the eye, the more prone the eye is to cataract development.[5] *Suggested Dosage:* Take as directed.

PYCNOGENOL (PROANTHOCYANIDINS) These compounds that are found in bioflavonoids which have powerful antioxidant activity and can help reduce the risk of eye damage. Clinical studies have shown that these compounds can protect against lipid peroxidation in the eye.[6] *Suggested Dosage:* Take as directed.

QUERCETIN AND NARINGIN These bioflavonoids inhibit the action of aldose reductase which results in a decrease in the

cataract-causing substances that accumulate in the lens tissue.[7] *Suggested Dosage:* Take as directed.

VITAMIN A WITH BETA CAROTENE This powerful antioxidant duo is especially beneficial for vision-related problems. When combined with vitamin C, these nutrients have proven their ability to significantly retard cataract formation.[8] Moreover, a lack of beta-carotenoids has been linked to increased risk for developing cataracts.[9] *Suggested Dosage:* 25,000 IU of vitamin A daily and take beta-carotene as directed.

VITAMIN B2 A deficiency of this vitamin can cause the formation of cataracts to occur rapidly.[10] *Suggested Dosage:* 50 mg daily.

SECONDARY NUTRIENTS

FOLIC ACID: A lack of folic acid is thought to be one of the causal factors in the development of cataracts.[12] *Suggested Dosage:* Take as directed.

ZINC: Proper doses of zinc sulfate can help stimulate lens tissue.[13] *Suggested Dosage:* Take as directed using picolinate products. Do not exceed recommended dosages.

CYSTEINE: This amino acid promotes the production of glutathione which protects the eye from age-related diseases like cataracts.[14] *Suggested Dosage:* Take as directed on an empty stomach with fruit juice.

Home Care Suggestions

◆ If you are in the early stages of cataract formation, use herbs and nutritional supplements to stop the progression of the disease in order to avoid surgery if possible.

◆ Do not use antihistamines if you have cataracts.

◆ Ask your doctor about eye drops that contain pantetheine; these may halt the progression of the disease.

◆ If you smoke, stop.

◆ If you drink alcoholic beverages, stop.

Other Supportive Therapies

HOMEOPATHY: Phosphorus, calcarea and silica are all used for varying stages of cataract development.

Scientific Facts-at-a-Glance

Various kinds of sugars can produce alcohol in the lens of the eye. These alcohols are not efficiently metabolized, resulting in tissue damage and swelling. The tissue can even rupture and cause obstructed vision. Studies which demonstrate this effect strongly suggest that a high-sugar diet, (especially the lactose found in milk sugar), can affect the course of cataract formation.[15]

Spirit/Mind Considerations

Cataracts are inevitably connected to aging and may add to the anxiety which usually accompanies the process of growing older. Today, there is plenty that can be done to alleviate the blindness than accompanies cataracts. The worse thing to do is to assume that blindness is inevitable and that life is over. Learning to deal with the many physical changes that accompany growing older is crucial to remaining active and emotionally positive. Monitoring our vision as we get older can help to prevent the depression that can result if we feel handicapped by limited vision. Cataracts can be prevented and successfully treated.

Prevention

- ◆ Make sure you wear UV-blocking sunglasses and hats when necessary.
- ◆ Take a good antioxidant and multiple vitamin and mineral supplement everyday.
- ◆ Take bilberry with a vitamin E supplement after the age of 50.
- ◆ Avoid excess dairy products and white sugar.
- ◆ Eat fresh fruits and vegetables naturally high in vitamin C and bioflavonoids.
- ◆ Protect your eyes from injury, ultraviolet light, steroids, x-rays and poisons.
- ◆ Keep your blood sugar at normal levels.
- ◆ Don't smoke or use alcohol.

Doctor's Notes

Your eye doctor can detect the initial stages of cataract formation long before you can perceive any visible sign. At this point, using a diet and nutritive supplement protocol designed to prevent or slow this condition is highly recommended.

Additional Resources

National Council on Aging
409 Third St. SW, 2nd floor
Washington, DC 20024
202-479-1200

National Association for the Visually Handicapped
3201 Balboa St.
San Francisco, CA 94121
415-221-3201

Endnotes

1. G. Bravetti, "Preventative medical treatment of senile cataract with vitamin E and anthocyanosides: Clinical evaluation," Ann Otalmol Clin Ocul, 1989, 115: 109.
2. P.F. Jacques and L.T. Chylack, "At the demiologic evidence of a roll for the antioxidant vitamins and carotenoids in cataract prevention,"Amer Jour Clin Nutr, 1991 53:352S-5S. See also S.M. Buton "Vitamin C and the aging eye," Arch Intern Med, 1939, 63:930-35.
3. O. Neuwirth-Lux and F. Billson, "Vitamin E and rabbit corneal endothelial cell survival," Aust Nzj Opthamol, 1987, 15(4): 309-14.
4. P. Wanger and P. Weswig, "Effects of selenium, chromium and antioxidants on growth eye cataracts, plasma cholesterol in blood glucose in selenium deficient vitamin E supplemented rats," Nutr Rup Int 1975: 12:345-58.
5. Alan H. Pressman, The GSH Phenomenon, Nature's Most Powerful Antioxidant and Healing Agent, Glutathione, St. Martin's Press, New York: 1997, 141.
6. M.T. Meunier, et al., "Free radical scavenger activity of procyanidolic oligomers and anthocyanosides with respect to superoxide anion and lipid peroxidation," Planta Med Phytother, 1989, 23(4): 267-74.
7. S.D. Varma, et al., "Diabetic cataracts and flavonoids" Science, 1977 195:205-06.
8. D. Atkinson, "Malnutrition as an etiological factor in senile cataract," Eye Ear Nose Throat Mon, 1952, 31: 79-83.
9. P.F. Jacques, and L.T. Chylack, "Epidemiologic evidence of a role for the antioxidant vitamins and carotenoids in cataract prevention," Amer Jour Clin Nutri, 1991, 53: 352S-55S.
10. American Journal of Opthamology, 1931, 14: 1005-09.
11. S.A. Mansore, et al., "Effect of antioxidant on the progress of cataracts in Emery mice," Abstract Invest Opthamol Vis Sci, 1984, 25:138.
12. P.H. Jacques, et al., "Vitamin intake and senile cataract," Abstract Jour Amer Coll Nutr 1987, 6(5): 435.
13. I.P. Chuistova, et al., ""Experimental morphologic foundation for the usage of zinc in the treatment of cataract" Opthamol ZH, 1985, 7:396.
14. H. Cole, "Enzyme activity may hold the key to cataract activity, "Jama 1985, 254(8):1008.
15. J.H. Kinoshita, Invest Opthalmol, 1965, 4: 786-99.

CHICKEN POX

Chicken pox is a common childhood disease caused by the herpes zoster virus. While most children will usually come down with chicken pox before the age of eight, a small percentage of adults contract the disease.

Chicken pox is characterized by a headache and a mild fever, followed by the eruption of small, red, itchy spots. The incubation period for chicken pox is between fourteen to seventeen days. Having chicken pox usually results in life-long immunity to the disease. However, the herpes zoster virus can live in the body and appear later as shingles.

A person with chicken pox is considered highly infectious from around two days before the rash appears until approximately a week later. Chicken pox occurs more often in the winter and spring, in temperate regions, and is seen year round in warmer climates.

Symptoms

From ten to twenty-one days after exposure, symptoms of chicken pox can occur. The severity of the disease is thought to be related to the extent of exposure.

A rash, which initially resembles a flat red splotch, generally appears on the trunk, the armpits, on the upper arms and legs, on the scalp, inside the mouth and occasionally in the throat and bronchial tubes (which can cause a cough). The "spots" eventually become fluid-filled blisters within a few hours of eruption. After several days, they will dry out and form scabs. After the sores have formed crusts, the fever usually disappears.

The eruption of the pox continues in cycles which can last from three days to one week. These blisters are considered infectious.

Children usually develop a slight fever with chicken pox. An adult with the virus typically experiences a high fever and can subsequently contract pneumonia. Adults can also experience flu-like symptoms with the disease.

The rash that accompanies chicken pox is extremely itchy and can be very miserable depending on the location of the sores. Once the scabs disappear, the child is no longer considered contagious.

Precautions

Although rare, possible serious complications of chicken pox can occur. Watch for a sudden, very high fever, vomiting, convulsions, severe headache, swollen lymph glands under the arms, neck or in the groin area and broken blood vessels, bruising or red streaking. If any of these symptoms suddenly appear, call your doctor immediately.

The older one is, the more severe chicken pox will be. In some cases, pneumonia and encephalitis can develop as secondary infections. Adults should avoid contact with exposed individuals. Women in their final stage of pregnancy should avoid exposure. If they do catch the disease, the newborn may develop a severe case of the virus.

Anyone taking cancer drugs or cortisone should immediately contact a physician if infected by chicken pox.

Never give a child aspirin if a viral infection is suspected because this can increase the risk of Reye's syndrome, a potentially fatal disorder. The combination of giving aspirin with the chicken pox virus, has an especially strong correlation with the incidence of Reye's syndrome.

Causes

Chicken pox is caused by a virus (varicella-zoster) that is spread from person to person through airborne droplets or through contaminated bedding or clothing. The disease is very contagious. Over 90 percent of siblings in a particular family will catch the disease.

Conventional Therapies

Complete recovery usually takes place within ten days. Acetaminophen is usually suggested for fever and discomfort, but some studies have indicated that using acetaminophen (Tylenol) prolonged the illness and was not that effective in relieving symptoms. Some physicians believe that we are too quick to try to lower a fever. If a fever is not too high, it can actually speed the recovery process. Calamine lotion is the standard medication used to relieve itchiness and irritation. In very severe cases, or when the immune system is weak, an antiviral drug, (Acyclovir) may be prescribed, although there is some evidence that the drug is not effective unless administered immediately after the rash appears. If the sores become infected, an antibiotic ointment can be prescribed. No vaccine against chicken pox is available at this time but one is in development. Most doctors will want to treat chicken pox without an office visit unless complications arise.

Dietary Guidelines

- ♦ Typically, sores in the mouth may interfere with eating, so nutritious milk shakes, liquid meal replacements, shakes, popsicles, etc., may be more appealing to the child.
- ♦ Oral numbing sprays can be used just prior to eating so ingesting food is easier. Check with your doctor or dentist for prescription varieties.
- ♦ Avoid salty or spicy foods and citrus fruits.
- ♦ Give plenty of liquids in the form of vegetable broths and mild fruit juices.
- ♦ Do not use sweets, chocolate or meat.
- ♦ Offer the child mild foods that are easy to eat and digest, such as creamy mashed potatoes, rice pudding, scrambled eggs, or milk shakes.

Recommended Nutritional Supplements

PRIMARY NUTRIENTS

BETA CAROTENE Helps to enhance the immune system and aids in healing tissue. *Suggested Dosage:* 4,000 IU daily or an age-appropriate dose. Interestingly, a vitamin A deficiency has been linked to diseases like measles and chicken pox.[1]

VITAMIN C Helps to control fever and is thought to be a natural an antiviral compound which also eliminates toxins and scavenges for free radicals. Vitamin C possesses properties that work similarly to interferon in helping the immune system fight off viral infections.[2] *Suggested Dosage:* Take as directed using liquid products that have been esterized. Add to juice, etc.

VITAMIN E Promotes healing, contributes to cell oxygenation and is an excellent antioxidant. Capsules can be opened and placed directly on sores to help minimize scarring. Vitamin E is useful for chicken pox in that it helps heal tissue while enhancing immune response.[3] *Suggested Dosage:* Take as directed.

LIQUID CHROLOPHYLL Helps to purify the blood of toxins released by viral invaders. *Suggested Dosage:* Take as directed. Can be added to juice, etc.

ELECTROLYTE REPLACEMENT LIQUID If heavy sweating occurs due to fever, use a product like Pedialyte as directed to replace minerals lost. *Suggested Dosage:* Take as directed.

ECHINACEA Helps to boost the immune system and has impressive antiviral properties.[4] *Suggested Dosage:* Try to find guaranteed potency liquid extracts.

ST. JOHN'S WORT The hypericin content of this herb has powerful antiviral actions against the herpes strain.[5] *Suggested Dosage:* Take as directed in age-appropriate doses.

GOLDENSEAL A natural antibiotic herb which contains berberine compounds that are beneficial for severe itching and stimulate immune defenses as well.[6] *Suggested Dosage:* Take as directed in age-appropriate doses. Do not use for longer than a week.

SECONDARY NUTRIENTS

GINGER AND BAYBERRY: These work together to help protect against viruses and to calm the digestive system. Ginger teas can help bring down a fever.

RED CLOVER: Helps to cleanse the blood of impurities. *Suggested Dosage:* Take as directed.

HOPS AND VALERIAN: Can be used to promote sleep and calm the nerves. *Suggested Dosage:* Take as directed for the appropriate age of the child.

TEA TREE OIL: Can be applied to sores to help facilitate healing and prevent infection.

Home Care Suggestions

♦ Wet compresses can be applied to the pox to ease itching. Use red raspberry, catnip and peppermint powder mixed in a base of diluted apple cider vinegar.
♦ Colloidal oatmeal baths have also been used with some success in controlling the itching. Aveeno is a brand of colloidal oatmeal which can be purchased at a pharmacy.

♦ Clothing should be light and nonconstrictive.
♦ Do not use cortisone-based ointments on the rash. These can increase the risk of infection.
♦ Keep the child's nails short and file them smooth to discourage scratching which can lead to infection and scarring. Wash the hands often to prevent secondary infections. For very young children, soft gloves or socks over the hands are recommended.
♦ For itching, use an aloe vera or comfrey salve. A black walnut tincture can also be used.
♦ Take a warm bath using one cup of baking soda and to 1/2 cup of apple cider vinegar.
♦ A cool bath can also ease itching, especially if pox are present in the genital area. Corn starch may be added to the water.
♦ Dyprotex cream, an over-the-counter preparation, can be used in pad or lotion form. It helps to relieve itching and is less drying than calamine-based medications.
♦ Using olive oil on the dried out scabs may cause them to drop off sooner.
♦ Witch hazel applied to the sores can help to calm itching and inflammation.

Other Supportive Therapies

HOMEOPATHY: Antimonium tart. 12C, Pulsatilla 12C and Rhus tox. 12C are typically used to treat the symptoms of chicken pox.

Scientific Facts-at-a-Glance

Although a chicken pox vaccine is available, considerable controversy surrounds its usage because adverse reactions have been documented. Because chicken pox is generally not considered a serious disease, caution should be exercised in using the vaccine.

Spirit/Mind Considerations

Anyone who comes down with chicken pox usually feels miserable and may assume they will be permanently scarred by the sores. Gentle support and patience with "itchy children" is important. Keeping a child busy with suitable activities helps to keep the mind off of the sores.

Prevention

♦ It is recommended that young, healthy children be deliberately exposed to chicken pox so that the disease will no be contracted as an adolescent or adult.
♦ Those who have never had the disease, are pregnant or taking immunosuppressant drugs, should avoid contact with groups of children who have had possible contact with the chicken pox virus.

Endnotes
1. Michael T. Murray, ND, Encyclopedia of Nutritional Supplements, Prima Publishing, Rocklin, CA: 24.
2. A. Bendich, "Vitamin C and immune response," Food Techol, 1987, 41: 112-14.

3. Plastic and Reconstructive Surgery, June, 1982, 69: 1029-30.

4. R Bauer, and H. Wagner, "Echinacea species as potential immunostimulatory drugs," Econ Med Plant Res, 1991, 5: 253-321.

5. G. Lavie, et al., "Antiviral pharmaceutical compositions containing hypericin or pseudohypericin," European Patent Application, 87111467, 8-8-87, European Patent Office.

6. M. Sabir and N. Bhide, "Study of some pharmacologic actions of berberine," Indian Jour Physiol Pharm, 1971, 15: 111-132.

CHRONIC FATIGUE SYNDROME (CFS)

Chronic fatigue syndrome (CFS) has become a common household term but it is still considered a somewhat baffling disorder. It is now also referred to as ME (myalgic encephalomyelitis) and PVFS (post-viral fatigue syndrome). It can cause varying degrees of malaise which have no single obvious cause.

CFS, also known as "the yuppie flu," is a persistent disease and can be unusually difficult to treat. For unknown reasons, 80 percent of those who suffer from CFS are women who are generally between the ages of 24 and 45.

The symptoms of CFS can be confusing and difficult to assess. Consequently, misdiagnosis is frequent. Experts believe the Epstein-Barr virus, unwittingly carried by thousands of people, is the cause of the disease. Some health care professionals dispute the involvement of this particular virus in CFS and consider this ailment as simply one of many syndromes caused by Western lifestyle and diet.

It may well be one of those disorders which is a result of compromised immunity. Chronic fatigue syndrome may persist for months or even years and its occurrence is on the increase.

Symptoms

CFS typically causes flu-like symptoms that persist and may include a low-grade fever, sore throat, muscles aches and pains, extreme fatigue, excess sleeping, minimal stamina, swollen glands, appetite loss, intestinal problems, anxiety, depression, irritability, sleep disturbances, mood swings, memory loss, headaches, sensitivity to light and heat, recurring upper respiratory tract infections and difficulty concentrating.

Precautions

Anyone suffering from any or some of these symptoms should see a doctor immediately. No one should assume that they have CFS. Many other conditions can cause feelings of fatigue or malaise.

People who have inadvertently contracted a parasitic infection may experience chronic fatigue syndrome and other related symptoms.

Causes

The Epstein-Barr virus, which is also involved in mononucleosis, is believed to cause CFS. However, unlike mononucleosis, CFS is not considered contagious. Significant controversy surrounds the notion that a virus causes this syndrome. There are some doctors who question viral involvement and regard the cause of CFS as an unsolved mystery. The notion that a human retro virus or a herpes virus causes CFS is unsubstantiated. Other theories suggest that vaccinations may eventually confuse the immune system, resulting in diseases like CFS.

Stress has been implicated as a possible cause in that highly motivated people seem more prone to develop the disease. Immune dysfunction can easily occur after periods of stress or trauma.

Other causes that have been linked to this disorder are food allergies, liver dysfunction, candida, mercury poisoning, hypoglycemia, anemia, hypothyroidism, sleep apnea, malnutrition, parasites, abnormal gut permeability and colon disease.

Conventional Therapies

The symptoms of CFS are sometimes treated with antibiotics which has no effect if the Epstein-Barr virus is involved. You can expect your doctor to run a battery of blood tests to check for elevated levels of antibodies to rule out other diseases such as cancer, diabetes, AIDS, endocrine disorders, anemia, leukemia, etc.

If the Epstein-Barr virus turns up in the blood, your physician will likely diagnose you with CFS. Doctors will usually prescribe a prescription vitamin and mineral supplement and recommend rest. To date, the medical profession considers CFS an incurable disease. Be careful not to become involved in drastic treatment protocols for CFS which can include radical approaches like hydrogen peroxide injections, cyclophosphamides, etc.

Dietary Guidelines

♦ Proper diet is crucial for anyone with an immune-related disease. First, avoid all caffeine, white sugar, alcohol and tobacco.
♦ Drink six to eight glasses of pure water daily.
♦ Emphasize whole grains, raw fruits and vegetables and protein sources in the form of legumes, lean white meats and fish.
♦ Use fresh seeds and nuts and make your own vegetable juices.
♦ Avoid empty calorie junk foods.
♦ If meals are a problem, use a good protein supplement drink to help boost energy and stamina.
♦ Make sure you are not suffering from a gluten, shellfish, sulfite or some other food allergy. As in any viral infection, the importance of susceptibility is often minimized by the medical profession. Strengthening the immune system is essential to build up resistance to infections from viruses like Epstein-Barr.

Recommended Nutritional Supplements

PRIMARY NUTRIENTS

VITAMIN AND MINERAL SUPPLEMENTS Take a good supplement every day that has a wide array of organic nutrients and is rapidly assimilated. *Suggested Dosage:* Take as directed.

VEGETABLE-BASED PROTEIN SUPPLEMENT Some evidence exists that rice protein may help to boost liver function and toxicity and treat abnormal gut permeability, which may be compromised in some cases of CFS.[1] *Suggested Dosage:* Look for quality vegetable-based products that taste good and mix easily in liquid.

VITAMIN A WITH BETA CAROTENE Enhances immune function and scavenges for damaging free radicals. Several clinical studies have found that this duo has the ability to boost immunological function.[2] Studies have found that taking a beta carotene supplement is even better absorbed than food sources.[3] *Suggested Dosage:* Use up to 25,000 of vitamin A per day for two weeks, then reduce to 10,000 IU per day. If you are pregnant, do not exceed 10,000 IU daily.

VITAMIN B12 Supplementation of this vitamin has been shown to improve the symptoms of this disease.[4] *Suggested Dosage:* Ask your doctor about vitamin B12 injections. Good oral forms include sublingual products. Take a directed.

GERMANIUM Clinicians have reported that between 20 and 50 percent of their patients who had CFS and received germanium supplements experience significant symptom relief.[5] *Suggested Dosage:* Take as directed. Only use this supplement with your doctor's approval and only take recommended dosages.

MAGNESIUM AND ZINC After six weeks of magnesium supplementation, 32 people with chronic fatigue syndrome experienced improved energy, better mood, and less pain.[6] Zinc also helps to stimulate better immune function and can boost a suppressed appetite as well. *Suggested Dosage:* Take as directed.

COENZYME Q10 Supplementation with this nutrient can help fight fatigue that is associated with this disease.[7] *Suggested Dosage:* Take as directed.

ESSENTIAL FATTY ACIDS Sixty-three patients who received EFAs from a combination of evening primrose oil and fish oil, experienced marked improvement in fatigue, depression and aches and pains with no apparent side effects.[8] *Suggested Dosage:* Take as directed.

ECHINACEA This herb contains special polysaccharides which can stimulate the immune system to fight against viral infections.[9] *Suggested Dosage:* Take as directed.

HERBAL COMBINATION This combination should include St. John's wort, kava kava, Siberian ginseng, gotu kola, kelp, astragalus, shiitake and reishi mushroom, and licorice root. *Suggested Dosage:* Four to eight capsules daily. Botanicals have been employed by many cultures to support and improve immune function. This formula contains some of the best herbs known to build and strengthen the body's resistance to disease. It is ideal for sufferers of chronic immune deficiency and may be used daily.

ST. JOHN'S WORT: One of the most impressive properties of this herb is its ability to fight viral infections. Interestingly, people who suffer from viral conditions such as chronic fatigue syndrome, mononucleosis, herpes simplex and AIDS are also often depressed. In these conditions, St. John's wort will provide mood elevation while it fights viral infection.[10] KAVA KAVA: Kava kava is used by people throughout the South Pacific where it is an important ceremonial drink. People who consume kava kava find a sense of well-being and happy contentment. After much clinical research, several European countries approved kava kava for the treatment of nervous anxiety and restlessness.[11] SIBERIAN GINSENG: Chronic stress can lead to illness by eroding immune function. Siberian ginseng has a clinically supported reputation as a stress fighter. It will also improve energy levels, and mental function and stamina, which are often lacking in chronically ill people. In the past ten years, research has demonstrated Siberian ginseng's ability to increase important T-lymphocytes of the helper variety. These lymphocytes are significantly reduced in HIV infections. Studies have confirmed the ability of this herb to improve and normalize immune system actions.[12] GOTU KOLA: Ayurvedic doctors use gotu kola as a central nervous system tonic to improve mental stamina and enhance memory. Its application in CFS is as a mental stimulant with anti-stress properties that also have a mild tranquilizing effect.[13] KELP: Kelp provides organic iodine which promotes healthy thyroid function. A dysfunctional thyroid has been associated with lethargy and general malaise. Kelp further provides trace elements that may be lacking in the diet, helping to provide chemical balance to the body.[14] ASTRAGALUS: Astragalus is one of the most popular herbs in Chinese medicine where it is regarded as a tonic, energizer and potent immune builder. Recent scientific studies have confirmed the benefits of astragalus for immune function. Astragalus has been shown to increase phagocytosis and interferon production. This herb can stimulate the production of interferon and has been used for centuries by the Chinese to enhance immune function.[15] SHIITAKE AND REISHI MUSHROOM: Shiitake mushrooms have received considerable attention for their immune system building effects. This mushroom has been scientifically studied and shown to stimulate interferon production and increase helper T-lymphocytes. This mushroom contains powerful immunostimulating polysaccharides. LICORICE ROOT: Licorice root is one of the most used plants in Chinese medicine and is referred to as the "Great Adjunct" because it increases the effectiveness of other herbs. However, animal studies have shown licorice to enhance the production of interferon and macrophage (a large phagocyte) activity and inhibits herpes-type viruses.[17] Licorice should not be used by anyone with high blood pressure, kidney disease or who is taking digitalis.

SECONDARY NUTRIENTS

VITAMIN C WITH BIOFLAVONOIDS: Studies have shown that these supplements can enhance resistance to fatigue while boosting immunity.[18] *Suggested Dosage:* 1,000 mg with each of three meals

GOLDENSEAL: Berberine and other alkaloids found in this herb can boost white cell activity and improve liver function.[19] *Suggested Dosage:* Take as directed, but do not use for more than one week consecutively.

ACIDOPHILUS: Replenishes friendly flora which can help to fight infections and restore vitality. *Suggested Dosage:* Take as directed using guaranteed bacterial count products with bifidobacteria. Check expiration date.

GARLIC: Garlic has proven itself as an effective antiviral agent and boosts the immune system.[20] *Suggested Dosage:* Take two capsules with all three meals during the day.

MILK THISTLE (SILYMARIN): Several theories suggest that liver toxicity or malfunction is intrinsically linked to CFS. This herb has the ability to stimulate liver tissue regeneration while detoxifying at the same time.[21] *Suggested Dosage:* Take as directed using standardized, guaranteed potency varieties.

PROTEOLYTIC ENZYMES: Improves the assimilation of nutrients and is recommended in cases where malabsorption is suspected. *Suggested Dosage:* Take before each meal as directed.

CARNITINE, TAURINE AND CYSTEINE: This trio of amino acids helps to support immune function. *Suggested Dosage:* Take as directed on an empty stomach with fruit juice.

DHEA: Low levels of this hormone have been linked to CFS. As with any hormonal supplement, check with your doctor first. *Suggested Dosage:* Take as directed.

Home Care Suggestions

- Keep a positive attitude by setting and achieving small goals each day.
- Very mild exercise has been suggested for CFS victims to increase stamina and oxygenate cells. Exercise also helps to facilitate better sleep.
- Get adequate amounts of sleep, including at least one daytime nap.
- Talk to others who suffer from the disease and share your feelings with your family and friends.
- Massage and exercise, in combination with elevation of the extremities, are believed to stimulate the lymphatic system which can, in turn, help strengthen the immune system.
- Stay away from allergens. CFS victims are often more sensitive to allergic reaction since their immune system is compromised.
- Make sure to rule out environmental pollutants, Candida, food allergies, parasites, or bowel disease as a possible cause of CFS. Check the section on food allergies for more information.

Other Supportive Therapies

ACUPUNCTURE: Specific points can be stimulated which will help to trigger better immune function.

MEDITATION OR YOGA: Learning to completely de-stress through these disciplines is very helpful and can foster feelings of true rest and well being.

Scientific Facts-at-a-Glance

While there has been much speculation that the human retro virus or chicken pox is somehow involved with CFS, there is not documented scientific data to back up these links. The notion, however, that food allergies may be involved is intriguing. If we are constantly battling certain foods as allergens, it would seem logical to assume that we may somehow confuse or "stress out" various immune functions. Likewise, the idea that certain vaccines may trigger unwanted immune responses that manifest themselves in CFS is rather engaging.

Spirit/Mind Considerations

It is interesting to know that there have been several occasions where CFS was diagnosed when the real problem was actually clinical depression (which can be successfully treated). Depression can cause significant feelings of fatigue as well as other symptoms and should be ruled out before any treatment plans are initiated. Anyone who does have CFS may easily feel that they are being patronized. In other words, they may feel sick but may also feel as though they do not have a legitimate disease. Frequently, family members, friends and even physicians don't fully understand the physical and emotional aspects associated with CFS. It can be very incapacitating and easily initiate feelings of confusion, impaired thinking and sadness. People with CFS usually are not just crying out for attention, they are victims of a syndrome that makes it difficult to function in all respects. All parties involved need to educate themselves in order to fully appreciate the magnitude of this disease and its disruption of daily routine. Marriages and other relationships can become very stressed by CFS. Family members need to be extremely supportive and never assume that anyone suffering from CFS is lazy or unproductive. The opposite is usually the case. Again, meditation can help to relieve stress which has been implicated as a major causal factor in immune-related disorders. Keeping a positive attitude is also very helpful.

Prevention

◆ Keep your colon healthy with high-fiber foods.
◆ Make stress reduction a part of your daily routine. Use counseling, relaxation techniques and exercise.
◆ Make sure to avoid exposure to parasites.
◆ There is some speculation that those who exercise regularly and are in good physical condition are more resistant to the Epstein-Barr virus.
◆ Keep the immune system healthy through proper diet, vitamin, mineral supplements and exercise.

Additional Resources

Chronic Fatigue and Immune Dysfunction (CFIDS) Foundation
PO Box 220398
Charlotte, NC 28222-0398
800-442-4347

Endnotes

1. J.S. Bland, et al., "A medical food-supplemented detoxification program in the management of chronic health problems," Altern Therap, 1995, 1: 62-71.

2. A. Bendich, "Beta-carotene and immune response," Proc Nutr Soc, 1991, 50: 263-74.

3. E.D. Brown, et al., "Plasma carotenoids in normal men after a single ingestion of vegetables or purified beta-carotene," Amer Jour Clin Nutr, 1989, 49: 1258-65.

4. C.W. Lapp, "Chronic fatigue syndrome is a real disease," North Carolina Family Physician, 1992, 43(1): 6-11.

5. G.R. Fallona and S.A. Lavine "The use of organic Germanium in chronic Epstine-Barr virus syndrome: An example of interferon, modulation of herpes reactivation" Jour Orthomol Med. 1988,3(1):29-31.

6. I.M. Cox et al "Red blood cell magnesium and chronic fatigue syndrome," Lancet, 1991,337:757-60.

7. A. Goldberg, CFIDS Chronicle, 1989 Summer/ Fall.

8. P.O. Behan et al "Effect of high doses of essential fatty acids on the post viral fatigue syndrome," Acta Neurol Scand, 1990 82(3):209-16.

9. J. Moz, "Effect of echinacin on phagocytosis and natural killer cells," Med Welt, 1983 34:1463-67.

10. G. Lavie, et al., "Hypericin as an inactivator of infectious viruses in blood components," Transfusion, 1995, 35: 392-400.

11. Rebecca Flynn, M.S., and Mark Roest. Your Guide to Standard Herbalized Products. One World Press, Prescott Arizona: 1995: 52-58.

12. B. Bohn, et al., "Flow-cytometric studies with Eleuterococcus senticosus extract as an immunomodulatory agent," Arzneimittel-Forsch, 1987, 37: 1193-96.

13. A.S. Ramaswamy, et al., "Pharmacological studies on Centella asiatica, Jour Res India Med, 1970, 4: 160-75.

14. Daniel B. Mowrey, Ph.D. The Scientific Validation of Herbal Medicine (Keats Publishing, Connecticut, 1986): 123

15. H. Yunde et al "Effect of radix astragalus on the interferon system," Chinese Medical Jour. 1981 94:35-40.

16. F. Fukucuoka, "Polysaccaride extract active against tumors," Chem Abstracts, 1971, 74:324-25.

17. N. Abe, et al., "Interferon induction by glycyrrhizin and glycyrrhetinic acid in mice," Microb Immunol, 1982, 26: 353-359.

18. E. Cheraskin, et al., "Daily vitamin C consumption and fatigability," Jour Amer Geria Soc, 1976, 24: 136-37.

19. Y. Kumazawa, et al., "Activation of perotenil macrophages by berberine alkaloids in terms of induction of cytostatic activity," Int Jour Immunofarmocal, 1984, 6: 587-92.

20. N.D. Weber, et al., "In vitro virucidal effects of Allium sativum (garlic) extract and compounds," Planta Medica, 1992, 58: 417-23.

21. H.A. Salmi and S. Sarna, "Effect of silymarin on chemical, functional, and morphologic alteration of the liver: A double-blind controlled study," Scand Jour Gastroent, 1982, 17: 417-21.

COLIC

Colic is a digestive condition that babies under the age of five months can experience from time to time. It is characterized by spasmodic intestinal pain that can come in waves of varying intensity and cause physical distress. It most commonly appears around three to four weeks of age and commonly disappears at twelve weeks. The dinner hour or from around 6 p.m. to 9 p.m. seems to be the worst time for a colicky baby. For generations, various home remedies have tried to relieve colic, although for some babies, a more mature digestive system seems like it may be the only complete cure. In other words, be patient. Colic will pass in time.

Symptoms

Episodes of colic are characterized by irritable screams or cries from the infant, accompanied by the drawing up of the legs and clenching of the fists. The infant's face may become red. Passing gas is a common cause. Intervals of quiet in-between cries is also typical of colicky babies. Colic tends to worsen in the evening and can be difficult to deal with if prolonged.

Babies with colic will often try to frantically feed, then pull away. Some theories have speculated that exposure to stressful situations or even to wind may induce colic.

Babies who experience colic are usually healthy otherwise. For some babies, having a bowel movement brings some relief.

Precautions

If your baby is experiencing diarrhea, fever, constipation or acts sick, see your physician immediately.

Causes

- Infantile colic occurs in one out of ten babies. The exact cause of colic is unknown.
- Some studies suggest that the incidence of colic is higher among bottle-fed babies.
- If nursing, it is thought that some foods the mother eats may cause colic in the infant. Foods to avoid are cabbage, onions, garlic, spicy foods and chocolate.
- There is also evidence to support that cow's milk can cause colic, not only in formula products but in breast milk itself (which results from the mother's ingestion of dairy products). It is recommended that nursing mothers avoid drinking cow's milk.
- Some studies have suggested that colic is an allergic reaction to certain kinds of protein. Changing your baby to a protein-treated formula may help you to assess if this is indeed the cause of the colic.
- Eating too rapidly, excessive swallowing of air have also been cited as possible causes of colic.
- Not burping your baby often enough.
- Excessive exposure to cold.

Conventional Treatments

Doctors seem at a loss to provide a successful treatment for colic. Other than strong antispasmodics or sedatives, treatment is minimal and not very effective. Typically, medical treatment is minimal. In very severe cases, an antispasmodic drug such as phenobarbital may be prescribed, although this form of treatment is not recommended for infants under the age of six months.

Dietary Guidelines

- Breast-feeding is generally recommended over bottle feeding and should optimally last for the first six months of the infant's life.
- If breast feeding is used, do not eat dairy products or cow's milk.
- Avoid onions, garlic, caffeine, cabbage, broccoli, ham, bacon, shellfish, bananas, nuts chocolate, strawberries, oranges, tobacco and alcohol.
- If using a formula, try one that has been protein treated or is not synthesized from cow's milk. Try 2 oz. of warm water to reduce the symptoms of colic and fill the baby's need to suck.

Recommended Nutritional Supplements

PRIMARY NUTRIENTS

Make sure to get the approval of your doctor before giving your baby any herbal supplements.

CATNIP, PEPPERMINT, FENNEL, OR ANISE TEA Make tea as usual and administer one tablespoon at a time to the baby. Tea may also be given in a bottle as long as it is not too concentrated. Never give honey to a baby that is less than one year old. Raw honey can harbor organisms which can cause infant botulism. *Suggested Dosage:* Take as directed.

HERBAL COMBINATION Also recommended is an herbal combination that includes peppermint, fennel, papaya and anise, ginger, catnip and chamomile. The herbal capsule can be opened and steeped in a small amount of boiling water, filtered through a cheesecloth and given by the teaspoon or in 2 oz. of pure water.

PEPPERMINT: The volatile compounds found in this herb are capable of relieving abdominal pain and distension, flatulence and nausea. In addition, peppermint can help to quiet stomach spasms by relaxing intestinal muscle.[1] FENNEL: The essential oils found in fennel work to enhance digestion and to eliminate the formation of gas and gripping pains.[2] GINGER: The anti-nausea properties of ginger are well documented. It has a carminative action which helps to stop stomach gripping, nausea and indigestion.[3] CATNIP: Gently eases stomach distress and promotes overall relaxation.[4] CHAMOMILE: A traditional herb used to treat children's ailments, chamomile helps to relieve acute stomach upset and calm an agitated nervous system.[5] PAPAYA AND ANISE: Papaya contains digestive enzymes that break down protein and other macronutrients. Anise seeds contain licorice-like volatile oils that prevent gas and promote digestion.

Home Care Suggestions

- Infant seats and crib mattresses can be purchased with motorized attachments which vibrate and gently coax a colicky baby to sleep.
- If mixing a formula with water make sure it is not too concentrated (it may cause intestinal irritation).
- Avoid formulas that have been iron-fortified. Excess iron in an infant's diet can cause intestinal problems. Iron-free formulas are sometimes hard to locate.
- Placing the infant on its stomach securely on top of a running dryer or washer (carefully supervise this activity) can help to soothe stomach pain and facilitate the movement of gas.
- Don't overfeed the baby. While the infant may appear hungry and take more breast milk or formula, this usually only serves to worsen the problem. Using certain weak herbal teas in pure water may help to pacify the baby and treat the spasms.
- Give the baby a warm bath in the evenings when the colic is at its worst.
- Taking the baby for a ride in the car can often help to bring about sleep.
- Make sure that your baby has been adequately burped after a feeding. Burp more than once during a feeding and keep the baby's head supported in a comfortable position while feeding.
- Place the baby on its stomach on your lap and gently swing the baby back and forth on your knees.
- Use a heating pad or hot water bottle on a comfortable setting under the infant's stomach. Watch for overheating or leaky hot water bottles.
- A mechanized baby swing may help to soothe the infant and provide a break for the parents also.
- If the baby must be held, carry the infant in a front sling or pouch so you still have your hands free. An activity like vacuuming may help to get the baby to sleep while in the sling.
- The use of pacifier may be helpful.
- Play music or try a neutral noise in the nursery, such as a fan, radio static, or an aquarium filter.
- Don't let your baby oversleep in the day. If naps go for longer than three hours, wake the baby for a bath, etc.
- Keep the baby's feet warm. Traditionally it has been believed that cold feet may cause abdominal pain in infants. Some traditional home remedies suggest putting the baby's feet in warm water.
- Never smoke around an infant. Some studies indicate that colic dramatically increases when infants are exposed to cigarette smoke.

Other Supportive Therapies

HOMEOPATHY: Colocynthis, chamamilla or dioscorea may be used. Check with your doctor before using with an infant.

MASSAGE: Rubbing oil of fennel gently on the baby's abdomen, followed by a warm bath, may offer some relief.

Scientific Facts-at-a-Glance

Research from British hospitals has found that many babies with colic are allergic to cow's milk. In addition, if they are nursing and their mothers drink cow's milk or dairy products, they can still experience allergic reactions. If you need to, try formulas which are lactose and gluten-free.

Spirit/Mind Considerations

Frequently, the caretaker of a colicky infant needs support from other family members so fatigue and exhaustion do not become overwhelming. Typically, new mothers believe that their fussy baby is an indication of their own inadequate mothering. Colic has nothing to do with successful mothering and will disappear within the first few months of infancy. Learning to relax is so important. Just remember that infants cry. It's as simple as that. Don't let yourself become tense or anxious. Know that colic can be a normal part of growing up and that the child will grow out of it.

Prevention

- Feed your baby in a relaxed atmosphere and in an upright position.
- Don't leave the baby with a propped bottle.
- Breast feed if possible and avoid eating food which may cause problems.
- Do not introduce new foods or juices until the baby is at least five months old and you have your doctor's approval.
- Experiment with different formulas. Predigested protein formulas can work better for colic/colic prevention.

Doctor's Notes

Colic is one of those conditions that appears for no apparent reason and disappears just as mysteriously. Although breast-fed babies seem less prone to colic, they can also become colicky. One must remember that the digestive system of a newborn has much adjusting to do and a few gastrointestinal upsets are normal. It is important to remember, however, that if any other symptoms accompany colic, you should see your doctor right away.

Endnotes

1. Alma E. Guiness, Family Guide to Natural Medicine, Reader's Digest, 1993: 300.
2. Mark Pederson, Nutritional Herbology, Wendall Whitman Co., Warsaw, Indiana: 1995, 90.
3. D.B. Mowrey, and D.E. Clayson, "Motion sickness, ginger and psychophysics," Lancet, 1982, I: 655-57.
4. Alma E. Guiness, Family Guide to Natural Medicine, Reader's Digest, 1993, 300.
5. Alma E. Guiness, Family Guide to Natural Medicine, Reader's Digest, 1993, 301.

COLITIS

Colitis refers to a condition characterized by inflammation of the colon or large intestine, which brings on episodes of diarrhea or constipation. It is also commonly reffered to as inflammatory bowel disease (IBD), and the terms are interchangeable. Colitis can be sporadic or can exist as a chronic disorder. It is considered unpredictable and may be linked to several factors, both physiological and psychological.

Colitis and irritable bowel syndrome are sometimes interchangeable terms and usually deal with inflammation that effects only the surface regions of bowel sections. Crohn's disease is characterized by inflammation that effects the total thickness of the bowel lining (it's also called enteritis). Ulcerative colitis typically affects the colon lining and is differentiated by the development of ulcers or sores that are difficult to heal. Colitis can effect anyone at any age but it typically occurs between the ages of 15 and 30 and females are slightly more prone than males.

Many natural health care experts have concluded that these bowel diseases are only one of many ailments which have developed due to typical western diets which are low in fiber and high in refined flours, white sugar, fats, meats and dairy products.

Symptoms

Colitis usually causes a number of symptoms which can all overlap, depending on the type of bowel disease present. Typical symptoms include diarrhea or constipation (with hard, dry, pellet like feces and the passage of stringy mucous in the stool), pain during a bowel movement, abdominal tenderness, hemorrhoids, weakness, fatigue, cold sweats, stomach cramps, bloating and gas, headache, fever, nausea, loss of appetite (anorexia), rectal bleeding (bloody, watery stools can occur in ulcerative colitis) and feeling sick during or right after eating. Joint pain which mimics arthritis can also be associated with colitis.

Precautions

Any of the above symptoms may indicate colon cancer and should be checked out by your doctor immediately. In addition anyone with colitis runs an increased risk of developing colon cancer. It's a good idea to have periodic colon examinations to make sure that cancerous tumors are caught in their early stages.

Causes

Several interesting theories have linked IBD to emotional and nutritional factors. Like any other disease that results from the inflammatory process, several causal components may be involved. Some of the more interesting ones deal with the effect of certain vaccines, undigested protein particles and food allergies. In addition, colitis may be also initiated by food allergies (especially gluten and cow's milk), genetic predisposition, deranged intestinal microflora, viral, bacterial or parasitic infection (giardia for example), prolonged use of an antibiotics, immune dysfunction, ischemia or impaired blood supply to the intestinal wall, faulty diet, constipation, eating too rapidly, drinking too much liquid with meals, ingesting excessive cathartics and emotional stress.

Conventional Therapies

Often an infection that causes colitis will resolve itself without treatment. However, once a pattern of diarrhea and irritation is established, bowel problems can persist indefinitely.

Antibiotics such as erythromycin are routinely used to treat campylobacter infections. If a parasitic infection is suspected, other antibiotics are commonly used. Ironically, the very use of antibiotics in treating certain forms of colitis can create more intestinal irritation and kill the friendly intestinal flora which are so crucial to colon heath.

Colitis often evades conventional medical approaches. If the diagnosis is ulcerative colitis, corticosteroid therapy is recommended either by mouth or by enema. Surgery to remove certain sections of the bowel may be advised. Diet modifications and vitamin therapy are also routine.

If constipation is present a mild, nonirritating laxative and a stool softener may be suggested. For cases with severe abdominal pain, an antispasmodic may be recommended.

When nervous tension is seen as a precipitating factor, a mild sedative or tranquilizer may be suggested.

Again, if you can avoid antibiotics or powerful tranquilizing drugs and use safer, natural therapies, you'll be not only targeting symptoms, but promoting the healing process itself. Moreover, medical treatments rarely address the cause of the condition in the first place. Often simple changes in diet and lifestyle are much more effective than drug protocols.

Dietary Guidelines

- ◆ It is vitally important when experiencing any IBD to eat the right foods and take a strong vitamin and mineral supplement daily.
- ◆ In some cases of IBD, where diarrhea is severe, a liquid diet is suggested for a short time. Using carrot juice, cabbage juice, green juices and herb teas is recommended to promote healing of the bowel lining.
- ◆ When eating solid food, chew thoroughly and do not drink liquids with meals. During a flare-up, avoid high-roughage foods which contain skins and seeds, especially popcorn.
- ◆ For some people, the inclusion of fibrous foods is not irritating and seems to promote healing. For example, some colitis sufferers cannot tolerate fresh peas while others find them perfectly digestible. Check with your physician and then experiment with certain foods.
- ◆ You may want to puree cooked vegetables until the condition clears up.
- ◆ Emphasize yellow fruits, cantaloupe, pears, watermelon, kelp, agar and cucumbers. Fruits with pectin, such as apples and pears, seem especially beneficial.

- It might be advantageous to peel all fruit and get rid of its fibrous parts.
- Avoid fruits that have been canned in sugar and dried fruits.
- Do not eat dairy foods. A lactose intolerance may be part of the problem.
- Use soups, especially vegetable broths. Make it a habit to eat fruit at the end of a meal. If fruit juices are too irritating, dilute them with pure water and don't eat fruit on an empty stomach.
- Zwieback toast and other mild foods such as rice cereal are recommended.
- Do not eat fried foods or any other food that seem to aggravate the disorder.
- Cold, sugary cereals can be particularly bad. Even corn flakes can be extremely irritating to the bowel.
- Keep a list of offending foods. Food allergies are strongly suspected as a major contributory factor to bowel disorders.
- Foods to avoid are coffee, dairy foods, eggs, wheat gluten and raw vegetables. Remove the skin from turkey or chicken. Too much meat increases bowel transit time and fails to properly clean the gastrointestinal tract.
- Too little fiber can lead to constipation, diverticulitis and other gastrointestinal tract disorders.
- White fish is an acceptable source of protein as are any soy foods, especially tofu.
- Do not smoke or drink alcohol.
- After an inflammatory episode has passed, emphasizing complex carbohydrates with high-fiber contents has been shown to be quite beneficial.
- Eating foods high in fiber is generally discouraged for people with colitis; however, certain fiber sources are considered very valuable.
- Stay away from wheat bran and consider using fiber supplements that contain healing herbs and can be mixed in liquid.
- Make sure not to eat fiber in excess. Start slowly and see how increasing fiber is tolerated. For some bowel conditions, adding fiber may aggravate symptoms and cause more bloating gas and possible diarrhea.

Recommended Nutritional Supplements

PRIMARY NUTRIENTS

ACIDOPHILUS Helps to replenish friendly bacteria in the bowel and works to control gas and bloating. Studies have found that symptoms associated with colitis and irritable bowel syndrome were relieved when lactobacillus was administered.[1] *Suggested Dosage:* Take as directed using milk-free, guaranteed bacterial count products with bifidobacteria. Check for expiration date. Take on an empty stomach.

DIGESTIVE ENZYMES These compounds help to more throughly digest food, help to avoid the retention of undigested protein particles which can initiate food allergies and ease inflammation. Bromelain, which comes from pineapple, has demonstrated some remarkable anti-inflammatory properties.[2] *Suggested Dosage:* Take as directed on an empty stomach 30 minutes before meals and before going to bed. Enteric-coated bromelain and other enzymes may be preferable for bowel treatment.

PEPPERMINT OIL Clinical studies have found that enteric-coated capsules relaxes gastrointestinal smooth muscle and can help to significantly reduce the symptoms of irritable bowel syndrome.[3] *Suggested Dosage:* Take two capsules 30 minutes before each of three meals per day.

SUPEROXIDE DIMUSTASE (SOD) Liposomal SOD, which is considered an effective free radical scavenger and antioxidant, has been used to successfully treat people with Crohn's disease. It helps to neutralize the damaging effects caused by excessive inflammatory reactions in the bowel.[4] *Suggested Dosage:* Take as directed using liposomal forms only. Other types may not be effective when ingested.

VITAMIN A Works to heal the mucus membranes of the bowel. In addition, a deficiency of vitamins A, E and K have been noted in a good percentage of people with IBD. These vitamins are important to proper metabolism of the intestinal mucosa. Clinical trials have found that vitamin A supplementation may help treat Crohn's disease.[5] *Suggested Dosage:* 25,000 IU daily. If you are pregnant, do not take over 10,000 IU.

VITAMIN D A vitamin D deficiency is also common in people that suffer from chronic colon disorders and should be supplemented.[6] A deficiency in this vitamin can lead to calcium loss from the bones. *Suggested Dosage:* Take as directed.

VITAMIN K Like vitamin D, people who suffer with IBD are very prone to developing vitamin K deficiencies.[7] This vitamin is vital for proper blood clotting. Eighteen patients with Chron's disease or ulcerative colitis who received vitamin K supplements were found to improve. *Suggested Dosage:* Blue-green algaes or liquid fat soluble chlorophyll preparations are an excellent source of vitamin K. Take as directed.

VITAMIN C WITH BIOFLAVONOIDS Bioflavonoid compounds, especially quercitin, help to inhibit the inflammatory response in the bowel.[8] *Suggested Dosage:* 6,000 mg divided with each of three meals.

VITAMIN E Promotes tissue healing of the bowel lining and acts to scavenge free radicals which can be produced by tissue trauma. Some studies have shown dramatic improvement with vitamin E therapy for ulcerative colitis.[9] *Suggested Dosage:* 400 to 800 IU daily.

ESSENTIAL FATTY ACIDS Both the omega-3 and omega-6 fatty acids are useful. Fish oil and evening primrose or flaxseed oil can provide these essential fatty acids which the body may be lacking when IBD is present. Studies using fish oil have found that its EPA and DHA content resulted in a 65 percent drop in inflammatory compounds found in the intestines and an 80 percent decrease in the number of cellular mutations found in diseased colons.[10] *Suggested Dosage:* Take as directed.

OMEGA-3 OILS These oils found in certain fish and plants help to normalize prostaglandin activity which is impaired in Crohn's disease.[11] *Suggested Dosage:* Take as directed. If you are using fish oil, take with a vitamin E supplement.

FOLIC ACID Supplementing folate can help to reduce the diarrhea associated with this disease. A folic acid deficiency is common in Crohn's disease.[12] *Suggested Dosage:* Take as directed.

MAGNESIUM, ZINC, VITAMIN A AND VITAMIN E Magnesium deficiency is very prevalent with people who have inflammatory bowel disorders.[13] A zinc deficiency has been found in almost half of all people suffering from Chron's disease.[14] *Suggested Dosage:* Take as directed. Use chelated zinc products and take with meals.

FIBER SUPPLEMENT WITH PSYLLIUM Supplements which contain psyllium or water soluble fiber have proven themselves invaluable for people with chronic recurrent diarrhea, pain and constipation. This seed helps to speed transit time and relieves both constipation and diarrhea. In addition, it helps to normalize colonic bacteria which are so crucial to bowel health.[15] *Suggested Dosage:* Take as directed before retiring to bed. Make sure to drink extra water all through the day when taking a fiber supplement.

HERBAL COMBINATION This combination should include includes astragalus, schizandra, goldenseal root, licorice root, papaya leaves, gentian root, myrrh gum, Irish moss, fenugreek seeds, ginger root, valerian root, kava and aloe vera gel. *Suggested Dosage:* Two to four capsules daily. Nausea and flatulence are common gastrointestinal problems of IBD. This formula will treat the most common of these disorders and help treat the symptoms of some gastrointestinal tract disorders that are genetically inherited.

GOLDENSEAL ROOT: Goldenseal has been used to restore the mucus lining of the gastrointestinal tract. Goldenseal promotes bile secretion, restores proper bowel transit time and removes excess water from the body. Its berberine content is effective in treating the majority of gastrointestinal infections which may be at the root of colitis.[16] LICORICE ROOT: Licorice has been recognized for its anti-inflammatory activity which can help in cases of gastritis and inflammatory bowel disease. It can inhibit the formation of inflammatory prostaglandins which promote bowel inflammation.[17] Licorice has a diuretic and mild laxative effect that cleanses toxins from the body. The licorice in this formula is true licorice, which is not used in most licorice candies in the United States. PAPAYA LEAVES: Both papaya fruit and leaves are a source of papain which is a mixture of protein-digesting enzymes. Studies have found that it can enhance the digestion of wheat gluten and inhibit its inflammatory response in the colon in people with celiac

disease.[18] GENTIAN ROOT: Gentian enjoys widespread use, particularly in Europe as a digestive aid. It increases saliva and is believed to increase secretion of gastric juices.[19] Some herbalists have used it to expel intestinal worms. Its anti-inflammatory effects are helpful with gastritis and IBD. It is considered a bitter tonic. MYRRH GUM: Myrrh gum is used to heal the gastric mucosa of the intestinal tract. Myrrh gum is carminative, reduces gas and bloating and calms the stomach. It also is a mild laxative.[20] IRISH MOSS: Irish moss is rich in trace mineral nutrients. It also contains large amounts of mucilage which soothes the gastrointestinal tract.[21] It is specifically used for dyspepsia, nausea, heartburn and diarrhea. FENUGREEK SEEDS: As much as 40 percent of the weight of fenugreek seeds is mucilage. Mucilage is a gelatin-like substance usually made up of proteins and polysaccharides which heal irritated intestinal tract lining to hold water. It also prompts pancreatic secretion, which boosts digestion.[22] GINGER ROOT: Ginger is one of the best herbs for the treatment of digestive disorders. Ginger prevents nausea, gas, bloating and vomiting. Ginger root is not a laxative, but it will tonify the intestinal muscle and provides a source of proteolytic enzymes to aid digestion.[23] ALOE VERA GEL: Aloe vera gel is a clear, jelly-like material called mucilage. Aloe has been successfully employed in treating irritable bowel syndrome. Aloe gel improves bowel transit time, reducing putrefaction in the intestinal tract and increases friendly bacteria like acidophilus.[24] If you have any gripping with this herb, add more ginger. This herb is usually part of combinations and if used single may cause cramping. VALERIAN ROOT AND KAVA: An important stress-management tool in cases of colitis. These herbs work to calm the central nervous system without the addiction or artificial sedative effects associated with tranquilizing drugs.

SECONDARY NUTRIENTS

GARLIC OIL (ENTERIC COATED): Garlic helps to get rid of any pathogens in the colon and also promotes the healing of tissue. *Suggested Dosage:* Take as directed.

ALFALFA: Can help to promote healing through its chlorophyll content. *Suggested Dosage:* Can be taken in liquid or capsule form. Take as directed.

CABBAGE JUICE OR POWDER: Compounds in cabbage have the ability to help in healing gastrointestinal ulcers. *Suggested Dosage:* You may have trouble finding cabbage powder. Juicing cabbage may be more practical. Take a 1/2 cup of juice in the morning and at night on an empty stomach.

HOPS AND VALERIAN ROOT: Both of these herbs are natural tranquilizers which can help with stress and promote relaxation. *Suggested Dosage:* Take as directed.

SLIPPERY ELM: Helps to control diarrhea and soothes irritated membranes. *Suggested Dosage:* Take as directed.

Home Care Suggestions

- ◆ Eat slowly and do not drink too much liquid with meals.
- ◆ Avoid belts or waistbands that are too restrictive.
- ◆ Use bistort drops for diarrhea. It acts as a natural anti-inflammatory in the colon.

- Incorporate a regular exercise program into your life to facilitate the removal of toxins through the lymph system.
- Learn to recognize the stress factor and as soon as you feel stress, use breathing or meditation to dispel its physical effects.
- Make a list of everything you eat and subsequent symptoms. Finding out if you are sensitive to offending foods is vital.
- If diarrhea is severe, avoid overusing Immodium AD and Lomitil. See your doctor. If ulcerative colitis is present do not use aspirin, ibuprofen, naprosyn, voltaren and feldene. These can cause further damage to the intestinal lining. Check with your doctor before taking any medication.
- Learn to use relaxation techniques such as yoga, biofeedback, controlled breathing, self-hypnosis, etc, to reduce daily tension and control stress.
- Have regular screenings for colon cancer. Chronic colitis can increase your risk.
- Incorporate a regular exercise program into your routine to help relieve stress.

Other Supportive Therapies

HOMEOPATHY: Podophyllum and arsenicum alb are typically used for bowel disease.

ACUPUNCTURE: The stimulation of certain points can help to promote the relaxation of bowel muscle.

MASSAGE: The overall de-stressing effects of a good massage is very beneficial for people with bowel disorders that are impacted by anxiety. In addition, massage helps to stimulate circulation and facilitates the removal of toxins from the body.

Scientific Facts-at-a-Glance

The notion that vaccinations may disrupt normal immune function and affect the bowel as well as other body systems is something worth considering. Some studies have suggested that those who have been vaccinated against measles were three times more likely to develop Crohn's disease or ulcerative colitis.[25] What studies like this do is to raise awareness that the mysterious development of autoimmune diseases may be due to immune dysfunction triggered by the abnormal introduction of foreign antigens.

Spirit/Mind Considerations

IBD is frequently linked to anxiety and stress. For this reason, herbs that help to calm the central nervous system may be of great value. People with these disorders often internalize stress which takes its toll on their gastrointestinal tracts. If you ask someone with IBD if they feel stressed out, they often reply in the negative. Many of these individuals are people pleasers, perfectionists and run at a fast pace. If their bowels are susceptible, this type of unexpressed stress can often manifest itself as chronic diarrhea, constipation, stomach bloating and continual inflammation. Learning to de-stress and to meditate can be of great value for anyone who suffers from these diseases. Moreover, if you have emotional issues that have not been resolved, do so.

Prevention

- Eating a diet that is low in hydrogenated fats and high in fiber and complex carbohydrates can help to minimize the risk of IBD. Consuming plenty of raw fruits and vegetables and whole grain foods are vital to colon health.
- Keep the colon active by eating foods that promote proper elimination. Constipation is a contributory factor to any bowel disease.
- Prevent colon irritations by avoiding irritating foods, such as heavy, rich junk foods, salt, sugar, fried foods, etc.
- Don't eat under high stress situations, when anxious or hurried or during high adrenalin times. Chew food thoroughly
- Don't overuse over-the counter laxatives which can irritate the colon.
- Stay away from smoking, fumes, chemical sprays and food additives.
- Drink plenty of pure water every day (six to eight glasses).

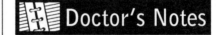 Doctor's Notes

While the addition of fiber can be helpful, too much fiber is not beneficial in most cases of IBD. Chinese herbal formulas that use combinations containing astragalus and schizandra are recommended.

My experience with a 16-year-old boy who had severe problems with ulcerative colitis supports the use of herbal therapies. He was losing weight and suffered from continuous bloody diarrhea. The medical advice he had previously received was to have bowel surgery, which consisted of taking the diseased part of the small intestine and replacing it with large intestine. His mother did not approve of this particular approach. He was put on all the herbs mentioned in this section in addition to treatments of acupuncture. He subsequently gained 30 pounds and is now in his second year of college with only an occasional flare up of his symptoms when under extreme stress.

Most IBD is closely tied with stress and diet. Stress may not be the actual cause of these diseases, but people who suffer from IBD usually have bowels that are very stress sensitive due to their inability to manage and channel stressful situations.

It is very important to remember to increase fiber. The colon is an organ that responds beautifully to natural treatments. Herbs that quiet digestion, ease anxiety and promote good bowel elimination are all very helpful.

Equally important for anyone with IBD is to begin a meditation program. I have found that it may be one of the single most important therapies you can incorporate into your life. If you need an extra boost in managing tension or in promoting relaxation, take valerian root, kava kava or other herbal blends designed to decrease anxiety. Combine them with the herbs and vitamins you need to heal the colon and facilitate better digestion. Increasing fiber intake is also vital and can be easily accomplished by eating more foods in their natural state and using fiber supplements if necessary. Acupuncture treatments have also been beneficial for IBD.

Additional Resources

Crohn's and Colitis Foundation of America
386 Park Avenue south, 17th Floor
New York, NY 10016-8804
800-343-3637
212-685-3440

Endnotes

1. L.F. Rettger, et al., Lactobacillus Acidophilus: Its Therapeutic Application, Yale University Press, New Haven: 1935.

2. S. Taussig and S. Batkin, "Bromelain, the enzyme complex of pineapple and its clinical application: An update," Jour Ethno Pharmacol, 1988, 22: 191-203.

3. W.D. Rees, et al., "Treating irritable bowel syndrome with peppermint oil," British Med Jour, 1979, 2(6194): 835-36.

4. Y. Niwa, et al., "Effect of liposomal encapsulated superoxide dimustase on active oxygen-related human disorders," Free Rad Res Commu, 1985, 1: 137-53.

5. M. Skogh, et al., "Vitamin A in Crohn's disease," Lancet, 1980, I: 776.

6. A.D. Harries, et al., "Vitamin D status in Crohn's disease: Association with nutrition and disease activity," Gut, 1985, 26: 1197-1203.

7. S.D. Krasinski, et al., "The prevalence of vitamin K deficiency in gastrointestinal disorders," Amer Jour Clin Nutr, 1985, 41: 639-43.

8. E. Middleton, "The flavonoids," Trends Pharmaceutical Science, 1984, 5: 335-38.

9. J.D. Bennet, "Use of a-tocopharyl-quinone in the treatment of ulcerative colitis," Gut, 1986, 27:695-97.

CORONARY HEART DISEASE

Coronary heart disease (CHD), also known as coronary artery disease or cardiovascular disease, refers to damage or malfunction of the heart that is usually caused by the narrowing or blockage of the coronary arteries resulting in decreased blood supply to the heart. Typically, the presence of angina or the occurrence of a heart attack indicates the presence of heart disease. Coronary heart disease (CHD) is extremely common in Western developed nations and causes more death in the United States than any other disorder.

Coronary heart disease can rightfully be considered a modern day plague. Like so many other diseases, it is directly linked to the way we live and the way we eat. Unfortunately, smoking, drinking and eating a diet high in saturated fats has created a coronary crisis in our country. The only good news about coronary heart disease is that if you start exercising and eat right, you can reverse the progress of this silent killer.

Thirty percent of all deaths in the United States are due to CHD. Most deaths from CHD occur in people over 65, although heart disease can strike middle aged men and women often without warning. The mortality rate from CHD in men between the ages of 35 and 64 has declined by 35 percent from 1968 to 1982. The improvement of surgical techniques and better control of high blood pressure is thought to be responsible for this decrease. Men are more susceptible to CHD than women; however, after menopause, women develop an increased risk for the disease. The incidence of CHD is much lower in underdeveloped countries probably due to their simpler diets. An estimated 50 million Americans suffer from heart disease. A great deal of these people will have no noticeable symptoms of the disorder.

Symptoms

In its early stages CHD may not have any perceivable symptoms. Unfortunately, in many cases the first sign of the disease may be a potentially fatal condition. Angina or periodic chest pain, a heart attack, pain in the left arm, shortness of breath while going up stairs or engaging in other activities, and irregular heartbeat can all be symptoms of the disease depending on its stage of advancement. Congestive heart failure results when the heart becomes fatigued due to artery constriction or mechanical problems. As a result, it cannot handle blood pumping requirements.

When the heart cannot carry its workload, fluid accumulation backs into the lungs, a condition referred to as pulmonary edema. It causes labored breathing, breathlessness, and fatigue, which can occur even after mild exertion. In some cases, congestive heart failure is misdiagnosed as simple pneumonia or asthma. Congestive heart failure should be suspected if the pneumonia or asthma do not respond to drug therapy. Swelling in the ankles and feet can also accompany this condition. Diuretics, vasodilators and in some cases, heart valve surgery are required to reverse this condition. Ideally, heart valve surgery should be done to prevent heart failure rather than to try to reverse it.

Causes

Fatty deposits can form in the arteries and gradually reduce blood flow to heart muscle, resulting in a lack of oxygen. Angina is a warning sign of this condition.

Factors that increase the risk of developing coronary heart disease are smoking (which can make you twice as susceptible as a non-smoker), high blood pressure, diabetes, genetic predisposition, obesity, sedentary lifestyle, taking birth control pills over the age of 35, stress and tension, periods of depression, or a high serum cholesterol level.

There is some speculation that the enzyme xanthine oxidase, found in homogenized dairy products, can cause artery and heart damage. In addition, some heart attacks, due to an arteriole spasm, have been linked with food allergies. A relatively new theory on a possible cause of CHD is that viruses present in the bloodstream may cause injury to blood vessels and can eventually lead to heart disease. Recent studies in Edinburgh, Scotland also linked a variant gene with atherosclerosis. This particular gene controls fibrinogen production.

Conventional Therapies

Drugs typically prescribed for heart disease do not actually treat the diseased heart and cannot replace damaged tissue. All they can do is to help a compromised heart function better, and in that respect they are very valuable to anyone suffering from CHD. Diagnosing CHD may require an angiography, a procedure in which radiopaque dye is injected into the arteries and a X-ray is taken. An echogram may be ordered by your doctor to check for any heart failure that might be in progress. Drugs that improve blood flow to the heart and reduce the workload of the heart include glyceryl trinitrate and other nitrates, beta-blockers, calcium channel blockers and vasodilators. If the heart has a weak pumping action, a vasodilator such as digoxin may be prescribed.

Commonly Prescribed Drugs

DIGITALIS (DIGOXIN, LANOXIN): Increases the force of heart muscle contraction, helping to reverse heart failure. This drug also helps to slow the heart in the case of flutters, fibrillations and tachycardia (when the heart beats too fast).

NITRATES: This class of drugs relaxes the blood vessels, putting less stress on the heart and facilitating better blood flow. Nitrates are commonly prescribed for angina. Nitroglycerine has recently been approved in spray form which can relieve symptoms of angina more readily than sublingual tablets.

CALCIUM CHANNEL BLOCKERS: Also considered blood vessel relaxants which lower blood pressure and, like nitrates help relieve angina. The effects of calcium channel blockers in this respect is longer in its duration than nitrates.

BETA-BLOCKERS: These drugs inhibit the action of adrenaline on the heart, stimulating the heart to beat faster and

work harder. These drugs are also used for angina, arrhythmias and high blood pressure.

LIDOCAINE, PROCAN AND PRONESTYL: These provide an anesthetic like effect on the heart to suppress abnormal heart rhythms.

In some cases, a coronary by-pass will be required to remove a clogged artery. Angioplasty is also an option.

The value of taking an aspirin a day to prevent stroke and heart attack is becoming more controversial and should be discussed with your doctor. Substituting omega-3 fatty acids can achieve similar blood thinning results without the complications of aspirin therapy and should be investigated.

Dietary Guidelines

- ◆ Do not use alcohol, tobacco or caffeine.
- ◆ Eat a diet that is high in fiber, lean meats, fresh fruits and vegetables.
- ◆ Use safflower and olive oil and supplement your diet with essential fatty acids found in primrose, flaxseed and black currant oil.
- ◆ Whole grains are highly recommended. Buckwheat helps to strengthen veins.
- ◆ Try to substantially increase your fiber content substantially.
- ◆ Avoid red meats, hydrogenated fats such as shortening and margarine, animal fats, white sugar products, rich dairy foods, eggs, and empty calorie foods that are high in fat, salt and sugar and low in nutrients.
- ◆ Avoid using salt. It can be hidden in MSG, baking soda, canned vegetables, canned soups, diet soft drinks, meat tenderizers, softened water, certain foods with sugar substitutes and preserved foods.

Recommended Nutritional Supplements

PRIMARY NUTRIENTS

GARLIC AND ONION Both of these extracts have successfully treated both hypertension and high cholesterol, both directly linked to CHD.[1] *Suggested Dosage:* Take 2 to 3 capsules with each meal.

COENZYME Q10 Helps to strengthen and oxygenate heart muscle and contributes to metabolic processes. Studies have conclusively proven its significant benefit in treating both cardiovascular disease and hypertension.[2] *Suggested Dosage:* Take 100 mg daily. For established serious cases of CHD, take 300 to 400 mg daily.

ESSENTIAL FATTY ACIDS Both of these fatty acids are found in fish oils and flaxseed and can contribute to decreased blood pressure and blood lipids. The fact that Eskimo cultures eat diets high in saturated fats but have low cardiovascular disease is attributed to the effect of coldwater fish consumption.[3] *Suggested Dosage:* Take as directed a blend of fish oil or flaxseed oil with oils like Borage or evening primrose. Keep refrigerated. If you use fish oil, take a vitamin E supplement.

VITAMIN E Works to scavenge for free radicals and helps to protect against heart disease and stroke by also reducing LDL cholesterol. Low levels of this vitamin are considered a primary predictor of heart disease.[4] *Suggested Dosage:* If you have a low risk of CHD, take 100 IU per day. If you are at high risk, take 400 to 800 IU per day.

VITAMIN C WITH BIOFLAVONOIDS These compounds act as free radical scavengers in the arteries and heart muscle. They have also been shown to lower blood pressure in clinical tests. Supplementation may actually reduce blood pressure.[5] *Suggested Dosage:* 1,000 to 3,000 mg per day.

CALCIUM This mineral is very important in maintaining or normalizing blood pressure and ensuring proper heart muscle function. Supplementation can actually modify hypertension in some people.[6] *Suggested Dosage:* 1,000 mg per day of the citrate or gluconate variety.

MAGNESIUM The proper balance of minerals like magnesium is vital for regulating blood pressure and for nourishing heart muscle.[7] *Suggested Dosage:* 400 to 800 mg per day. Use chelated products.

SELENIUM Keeping selenium levels high may be linked to lowblood pressure levels. Studies have found a direct correlation and due to the fact that many American diets are selenium deficient, supplementation may be vital.[8] *Suggested Dosage:* Take as directed.

POTASSIUM The ratio of sodium to potassium is considered a profound determiner of blood pressure. Supplementation may be of value.[9] In addition, potassium is considered an electrolyte which helps regulate heart contraction. *Suggested Dosage:* Take only as directed.

NICOTINIC ACID A compound contained in niacin, this substance has the ability to substantially lower blood cholesterol and triglyceride levels.[10] *Suggested Dosage:* Take as directed.

HAWTHORN The proanthocyanidins found in this herb actually inhibit angiotensin-converting enzymes in much the same way as some prescription high blood pressure medications.[11] *Suggested Dosage:* Take as directed. Combining with rosemary can also be helpful.

FIBER SUPPLEMENT Boosting fiber intake can be one of the single most effective treatments of hypertension and can also significantly lower blood cholesterol levels.[12] *Suggested Dosage:* Take first thing in the morning and before going to bed. Use products that can be mixed in liquid.

FOLIC ACID WITH VITAMIN B6 Very recent data suggests that taking more than RDA recommended requirements of these two vitamins can prevent heart disease. *Suggested Dosage:* Take as directed; however, ask your doctor about upping dosages.

POLYUNSATURATED LECITHIN Can help with the proper emulsifying of fats in the blood stream. Animal studies indicate that lecithin facilitates the breakdown and elimination of cholesterol. *Suggested Dosage:* Take as directed.

PHOSPHATDITYL CHOLINE Helps to reduce fat and triglyceride levels in the blood. *Suggested Dosage:* Take as directed.

HERBAL COMBINATION This combination should include hawthorn berries, motherwort, rosemary leaves, cayenne, kelp, wood betony and shepherd's purse. *Suggested Dosage:* Four to six capsules daily.

HAWTHORN BERRY: Next to digitalis, hawthorn is probably the most recognized herb for positively affecting the heart. As demonstrated by scientific studies, hawthorn supports metabolic processes in the heart, dilates coronary vessels, reduces peripheral resistance, lowers blood pressure, reduces tendency for angina attacks and strengthens damaged or weakened heart muscles.[13] MOTHERWORT: The use of motherwort as a cardiotonic spans centuries. Motherwort is especially beneficial in cases of nervous heart conditions that can cause, among other things, palpitation or abnormally rapid or fluttering heart beats.[14] ROSEMARY: A powerful antioxidant herb that supports the integrity of the veins. Rosemary has also exhibited cardiotonic capacity which helps with normal heart function. It also causes mild perspiration, releasing toxins from the body and improving health.[15] CAYENNE: Cayenne supports and improves circulation. Cayenne is considered an herb activator that increases the effectiveness of other herbs. It stimulates digestion and promotes perspiration. Cayenne has been shown to reduce blood pressure, especially in conjunction with garlic. KELP: Kelp is a powerhouse of micronutrients that assist with various metabolic processes. Kelp has been considered a blood vessel cleanser and a treatment for atherosclerosis.[16] WOOD BETONY: Wood betony is carminative, diuretic, and nervine. These three actions support a healthy cardiovascular system. SHEPHERD'S PURSE: Shepherd's purse is a common weed that grows all over the United States. It is a diuretic and has an ability to regulate blood pressure and heart action.

SECONDARY NUTRIENTS

L-CARNITINE: Helps to sustain cardiac muscle and is involved in caloric conversion of macronutrients to muscle. A deficiency of carnitine has been linked with heart disease. *Suggested Dosage:* Take as directed on an empty stomach with fruit juice.

GINKGO: This herb works to boost circulation and can help protect heart muscle by enhancing oxygenation. *Suggested Dosage:* Take as directed using standardized products.

POTASSIUM: Potassium helps to keep heart muscle in proper contraction and rhythm. A lack of potassium can cause abnormal heartbeats. *Suggested Dosage:* Take with your doctor's approval as directed.

VITAMIN B-COMPLEX: These vitamins are necessary for healthy heart function. *Suggested Dosage:* Take as directed.

Home Care Suggestions

+ After receiving proper medical attention, the best thing you can do for yourself is to restructure your lifestyle and eating habits. While it may seem discouraging at first, thousands of people have successfully done it and have received a new lease on life. Regular exercise (that has been approved by your doctor, of course) along with a diet that is outlined in the nutritional section of this chapter can literally work miracles.
+ Learn to relax and enjoy life. Open your mind to relaxation techniques such as biofeedback, yoga, meditation etc. These can really help to relax the entire body and counteract the bad effects of stress.
+ Join others in exercising. Walk the malls or buy a treadmill.
+ Purchase the latest cookbooks with wonderful low-fat recipes and learn to read ingredient labels in the grocery store. There are more and more low-fat products available and some of them even taste good. Learn to cook with olive oil.

Other Supportive Therapies

ACUPUNCTURE: Helps to boost circulation and prompt relaxation.

HOMEOPATHY: Arnica and kali mur 6x are used for heart conditions.

MASSAGE THERAPY: Massage helps to loosen tense muscles and alleviate stress.

Scientific Facts-at-a-Glance

Drinking alcohol can have a very devastating effect on the heart in a number of ways. First, alcohol directly injures heart muscle. Moreover, it contributes to a number of nutritional deficiencies that also damage the heart. In addition, many of us are completely unaware that most alcoholic beverages also contain toxic metabolites or metals like cobalt that contribute to heart disease.[17]

Spirit/Mind Therapies

Anytime we are dealing with cardiovascular disease, the mind/body connection must be addressed. Years of data tells us that if you are a person who internalizes stress, you may be at a much higher risk for developing CHD. Moreover, if you are stressed out and smoke, your cardiovascular system can rapidly age and deteriorate before its time. Stress causes adrenal hormones that, when combined with nicotine and alcohol, dramatically raise cholesterol levels and predispose the human body to all kinds of disease. All of us need to pay attention to managing stress constructively rather than destructively. Those of us who fit the Type A personality profile need to be particularly aware of how we construe stress and what we do with it.

Prevention

+ Do not consume caffeine and alcohol.
+ Reduce your serum cholesterol levels if too high by eating a high-fiber, low-fat diet that avoids rich dairy foods, animal fats, saturated fats such as shortening, high-sugar foods, and red meats.
+ Emphasize fresh fruits and vegetables, garlic and onions, almonds, broiled fish, tuna, pink salmon, white skinless turkey and chicken meat, whole grains such as whole wheat or oat bran, olive oil and safflower oil.
+ Do not smoke: It cuts your chances of developing heart disease by half.
+ Exercise regularly. Walking for twenty minutes five times a week is considered excellent aerobic exercise and promotes a stronger and healthier heart.
+ Check your pulse first thing in the morning before getting out of bed. If your pulse rate is 60 or below and is strong and steady you can assume that your heart is functioning efficiently. If the rate is above 80, you may need to change your diet and incorporate a good aerobic exercise plan into your life. Use this pulse check to keep tabs on your cardiovascular health.
+ Keep your weight at an optimum level.
+ Take daily supplements of omega-3 oils, vitamins C and E, calcium citrate and magnesium
+ Get stress levels in your life under control. Stress causes adrenalin surges in the body which can strain the heart. In addition, there is evidence to suggest that prolonged stress can raise cholesterol levels and contribute to the development of coronary heart disease.

Doctor's Notes

Today, we know that deficiencies in vitamin E, the B vitamins and folic acid can all be linked with an increase of coronary artery disease. Dr. Dean Ornish points out that even if you have coronary artery disease, if you change your eating habits and limit saturated fat intake to less than 10 percent of your total caloric consumption, you can reverse the disease process. The addition of mild meditative exercises such as walking on the beach can also significantly reduce symptoms of CHD.

One of the very best herbs available for treating heart conditions is hawthorn berry. It has the ability to help dilate coronary arteries and improve the metabolic function of heart muscle. After you have taken this herb for four to six weeks you will probably notice that your need for nitroglycerine pills decreases. Why? Because blood flow to the heart has been improved, and the efficiency of the heart muscle is increasing. Motherwort and coenzyme Q10 help to enhance these same functions. The average heart beats over 100,000 times a day and about 38 million times per year. To illustrate, this remarkable organ raises the equivalent of one ton to a height of 41 feet every 24 hours. Fortunately there are many herbs that support the function of the heart.

The highly effective heart medicine "digitalis" is actually a derivative of a botanical commonly known as fox glove, or

Digitalis purpurea. While the herb is associated with a narrow safety margin and not found in this formula, the other botanicals described are quite safe and effective. The above nutrient and herbal formula can strengthen a weak heart, restore proper heart rhythm, reduce blood pressure and prevent angina.

Additional Resources

American Heart Association
7272 Greenville Avenue
Dallas, TX 75231
(214) 373-6300

Endnotes

1. D. Louria, et al., "Onion extract in treatment of hypertension and hyperlipidemia: A preliminary communication," Curr Ther Res, 1985, 37(1):127-31.

2. T. Yamagami, et al., "Bioenergetics in clinical medicine: Studies on coenzyme Q-10 and essential hypertension," Res Commun Chem Pathol Pharmacol, 1975, 11:273.

3. P. Singer, "Blood pressure-lowering effect of w-3 polyunsaturated fatty acids in clinical studies," in A.P. Simopoulos et al., eds. "Health effects of w-3 polyunsaturated fatty acids in seafoods," World Rev Nutr Diet, 1991, 66:329-48.

4. K.F. Gey, et al., "Inverse correlation between plasma vitamin E and mortality from ischemic heart disease in cross-cultural epidemiology," Amer Jour Clin Nutri, 1991, 53: 326S-334S.

5. O. Osilesi. et al., "Blood pressure and plasma lipids during ascorbic acid supplementation in borderline hypertensive and normotensive adults," Nutr Res, 1991, 11:405-12.

6. D. McCarron, et al., "Dietary calcium and blood pressure: Modifying factors in specific populations. Am J Clin Nutr, 1991, 54:215S-19S.

7. T. Moore, "The role of dietary electrolytes in hypertension," J Am Coll Nutr, 1989, 8: Suppl S:68S-80S.

8. J. Salonen, et al., "Blood pressure, dietary fats, and antioxidants," Am Jour Clin Nutr, 1988, 48:1226-32.

9. A. Sianin, et al., "Controlled trial of long term oral potassium supplements in patients with mild hypertension," Bri Med Jour, 1987, 294:1453-56.

10. J.R. DiPalma and W.S. Thayer, "The use of niacin as a drug," Ann Rev Nutr, 1991, 11: 169-87.

11. S. Uchida, et al., "Inhibitory effects of condensed tannins on angiotensin converting enzyme," Jap Jour Pharmacol, 1987. 43:242-5.

12. P. Little, et al., "A controlled trial of a low sodium, low fat, high fiber diet in treated hypertensive patients: the efficacy of multiple dietary intervention," Postgraduate Medical Journal, 1990, 66(778): 616-21. F.L. Shinnick, et al., "Dose response to a dietary oat bran fraction in cholesterol-fed rats," Jour Nutri. 1990, 120(6): 561-68.

13. R. Blesken, "Crataegus in cardiology," Fortsc Med, 1992, 110(15): 290-92.

14. F. Arustamova, " Hypotensive effect of leonarus cardiaca on animals in experimental chronic hypertension," Uzvestuta Akad Nauk Arm SSR Biol Nauki, 1963, 16(7): 47-52.

15. A. Boido, et al., "N-substituted derivatives of rosmaricine," Stu Sass Sez 2, 1975, 53(5-6): 383-93.

16. P. Searle, et al., "Study of a cardiotonic fraction from an extract of the seaweed undaria pinnatifida," Procee West Pharmacol Soc, 1981, 24: 63-65.

17. G. Burch and T. Giles, "Alcoholic cardiomyopathy" in B Kissin, The Biology of Alcoholism, vol.3, (Plenum Press, New York: 1974).

CROHN'S DISEASE

SEE "COLITIS"

CYSTS, BREAST

SEE "FIBROCYSTIC BREAST DISEASE"

DERMATITIS

SEE "ECZEMA"

DIARRHEA

All of us have experienced the misery of diarrhea, a common malady characterized by the increased frequency, or fluidity of bowel movements. Diarrhea is not considered a disorder in itself, but is, rather, a symptom of another physiological or emotional problem. Diarrhea usually resolves itself within a couple of days without treatment. Chronic diarrhea may indicate the presence of a serious intestinal condition. Diarrhea in babies, small children and the elderly is more serious than in adults due to the risk of dehydration.

Symptoms

Adult diarrhea is characterized by runny stools, cramping, gas, nausea, weakness, cold sweats, increased frequency of bowel movements, thirst, abdominal pain, vomiting and fever (some cases).

The unusual loss of fluids through the bowel can lead to dehydration where electrolytes (minerals) are lost.

Precautions

See your physician immediately if there is blood in the stools, the stool appears unusually dark (some medications which contain bismuth subsalicylate such as pepto-bismol, or iron may turn the stool black), if there is severe abdominal or rectal pain, if urination has stopped or if you have a fever above 101° F. If the diarrhea lasts for more than two days, a serious ailment may exist. Consult your physician immediately.

If you suspect that an infant may be dehydrated, look for symptoms like glazed eyes, sunken eyes, unresponsiveness, a dry tongue, depressed fontanelle at the upper front part of the head, loose skin or drowsiness. Any infantile diarrhea that does not stop within 48 hours should be investigated by a doctor.

Causes

Diarrhea occurs when too much water is passed along with the stool during a bowel movement due to decreased absorption of the intestinal tract walls. The most common causes of diarrhea include eating contaminated food, drinking impure water, food poisoning (usually indicates the presence of *Staphylococcus* or *Clostridium* bacteria in the food), *Salmonella* or *Campylobacter* bacteria (occurs 12 to 48 hours after eating), Norwalk virus, gastroenteritis, food allergies, typhoid, drug toxicity, amoebic dysentery, shigellosis, giardia or a lack of hydrochloric acid in the stomach.

Chronic diarrhea, which commonly occurs as random attacks of loose stools, can be brought on by Crohn's disease, colitis, diverticulosis, colon cancer, irritable bowel syndrome, emotional anxiety, incomplete digestion of certain foods, overuse of laxatives, antacids, intolerance to caffeine, excessive consumption of fruit or of green fruit or rancid foods, and parasites.

Infant diarrhea commonly results from viral infections. Breast-fed babies are less likely to contract these infections. A lactose intolerance may also cause infant diarrhea.

Conventional Therapies

Water and minerals lost during severe diarrhea need to be replenished immediately. Your doctor may suggest a product such as Pedialyte, Resol, or Lytren for infants and small children. For adults, electrolyte mixtures such as Gatorade may be recommended. Antidiarrheal drugs may be required, but they should not be taken to treat diarrhea that results from infection. If the diarrhea persists, your physician may require a stool culture, a barium x-ray, sigmoidoscopy or biopsy of the rectum. Your physician may recommend over-the-counter remedies such as Immodium which causes the bowel to tighten up. Other products such as Pepto-Bismol, and Kaopectate may be effective if the diarrhea is not too severe.

Dyphenoxylate may be used by your physician if symptoms are more persistent. Narcotic preparations such as paregoric, parepectolin or parelixir may be prescribed for adults. Lomotil, a narcotic-like preparation may also decrease the frequency of bowel movements in adults. If dehydration is severe enough, intravenous fluids may be administered either at the doctor's office or in the hospital. The availability of intravenous fluid administration can prevent dehydration and diarrhea in small children and infants, a condition that used to be fatal in the early 1900s.

Dietary Guidelines

◆ Drinking rice water until the diarrhea subsides is always good.
◆ Foods like rice cereal, bananas, applesauce, mashed cooked carrots, active culture yogurt, plain dry crackers, and steamed chicken without the skin are ideal for those suffering from diarrhea.
◆ Carrot soup is an old remedy especially good for children.
◆ Avoid all dairy products, pulpy citrus juices and limit intake of fats and wheat.
◆ Do not consume alcohol, caffeine and artificial sweeteners.
◆ A clear diet which consists of broths, apple juice, Jello, etc., is recommended to give the bowel a rest.
◆ Avoid carbonated beverages or make them go flat by shaking them.
◆ Drink plenty of fluids. Use popsicles, iced fruit bars or flat sodas to encourage children to increase their fluid intake.

Recommended Nutritional Supplements

PRIMARY NUTRIENTS

ACIDOPHILUS Frequently, diarrhea is caused by a lack of friendly bacteria in the bowel. Taking antibiotics or eating poor diets can result in a predominance of bad bacteria which can cause flatulence and other lower bowel problems.[1] *Suggested Dosage:* Take as directed on an empty stomach in the morning using liquid or tablet varieties with guaranteed bacterial count, and bifidobacteria. Check expiration date.

FOLIC ACID Studies have found that this nutrient can help to control infant diarrhea.[2] It is also part of the B-vitamin array which helps to prompt good intestinal absorption of nutrients. *Suggested Dosage:* 50 mg per day.

VITAMIN A If your child has chronic diarrhea, it may indicate a vitamin A deficiency.[3] *Suggested Dosage:* Take as directed according to instructions for the child's age and weight. If you are an adult, take 10,000 IU per day. Pregnant women should not take over 10,000 IU per day.

VITAMIN C WITH BIOFLAVONOIDS Continual diarrhea can deplete body stores of ascorbic acid and may result in low plasma levels.[4] Vitamin C and bioflavonoids also help to promote tissue healing in the intestines. *Suggested Dosage:* You may want to use mild doses to begin with and remember that excessive consumption of vitamin C can cause diarrhea. Take 500 mg twice a day with meals using a buffered or esterized product.

ZINC Clinical tests showed that taking zinc can help to prevent the type of malnutrition that can result with uncontrolled diarrhea.[5] It also contributes to mucus membrane repair and fortifies immune function if an infection is present. *Suggested Dosage:* 50 mg per day. Use picolinate or gluconate products. Lozenges can be used. Do not take more than 100 mg of zinc per day.

OMEGA-6 FATTY ACIDS These compounds can actually help to bind the type of pathogenic bacteria that are sometimes responsible for diarrhea.[6] Essential fatty acids also help to form stool. *Suggested Dosage:* Take as directed using a variety of oils.

DIGESTIVE ENZYMES Boosting the ability to break down the food components we ingest can be of great value in controlling diarrhea caused by faulty digestion or even stress. *Suggested Dosage:* Take as directed 30 minutes before eating.

GUAR GUM, PECTIN AND PSYLLIUM Helps in forming stool and works to clean out residue trapped in the bowel, which may cause diarrhea due to continual irritation and putrefaction. Fiber also helps restore normal flora in the intestines which is vital to proper stool formation and elimination.[7] *Suggested Dosage:* Take as directed using powdered products that are mixed with pure water or juice just before going to bed on an empty stomach. High-fiber products can sometimes aggravate diarrhea and gas. Adjust your dosage until your system becomes used to these bulking agents, and then continue to take them indefinitely.

GARLIC Can help kill any bacterial or viral infection that may be causing diarrhea. Also fights parasitic infestation and boosts immunity[8]. *Suggested Dosage:* Take two capsules with each of three meals using enteric-coated products that do not dissolve until they reach the large intestine.

SLIPPERY ELM The high mucilage content of this herb soothes the irritated mucus membranes of the bowel and decreases transit time while absorbing intestinal toxins.[9] *Suggested Dosage:* Take as directed. This herb may be taken by capsule or mixed into mashed bananas or applesauce for children.

PEPPERMINT OIL Soothes the lower bowel and helps to control gas and bloating associated with diarrhea by relaxing bowel spasms.[10] *Suggested Dosage:* Take as directed. Enteric coating is vital so the oil is not released in the stomach.

TUMERIC AND ARTICHOKE These herbs help to stimulate bile flow which facilitates better lipid digestion. Compounds in turmeric can inhibit gas and calm colonic spasms.[11] Anyone who has gallbladder trouble or has had their gallbladder removed should take these herbs. *Suggested Dosage:* Take as directed, just prior to eating.

HERBAL COMBINATION This combination should include goldenseal, papaya leaves, fenugreek seeds, gentian root, Irish moss, myrrh gum and ginger root. *Suggested Dosage:* Take as directed.

GOLDENSEAL: This herb contains berberine which helps to control acute diarrhea brought on by intestinal bacterial infections. In addition to its direct antimicrobial activity, it can inhibit the metabolic function of infective organisms and the toxins they form in the bowel.[12] PAPAYA LEAVES: Both papaya fruit and leaves are a source of papain which is a mixture of protein-digesting enzymes. Studies have found that it can enhance the digestion of wheat gluten and inhibit its inflammatory response in the colon in people with celiac disease or chronic diarrhea.[13] GENTIAN

ROOT: Gentian enjoys widespread use particularly in Europe as a digestive aid. It increases saliva and is believed to increase secretion of gastric juices.[14] Some herbalists have used it to expel intestinal worms. Its anti-inflammatory effects are helpful with gastrointestinal disorders like diarrhea. MYRRH GUM: Myrrh gum is used to heal the gastric mucosa of the intestinal tract. Myrrh gum is carminative, reduces gas and bloating, and calms the stomach.[15] IRISH MOSS: Irish moss is rich in trace mineral nutrients. It also contains large amounts of mucilage which soothes the gastrointestinal tract.[16] It is specifically used for dyspepsia, nausea, heartburn and diarrhea. FENUGREEK SEEDS: As much as 40 percent of the weight of fenugreek seeds is mucilage. Mucilage is a gelatin-like substance usually made up of proteins and polysaccharides which heals irritated intestinal tract lining and helps to hold water. It also boosts digestion by prompting pancreatic secretion.[17] GINGER ROOT: Ginger is one of the best herbs for the treatment of digestive disorders. Ginger prevents nausea, gas, bloating and vomiting. Ginger root helps to tonify the intestinal muscle and provides a source of proteolytic enzymes to aid digestion.[18]

SECONDARY NUTRIENTS

POTASSIUM: Potassium is lost in watery stools and needs to be replaced. Calcium, magnesium and zinc should also be replenished. *Suggested Dosage:* Take only as directed. Electrolyte drinks can be a good source of potassium during episodes of diarrhea.

CAROB POWDER: Helps to normalize the bowels and control diarrhea. *Suggested Dosage:* Take as directed. Carob can be mixed with juices or put into applesauce, etc.

VITAMIN E: Promotes healing of damaged tissued and protects the membranes of the bowel lining. *Suggested Dosage:* 400 to 800 IU per day.

ECHINACEA: Helps to control diarrhea that is caused by an infectious organism by boosting immune response. *Suggested Dosage:* Take as directed. Do not use for more than two weeks at a time. Look for guaranteed potency or standardized products.

Home Care Suggestions

- If an electrolyte fluid is not available, sugar and salt can be added to water. (One teaspoon of sugar and a pinch of salt to one quart of water). Measure the salt accurately. An excess of salt can cause additional dehydration.
- Adding a teaspoon of sugar to juice or water enables the intestines to absorb more of the water content.
- Another good fluid replacement can be made from mixing one teaspoon of honey and a pinch of salt in 8 ounces of a clear fruit juice.
- Over-the-counter drugs such as antacids, antibiotics and quinidine can cause diarrhea. In addition, some nonsteroidal, anti-inflammatory drugs (such as Meclomen), some blood pressure medications, gold compounds and digitalis may also cause diarrhea. If you are undergoing cancer treatment, diarrhea can be a common side effect. Check with your physician to see if anything you might be taking could be the cause.

Other Supportive Therapies

HOMEOPATHY: Arsenicum alb. 6C and Pulsatilla 6C are traditional homeopathic medicines for diarrhea.

MASSAGE: Massage can help to dispel and alleviate stress-related diarrhea.

ACUPUNCTURE: Working the body on this level can also facilitate better relaxation in cases of emotionally-caused diarrhea.

MEDITATION: Learning to meditate can be an invaluable way to de-stress even when on the job.

Scientific Facts-at-a-Glance

The possibility of a hydrochloric acid deficiency should be ruled out in cases of unexplained diarrhea. Apparently, many people are prone to this little-known disorder which can cause all kinds of gastrointestinal problems that are often misdiagnosed as colitis, Crohn's disease, etc. One study published in *JAMA* in 1902 found that cases of unexplained chronic diarrhea were completely relieved when hydrochloric acid supplements were given. Although its scientific findings may be a bit dusty, it's suggestions are certainly worth reviewing.[19] Milk allergies can also be an overlooked cause of chronic diarrhea and interestingly, artificial sweeteners like mannitol and sorbitol can produce diarrhea in some people.[20]

Spirit/Mind Considerations

Nervous diarrhea is brought on during periods of high emotional stress. Psychological counseling centered on biofeedback, meditation, or relaxation techniques may help to control this type of diarrhea. As is the case with any stress-related disorder, the management of stress is crucial. If you have a sensitive colon, you may be prone to bouts of this type of diarrhea. The first thing to do is to recognize the fact that your diarrhea is stress related.

Prevention

To Prevent Infant Diarrhea

- Breast-feed instead of bottle feed your baby.
- Do not introduce dairy products, citrus fruits or wheat into you baby's diet too early.
- Wash your hands with soap and water after each diaper change.
- Try not to overuse antibiotics as these can cause chronic diarrhea.

To Prevent Adult Diarrhea

- When traveling, drink only bottled or canned beverages. Don't use ice unless you make it yourself from bottled water.
- Stay away from raw food. Cook all foods thoroughly and peel all local fruits.
- Don't drink out of any mountain stream or natural water supply no matter how clean it looks. Most of the time, when water from a pure source (like a mountain stream) looks clean, it is loaded with bacteria.
- Use good hygiene when preparing food. Wash hands frequently, keep dishes, glasses and silverware well-cleaned. Disinfect areas where bacteria can grow.
- Avoid using wood cutting boards which can harbor bacteria.
- Refrigerate foods immediately after eating. Don't let leftovers sit out, especially foods containing dairy products.
- Make sure that hamburger, poultry and pork are cooked all the way through.
- Do not let other foods such as salad greens become contaminated by coming in contact with raw poultry, pork, etc.
- Eating dill has long been accepted in folk medicine as a way to prevent diarrhea. It is believed to kill intestinal bacteria that cause diarrhea.

Doctor's Notes

Diarrhea can be caused by numerous things. Drinking nothing but rice water until it is controlled can be helpful. Boil rice in two to three times as much water. When the rice is cooked, drain the water and keep it. Add some flavoring to the water and drink as much as you can throughout the day. When the flu is involved, eating fat or protein will only serve to aggravate diarrhea and should be avoided. When you do begin to add back these foods, make sure to take a good digestive enzyme product to boost the breakdown of these macronutrients. In addition, using herbs which increase bile acid flow such as tumeric or artichoke help to break down fats, which makes it easier to avoid another bout with diarrhea. I have found that some people seem to suffer with chronic diarrhea after having their gallbladders removed. Using the appropriate herbs and enzymes we've mentioned has successfully controlled their diarrhea. Remember, it is crucial to find out what is causing your diarrhea in order to treat it effectively. Infectious agents such as amoebas and parasites must be diagnosed before treatment can begin.

Endnotes

1. See "Lactobacilli as dietary supplements and manifestations of their functions in the intestines," in B. Hallgren, Ed. Nutrition and the Intestinal Flora, (Stockholm, Almqvist and Wiksell International, 1983), 93-98.
2. I.E. Haffejee, "Effect of oral folate on duration of acute infantile diarrhea," Letter, Lancet, 1988, 2:334-35.
3. N. Usha, et al., "Early detection of vitamin A deficiency in children with persistent diarrhea," Letter. Lancet, 1990,1:422.
4. F.H. Gardner, "Nutritional management of chronic diarrhea in adults," JAMA, 1962, 180:147-52.
5. R.H. Behrens, et al., "Zinc supplementation during diarrhoea, a fortification against malnutrition?" Letter, Lancet, 1990, 336:442-423.
6. H.Chart H, B.Siad and B. Rowe, "Linoleic acid adhesion of enteropathogenic Escherichia coli to hep-2 cells," Letter, Lancet, 1991, 338:126-7.
7. David Kritchevsky, and Charles Bonfield, Dietary Fiber in Health and Disease, (Eagan Press, St. Paul, Minnesota: 1995).

8. H. Barowski, and L Boyd, "The use of garlic (allistan) in gastrointestinal disturbances," Rev Gastroenterol, 1944, 11: 22-26.

9. Mark Pederson, Nutritional Herbology, (Wendell Whitman Co., Warsaw, Indiana: 1987): 160.

10. R. Leicester and R. Hunt, "Peppermint oil to reduce colonic spasm during endoscopy," Lancet, 1982, II: 989.

11. H. Ammon and M. Wahl, Pharmacology of Curcuma longa, Planta Medica, 1991, 57: 1-7.

12. Y.H. Tai, et al., "Antisecretory effects of berberine in rat ileum," Amer Jour. Physiol, 1981, 241: G253-8.

13. M. Messer, C.M. Anderson and L. Hubbard, "Studies on the mechanism of destruction of the toxic action of wheat gluten in celiac disease by crude papain," Gut, 1964, 5: 295-303.

14. H. Glatzel and K. Hackenberg, "Roentgenological studies of the effect of bitters on digestive organs," Planta Medica, 1967, 15(3): 223-32.

15. F. Ellingwood, American Materia Medica, Therapeutics and Pharmacognosy, (Eclectic Medical Publication, Portland, Oregon: 1983).

16. W. Szturma, "Method for treating gastro-intestinal ulcers with extract of herb cetaria," US Patent 4150123, issued April 17, 1979.

17. G. Ribes, et al., "Effect of fenugreek seeds on endocrine pancreatic secretions in dogs," Annals of Nutrition and Metabolism, 1984, 28: 37-43.

18. E.H. Thompson, et al., "Ginger rhizome: A new source of proteolytic enzyme," Journal of Food Science, 1973, 38(4): 652-55.

19. Bulletin Gen di Therapeutique, Paris, abstracted in JAMA, 1902, 39:55.

20. E. Rubenstein and D. Federman, Scientific American Medicine, New York: 1988.

DIVERTICULITIS

Diverticulitis occurs when small grape-like sacs found along the wall of the colon become inflamed. The development of these sacs is referred to as diverticulosis and can occur without any perceivable symptoms. More than half of people over the age of 60 suffer from diverticulosis. These sacs may occur anywhere along the intestinal tract, but they usually form toward the end of the large intestine. Chronic constipation can cause the formation of these pouches due to added strain on the colon. Divertitculitis results when these sacs become inflamed from extra intestinal matter present in the colon. These sac-like swellings can harbor bacteria and infection, causing various symptoms of intestinal distress. Of those who have diverticulosis only about 10 percent will develop diverticulitis. Severe diverticulitis can cause a perforation in the intestinal wall, which may lead to an abscess or peritonitis.

Symptoms

Divertuculitis is characterized by cramping pains, tenderness in the left side of the abdomen, rigidity in the abdomen, severe abdominal pain, nausea, constipation, fever, and passage of blood in the stool due to diverticula that have bled.

See your doctor immediately if you have severe pain in the lower left area of the abdomen in tandem with a fever. The symptoms of diverticulitis can mimic those of appendicitis; however, pain in diverticulitis is usually centered on the left side of the lower abdomen.

Causes

Some studies indicate that diverticulitis is linked to the Western dietary habits, which are usually low in fiber and high in processed, fatty foods. Interestingly, diverticulitis is rarely found in Asia and Africa, where fiber consumption is much more routine.

Constipation, which results from lack of roughage in the diet, can cause the formation of the diverticula. The colon can be weakened when you have to force feces out of your system. Stress has also been linked to the disease. A family history of diverticulitis, gallbladder disease, obesity and coronary heart disease could increase the probability of developing the disorder.

Conventional Therapies

Like other colon-based diseases, by the time a doctor deals with the problem, the damage has been done. Therefore, preventative medicine is a much better approach in the case of disorders like diverticulitis.

Once diverticulitis occurs, however, treatment is centered on fighting the infection with antibiotics and preventing more serious complications. Your physician will check for abdomen rigidity and for any lumps which could indicate the presence of an abscess. Bed rest and antibiotics are routinely prescribed to clear up any infection contained within the diverticula. If the symptoms are especially severe, your doctor may suggest a liquid diet or intravenous fluids. Five percent of diverticulitis cases require surgery, especially if any perforation occurs in the intestinal wall. In rare cases, a tight stricture can form around the areas of infection and must be surgically removed.

Dietary Guidelines

- ◆ Avoid seedy foods, nuts, and dairy products.
- ◆ Red meats, sugar products, fried foods, and spicy foods should not be consumed.
- ◆ Eat raw vegetables until the inflammation subsides. Steamed vegetables can even be blended before eating if symptoms are severe.
- ◆ Emphasize a low-carbohydrate, low-fat diet high in vegetables and fish until the inflammation is under control. Then increase complex carbohydrates and fiber.
- ◆ Take fiber and acidophilus right after getting up in the morning to help establish regular morning bowel movements.
- ◆ Fiber supplementation couples with drinking plenty of pure water is the key to controlling diverticulitis.
- ◆ Carrot and cabbage juice have beneficial anti-inflammatory properties.

Recommended Nutritional Supplements

PRIMARY NUTRIENTS

ACIDOPHILUS Helps to replenish friendly bacteria in the bowel and works to control gas and bloating. Studies have found that symptoms associated with diverticulitis and irritable bowel syndrome were relieved when lactobacillus was administered.[1] *Suggested Dosage:* Take as directed using milk-free, guaranteed bacterial count products with bifidobacteria. Check for expiration date. Take on an empty stomach.

DIGESTIVE OR PROTEOLYTIC ENZYMES These compounds help to more throughly digest food, help to avoid the retention of undigested protein particles which can initiate food allergies and ease inflammation. Bromelain, which comes from pineapple has demonstrated some remarkable anti-inflammatory properties.[2] *Suggested Dosage:* Take as directed on an empty stomach 30 minutes before meals and before going to bed. Enteric-coated bromelain and other enzymes may be preferable for bowel treatment.

PEPPERMINT OIL Clinical studies have found that enteric-coated capsules relax gastrointestinal smooth muscle and can help to significantly reduce the symptoms of bowel inflammation.[3] *Suggested Dosage:* Take two capsules 30 minutes before each of three meals per day.

SUPEROXIDE DIMUSTASE (SOD) Liposomal SOD which is considered an effective free radical scavenger and antioxidant has been used to successfully treat people with Crohn's disease. It helps to neutralize the damaging effects excessive inflammatory reactions in the bowel.[4] *Suggested Dosage:* Take as directed using liposomal forms only. Other types may not be effective when ingested.

VITAMIN A Works to heal the mucus membranes of the bowel. In addition, a deficiency of vitamin A, E and K have been noted in a good percentage of people with colon disorders. This vitamin is important to proper metabolism of the intestinal mucosa. Clinical trails have found that vitamin A supplementation may help treat Crohn's disease.[5] *Suggested Dosage:* 25,000 IU daily. Caution: If you are pregnant, do not take over 10,000 IU.

VITAMIN D A vitamin D deficiency is also common in people that suffer from chronic colon disorders and should be supplemented.[6] A deficiency in this vitamin can lead to calcium loss from the bones. *Suggested Dosage:* Take as directed.

VITAMIN K Like vitamin D, people who suffer with chronic bowel irritation are very prone to developing vitamin K deficiencies.[7] This vitamin is vital for proper blood clotting. Eighteen patients with colon diseases received vitamin K supplements were found to improve. *Suggested Dosage:* Blue-green algae or liquid fat-soluble chlorophyll preparations are an excellent source of vitamin K. Take as directed.

VITAMIN C WITH BIOFLAVONOIDS Bioflavonoid compounds help to inhibit the inflammatory response in the bowel.[8] *Suggested Dosage:* 6,000 mg divided with each of three meals.

VITAMIN E Promotes tissue healing of the bowel lining and acts to scavenge free radicals which can be produced by tissue trauma. Some studies have shown dramatic improvement with vitamin E therapy for ulcerative colitis.[9] *Suggested Dosage:* 400 to 800 IU daily.

ESSENTIAL FATTY ACIDS Both the omega-3 and omega-6 acids are useful. Fish, evening primrose or flaxseed oil can provide these essential fatty acids which the body may be lacking when colon irritation is present. Studies using fish oil have found that its EPA and DHA content resulted in a 65 percent drop in inflammatory compounds found in the intestines and an 80 percent decrease in the number of cellular mutations found in diseased colons.[10]

OMEGA-3 OILS These oils found in certain fish and plants help to normalize prostaglandin activity which is impaired in many people prone to colon problems.[11] *Suggested Dosage:* Take as directed. If you are using fish oil, take with a vitamin E supplement.

FOLIC ACID Supplementing folate can help to reduce the diarrhea associated with this disease. A folic acid deficiency is common in people with colon disease.[12] *Suggested Dosage:* Take as directed.

MAGNESIUM, ZINC, VITAMIN A, VITAMIN E Magnesium deficiency is very prevalent with people who have inflammatory bowel disorders.[13] A zinc deficiency has been found in almost half of all people suffering from Crohn's disease.[14] *Suggested Dosage:* Take as directed. Use chelated zinc products and take with meals.

PSYLLIUM SEEED Supplements which contain psyllium or water soluble fiber have proven themselves invaluable for people with chronic recurrent diarrhea, pain and constipation. This seed helps to speed transit time and relieves both constipation and diarrhea. In addition, it helps to normalize colonic bacteria which are so crucial to bowel health.[15] *Suggested Dosage:* Take as directed before retiring to bed. Make sure to drink extra water all through the day when taking a fiber supplement.

HERBAL COMBINATION This combination should include goldenseal root, licorice root, papaya leaves, gentian root, myrrh gum, Irish moss, fenugreek seeds, ginger root, aloe vera gel, and a combination of valerian root and kava. Nausea and flatulence are common gastrointestinal tract problems with diverticulitis. This formula contains herbs that will treat the most common of these disorders and help treat the symptoms of some gastrointestinal tract disorders that are genetically inherited. *Suggested Dosage:* Two to four capsules daily.

GOLDENSEAL ROOT: Goldenseal has been used to restore the mucus lining of the gastrointestinal tract and keep it from being easily disrupted by strengthening the cross-linking of proteins in the mucus. Goldenseal promotes bile secretion, restores proper bowel transit time and removes excess water from the body. Its berberine content is effective in treating the majority of gastrointestinal infections which may be at the root of diverticulitis.[16] LICORICE ROOT: Licorice has been recognized for its anti-inflammatory activity which can help in cases of gastritis and inflammatory bowel disease. It can inhibit the formation of inflammatory prostaglandins which promote bowel inflammation.[17] Licorice has a diuretic and mild laxative effect that cleanses toxins from the body. The licorice in this formula is true licorice, which is not used in most licorice candies in the United States. PAPAYA LEAVES: Both papaya fruit and leaves are a source of papain which is a mixture of protein-digesting enzymes. Studies have found that it can enhance the digestion of wheat gluten and inhibit its inflammatory response in the colon in people with celiac disease.[18] GENTIAN ROOT: Gentian enjoys widespread use in Europe as a digestive aid. It increases saliva and is believed to increase secretion of gastric juices.[19] Some herbalists have used it to expel intestinal worms. Its anti-inflammatory effects are helpful with gastritis and IBD. It is considered a bitter tonic. MYRRH GUM: Myrrh gum is used to heal the gastric mucosa of the intestinal tract. Myrrh gum is carminative, reduces gas and bloating, and calms the stomach. It also is a mild laxative.[20] IRISH MOSS: Irish moss is rich in trace mineral nutrients. It also contains large amounts of mucilage which soothes the gastrointestinal tract.[21] It is specifically used for dyspepsia, nausea, heartburn, and diarrhea. FENUGREEK SEEDS: As much as 40 percent of the weight of fenugreek seeds is mucilage. Mucilage is a gelatin-like substance usually made up of proteins and

polysaccharides which heals irritated intestinal tract lining and helps to hold water. It also prompts pancreatic secretion which boosts digestion.[22] GINGER ROOT: Ginger is one of the best herbs for the treatment of digestive disorders. Ginger prevents nausea, gas, bloating, and vomiting. Ginger root is not a laxative, but it will tonify the intestinal muscle and provides a source of proteolytic enzymes to aid digestion.[23] ALOE VERA GEL: Aloe vera gel is a clear jelly-like material that has been successfully employed in treating irritable bowel syndrome. Aloe gel improves bowel transit time, reducing putrefaction in the intestinal tract, and increases friendly bacteria like acidophilus.[24] If you have any gripping with this herb, add more ginger. This herb is usually part of combinations and if used single may cause cramping. COMBINATION OF VALERIAN ROOT AND KAVA: For stress management which is very important in most cases of colon irritation. These herbs work to calm the central nervous system without addiction or artificial sedative effects found with tranquilizing drugs.

Secondary Nutrients

GARLIC OIL (ENTERIC COATED): Garlic helps to get rid of any pathogens in the colon and also promotes the healing of tissue. *Suggested Dosage:* Garlic oil can be taken in enteric-coated capsules. Take one with each meal.

ALFALFA: Can help to promote healing through its chlorophyll content. *Suggested Dosage:* Can be taken in liquid or capsule form. Take as directed.

CABBAGE JUICE OR POWDER: Compounds in cabbage have the ability to help in healing gastrointestinal ulcers. *Suggested Dosage:* You may have trouble finding cabbage powder. Juicing cabbage may be more practical.

Home Care Suggestions

◆ Controlling diverticulitis involves four primary areas of focus: increasing dietary fiber, controlling emotional stress and avoiding certain culprit foods and habits.

◆ Standing up and stretching the arms high above the head can help relieve pain.

◆ A short fast can help to alleviate some of the symptoms of diverticulitis by resting the digestive system.

Other Supportive Therapies

MASSAGE: This can help to ease constipation and control pain.

ACUPUNCTURE: Helps to stimulate the immune system and to facilitate better digestion and elimination.

Scientific-Facts-at-a-Glance

Many experts in the field of nutrition have concluded that diverticulitis is a disease that is directly linked to low fiber consumption. There is much statistical data to back this claim. For example, the mortality rate due to colon disease drastically dropped in World War II England when citizens were forced to stop eating processed foods in favor of a more natural, fiber-rich diet.[25]

Spirit/Mind Considerations

As in the case of most colon disorders, stress is considered a major cause. Anxiety, fatigue, hostility, sleep disorders and depression must be addressed in order to avoid several intestinal diseases. The use of biofeedback, counseling, physical exercise, relaxation techniques and meditation therapies such as yoga should be considered. For many people with stress-related illness, a brisk daily walk can be invaluable.

Prevention

◆ Modify your diet. Eat plenty of whole grain breads, cereals, and foods high in fiber, (at least 30 to 35 grams every day), fresh fruits and vegetables with their peelings left on.

◆ Eating fiber through oat bran, etc. and drinking at least 6 six glasses of water per day helps to prevent constipation. Consequently, accumulation of intestinal matter in the diverticula is minimized, therefore the infection which causes diverticulitis is avoided.

◆ Diverticulitis may well be a disease of lifestyle. People who eat healthy and exercise regularly seem to rarely suffer from diverticulitis.

◆ Do not overuse laxatives if constipated, especially suppositories. Laxatives can be habit forming and can cause bowel irritation. Constipation itself can cause the formation of diverticula and should be minimized through diet and exercise.

◆ If you have diverticula already, avoid seedy foods like raspberries, nuts and popcorn. These foods can easily become lodged in the diverticula and cause inflammation which results in diverticulitis.

Doctor's Notes

Our emphasis on eating high-protein (meat), low-fiber diets can lead to diverticulitis. If dietary adjustments are not made, the diverticular sacs that form can become infected, requiring antibiotics or even surgery. The best advice for anyone with diverticulitis is to drink lots of water and dramatically increase your fiber intake. Fiber supplements can work wonders if they are taken consistently. Eating the right foods in their natural state can help to clean out these sacs and to eventually cause them to shrink.

Endnotes

1. L.F. Rettger, et al., Lactobacillus Acidophilus: Its Therapeutic Application, Yale University Press, New Haven: 1935.
2. S. Taussig and S. Batkin, "Bromelain, the enzyme complex of pineapple and its clinical application: An update," Jour Ethno Pharmacol, 1988, 22: 191-203.
3. W.D. Rees, et al., "Treating irritable bowel syndrome with peppermint oil," British Med Jour, 1979, 2(6194): 835-36.
4. Y. Niwa, et al., "Effect of liposomal encapsulated superoxide dimustase on active oxygen-related human disorders," Free Rad Res Commu, 1985, 1: 137-53.
5. M. Skogh, et al., "Vitamin A in Crohn's disease," Lancet, 1980, I: 776.
6. A.D. Harries, et al., "Vitamin D status in Crohn's disease: Association with nutrition and disease activity," Gut, 1985, 26: 1197-1203.
7. S.D. Krasinski, et al., "The prevalence of vitamin K deficiency in gastrointestinal disorders," Amer Jour Clin Nutr, 1985, 41: 639-43.
8. E. Middleton, "The flavonoids," Trends Pharmaceutical Science, 1984, 5: 335-38.
9. J.D. Bennet, "Use of a-tocopherol-quinone in the treatment of ulcerative colitis," Gut, 1986, 27:695-97.
10. W.F. Stenson, "Dietary supplementation with fish oil in ulcerative colitis," Ann Int Med, 1992, 116: 609-14.
11. "Dietary fish oil alters Leukotrine generation and neutrophil function," Nutrition Review, 1986, 44:137-9.
12. P. Hoges, et al., "Vitamin and iron intake in patients with Chron's Disease," Journal of the American Dietetic Association, 1984, 84(1):52-58.
13. I.H. Rosenberg et al., "Nutritional aspects of an inflammatory bowel disease," Ann Rev Nutr, 1985, 5:463-84.
14. C.R. Fleming, et al., "Zinc nutrition in Chron's disease," Dig Dis Sci, 1981, 26:865-70.
15. L.O. Soifer, et al., "Effects of medicinal fiber on colic transit in patients with irritable bowel syndrome," Acta Gastroenter Latinum, 1987, 17(4): 317-23. See also B. Morseon, "Pathology of diverticular disease of the colon," Clin Gastro, 1975, 4(1): 37.
16. Y. Kaneday, et al., "In vitro effects of berberine sulfate on the growth of Entamoeba histolytica, Giardia lamblia and tricomanons vaginalis," Ann Trop Med Parasitol, 1991, 85: 417-25.
17. E. Okimasa, et al., "Inhibition of phospholipase A2 by glycyrrhizin, an anti-inflammatory drug," Acta Med Okayama, 1983, 37: 385-91.
18. M. Messer, C.M. Anderson and L. Hubbard, "Studies on the mechanism of destruction of the toxic action of wheat gluten in celiac disease by crude papain," Gut, 1964, 5: 295-303.
19. H. Glatzel and K. Hackenberg, "Roientgenological studies of the effect of bitters on digestive organs," Planta Medica, 1967, 15(3): 223-32.
20. F. Ellingwood, American Materia Medica, Therapeutics and Pharmacognosy, (Eclectic Medical Publication, Portland, Oregon: 1983).
21. W. Szturma, "Method for treating gastro-intestinal ulcers with extract of herb cetaria," US Patent 4150123, issued April 17, 1979.
22. G. Ribes, et al., "Effect of fenugreek seeds on endocrine pancreatic secretions in dogs," Annals of Nutrition and Metabolism, 1984, 28: 37-43.
23. E.H. Thompson, et al., "Ginger rhizome: A new source of proteolytic enzyme," Journal of Food Science, 1973, 38(4): 652-55.
24. J. Bland, "Effect of orally-consumed Aloe vera juice on human gastrointestinal function," Natural Foods Network Newsl, August, 1985.
25. A. Brodribb, "Dietary fiber in diverticular diseases of the colon," in Medical Aspects of Dietary Fiber, G. Spiller and R. Kay, (Plenum Medical, New York: 1980): 46.

DYSMENORRHEA

SEE "MENSTRUAL CRAMPS"

EARACHE

The estimated cost of treating earaches alone is over $1 billion annually. Children are the most susceptible to ear infections, and there is some controversy surrounding the best way to treat them. Over 25 million prescriptions with over 1 billion individual doses of antibiotics are given to children in the space of a year. Technically, a middle ear infection also known as otitis media is the most common kind of earache. This disorder affects 20 to 40 percent of children under the age of six and is the most frequently diagnosed childhood disorder. An estimated 30 million doctor's office visits per year are for middle ear infections. Most children will outgrow their tendency for ear infections by age three. An earache can be characterized by a dull, throbbing or stabbing pain in the ear. Middle ear infections can cause the eardrum to burst, which causes a discharge of fluid and an immediate sense of relief caused by fluid pressure. A perforated eardrum should always be examined by a doctor. It will usually heal on its own. Higher altitudes and cold climates seem to increase the risk of ear infections.

Symptoms

External ear infections can cause itching, burning pain, and discharge. Middle ear infections can cause earache (sharp, dull, throbbing or stabbing pain), fever, chills, irritability, red, swollen eardrum, hearing loss, vertigo, nausea, buzzing or ringing sounds and/or a blocked sensation. In babies, agitation or pulling at the ear and sleeplessness may be present.

Precautions

An ear infection can be a serious medical condition. Anyone with the above symptoms should see their physician immediately. An untreated middle ear infection can lead to hearing loss or deafness, mastoiditis (an infection of the bone behind the ear), or a brain abscess. A viral infection of the inner ear may lead to labyrinthitis which causes severe vertigo and sudden hearing loss.

Causes

Several factors may be involved in why the inner ear feels tender or inflamed.

There are three main conditions which can cause an earache. These are infections of the external ear, referring to the canal which leads to the eardrum; infections of the middle ear which is the area beyond the eardrum; or a blockage of the eustachian tube, which usually causes both ears to hurt.

Middle ear infections, which constitute the most common kind of earache, are usually brought on by abnormal eustachian tube function. This tube clears fluid from the middle ear and regulates pressure. In infants and small children, it is much smaller in diameter and can easily become blocked. Once an obstruction is present, fluid will build up in the tube providing an excellent environment for bacterial growth. The organisms most commonly responsible for ear infections is the streptococcus pneumonia and the hemophilus influenza.

Occasionally, a viral infection may be present in the inner ear. Conditions that can cause a blockage of the eustachian tube are weak tissue support around the tube causing it to collapse and an abnormal opening to the tube and chronic allergies or infections.

Swimmer's ear, which only affects the canal in front of the ear drum, is caused when water becomes trapped in the ear canal and breaks down the skin lining. As a result, bacterial infection can spread. The decompression that can occur in air travel can also trigger an earache. In addition, childhood diseases such as measles and chicken pox along with throat infections can also cause earaches. Contamination of the middle ear can also occur during vigorous nose blowing, sneezing or if the nose is plugged. Earaches usually clear up within three to five days.

Bottle feeding babies has been linked to the incidence of ear infections as compared with breast fed babies and may be associated with the advantages of the built-in immunity builders contained in breast milk. In addition, possible allergies to cow's milk can be avoided by breast feeding. If you do bottle feed, make sure your child is propped up when feeding.

Conventional Therapies

Antibiotic therapy is the most common treatment for ear infections. Amoxicillin is usually the drug of choice because it specifically targets the bacteria commonly involved. If an allergy to penicillin exists, trimethoprim-sulfamethoxazole (bactrim or septra) can be prescribed. Antibiotic therapy usually lasts for ten to fourteen days.

Occasionally, some doctors may recommend a decongestant, assuming that it may help relieve any congestion which has blocked the eustachian tube. When the pain of an earache is particularly severe, anesthetic eardrops may also be prescribed.

Antibiotic eardrops are used to treat infections of the external ear. Frequently, this type of ear infection will clear up with drops only (although antibiotics often are prescribed when they're not necessary).

A myringotomy involves placing tiny tubes through the ear drum to increase fluid drainage from the eustachian tube. It has become a popular form of treatment for children with chronic ear infections. It is the number one surgical procedure performed in the U.S. Recently, it was discovered that up to 50 percent of myringotomies are unnecessary. Another controversy is whether the existence of these tubes may, in fact, increase susceptibility to ear infection.

Analgesics are also routinely prescribed for earaches. While the use of antibiotics has been very effective in clearing up the majority of ear infections, new strains of bacteria resistant to present antibiotics have appeared. They require the synthesis of new antibiotics, like augmentin (which is designed to destroy the B-cat bacterium). Some studies suggest that the majority of earaches will resolve themselves within three days. The incidence of chronic middle ear disease in children has actually increased since the advent of antibiotics. While antibiotics may be required they should be used judiciously.

Dietary Guidelines

- If you have a child that suffers from recurring ear infections, it is important to concentrate on building up his or her immune system.
- Incorporate a diet with plenty of fresh fruits, vegetables and whole grains.
- Avoid dairy products which encourage the production of mucous.
- Avoid a diet high in empty calories, junk foods, fats and meats.
- Drink the juice of an orange or lemon diluted with 25 percent water. A little pure maple syrup may be added.
- Emphasize fresh juices, both fruit and vegetable. To decrease their sugar content, however, dilute them with pure water.
- Food allergies, especially those to milk or wheat products, can cause recurring ear infections in children. Make sure to rule out this possibility by following the food elimination guide contained in the Food Allergy section of this book. The most common allergy-producing foods include dairy products, wheat, oranges, corn, nuts (peanut butter) and various fruits.

Recommended Nutritional Supplements

PRIMARY NUTRIENTS

ACIDOPHILUS Restores friendly flora that help to boost immunity. If your child has been on antibiotics, replacing lost bacteria is essential.[1] Some controversy exists over whether taking acidophilus during antibiotic therapy is effective or not. *Suggested Dosage:* Take liberally, using active culture yogurts and bifido bacteria-containing supplements. Antibiotics kill friendly bacteria which, in turn, increases susceptibility to future infections. Use milk-free products with guaranteed bacterial count. Check expiration date.

VITAMIN A WITH BETA-CAROTENE Even in 1931, studies found that a diet rich in carotenes correlated with the number of days missed by school children.[2] In addition, vitamin A boosts immunity and is especially important during infections.[3] *Suggested Dosage:* 10,000 IU of vitamin A (or an age-appropriate dose) and 20,000 IU of beta carotene daily.

VITAMIN C WITH BIOFLAVONOIDS Fights infection by boosting immune function. In addition, the presence of an infection can deplete vitamin C stores.[4] *Suggested Dosage:* 1,000 mg with each of three meals (or an age-appropriate dose). Use esterized or buffered products if stomach upset is a problem. Powdered ascorbic acid, which can be measured into drinks, is practical for treating children.

ZINC Boosts immune response which may shorten the length of the ear infection or lessen its severity. Moreover, children who suffer from zinc deficiencies are more susceptible to infection.[5] *Suggested Dosage:* Take as directed.

HERBAL COMBINATION Also recommended is an herbal combination that includes echinacea, goldenseal root, myrrh gum, garlic, licorice root, blue vervain, butternut root bark and kelp. *Suggested Dosage:* Six to twelve capsules daily. This formula should not be used for more than three weeks at a time.

ECHINACEA: In Germany, this herb is routinely used to treat infections of the head, nose and throat. Immune stimulation is a well-known property of echinacea. It stimulates the ingestion and digestion of foreign bacteria and matter by cells called phagocytes. It also improves mobility of infection-combating leukocytes (white blood cells).[6] As a point of caution, some herbs like *Parthenium integrifolium* have been substituted for the true echinacea and labeled as echinacea. Don't accept substitutes and insist on the real plant. GOLDENSEAL ROOT: The berberine content of this herb is recognized by many herbalists and natural healers as possessing the ability to strengthen mucus linings, making it harder for pathogens to penetrate. Two of goldenseal's more active compounds, hydrastine and berberine, have demonstrated effectiveness in treating various bacterial and viral infections, especially those of the respiratory tract.[7] MYRRH GUM: Myrrh gum has some similar properties as found in echinacea and goldenseal root. Myrrh gum stimulates phagocyte activity and reduces inflammation of the mucus secreting mucosa.[8] Myrrh is officially recognized in Britain, France and Germany for its medicinal value. GARLIC: Garlic is another herb that can be considered a tonic. It is a powerful agent against infections of various types and origins. Garlic can increase the number of leukocytes (white blood cells) which help fight infections.[9] In addition, garlic increases perspiration, which further cleanses the body. LICORICE ROOT: Licorice root contributes in several important ways to this formula. It stimulates secretion of the hormone aldosterone from the adrenal cortex, producing a higher energy level which is usually needed when combating infections. It is also an impressive immune system booster.[10] Long-term consumption of licorice is not recommended as it may cause weakness, electrolyte imbalances, water retention and hypertension. Licorice is officially recognized for therapeutic activity in Britain, France, Germany, Belgium, China and many other countries. BLUE VERVAIN: This herb helps to break the cycle of chronically occurring infections. It has been used for colds and flu and has an ability to reduce fever. BUTTERNUT ROOT BARK: Butternut is a laxative that is used to treat dysentery and diarrhea. It also has an ability to expel worms. While it is a laxative, it does not produce the sometimes painful gripping associated with other laxatives. Butternut improves liver function and stimulates bile production and flow. KELP: Kelp's function in this formula is to provide needed trace elements important in many metabolic processes in the body. These nutrients may further support the healing process and return the body to normal function. Kelp contains a soluble fiber called algin which is soothing to the gastrointestinal tract and improves bowel function.

SECONDARY NUTRIENTS

ASTRAGALUS: A Chinese herb well-known for its ability to enhance immune function when fighting an infection. *Suggested Dosage:* Take as directed using standardized products.

Home Care Suggestions

- No type of ear drop should be used if a ruptured ear drum is suspected. See your physician.
- Using saline gargles at the first sign of an earache can help to bring more blood to the eustachian tube and help to fight infection.
- Ear drops can be warmed prior to using by placing the bottle in a cup of hot water.
- Garlic oil drops placed in the ear can help to fight any infection present. Use an eyedropper to apply oil.
- If you have swimmer's ear, don't scratch it. You should make a solution of one part white vinegar to one part rubbing alcohol and place one to two drops in the ear three times a day. Some studies have indicated that this drop solution can cure up to 75 percent of external ear infections.
- Placing hygroscopic anhydrous glycerine into the ear can help to draw out fluids and reduce pressure.
- Apply heat locally as a hot, moist pack to the outer ear. A warm towel that has been soaked in chamomile tea and placed behind the ear can help with pain. Resoak and use as often as needed.
- An old remedy consists of roasting a lemon in the oven and using the juice as eardrops.
- Don't blow your nose during an earache or if you must, do it very gently.
- Keep the ear canal dry by placing cotton plugs in the ears when showering or washing your hair.
- Use acetaminophen for pain. Do not give aspirin to anyone under 21 because of the risk of Reye's syndrome.
- Prop your head up when sleeping which helps promote drainage of the eustachian tubes.
- For adults who suffer from chronic ear infections, using a decongestant nasal spray or an over-the-counter oral decongestant may help dry up any fluid present. You need to be careful; do not overuse nasal sprays, as they can become habit forming and can cause a rebound effect where congestion is actually increased. Also, a homemade nasal spray made out of one teaspoon of glycerine in one pint of warm water can be used to relieve congestion.

Scientific Facts-at-a-Glance

Statistics tell us that natural therapies may be more effective than continual drug treatments for earaches. There may be no long term benefits to routine antibiotic and surgical treatment of ear infections. Studies point out that children treated with antibiotics have a higher incidence of repeat ear infections when compared to those who have not received antibiotics.[10] While earaches should be seen by a doctor, perhaps focusing on diet, the elimination of allergy-producing foods and nutrient deficiencies would be more productive overall.

Spirit/Mind Considerations

For children, dietary factors may be the principle causes of repeated ear infections. For adults, however, continual infections signals a depressed immune system which must be fortified through diet, supplements and stress management.

Prevention

- Choosing to breast-feed your baby may be the one most effective way to prevent the incidence of ear infections. Breast milk provides the baby with antibodies for the first six months. It has anti-inflammatory properties and protects the child from allergies to certain foods, especially cow's milk.
- The role of food allergies as a major cause of earaches is strongly documented in medical publications. Any allergic reaction will cause swelling and inflammation of the eustachian tube and nose, which can encourage infection.
- If you bottle-feed your baby, do not prop the bottle. This can cause a regurgitation of the fluid into the middle ear and may increase the risk of infection.
- Do not introduce foods such as citrus fruits, wheat or cow's milk into your babies diet too early, which could increase the risk of developing food allergies.
- Try to protect your baby or small child from exposure to colds and flu.
- If you have trouble with earaches cover your ears when its windy or wear ear plugs.
- When flying, chew on gum or candy which helps keep the eustachian tube open during changes in air pressure
- Do not smoke. Tobacco smoke can irritate mucous-secreting canals for you and anyone around you, especially children.
- When swimming, wear ear plugs to avoid trapping water in the ear. After swimming, shake your head to remove any excess water and dry the ear as thoroughly as possible. A preventative home remedy for those prone to swimmer's ear is to insert one or two drops of a solution made from one part white vinegar and one part rubbing alcohol in each ear. This helps to dry out the canal and maintains the normal acid balance of the area.

Doctor's Notes

There are several very good immune-stimulating herbs which help to boost resistance and fight infection. At the top of the list are echinacea, goldenseal, myrrh gum and garlic. This herbal formula includes these four ingredients and is designed to fight viral and bacterial infections, enhance and support immune response, reduce fevers, cleanse the body and improve health. This formula is not just for those suffering from ear infections. It is for infections of varying types and origins.

With children, dietary changes are often profoundly significant in controlling ear infections. Milk allergies and sugar sensitivities can be major contributing factors to recurring infections. Building up your child's resistance is far better than having to treat symptoms.

Watch out for culprit foods and tell your doctor that you want to use antibiotics only when absolutely necessary. If you do, always supplement your child's diet with acidophilus.

Endnotes

1. G. Zoppi, et al., "Oral bacteriotherapy in clinical practice: The use of different preparations in the treatment of acute diarrhea," Euro Jour Pedia, 1982, 139: 22-24.

2. A. Bendich, "Betacarotene and immune response," Proc Nutri Soc, 1991, 50: 263-74.

3. R.D. Semba, "Vitamin A immunity and infection," Clin Info Dis, 1994, 19: 489-99.

4. J.J. Aleo, and H. Padh, "Inhibition of ascorbic acid uptake by endotoxin: evidence of mediation by serum factors," Proc Soc Exp Biol Med, 1985, 179(1): 128-31.

5. I. Lombeck, et al., "Hair zinc of young children from rural and urban areas in North Rhine-Westphalia, Germany," Euro Jour Pedia, 1988, 147(2): 179-83.

6. R. Bauer and H. Wagner, "Echinacea species as potential immunostimulatory drugs," Econ Med Plant Res, 1991, 5: 253-321.

7. D. Sun, et al., "Berberine sulfate blocks adherence of streptococcus pyogenes to epithelial cells, fobronectin and hexadecane," Antimivrob Agents Chemo, 1988, 32: 1370-74.

8. Encyclopedia of Chinese Drugs, 1977, Shanghai Scientific and Technical Publications, People's Republic of China.

9. H.P. Koch, "Garlicin, Fact or Fiction," Phytother Res, 1993, 7: 278-80.

10. Melvyn R. Werbach and Michael T. Murray, Botanical Influences on Illness, (Third Line Press, Tarzana, Ca: 1994).

11. Noel Peterson, ND, "Otis Media Fact Sheet," Health World.

EAR INFECTION

See "Earache"

ECZEMA

Eczema (also known as dermatitis) is a chronic skin disorder that is characterized by dry, itchy skin. The first sign of eczema in a small child may be the presence of red, chapped cheeks. Tiny red pimples may appear on the child's buttocks, the inner creases of the elbows or behind the knees. With time, eczema can spread and is commonly found on the backs of legs, fronts of arms and especially on the hands. Persistent scratching of these affected areas subsequently causes weepy, infected irritations. As areas of eczema dry, they produce crusts. Prolonged scratching and infection will eventually produce areas of skin that are rough and thickened.

Fifty percent of infant eczema cases clear up by eighteen months of age. Adult eczema is usually persistent and often resists treatment. Eczema is an inflammatory disease of the skin that is associated with asthma and is considered, at least to some extent, an allergic disorder. Eczema is a common condition which affects between 2 and 7 percent of the population.

Symptoms

Eczema produces oozing, red scaly, itchy patches of skin that blister and itch. In severe cases lesions may form and can become so irritated that they bleed. Eczema causes the water-holding capacity of the skin to decrease. People who suffer from this disorder have a higher-than-normal tendency to itch and to scratch. In several cases of eczema, the skin seemed to be more susceptible to bacterial growth, especially the *Staphylococcus aureus* bacteria.

Often intense itching can occur before any irritation is visible. Consequently, continual scratching can cause the visible symptoms of eczema.

Precautions

For severe infections where skin is weeping, etc., antibiotics may be required. See your physician.

Causes

Like allergic disorders, eczema runs in families. Two-thirds of people who suffer from eczema have family members with the same condition. Some of the factors that can lead to a breakout of eczema include emotional stress, food allergies, excessive sweating, continual contact with water or detergent agents and certain chemicals and contact allergens, such as wool or nickel.

Make sure to rule out a gluten sensitivity, milk allergies, or a hydrochloric acid deficiency.

Conventional Therapies

Most physicians will treat eczema with topical steroid ointments and lotions. If the skin infection is severe, antibiotics will be prescribed. For severe night itching, an antihistamine may be recommended. Cortisone can dramatically decrease inflammation and itching, but it also suppresses cell activity and growth. If used over a long period of time, the skin can become fragile and weak which increases its susceptibility to infection and damage. The risks of prolonged use of these preparations is particularly risky when facial skin is involved due to its delicate nature. Physicians will often ask a person suffering from eczema not to scratch, which is a totally unrealistic request. The best therapy medical science can offer the victim of eczema is the use of corticosteroid preparations and antibiotics if the infection is severe enough.

Dietary Guidelines

◆ Emphasize parsley, green leafy vegetables, sprouts, celery, pineapples, grapes, melons, kelp, unsalted seeds, onions, papayas, and pears in the diet.

◆ Do not consume dairy products. This is particularly important for young children. Allergies to cow's milk can severely aggravate eczema.

◆ If you know you are allergic to wheat, avoid foods from the same family which will probably also cause eczema. For example, rice, rye, millet and barley may cause eczema to flare up. Experiment and see if you can find a correlation between your diet and outbreaks of eczema.

◆ Keep a journal of your food intake and make note if and when eczema occurs.

Recommended Nutritional Supplements

PRIMARY NUTRIENTS

ESSENTIAL FATTY ACIDS People who suffer from eczema are often deficient in these fatty acids.[1] Supplementing the diet with evening primrose oil has resulted in marked improvement.[2] *Suggested Dosage:* Take as directed using a product with a variety of oils containing both omega-3 and omega-6 fatty acids.

VITAMIN E WITH SELENIUM Studies have shown that people with dermatitis and other skin conditions may be suffering from reduced selenium.[3] *Suggested Dosage:* 800 IU of vitamin E and suggested dosage for selenium.

ZINC When zinc levels become reduced in the epidermal skin layers, eczema can develop. Studies have shown that epidermal zinc concentrations play a very significant role in preventing dermatitis or eczema.[4] *Suggested Dosage:* No more than 100 mg per day. Lozenges may be used. Look for gluconate of picolinate products.

PABA PABA supplement significantly improved symptoms of dermatitis in test cases even when it was caused by a gluten allergy.[5] *Suggested Dosage:* 200 mg three time daily.

VITAMIN C WITH BIOFLAVONOIDS Bioflavonoids are powerful natural anti-inflammatory agents that can stabilize cell membranes of skin tissue. They also boost the function of vitamin C in the body.[6] *Suggested Dosage:* 3,000 to 5,000 mg of vitamin C per day. Take with meals.

VITAMIN A WITH BETA-CAROTENE Compounds found in vitamin A are crucial for proper skin maintenance. A vitamin A deficiency can cause a wide variety of diseases including eczema.[7] *Suggested Dosage:* 10,000 IU per day. If you are pregnant, do not exceed 10,000 IU daily. Take 25,000 IU of beta carotene daily.

GLUCOSAMINE The glycosaminoglycans contained in this natural compound help to synthesize collagen, which helps skin tissue to regenerate. *Suggested Dosage:* Take as directed.

LICORICE ROOT Helps to inhibit the excess histamine release which characterizes eczema.[8] Ointments made from licorice and chamomile have also been known to be equal or superior to cortisone-based ointments.[9] *Suggested Dosage:* Take as directed, using topical products, or make your own decoction and use it directly on the skin.

HERBAL COMBINATION This combination should include burdock root, gotu kola, yellow dock, dandelion root, milk thistle seeds, Irish moss, red clover blossoms, kelp, cayenne and sarsaparilla root. *Suggested Dosage:* Two to six capsules daily. For chronic conditions, use the maximum dosage of six capsules per day for a prolonged period. For best results use every day.

BURDOCK ROOT: In Europe, this herb is well known for its ability to treat skin disorders.[10] It is especially good for scaling eczema and has a long history of use for this condition. It also has an anti-inflammatory effect due to a compound called inulin which helps to normalize the inflammation caused by immune dysfunction in people with eczema. Burdock also helps to control staph infections, which can accompany eczema. It can be used in powdered form directly on the affected areas and taken internally as well. GOTU KOLA: Also known as *Centella asiatica,* this herb is supported by tremendous clinical research conducted in Europe which supports its effectiveness in the treatment of various skin disorders associated with cellulitis and even leprosy.[11] It also possesses wound healing properties and has been shown to decrease scarring.[12] YELLOW DOCK: Yellow dock root is a reputed blood purifier and has been prescribed for all types of skin problems including leprosy, boils and eczema. It has also been reported to clear a congested liver. Its laxative effect is well documented and supports the body's detoxifying ability.[13] DANDELION ROOT: This common yard weed has a long history of use in herbal medicine. It is part of this formula for its ability to strengthen the liver, improve bile formation, regulate the bowels, purify the blood and tonify the skin.[14] MILK THISTLE: There is probably not a person alive who could not benefit from milk thistle. This wonderful herb cleanses, strengthens and protects the liver and its functions and has proven itself valuable for skin disorders like psoriasis. Time-tested and proven in hospitals and clinics all over Europe, milk thistle is one of the only herbs known to treat some forms of psoriasis.[15] IRISH MOSS: The contribution of Irish moss is very simple. It provides a demulcent and soothing source of mucilage and improves intestinal function. RED CLOVER BLOSSOM: Red clover blossoms are a reputed blood purifier and officially recognized in the United Kingdom for treatment of skin conditions such as psoriasis, eczema and rashes. KELP: Kelp serves a similar function as Irish moss, but kelp is thought to be a blood purifier with the ability to alleviate skin problems, burns and insect bites. CAYENNE: Cayenne is a stimulant that helps to make all the other herbs function better. Such herbs are referred to as activators or catalysts. SARSAPARILLA ROOT: Sarsaparilla root has many benefits including the treatment of psoriasis and eczema. As a result of its diuretic and diaphoretic action sarsaparilla cleanses the body. This herb has received official recognition in European countries.

SECONDARY NUTRIENTS

VITAMIN D: Helps promote skin healing. *Suggested Dosage:* 500 IU daily.

VITAMIN B-COMPLEX: Yeast-free formulas are needed for the regeneration of skin cells. *Suggested Dosage:* 50 mg with each of three meals per day.

KOCHIA OIL: Used medicinally in China for a variety of disorders. Applied externally, it can help to minimize eczema. Purchasing this oil may prove difficult and might have to be special ordered through heath food stores or herbal distributors. *Suggested Usage:* Use as directed.

ST. JOHN'S WORT OIL: This is an old herbal remedy for skin irritations that promotes healing. *Suggested Usage:* Use as directed.

CHAMOMILE: Extracts of this herb exerted anti-inflammatory effects when applied topically in animal models of skin inflammation.[16] *Suggested Dosage:* Use topically as directed. You can make your own decoctions and apply the liquid directly to the skin.

GINKGO: New studies have found that the terpene compounds in this herb can help to inhibit the specific inflammatory response typically seen in eczema. *Suggested Dosage:* Take as directed.

HEARTSEASE: Particularly beneficial for weeping eczema if used externally as an ointment or cream. *Suggested Usage:* Use as directed. A wet compress can also be made by soaking a towel in heartsease tea and applying it to affected areas of skin.

Home Care Suggestions

- Use baking soda as an after-bath powder to help dry the skin.
- Be careful that your detergent or fabric softener sheets are not causing an allergic skin reaction. Rinse your sheets and towels twice. Using soap to launder your clothes is preferable. Avoid bleach or fabric softeners.
- Some physicians recommend using petroleum jelly to keep drying and scaling in control. Petroleum jelly helps to trap moisture on the skin.
- Antihistamines reduce itching but should be used with caution.
- The use of a non-oily zinc ointment can be used to control severe itching.
- Oatmeal baths can help relive the itching associated with eczema. An oatmeal bath can be made by using a powder such as Aveeno in the bath water.
- Use skin emollients that contain urea or lactic acid such as ultra-mild 25 and lac-hydrin 5.
- Avoid wearing wool, silk or synthetics which may aggravate itching.
- Never handle certain substances such as insulation (which is made of fiber glass), household cleaners or any caustic chemical without proper skin protection. If you suffer from hand eczema don't wash the dishes without protection. Use rubber gloves worn over cotton gloves.
- Keep your environment moist. Use a cool mist vaporizer or attach a humidifier to your furnace system.
- Buy and use cosmetics judiciously. Experiment with hypoallergenic varieties and use as little as possible. Usually, high priced cosmetics are no more or less likely to cause an allergic reaction. Unfortunately, a product that you have used for years with no problem can become an irritant. Often ingredients are revised or fragrances added, and eczema can result.
- Keep short fingernails on small children and put gloves or socks on their hands at night.
- Avoid the use of soap which has a tendency to dry out the skin. Use non-lipid containing cleansers. Cetyl alcohol preparations, such as cetaphil lotion, may be beneficial. Moisturel is another non-irritating skin cleanser. If you must use soap, purchase a very mild type of soap bar such as Dove.
- Bath and shower quickly and perhaps not so often. Dry yourself totally and use a cream to moisten your skin.
- Makes sure to rinse yourself thoroughly after using a hot tub or swimming pool. Chlorine residue on the skin may cause or aggravate eczema.
- Clothing that comes in direct contact with the skin should be cotton only, especially in the case of infants and children.
- Do not overdress children. Becoming too hot causes sweating which aggravates eczema.

Other Supportive Therapies

HOMEOPATHY: Sulfur, graphite, petroleum and rhus tox.

HYDROTHERAPY: Using hot and cold water treatments can help inflammation and itching. Sodium bicarbonate added to the water can enhance its anti-inflammatory effect.

ACUPUNCTURE: Acupuncture can help to stimulate circulation and facilitate the removal of toxins from the blood.

Scientific Facts-at-a-Glance

The liver's role in skin disorders is rarely addressed. Detoxifying and boosting liver function can help to promote skin health. In addition, numerous reports suggest that *Staphylococcus aureus* contributes to outbreaks of eczema. This bacterium has been isolated from affected skin in more than 90 percent of eczema patients.[17] For this reason, using an antibacterial agent directly on the skin may be helpful. Several herbs have the ability to heal while killing bacteria.

Spirit/Mind Considerations

Emotional stress can provoke eczema and increase the intensity of its symptoms. Some studies have shown that people who suffer from this condition manifested higher-than-normal levels of anxiety, hostility and psychological neurosis than the general public. Learning to diffuse stress by meditating or using controlled breathing can be highly beneficial. If you find that you need help to fall asleep or feel calm during the day, the nervine herbs which include passionflower, kava, valerian, skullcap and hops may be of value.

Prevention

◆ Using artificial fingernails or eyelashes may also cause an allergic skin reaction.
◆ Switch from antiperspirants to deodorants. An antiperspirant contains aluminum chloride, aluminum sulfate and zirconium chlorohydrates which can irritate sensitive skin. Watch out for strong deodorant soaps, also.
◆ Do not introduce foods such as citrus fruits, cow's milk and wheat into your baby's diet too soon. This may increase the child's susceptibility to allergic disorders.
◆ Cats and dogs that are kept in the house may also aggravate eczema.
◆ Baby lotions or any skin preparation that contain lanolin or a fragrance. Look for the hypo-allergenic label
◆ Also avoid metallic jewelry. Nickel allergies can cause severe eczema. Use stainless steel or gold posts on pierced earrings, cloth watch bands and make sure rings and necklaces are not made of nickel.
◆ Try to wash your hands in cold water rather than hot, which is much more drying.

Doctor's Notes

There are many different kinds of skin rashes which can result from infections, allergic reactions, sensitivities, etc. If you have a rash that does not clear up, you need to see your doctor to establish exactly what is causing it. Many rashes that are caused by allergy or sensitivity (acne for example) will clear up with homeopathic preparations like sulfur. Local creams made from calendula are good, and poultices can be made from gotu kola tea. Eczema responds well to zinc in supplements. Colon cleansing can also be helpful.

The skin is the largest and one of the most important organs of the body. It performs many vital functions including cleansing toxic substances from the body, keeping the body's temperature in check and providing a barrier to pathogenic bacteria and viruses. The condition of the skin is often a reflection of the health of the body. Imbalances and toxic buildup due to a dysfunctional liver or improper elimination may reveal themselves in the skin as eczema, psoriasis, rashes, acne, dermatitis, or a number of other disorders. By improving the internal health of the body, the skin's functionality and appearance will be positively affected. The herbal formula listed is designed to cleanse the body by activating all its methods of elimination which include cleansing, strengthening and supporting liver function. This formula will assist with a wide range of skin disorders including eczema, cellulitis, acne, psoriasis, burns and insect bites. Longer-lasting and more wide-ranging results can be achieved by improving the diet and abstaining from chocolate, nuts and stimulants such as caffeine.

Endnotes

1. A. Hansen et al., "Eczema and essential fatty acids," A.J. Dis Scild., 1947, 73:1-18.S.
2. J. Wright and J. Burton, "Oral evening primrose oil improves eczema," Lancet, 1982, vol. 2, 1120.
3. L. Juhlin et al., "Blood glutathione peroxidase levels in skin disease: Effect of selenium and Vitamin E treatment," Acata Derma (Stockholm), 1982, 62: 211-14.
4. G. Michmalsson and K. Ljunghall, "Patients with dermatitis, herpetiformis, acne, psoriasis and Darier's disease have low epidermal zinc concentrations," Acta Derm Venerol (Stockholm), 1990, 70(4):304-8. See also C.J.D. Zerafonetis, "Para amino benzoic acid in dermatitis hepitiformis,"Arch Dermatol, 1951, 63:115-32.
5. C.J.D. Zarafonetis et al., "PABA in dermatitis herpetiformis," Arch Derma Syphil, 1951, 63:115-132.
6. F. Pierce, et al., "Mucosal masted cells: The effect of quercitin and other flavonoids on antigen-induced histamine secretion from rat intestinal masted cells." Jour Allergy Clin Immunol, 1984, 73:819-23.
7. M.H. Zile and M.E. Collum, "The function of vitamin A: Current concepts," Proc Soc Exb Biol Med, 1983, 172:139-52.
8. T. Nikadio et al., "Inhibitors of cyclic AMP Phospho ciesterase in medicinal plants," Jour Med Plant Res, 1981, 43:18-23.
9. F.Q. Evans, "The rationale use of glycyrrhetinic acid in dermatology," Brit Jour Clin Prac, 1958, 12: 269-74.
10. F. Ellingwood, American Materia Medica, Therapeutics and Pharmacognosy, (Eclectic Medical Publications, Portland:1983).
11. T. Chakrabarty, et al., "Centella asiatica in the treatment of leprosy," Sci Culture, 1976, 42:573.
12. J.P. Bosse, et al., "Clinical study of a new antikeloid drug," Ann Plastic Surgery, 1979, 3: 13-21.
13. H.W. Felter, The Eclectic Materia Medica: Pharmacology and Therapeutics, (Eclectic Medical Publications, Portland: 1983).
14. K. Bohm, "Choleretic action of some medicinal plants," Arzneimittel-Forsch, 1959, 9:376-78.
15. G. Weber and K. Galle, "The liver, a therapeutic target in dermatoses," Med Welt, 1983, 34:108-111.
16. Della, Loggia R. et al., "Evaluation of the anti-inflammatory activity of chamomile preparations," Planta Med, 1990, 56:657-8.
17. Donald M. Leung, M.D. "Atopic Dermatitis," Medical Scientific Update, Feb. 1994, vol. 12.

ENDOMETRIOSIS

Endometriosis is still a fairly misunderstood condition that occurs when displaced fragments of the uterine lining become engorged with blood every month and inadvertently lodge in areas other than the uterus, such as the ovaries. Endometrium tissue can also form in the fallopian tubes, the vagina, the pelvic floor, the bowel or in scar tissue that has grown in the abdominal wall after surgery. A recent study disclosed that the most common site of endometriosis is in the deep peritoneal cavity of the pelvis.

During each menstrual cycle, these tissue fragments bleed in the same way that the uterine lining does. Because blood cannot escape these abnormal locations, blisters can form that cause irritation and scarring of surrounding tissue. Consequently, a fibrous cyst can develop around each blister. These cysts can burst causing abnormal bleeding of dark, brown blood accompanied by pain. Because endometriosis is connected with the menstrual cycle it commonly occurs between the ages of 25 and 40. Endometriosis is more frequent in women who have not had children. It is estimated that 40 to 60 percent of women who undergo hysterectomies have had some form of endometriosis. Endometriosis affects approximately 12 million American females.

Symptoms

Endometriosis is characterized by severe abdominal pain and back pain, especially during or after menstrual periods, heavy periods (including the passage of clots and tissue), irregular periods, painful sexual intercourse, nausea, vomiting, and/or diarrhea or constipation during periods.

In most cases, endometriosis causes no perceivable symptoms or the symptoms are so mild, they are dismissed as inconsequential.

In some cases, pregnancy and breast feeding can decrease the symptoms of endometriosis. Women with the disorder do conceive at a lower rate and have a higher incidence of miscarriage and ectopic pregnancy. After childbirth, the symptoms of the disorder may return. In cases of endometriosis where periods are particularly heavy, an iron deficiency can occur.

Causes

One theory used to explain this disorder called "reflux menstruation" suggests that uterine contractions during heavy periods may force the lining upward, through the fallopian tubes. Another theory proposes that endometrial tissue can develop from undifferentiated cells in the abdomen. Spreading endometrial cells through the blood and lymph channels is also considered a possible cause of the disorder.

Other possible causes of the endometriosis include cauterization of the cervix, using IUD's or as a complication of a laparoscopy.

A relatively new theory suggests that endometriosis is a congenital birth defect resulting from the migration of endometrial cells.

Conventional Therapies

Your physician may choose to prescribe hormones which are contained in birth control pills along with Danazol. When taken over a period of months, these hormones reduce the flow of blood in menstruation. This reduction of blood allows for the destruction of existing abnormal tissue. Progesterone therapy or synthetic male hormones may also be used in more severe cases, which stop the menstrual cycle completely. In difficult cases, radiation therapy or surgery may be necessary. Nafarelin (in nasal spray) helps to shrink lesions but has some unpleasant side effects. Injections of leuprolide are also used but like nafarelin, cause a number of negative side effects. If drug therapy fails, a hysterectomy may be recommended.

Endometriosis is difficult to diagnose and a laparoscopy may be recommended. A small abdominal incision is made which allows the doctor to insert a lighted viewing device to examine the pelvic cavity. Laser surgery through a laparoscopy may be able to find and destroy adhesions and cysts. Some new options include a procedure called a near-contact laparoscopy which has had some dramatic success. In this procedure, all suspected growths or adhesions are removed from the entire pelvic cavity. Surgical techniques can help control the symptoms of this disorder, but the disease has a tendency to recur. The use of analgesics for pain and hormonal therapy are limited in their usefulness and can have significant side effects. There is no known accepted cure for endometriosis in the medical community.

Dietary Guidelines

- Concentrate on foods rich in natural bioflavonoids and cruciferous compounds like grapes, apricots, broccoli, cauliflower, peppers, cherries and cabbage.
- Eat a diet low in animal fats and high in linolenic acids found in vegetable sources and in essential fatty acid supplements.
- Use soy-based foods like tofu for their isoflavone content.
- Avoid meats and dairy products. Increase your intake of fish, which is a natural antiprostaglandin and can help control cramping.
- Some theories maintain that hormones routinely given to fatten poultry and cattle collect within the human system and may cause hormonal disorders.
- Avoid caffeine. Some women claim that caffeine increases the pain associated with endometriosis. It has also been implicated as a major contributor in the development of fibrocystic breast disease.

Recommended Nutritional Supplements

PRIMARY NUTRIENTS

EVENING PRIMROSE OIL This oil contains essential fatty acids that help to control the period cramping that accompanies endometriosis.[1] *Suggested Dosage:* Take as directed using either capsulized or liquid forms. Keep refrigerated.

VITAMIN E Helps to normalize hormones and to control symptoms associated with difficult periods. Clinical studies have found that women with endometrial bleeding were significantly improved after ten weeks of vitamin E therapy.[2] *Suggested Dosage:* 400 to 800 IU per day.

VITAMIN A Some studies have found that vitamin A helped to normalize heavy periods, with blood loss significantly reduced. In addition, women who suffer from heavy periods may develop a vitamin A deficiency.[3] *Suggested Dosage:* Take as directed.

VITAMIN C WITH BIOFLAVONOIDS Assists in the healing process and strengthens capillary walls. Vitamin C also increases the absorption of iron. Studies where women with heavy periods were treated with vitamin C with bioflavonoids saw significant improvements in the women.[4] *Suggested Dosage:* 500 mg with each of three meals per day.

VITAMIN K Works to keep blood clotting normally. The notion that heavy bleeding may be linked to a vitamin K deficiency should be considered.[5] *Suggested Dosage:* 200 mg per day. Liquid, fat-soluble chlorophyll is an excellent source of vitamin K. Alfalfa is also a good source of this vitamin.

IRON If menstrual periods are consistently heavy, a deficiency of iron may occur. In addition, a lack of iron may actually contribute to heavy periods.[6] *Suggested Dosage:* Take as directed using organic varieties and do not exceed suggested doses. One hundred mg daily is the normal dosage. Too much iron can be hazardous. Certain herbs like gentian and nettle are naturally high in iron.

VITAMIN B-COMPLEX Boosts blood cell production and contributes to hormonal balance while it also helps the body cope with stress. *Suggested Dosage:* Take as directed.

CALCIUM/MAGNESIUM Some theories claim endometriosis is related to the body's inability to absorb calcium. *Suggested Dosage:* 1,500 mg of calcium and 1,000 mg of magnesium per day. Use gluconate or chelated products.

WILD YAM (CREAM OR TOPICAL FORM) As a natural source of progesterone, wild yam is better absorbed and utilized through the skin than through oral ingestion. Raising progesterone can help to treat heavy bleeding and irregular periods.[7] *Suggested Dosage:* Use as directed. Make sure not to take the treatment while in the midst of the menstrual cycle.

HERBAL COMBINATION This combination should include black cohosh root, dong quai, passionflower, red raspberry leaves, fenugreek seeds, licorice root, chamomile, black haw bark, saw palmetto berries, wild yam root, kelp and butternut root bark. *Suggested Dosage:* Four to six capsules daily. For chronic conditions and imbalances, the maximum dosage of six capsules per day should be taken for several months or until normal function is restored. Best if used daily throughout the month. Consult a health care professional before using this formula if you are pregnant or lactating.

BLACK COHOSH ROOT: Black cohosh root was so highly valued by the American Indian for female disorders that it was named "squaw root." Today black cohosh has been proven to be such an effective remedy for painful menstrual cramps, dysmenorrhea, menopausal disorders and premenstrual complaints, it has received official recognition in Britain and Germany. Studies have shown black cohosh root has endocrine activity which mimics estrogen.[8] DONG QUAI: Also known as "angelica," there is no other herb used more widely in Chinese medicine for treatment of gynecological ailments than dong quai. Dong quai relieves menstrual cramps, corrects irregular or retarded menstrual flow and alleviates unpleasant symptoms associated with menopause due to its mild estrogenic effect.[9] PASSIONFLOWER: Many women experience anxiety prior to and during menses and other hormonally related complaints. Passionflower has a mild sedative action which is good for anxiety. It also helps to relieve uterine spasms and cramping.[10] RED RASPBERRY LEAVES: This herb has been used for various female afflictions including pregnancy and childbirth problems. It specifically strengthens and tonifies the uterus, stops hemorrhages, decreases excess and increases deficient menstrual flow and relieves painful menstruation by relaxing the smooth muscles.[11] FENUGREEK SEEDS: Although fenugreek seed has been used to assist proper menstruation and promote lactation, its main role in this formula stems from its other properties. Fenugreek is a tonic herb, a mild diuretic and a source of mucilage, which provides soothing demulcent effects. LICORICE ROOT: Licorice root is incorporated into about a third of all Chinese herbal formulas and in a majority of herbal blends designed to treat female reproductive problems. Licorice not only contains hormonal precursors but stimulates the production of estrogen which decreases the symptoms associated with hormone fluctuation. It is also prized for its demulcent and mild laxative properties. It also has significant anti-inflammatory and antispasmodic properties.[12] CHAMOMILE: Aside from chamomile's carminative and tonic properties, this herb has gained world recognition for its anodyne (pain relieving), antispasmodic, and antianxiety properties. BLACK HAW BARK: Another name for black haw bark is cramp bark which aptly suggests its inclusion in any formula designed to alleviate menstrual difficulties. Historical and folkloric use as well as scientific evidence have proven this bark to be effective against muscle spasms and menstrual dysfunction, especially inconsistent or irregular cycles.[13] SAW PALMETTO BERRIES: This herb has been scientifically and clinically proven effective for male and female genitourinary problems. One study has shown it to be many times more effective than prescription anti-inflammatory medication in the treatment of pelvic congestion associated with menstrual dysfunction.[14] As an interesting side note, saw palmetto can help to prevent the growth of unwanted facial hair in women. WILD YAM ROOT: Wild yam root contains the steroidal saponins, which are precursors to hormones like progesterone. Wild yam has antispasmodic effects and is soothing to the nerves. It is also diuretic and helps to eliminate painful urination. It is highly recommended for cramping. KELP: Kelp provides important trace elements which are often missing or deficient in Western diets. Trace elements assist with many metabolic processes in the body, without which may lead to various problems.

SECONDARY NUTRIENTS

CRANESBILL: Cranesbill is considered by many herbalists to possess a powerful astringent effect, which means it will have a profound ability to shrink or constrict tissue. The obvious result is a reduction in blood flow and prevention of hemorrhage. *Suggested Dosage:* Take as directed.

SIBERIAN GINSENG: Helps to control abnormal bleeding and is considered a female tonic. *Suggested Dosage:* Take as directed using guaranteed potency products.

SHEPHERD'S PURSE: An antihemorrhagic herb used traditionally for obstetric and gynecological purposes. *Suggested Dosage:* Take as directed.

Home Care Suggestions

◆ Exercise has been found to reduce estrogen levels which can aggravate the progression of endometriosis. Regular brisk walking is recommended as the best type of exercise.

◆ Acupuncture and acupressure are routinely used by the Chinese for endometriosis and should be investigated as a viable option.

◆ Use a warm, moist heat on your abdomen and lower back.

◆ Try using a lubricant if sexual intercourse is painful. A change of position may also eliminate pain.

◆ Use over-the-counter drugs that also act as anti-prostaglandins. Prostaglandin is the hormone that causes uterine contraction, which can sometimes result in menstrual cramping. Such drugs contain ibuprofen and are found in Advil, Medipren or Nuprin. However their long-term use can be associated with significant side effects, including damage to the gastrointestinal tract and the liver.

Other Supportive Therapies

YOGA: Yoga positions such as the cobra, bow or cat hump can help to control the pain associated with periods.

HOMEOPATHY: Chamomile is a traditional medicine for menstrual irregularities.

ACUPUNCTURE: Can help to stimulate and normalize hormone levels.

Scientific Facts-at-a-Glance

Dr. David Redwine of the St. Charles Medical Center in Bend, Oregon, does not believe that reflux menstruation is responsible for endometriosis. He has a theory which proposes that the condition results from a type of birth anomaly in which cells which should have become part of the uterus become misplaced and grow. Later in life, due to hormonal stimulation, these cells become darkened endometrial tissue. Dr. Redwine uses very closely-monitored laser scopes to carefully search for these cells and removes them. He says that many of the lesions which are endometrial are not typically dark, but must still be removed or the disease will recur. He has an impressive success rate which suggests that his methods are based on fact.

Spirit/Mind Considerations

Endometriosis is a serious condition and a very real disease. It can be debilitating for some women and put an enormous strain on relationships. Having to face a very difficult and incapacitating period every month can be both physically and emotionally taxing. It is important for any woman who suffers from difficult menstrual periods to inform her family so they will know what to expect. In addition, becoming aware of your cycle and learning to recognize cues can help. Endometriosis is not a normal condition and should be respected as a serious ailment that needs proper treatment. Make sure to find a doctor who has successfully treated this disease and will offer you the emotional and physical support you need.

Doctor's Notes

While hormonal dysfunction may not be the primary cause of endometriosis, regulating estrogen/progesterone levels is very useful. The herbs listed in this section work together to modulate female hormones. They treat anxiety and the painful cramping associated with endometriosis. Surgical treatment of this condition may become necessary if it is severe enough. While menopause usually ends endometriosis, estrogen replacement therapy may reactivate endometrial tissue. If you have had a hysterectomy, you may want to wait three to nine months before initiating replacement hormone therapy.

Additional Resources

Endometriosis Association, International Headquarters
Box RD 8585 N 76th Place
Milwaukee, WI 53223
800-992-3636

For more on Dr. Redwine's approach:
Endometriosis Treatment Program
St. Charles Medical Center
2500 NE Neff Road
Bend, OR 97701-6015
503-382-4321

Endnotes

1. Michael T. Murray, Encyclopedia of Nutritional Supplements, (Prima Publishing, Rocklin, Ca: 1996), 247-48

2. P. Dasgupta, et al., "Vitamin E (alpha tocopherol) in the management of menorrhagia associated with the use of intrauterine contraceptive devices," Inter Jour Fertility, 1983, 28: 55-56.

3. D.M. Lithgow and W.M. Politzer, "Vitamin A in the treatment of menorrhagia," So Afric Med Jour, 1977, 51: 191-93.

4. J.D. Cohen and H.W. Rubin, "Functional menorrhagia: treatment with bioflavonoids and vitamin C," Curr Ther Res, 1960, 2: 539.

5. R. Ubner and H. Ungerleider, "Vitamin K therapy in menorrhagia," South Med Jour, 1944, 37: 556-58.

6. B. Arvidsson, et al., "Iron prophylaxis in menorrhagia," Acta Ob Gyn Scand, 1981, 60: 157-60.

7. John R. Lee, Natural Progesterone: The Multiple Roles of a Remarkable Hormone, revised. (BLL Publishing, Sebastopol, California: 1993), 4. See also U.S. Barzel,"Estrogens in the prevention and treatment of postmenopausal osteoporosis: a review." Am Jour Med, (1988), 85: 847-850 and D.R. Felson, Y. Zhang, M.T. Hannan, et al., "The effect of postmenopausal estrogen therapy on bone density in elderly women." The New England Journal of Medicine. (1993), 329: 1141-1146.

8. E.M. Duker, et al., "Effects of extracts from Cimicifuga racemosa on gonadotropin release in menopausal women and ovariectomized rats," Planta Medica, 1991, 57(5): 420-24.

9. D. Zhy, "Dong quai," Amer Jour Clin Med, 1987, 15(3-4): 1987.

10. E. Speroni and E. Minghetti, "Neuropharmocological activity of extracts from Passiflora incarnata," Planta Medica, 1988, 54(6): 488-91.

11. Mark Pederson, Nutritional Herbology, (Wendell Whitman, Warsaw, In: 1995), 145.

12. C.H. Costello, E.V. Lynn, "Estrogenic substances from plants: Glycyrrhiza," Jour Amer Pharm Soc, 1950, 39: 177-80.

13. P.H. List, et al., Hagers Hanbuch der Pharmazeutischen Praxis, vols. 2-5, Springer-Verlag, Berlin.

14. Rebecca Flynn, M.S. Your Guide to Standardized Herbal Products, (One World Press, Prescott, AZ: 1995), 67-69.

EPILEPSY

George Frederick Handel, as well as many other famous individuals, were known epileptics and had to suffer from the stigma that used to be associated with this disease.

Epilepsy is a term that encompasses a number of different symptoms which are all linked to the dysfunction of brain electrical activity. Epilepsy occurs when brain cells send out signals that are abnormally strong for no apparent reason. As a result, this sudden excess electrical discharge brings on an epileptic seizure. During a seizure, the electrical impulses of the brain become chaotic and unregulated. Epilepsy usually begins in childhood or adolescence and is outgrown by one-third of its victims.

There are several forms of epilepsy and the type of seizure that occurs is dependent on its place of origin in the brain and how extensively it affects surrounding areas. Generalized seizures, which cause a loss of consciousness, affect the entire brain and body. Grand mal seizures fall into this classification. Partial seizures include simple seizures where consciousness is maintained and complex seizures where it becomes lost. Absence seizures refer to a condition where a momentary loss of consciousness occurs with no other sign of abnormal movement. Petit mal seizures fall into this category. This type of epilepsy is more common in children and this absence of consciousness can last from just a few seconds to a minute. The child may appear to be daydreaming. This type of seizure can occur several times a day and hinder school work and activity. Approximately, one person in 200 suffers from epilepsy. There are close to one million epileptics in the United States

Symptoms

GRAND MAL SEIZURES

Grand mal seizures are characterized by a sudden and complete loss of consciousness, falling down, a high-pitched cry, a stiffening of the arms and legs, rhythmic muscle jerking, incontinence, cessation of breathing which causes bluish skin, and/or clenched teeth or tongue biting.

Following the seizure which usually lasts two minutes, a relaxed state occurs in which the victim will feel sleepy, confused, and uncooperative for a period from 15 minutes to several hours. During this time, if you try to physically move or restrain the person, they may become combative. It's best to keep them warm and safe, until they can be moved.

PETIT MAL SEIZURES

Petit mal seziures are just that: petite. They are still aggravating, however, and are characterized by brief lapses of consciousness, staring, rhythmic twitching of face muscles or eyelids, and a complete cessation of whatever activity the person was engaged in prior to the episode.

After the seizure is over, normal activity is resumed. The person usually has no recollection of the seizure which can occur up to several hundred times a day.

COMPLEX PARTIAL SEIZURES

This type of epilepsy can vary in its symptoms. An aura or warning can sometimes precede an attack which may include a feeling of apprehension, an unusual smell, a distortion in visual perception, or an abdominal sensation. After the aura, consciousness is impaired with loss of speech and repetitive movements such as swallowing, hand movements, or gestures. Confusion is also common, as is forgetting the episode even happened.

Precautions

- Move anything away from the victim that could cause injury. Gently place the person on a bed on the floor.
- Loosen tight clothing around the neck.
- If possible, turn the victim on his or her side.
- Call an ambulance.
- Stay calm. A seizure can be very frightening to eyewitnesses. Often the victim's face will turn blue and stop breathing. Seizures are usually brief and the incidence of death during a seizure is very low.
- Do not try to restrain the victim or put anything in the mouth.
- Do not attempt to move the victim unless there is the danger of further injury.
- The most important things to consider when caring for someone who has a seizure is to let the convulsion run its course and to make sure the victim can breathe and will not be injured by furniture, etc.

Causes

The exact cause of an epileptic seizure remains somewhat of a mystery. While certain injuries to the head can cause the onset of epilepsy, in two out of three individuals suffering from the disorder, no structural abnormalities or scar tissue is present. In one third of epileptics, epilepsy is a secondary complication precipitated by physical damage to the brain through traumatic birth, bacterial meningitis, malaria, rickets, rabies, tetanus, malnutrition, poisoning, cerebral palsy, mental retardation, brain tumors, hydrocephalus, stroke, lack of oxygen, injury to the head and heredity.

New theories also point to chemicals found in aerosols, pesticides, diesel emissions and solvents as possible substances involved in triggering a seizure. In addition, the notion of food allergies cannot be dismissed in epilepsy. Links between celiac disease and epilepsy have been made. In other words, a food intolerance to gluten, oats, wheat or barley may be associated with epileptic seizures.

Seizures can be caused by a number of conditions such as fever, head trauma, infectious diseases or poisoning. Anyone who has suffered a seizure of any type should immediately see a physician.

Conventional Therapies

An electroencephalogram (EEG test) will be ordered by your doctor. It is a painless procedure and involves tracking brain wave patterns through electrodes that are positioned on the head. A skull x-ray may also be required if a possibility exists that the seizures are being caused by infection or injury. In some cases, a CAT scan of the brain will prove helpful in making an accurate diagnosis. The possibility of a brain tumor must be ruled out. Anticonvulsant drugs will be prescribed. A period of experimentation with several drugs may be necessary. Phenytoin (dilantin) has been widely prescribed in the past for epilepsy. It targets the motor cortex of the brain and inhibits the electrical brain waves that cause seizure activity. Phenobarbital, carbamazepine (Tegretol), valproate (Depakote), and ethosuximide (Zarontin) are other drugs commonly prescribed for epilepsy. Epileptics need to see their doctor regularly for blood tests that can determine whether anticonvulsant drugs are effective. Surgery is considered an option only in rare cases of epilepsy where a single area of brain damage exists such as scar tissue in the temporal lobe that could be removed.

Anyone who is taking anticonvulsant drugs should never stop taking them suddenly. The dose must be cut gradually to avoid bringing on seizures. This should be done only under a doctors supervision. The negative side effects of anticonvulsant can be decreased by careful attention to diet and exercise.

Dietary Guidelines

- Rule out food allergies (especially gluten) as a possible contributing factor.
- Eat a diet high in dark green leafy vegetables, carrots, raw fruits, fresh juices, whole grains, low-fat cheeses and low-fat meats.
- Avoid alcohol (which usually interacts with anticonvulsant drugs and can be lethal if mixed with phenobarbital), caffeine, coffee, tea, chocolate and artificial sweeteners, nicotine, refined sugars and flours.
- Eat regular, nutritious meals. Low blood sugar has also been linked to seizures, so avoiding high-glycemic foods that are low in fiber is crucial.
- Remember that antiseizure drugs such as Dilantin and Depakote can destroy nutrients such as most of the B-vitamins, suggesting that supplementation is vital for anyone taking these medicines.
- Eating foods like yogurt with active cultures is also recommended.
- Juicing green vegetables is also recommended. Use olive oil and stay away from artificial sweeteners.

Recommended Nutritional Supplements

Herbs, vitamins or minerals should never be used to take the place of anticonvulsant medication that is being taken for epilepsy. Herbal treatments can only help to eventually decrease the dosage or to counteract drug-induced side-effects.

PRIMARY NUTRIENTS

FOLIC ACID AND PANTOTHENIC ACID Some studies have found that supplementation of these nutrients can affect the frequency of epileptic seizures.[1] Both of these are vitally important for normal nerve cell behavior. *Suggested Dosage:* Take 400 mg of folic acid and 500 mg of pantothenic acid per day.

VITAMIN D Danish medical studies done on a small scale indicate that when vitamin D supplements were given to epileptics being treated by anticonvulsant drugs, the incidence of seizures was significantly reduced. Some epileptic medications interfere with the metabolism of vitamin D.[2] *Suggested Dosage:* Take as directed.

VITAMIN B3 OR NIACIN Studies have found that taking niacin can help to potentiate the pharmacological activity of certain anticonvulsant drugs like phenobarbital.[3] *Suggested Dosage:* 50 mg per day.

VITAMIN B1 OR THIAMINE Recent studies strongly suggest that epileptics have low blood levels of this vitamin. While this may be a residual effect of medication, the exact cause remains unknown.[4] *Suggested Dosage:* Take as directed.

VITAMIN B6 Essential for normal brain function. Due to the fact that anticonvulsant drugs deplete the body of B-vitamins, supplementation is vital. This vitamin has been used to treat a variety of brain disorders.[5] *Suggested Dosage:* Take as directed with your physician's knowledge.

VITAMIN E The use of natural vitamin E has been used in clinical double-blind studies and is thought to help reduce the incidence of seizures under certain circumstances.[6] *Suggested Dosage:* 400 to 800 IU daily.

MAGNESIUM A lack of this mineral has been found in epileptics.[7] It is needed to ensure proper nervous system function. *Suggested Dosage:* 500 mg per day in divided doses on an empty stomach. If you suspect you may be deficient in hydrochloric acid, take a supplement with your magnesium. Use chelated products.

MANGANESE Studies using this nutrient have concluded that supplementation may help to control both major and minor epileptic seizures.[8] *Suggested Dosage:* Take as directed.

SELENIUM Supplementation may be beneficial for early childhood seizures.[9] *Suggested Dosage:* Take as directed.

L-TAURINE AND L-TYROSINE These amino acids are important for the proper functioning of brain cells. Taurine is a neuroinhibitory amino acid.[10] *Suggested Dosage:* Do not take tyrosine if you are taking a MAO-inhibiting drug. Take as directed on an empty stomach with fruit juice.

GINKGO Ginkgo helps to stimulate brain function and can boost memory capacity which may be impaired by anticonvulsant drugs by enhancing oxygenation.[11] *Suggested Dosage:* Take as directed using standardized products.

HERBAL COMBINATION This combination should include kava kava, valerian root, hops, skullcap, and passionflower.

Suggested Dosage: Take two capsules with each meal and two before bedtime. If you feel drowsy, cut down your dosage.

KAVA KAVA: This herb contains kavalactones which have distinct anticonvulsant and muscle relaxant properties which act on the limbic system of the brain, which is the seat of brain activity and contributes to inducing sleep. Unlike narcotic drugs, kava is not addictive, nor does it lose its effectiveness over time.[12] VALERIAN ROOT: Compounds contained in this herb interact with various brain receptor sites to promote sedation much in the same way that barbiturates like phenobarbital do but without the dangerous side effects associated with hypnotic and tranquilizing drugs.[13] HOPS: Hops has natural calmative, sedative and hypnotic properties which contribute to controlled brain activity by promoting sleep and relaxation.[14] Hops has traditionally been used to treat insomnia and is added to this formula for its ability to act synergistically with other nervine herbs. SKULLCAP: This botanical is considered an anticonvulsant with distinct antispasmodic properties that was historically used to treat convulsions, hysteria, muscle twitching and delirium.[15] PASSIONFLOWER: Considered a natural CNS depressant and antispasmodic, this herb contains alkaloids and flavonoids which have non-addictive narcotic effects which quiet the brain and promote sleep and relaxation.[16]

SECONDARY NUTRIENTS

ACIDOPHILUS: Important when taking any prolonged drug therapy. Helps to replace friendly bacteria essential for good health. *Suggested Dosage:* Take as directed in the morning or just before retiring on an empty stomach using milk-free products with guaranteed bacterial count. Check expiration date.

CALCIUM: Works to ensure the proper function of nerve transmission in the brain and spinal cord. *Suggested Dosage:* Take as directed with magnesium using gluconate or citrate products if possible.

ZINC: Works to protect brain cells. In addition, anticonvulsant drugs can cause zinc depletion. *Suggested Dosage:* 50 mg per day using gluconate or picolinate varieties. Lozenges are acceptable. Caution: Do not exceed over 100 mg of zinc per day.

CHOLINE: Important as a protective agent for nerve cells in the brain. *Suggested Dosage:* Take as directed.

Home Care Suggestions

- ◆ Wear a tag or keep a card in your wallet which identifies you as a epileptic and carry it with you at all times.
- ◆ The possible value of hyperbaric therapy which involves high pressure oxygen should be investigated.
- ◆ One of the best things an epileptic can do is to exercise on a regular basis. While water sports and high-risk activities might be discouraged, walking, jogging, or playing tennis can help to keep the mind alert and help counteract the side effects of drug therapy.
- ◆ Make sure you get adequate sleep every night. A lack of sleep can increase your risk for a seizure. Interrupted sleep patterns can also cause fatigue which, if severe enough, can result in seizure activity.

◆ Get involved with various epileptic associations located throughout the country.

Other Supportive Therapies

BIOFEEDBACK: Several studies have suggested that with practice, epileptics can learn to control their seizures through visualization and biofeedback, which is the ability to actually direct biological events with the mind.

ACUPUNCTURE: Stimulating certain pressure points can help to relieve cranial problems and may help to discourage seizures.

BACH FLOWER REMEDIES: Clematis is used to restore clear thinking after a seizure and Rescue Remedy for attacks is also suggested.

MEDITATION: "Destressing" and clearing the mind of all conscious thought can be very helpful for anyone with epilepsy.

Scientific Facts-at-a-Glance

Recent studies have found that there may be a link between DPT and MMR vaccine and an increased risk for seizures. Allergies to milk products and gluten may also trigger seizures.[16] Unfortunately, when someone has a seizure, so many factors may be involved that care must be taken to arrive at a conclusive diagnosis of epilepsy, which is usually confirmed by altered brain waves as seen on an EEG reading. The link between colon congestion and epilepsy has also been suggested and should be considered.

Spirit/Mind Considerations

Epileptics have a tendency to feel that their condition is something to be ashamed of. In the past, the disease may have been viewed as a social stigma, but present knowledge and treatment of the disease provide a much more positive outlook for epileptics. With medication, most epileptics lead a perfectly normal life. Being over-protective of epileptics can create more psychological stress than anything else. Children with only minimal restrictions should be able to participate in sports and other activities, although increased supervision is encouraged. Adults with active seizures should avoid high-risk jobs such as construction, driving or operating dangerous machinery.

Anyone suffering from epilepsy should inform his or her co-workers and friends of the condition with instructions on what to do if a seizure occurs. In addition, keeping the mind calm by utilizing meditation and relaxation are invaluable tools for controlling seizures. Often, epileptics are more vulnerable to problems if they are nervous or afraid. Adrenaline surges may aggravate the abnormal electrical brain activity which brings on a seizure.

Prevention

◆ Take your medication at the same time each day and in the exact prescribed dose.

◆ Do not attempt to blow up balloons. For some epileptics this activity can precipitate a seizure.

◆ Do not become overly fatigued or stressed. Use exercise, biofeedback and relaxation techniques, including meditation to relax.

◆ Be more careful if you have an infectious illness, especially if a fever is present. This type of situation may increase your susceptibility to a seizure.

◆ Don't get up too quickly in the morning. Allow your body to slowly adjust to waking up. Perform stretching exercises while still in bed and take some deep breaths.

◆ Some epileptics have used biofeedback and have actually been able to avoid a seizure that they feel coming on through some mental distraction. While this is not recommended alone, its possible value should be explored.

Doctor's Notes

Epilepsy still perplexes doctors and the exact mechanisms which trigger a seizure are not completely understood. One thing is certain: Anxiety, lack of sleep and poor nutrition directly affect the incidence of seizures. Your optimal goal should be to remain seizure-free on the least possible amount of medication. If you want to try supplements, tell your doctors and then slowly lower your dosages and monitor yourself closely. During this time period, you will want someone else to drive you and stay in safe environments. While you may not find it possible to completely eliminate all anticonvulsant drugs, you may be able to function on much smaller dosages than was originally assumed.

Additional Resources

The Epilepsy Foundation of America
4351 Garden City Drive, Suite 406
Landover, MD 20785
301-459-3700

Epilepsy Concern International Service Group
Executive Director
1282 Wynnewood Drive
West Palm Beach, FL 33417
407-683-0044

Endnotes

1. F.B.Givverd, et al., "The influence of folic acid on the frequency of epileptic attacks," Eur J Clin Pharmacol, 1981, 19(1):57-60.

2. N.W. Flodin, "Anticonvulsant drugs interfere with vitamin D and calcium metabolism," Pharmacolgy of Micronutrients, (Alan R. Liss Inc., New York, 1988).

3. N.D. Bourgeois, et al., "Potentiation of the antiepileptic activity of phenobarbital by nicotinamide," Epilepsia, 1983, 24:238-44.

4. K.H. Krause, et al., "B-vitamins in epileptics," Biblthca Nutr Dieta, 1986, 38:154-67.

5. A. Sholer, and C. Pfeiffer, "Vitamin B6 and the treatment of mental disease," Int Clin Nutr Rev, 1988, 8(3).

6. C. Sullivan, et al., "Seizures and natural vitamin E," Letter. Med Jour Aust 1990, 52:613-14.

7. P.L. Jooste, et al., "Epileptic-type convulsions and magnesium deficiency," Aviat Space Environ Med, 1979, 50(7):734-35.

8. C. Pfeiffer and S. LaMola, "Zinc and manganese in the schizophrenias," JAMA, 1977, 238:1805.

9. G.F. Weber, et al., "Glutathione peroxidase deficiency and childhood seizures," Lancet, 1991, 337:1443-4.

10. L. Durelli L and R. Tutani. "The current status of taurine in epilepsy," Clin Neuropharmacol, 1983, 6(1):37-48.

11. J. Kleijnen and P. Knipschild, "Ginkgo," Lancet, 1992, 340: 1136-39.

12. E. Holm, et al., "Studies on the profile of the neurophysiological effects of D,L Kavain: Cerebral sites of action and sleep-wakefulness-rhythm in animals," Arzneimittel-Forsch, 1991, 41: 673-83.

13. T. Mennini, et al., "In vitro study on the interaction of extracts and pure compounds from Valeriana officinalis roots with GABA. Benzodiazepine, and barbiturate receptors in rat brain," Fitoterapia, 1993, 54(4): 291-300.

14. Michael T. Murray, The Healing Power or Herbs, 2nd ed. (Prima Publishing, Rocklin, CA., 1992): 371.

15. N. Sopranzi, et al., "Biological and electroencephalographic parameters in rats in relation to Passiflora incarnata," Clin Ter, 1990, 132(5): 329-33.

16. K.L. Reichelt, et al., "Gluten, milk proteins and autism: Dietary intervention effects on behavior and peptide secretion," Jour Appl Nutr, 1990, 42(1):1-11.

FEVER

A fever is not a disease. It's a symptom that indicates the presence of a disease. Fever occurs when there is an elevation in body temperature. The presence of a fever usually indicates that the body is fighting some type of infection. The normal body temperature ranges from 98 to 99° F. Temperature is generally at its lowest in the morning. Generally speaking, children have higher body temperatures than adults. Elevating the body's temperature is a natural reaction of the immune system to destroy bacteria and viruses.

Symptoms

Fevers are usually associated with hot or clammy skin, sweating, headache, shivering (a sensation of being cold can be experienced either by lowering the temperature of the surrounding environment or by raising the body temperature), goose bumps, increased hunger and thirst, rapid breathing, confusion, delirium, seizures and possible death with a very high fever.

How high a fever climbs is not necessarily indicative of how serious the condition is that caused it.

Precautions

A doctor should be consulted immediately for any fever that goes above 102° F in adults, 101° F if over the age of 60, and 102° F in a child. In addition, see a physician for any fever present in babies less than three months old, fevers that linger more than three days, fevers accompanied by rash, headache, stiff neck, back pain or painful urination, or any fever that accompanies diabetes, heart or lung disease. Chronic recurring fevers should also be checked out. A prolonged high fever can cause brain damage or dehydration. A fever may indicate the presence of a serious condition. Remember that a rectal temperature can be up to a degree higher than one taken by mouth or under the arm.

Never administer aspirin to anyone under 21 who is feverish. If a viral infection is present, using aspirin increases the risk of Reye's syndrome, a potentially fatal condition. Aspirin may also cause gastrointestinal upset or even damage. It is also important to carefully read dosage recommendations on products like infant Tylenol. These drops are actually stronger than solutions for older children. If given round the clock, toxicity can occur and liver damage is a possibility. Make sure your doses are completely accurate and that the amount recommended by your doctor corresponds to the actual product you buy.

Causes

Bacterial and viral infections are the most common cause of a fever and are present in colds and flu sore throats, tonsillitis, typhoid, earaches, diarrhea, urinary tract infections, childhood diseases such as roseola, chicken pox, mumps, measles, pneumonia, appendicitis and meningitis.

When certain infections are present, proteins referred to as pyrogens are released which act on the temperature-controlling center of the brain. Other conditions that can cause a fever are dehydration, heat exhaustion, sunburn, heart attack, drug withdrawal and tumors of the lymphatic system.

Overdressing a baby or small child or leaving a child in a hot car can actually cause overheating.

Conventional Therapies

Your doctor will want to find out if an infection is causing the fever. The eyes, throat, skin, lungs, glands and abdomen will be examined. Blood and urine tests may be ordered. In certain cases, a chest x-ray or spinal tap may be necessary to rule out pneumonia or spinal meningitis. If a bacterial infection is present, antibiotics will be prescribed. Antipyretic drugs to lower temperature are routinely recommended and are usually over-the-counter preparations.

Dietary Guidelines

- The value of "starving a fever" has been questioned. The presence of a fever actually increases the body's need for calories.
- Foods that are recommended are those high in liquid content such as fresh fruits and vegetables.
- In addition, mild foods are encouraged in the form of whole grains, yogurt, etc.
- If a child with a fever refuses to eat, encourage drinking instead. Fluid intake is extremely important when a fever is present.
- Fruit and vegetable juices that are low in sodium are excellent.
- Fresh lemon juice in water is also recommended.

Recommended Nutritional Supplements

PRIMARY NUTRIENTS

VITAMIN A Fights infection and boost the functions of the immune system by increasing white blood cell count and enhancing antibody activity.[1] *Suggested Dosage:* Adults should take 25,000 IU daily . Children's dosages should be adjusted according to age and weight. Pregnant women should not take over 10,000 IU of vitamin A per day. Emulsion formulas may be more convenient for children than gel caps.

PROTEIN SUPPLEMENT Necessary for tissue repair. During periods of fever, tissue damage can occur. Taking extra protein can help supply the body with the extra boost it needs to recover from the effects of a fever. *Suggested Dosage:* Use as directed. Powders designed to mix with liquid are good and can be put in the blender with ice and fruit. Soy sources of protein are recommended.

VITAMIN C WITH BIOFLAVONOIDS Helps to reduce fevers and facilitates the elimination of toxins. Ascorbic acid has well

documented antibacterial and antiviral properties.[2] *Suggested Dosage:* 10,000 mg per day in divided doses with meals. Children's doses should be calculated according to age. Use esterized or buffered vitamin C if stomach problems occur. Calcium ascorbate forms of vitamin C are also good for children. If diarrhea occurs, lower the dosage. Vitamin C powder can be mixed in water and taken as a fluid supplement as well.

GARLIC A natural antibiotic and natural immunostimulant. Garlic has some remarkable anti-infection properties.[3] *Suggested Dosage:* Two capsules with each of three meals per day.

BARLEY WATER Helps to keep fever down. Barley water can be made by covering barley with water and steeping it for thirty minutes and then draining off the liquid. *Suggested Dosage:* One-half cup every two hours.

ACIDOPHILUS Keeps the bowel supplied with friendly bacteria which help to fight infection and keep immunity fortified. In addition, if you or your child has been on antibiotics for an infection, replacing good flora in the intestinal ecosystem is vital.[4] *Suggested Dosage:* Take as directed using guaranteed bacterial count products with bifidobacteria. Use milk-free varieties and check expiration date.

HERBAL COMBINATION This combination should include echinacea, goldenseal root, myrrh gum, garlic, licorice root, blue vervain, butternut root bark and kelp. *Suggested Dosage:* Six to twelve capsules daily. Should not be used for more than three weeks at a time. For a child, use appropriate age and weight dosage adjustments. Do not use this formula for more than two weeks consecutively.

ECHINACEA: A tremendous amount of scientific documentation is mounting supporting its various uses. In the United Kingdom it is used to fight chronic, viral and bacterial infections, pathogenic organisms in the blood, boils, various skin complaints, colds and influenza. In Germany it is used to treat infections of the head, nose and throat.[5] Some herbs like *Parthenium integrifolium* have been substituted for the true echinacea and labeled as echinacea. Don't accept substitutes and insist on the real plant. GOLDENSEAL ROOT: Infection-susceptible tissues of the body are protected by a mucus lining, which helps to keep out viruses and bacteria. When the mucus lining is weak or disrupted, pathogens can more easily enter and cause infection and subsequent fever. Goldenseal root is recognized by many herbalists and natural healers as possessing an ability to strengthen the mucus lining, making it harder for pathogens to penetrate. Two of goldenseal's more active compounds, hydrastine and berberine, have demonstrated effectiveness in treating various bacterial and viral infections, especially those of the respiratory tract.[6] MYRRH GUM: Myrrh gum has some similar properties as found in echinacea and goldenseal root. Myrrh gum stimulates phagocyte activity and reduces inflammation of the mucus secreting mucosa.[7] Myrrh gum also helps with skin problems, ulcers, and acts as an antiseptic and anti-inflammatory. GARLIC: Garlic is another herb that can be considered a tonic. Garlic can increase the number of leukocytes (white blood cells) which help fight infections. In addition, garlic increases perspiration which further cleanses the body, which is especially helpful when a fever is present.[8] LICORICE ROOT: Stimulates secretion of the hormone aldosterone from the adrenal cortex. This can produce a higher energy level which is usually needed when combating infections which cause fevers to occur. Licorice also has antiviral and antibacterial activity.[9] Long-term consumption of licorice is not recommended as it may cause weakness, electrolyte imbalances, water retention and hypertension. BLUE VERVAIN: Blue vervain has an ability to break the cycle of chronically occurring infections. It has been used for colds and flu and has the ability to reduce fever.[10] BUTTERNUT ROOT BARK: Butternut is a mild laxative and is included to improve liver function and stimulates bile production and flow, which helps to fight infection and also lowers fever.[11] KELP: Provides needed trace elements important in many metabolic processes in the body. These nutrients may further support the healing process and return the body to normal function.

SECONDARY NUTRIENTS

ASTRAGALUS: A Chinese herb which contains specific compounds that have impressive immuno-stimulatory properties. *Suggested Dosage:* Take as directed using standardized products.

BLACK ELDER: A traditional herbal treatment for fevers. *Suggested Dosage:* Take as directed using standardized products.

ELDER FLOWER, CATNIP AND PEPPERMINT TEA: When taken together, these herbs help to induce sweating and lower body temperature. *Suggested Dosage:* Take as directed. A tea or decoction is the easiest method and can be made from steeping dried herbs in boiling water.

WILLOWBARK: A natural analgesic rich in saliclylates which are aspirin-related compounds. Use for adults only. Do not give to children to avoid the risk of Reye's syndrome. *Suggested Dosage:* Take as directed using standardized products.

Home Care Suggestions

- ◆ Drink plenty of fluids. Fever can cause excessive sweating and loss of water. Keeping your fluids up can make it easier to bring a temperature down.
- ◆ Change clothing and bedding often if sweating is increased.
- ◆ Do not use a cold bath or an alcohol rub to bring down a fever. Tepid or warm baths are recommended so that body temperature is not brought down too quickly which can result in chills. Sponging the limbs with tepid or warm water is also effective.
- ◆ Keep your activity down. Although increasing exercise is accepted by some as a way to promote sweating and eliminate toxins, the presence of a fever and exercise both can stress the heart.
- ◆ Keep clothing appropriate. Do not overdress infants or small children.

Other Supportive Therapies

HYDROTHERAPY: Taking baths in tepid water that is just room temperature can help to bring down a fever and may be beneficial if chilling does not occur. Avoid using cold water.

HOMEOPATHY: Aconite 30C, Belladonna, 30C, Ferrum phos. 6C, Nux vomica 30C and Pulsatilla 12C are all used for fevers.

MASSAGE: Foot massage in which the big toe is stimulated can be helpful.

Scientific Facts-at-a-Glance

It can be very frightening for a parent to witness a seizure brought on by the presence of a fever. Contrary to popular notion, convulsions are usually not related to how high a fever is but rather how rapidly it rises. Some children can experience a febrile convulsion with a relatively low fever. Doctors will often place a child with febrile seizures on phenobarbital therapy until they reach a certain age. This practice is considered rather controversial. The potential liabilities of this approach as compared to its possible benefits should be discussed with your doctor.

Spirit/Mind Considerations

Fevers can initiate some very interesting brain mechanisms which may result in nightmares or fever deliriums. These experiences can be very frightening for children and should be managed with comfort and understanding. Some children are very prone to night terrors with fevers. Parents should be aware of these frightening episodes so they can be prepared to offer security. The clinginess that most children demonstrate when they have a fever indicates their need for extra physical comfort. Take the time to hold your child and reassure them with gentle touching or rocking.

Prevention

- ◆ A fever is a normal reaction of the body's immune system and is an integral part of combating infection. A fever should not be prevented. It should be watched and not allowed to climb too high.
- ◆ Fortifying the immune system so that resistance to infection is high and avoiding environments where exposure to infection is great can help avoid the illnesses commonly associated with fevers.

Doctor's Notes

Many physicians and health practitioners believe that a mild fever (under 100° F) can actually speed recovery from infection and should not be suppressed. By taking aspirin, ibuprofen or acetaminophen, fevers can be reduced. At the same time, the immune system can become suppressed to a certain extent by these medicines. This formula is not just for those suffering colds and flu, but it is for infections of varying types and origins.

Endnotes

1. R.D. Semba, "Vitamin A, immunity and infection," Clin Info Dis 1994, 19: 489-99.

2. R.E. Cathcart, "The third face of vitamin C," Jour Orthomol Med, 1992, 7: 197-200.

3. M.A. Adetumbi and B.H. Lau, "Allium sativum (garlic): a natural antibiotic," Med Hypoth, 1983, 12: 227-37.

4. G. Zoppi, et al., "Oral bacteriotherapy in clinical practice, I: The use of different preparations in the treatment of acute diarrhea," Euro Jour Ped, 1982, 139: 22-24.

5. R. Bauer and H. Wagner, "Echinacea species as potential immunostimulatory drugs," Econ Med Plant Res, 1991, 5: 253-321.

6. D. Sun, et al., "Berberine sulfate blocks adherence of streptococcus pyogenes to epithelial cells, fobronectin and hexadecane," Antimivrob Agents Chemo, 1988, 32: 1370-74.

7. Encyclopedia of Chinese Drugs, 1977, Shanghai Scientific and Technical Publications, People's Republic of China.

8. H.P. Koch, "Garlicin, Fact or Fiction," Phytother Res, 1993, 7: 278-80.

9. C.H. Costello, E.V. Lynn, "Estrogenic substances from plants: Glycyrrhiza," Jour Amer Pharm Soc, 1950, 39: 177-80.

10. S. Sakai, "Pharmacological actions of verben officinalis," Gitu Ika Daigaku Kiyo, 1963, 11 (1): 6-17.

11. J.D. Gunn, Domestic Physician or Home Book of Health, (Moore, Wilstach, Keys, Cincinnati: 1971).

FIBROCYSTIC BREAST DISEASE

While it is vital to have any lump or mass checked by your doctor, chances are that the breast lump you discover is one of several kinds of harmless lumps that typically occur in breast tissue. For that very reason, a woman should never be afraid to see her doctor, fearing the worst. The majority of breast lumps are not cancerous. A breast lump refers to any mass, cyst, swelling or thickening of the breast tissue. Breast tissue is very sensitive to hormonal changes and can enlarge, thicken and shrink as much as 50 percent throughout the menstrual cycle. Seventy-five percent of breast lumps are not cancerous, and the majority of lumps that cause pain are not malignant. All breast lumps need medical assessment. Fibrocystic breast disease is typically found in women of childbearing age. It usually involves the presence of lumps which are round and move about freely. They can be either firm or soft.

Symptoms

Fibrocystic disease is the most common cause of breast lumps and occurs when cysts and thickening of the milk glands develops. It usually affects women between the ages of 30 and 50 and can cause one or both breasts to become lumpy and tender to the touch, particularly just prior to a menstrual period. Symptoms include tenderness and lumpiness in the breasts. The discomfort is usually most pronounced before menstruation. Breast cysts may change in size, but they are benign. A cyst is tender and moves freely—it feels like an eyeball behind the eyelid. In contrast, a cancerous growth usually does not move freely, is most often not tender, and does not go away.

Causes

Normally, fluids from breast tissues are collected and transported out of the breasts by means of the lymphatic system. However, if there is more fluid than the system can cope with, small spaces in the breast may fill with fluid forming cysts. Many breast cysts swell before and during menstruation and the resulting pressure causes pain. Cysts may even beget more cysts. A breast lump pressing against a milk gland can stimulate production of the pituitary hormone prolactin, which in turn results in milk secretion. The milk-producing glands may multiply and carry milk into the supporting fibrous tissue, causing further cyst formation.

TYPES OF CYSTS/BREAST LUMPS

Fibroadenomas

Firm, rubbery, mobile and painless masses of tissue detected in the breast are usually benign fibroadenomas, which are commonly found in women from 20 on up. A fibroadenoma is usually a single lump that is commonly found on the upper section of the breast.

Lipoma

A lipoma is a benign, painless tumor that is comprised of fatty tissue and can sometimes cause the breast to change in shape and size. A intraductal papilloma is a wart-like growth that forms within a milk duct and can cause a nipple discharge that is either clear or dark and bloody. A pea sized lump may be detected just beneath the nipple. While this type of breast lump is considered harmless, it can become malignant.

Cystosarcoma

A cystosarcoma is a tumor that grows in the connective tissue of the breast and can become quite large very rapidly. It is usually benign but can, in rare instances, become malignant.

Cancerous Breast Lump

A cancerous breast lump is usually located on the upper, outer part of the breast. The lump is usually felt instead of seen and in most cases, is not painful. Most malignant breast lumps are the size of a pea and feel hard to the touch, although this is not always the case. Other symptoms of a malignant breast lump include a dark discharge form the nipple, a retraction or indentation of the nipple, and a dimpled area of crease skin which can be seen over the lump. In 90 percent of cases, only one breast is affected with a malignant lump.

CAUTION: Any change in the breast, nipple discharge or lump needs immediate medical attention.

Conventional Therapies

NOTE: Mammograms alone are not considered an effective way to diagnose a breast lump. Using aspiration or lump biopsies in combination with a mammogram is the best way to evaluate a breast lump.

Today aspiration, in which a needle is inserted into the lump and a sample of the fluid is retrieved, is a common way to evaluate breast cysts. Often, just aspirating the fluid out of the cyst will prevent its return in the future. Fibroadenomas, intraductal papillomas and other benign breast lumps are usually surgically removed to confirm that they are not malignant. These types of lumps may continue to grow if not removed. Very small lipomas or calcium deposits are not usually surgically removed. Lump biopsies are also routinely done as out-patient procedures in which a local anesthetic is used and a sample of the lump tissue is surgically removed for laboratory analysis. If cancer is discovered, blood tests, x-rays and other methods of scanning will be ordered to determine whether the disease has spread to other areas of the body.

After mammography, a new ultrasound technique can help to reduce uncertainty about whether a breast mass is malignant or not. Using high-definition digital ultrasound imaging can help to reduce unnecessary biopsies according to Kenneth Taylor, MD, Ph.D., at Yale University. The drug danocrine (Danazol), a hormone which acts through the pituitary gland, can reduce the function of the ovaries. This in turn decreases the amount of estrogen in the breast, shrinking the lumps. Danocrine is not effective for all women, but about 60 percent notice results within a few weeks. Many report less pain or tenderness. The drug may have some unpleasant effects. Natural therapies may be just as effective and infinitely safer.

Dietary Guidelines

- ◆ Eat a low-fat, high-fiber diet.
- ◆ Eat plenty of raw foods, including seeds, raw nuts, and grains. Emphasize fresh bananas, apples, grapes, grapefruit, fresh vegetables, and active-culture yogurt.
- ◆ Soy-based foods like tofu are highly recommended for their isoflavone content which helps to bind bad estrogen.
- ◆ Cruciferous vegetables like cabbage, broccoli, and Brussels sprouts contain indoles which also work to protect breast tissue from estrogen metabolites.
- ◆ Liberally consume whole grains and legumes.
- ◆ Therapeutic foods like garlic, onions and shiitake mushrooms are also good.
- ◆ Do not consume coffee, tea, caffeine drinks or alcohol.
- ◆ Avoid dairy products and animal meats.
- ◆ Do not eat hydrogenated fats found in margarine and minimize fried foods, salt, sugar and all white flour products.

Recommended Nutritional Supplements

PRIMARY NUTRIENTS

VITAMIN E Protects breast tissue due to its antioxidant ability and helps to modulate hormones. Clinical studies have found that breast tenderness and cystic lesions dramatically improved with vitamin E therapy.[1] *Suggested Dosage:* 800 to 1,200 IU daily. NOTE: Taking lipoic acid with vitamin E can help to sustain its effects for longer periods of time.

EVENING PRIMROSE OIL This oil has essential fatty acids which have natural antiprostaglandin agents which may help to reduce breast lumps. Studies have found that breast tenderness responded well to evening primrose oil therapy.[2] *Suggested Dosage:* 1,500 mg twice daily.

ISOFLAVONES These compounds which are considered phytoestrogens are found in soy-based foods and have the ability to protect breast tissue from the formation of tumors in a variety of beneficial ways.[3] *Suggested Dosage:* Take as directed.

INDOLES These phytochemicals are found in cruciferous vegetables like cabbage. Indole-3 carbinol can help to negate the effect of bad circulating estrogen so that it does not prompt the growth of breast tumors. The high intake of cabbage in Asian cultures is thought to be partially responsible for low rates of breast cancer. *Suggested Dosage:* Take as directed looking for indole-3-carbinol content.

WILD YAM CREAM This herb contains diosgenin which is a precursor to progesterone. It can help to raise progesterone levels and balance out estrogen which causes breast tissue to enlarge and become painful. Dr. Lee, who has done extensive research on natural progesterone believes that it can dramatically reduce fibrocystic disease.[4] *Suggested Dosage:* Take as directed for two weeks prior to the menstrual period rotating sites and taking a break during menstrual period days.

VITAMIN A Helps to keep breast ducts functioning properly and scavenges for free radicals in breast tissue. Using this vitamin has proven its ability to reduce breast pain.[5] *Suggested Dosage:* 15,000 IU daily. If you are pregnant, do not exceed 10,000 IU daily.

HERBAL COMBINATION This combination should contain the following herbs: black cohosh root, blue cohosh, dong quai, passion flower, red raspberry leaves, fenugreek seeds, licorice root, chamomile, black haw bark, saw palmetto berries, wild yam root, kelp, butternut root bark. *Suggested Dosage:* Four to six capsules daily. For chronic conditions and imbalances maximum dosage of six capsules per day should be taken for several months. CAUTION: Do not take these herbs if pregnant or lactating.

BLACK COHOSH ROOT: Black cohosh has been proven to be an effective remedy for painful menstrual cramps and other hormonally induced disorders and has received official recognition in Britain and Germany. Studies have shown black cohosh root to have endocrine activity with the ability to mimic estrogen.[6] BLUE COHOSH: This herb was used so extensively by Native American women, it also became known as squaw root. It is effective for menstrual cramps and PMS-related symptoms. It acts as a natural antispasmodic which helps to relax uterine muscle. DONG QUAI: There is no other herb used more widely in Chinese medicine for treatment of gynecological ailments than dong quai. Dong quai relieves menstrual cramps, corrects irregular or retarded menstrual flow, and alleviates unpleasant symptoms associated with menopause. Dong quai is said to have analgesic properties but this is probably due, in part, to its antispasmodic effect.[7] PASSION FLOWER: Many women experience anxiety prior to and during menses, and discomforts such as hot flashes when adjusting to menopause. Passion flower contributes a sedative action for anxiety and relieves spasms and cramps.[8] It has an overall calming effect. RED RASPBERRY LEAVES: Red raspberry leaves have long been used for various female afflictions during pregnancy and child birth in addition to those associated with menses. More specifically it strengthens and tonifies the uterus, stops hemorrhages, decreases excess and increases deficient menstrual flow, and relieves painful menstruation by relaxing the smooth muscles.[9] FENUGREEK SEEDS: Although fenugreek seeds have been used to assist proper menstruation and promote lactation, its main role in this formula stems from its other properties. Fenugreek is a tonic, mild diuretic, and a source for mucilage which provides soothing demulcent properties. Like many other seeds, fenugreek is nutritious and restorative, strengthening those recovering from illness or imbalances. LICORICE

ROOT: Licorice root is incorporated into about a third of all Chinese herbal formulas and a majority of the formulas dealing with female reproductive problems. This is an indication that it has tremendous versatility. Indeed, licorice supports the effects of all the other herbs of the formula. Licorice not only contains hormonal precursors but stimulates the production of estrogen.[10] This has been shown to decrease the symptoms associated with hormone fluctuation. CHAMOMILE: Aside from chamomile's carminative and tonic properties, this herb has gained world recognition for its anodyne (pain relieving), antispasmodic, and antianxiety properties. Chamomile has demonstrated its worth in many clinical studies, officially monographed in Britain, Belgium, France, and Germany. BLACK HAW BARK: Historical and folkloric use as well as scientific evidence have proven this bark to be effective against muscle spasms and menstrual dysfunction, especially inconsistent estrus cycles and menstrual cramping.[11] SAW PALMETTO BERRIES: One study has shown this herb to be many times more effective than prescription anti-inflammatory medication in the treatment of pelvic congestion associated with menstrual dysfunction.[12] As an interesting side note, saw palmetto can prevent the growth of unwanted facial hair in women. WILD YAM ROOT: Wild yam root contains the steroidal saponins botogenin and diosgenin. These are precursors to cortisone and other hormones like progesterone.[13] Wild yam has antispasmodic effects and is soothing to the nerves. It is also diuretic and helps to eliminate painful urination. It is highly recommended for cramping. KELP: Kelp provides important trace elements which are often missing or deficient in Western diets. Trace elements assist with many metabolic processes in the body, without which may lead to various problems. Kelp contains algin which provides soothing benefits to the GI tract. BUTTERNUT ROOT BARK: Butternut is a soothing laxative which helps to restore general health and sense of well-being. Its laxative effect in this formula may be too gentle for it to be obvious.

SECONDARY NUTRIENTS

VITAMIN B-COMPLEX: B-complex vitamins are important for all enzyme systems in the body. *Suggested Dosage:* 50 mg 3 times daily, with meals.

VITAMIN C: Needed for proper immune function, tissue repair, and adrenal hormone balance. *Suggested Dosage:* 2,000 to 4,000 mg daily, in divided doses.

ZINC: Helps to boost immunity. *Suggested Dosage:* 50 mg daily. Do not exceed a total of 100 mg daily from all supplements. Used for repair of tissues and immune function. Use zinc gluconate lozenges for best absorption.

PROTEOLYTIC ENZYMES (BROMELAIN): These enzymes are used to reduce inflammation and soreness in breast tissue due to swelling. *Suggested Dosage:* Use as directed on the label. Take with meals and between meals.

KELP: A rich source of iodine. Iodine deficiency has been linked to this disease. *Suggested Dosage:* 1,500 to 2,000 mg daily, in divided doses.

GOTU KOLA AND BUTCHER'S BROOM: These herbs help to counteract the inflammatory processes that sometimes occur in breast tissue. *Suggested Dosage:* Take as directed using guaranteed potency products.

Home Care Suggestions

- ◆ Hot, moist packs can help relieve breast tenderness.
- ◆ Make sure that bras are the right size for support and are not too small or constricting.
- ◆ Drink 8 to 10 glasses of pure water per day.

Other Supportive Therapies

HYDROTHERAPY: Hot moist packs or baths can help to ease breast pain and swelling.

Prevention

- ◆ Have a mammogram yearly after the age of 35.
- ◆ Do not become obese: Too much body fat increases estrogen levels which can cause breast disorders and lumps.
- ◆ Do not consume caffeine: The regular consumption of caffeine has been linked with the development of fibrous cysts in the breasts.
- ◆ Eat a diet that is low in animal fats and high in fiber.
- ◆ Learn to give yourself a breast examination and do it regularly. Refer to the cancer section for instructions on how to do a breast self-exam.
- ◆ Good results have been achieved using primrose oil to reduce the size of cysts.
- ◆ Thyroid function is important in fibrocystic disease; iodine deficiency can cause an underactive thyroid and has also been linked to fibrocystic disease.
- ◆ Drink plenty of water every day.
- ◆ Eat soy-based foods like tofu in abundance.
- ◆ Take a strong multiple vitamin and mineral supplement with extra vitamin E.
- ◆ Use essential fatty acids and take extra evening primrose oil.
- ◆ Eat a diet higher in protein (cottage cheese, tofu, beans, lean fish) and lower in fat.
- ◆ Do not consume alcohol.

Scientific Facts-at-a-Glance

Research shows that women who eliminate caffeine-containing substances from their diets, have a high rate of success in eliminating cysts. In addition, it is thought that more women suffer from an estrogen dominance than may be assumed. When the estrogen/progesterone ratio is impaired, symptoms of excess estrogen always include breast swelling, pain and fibrocystic disease. Estrogen directly affects the behavior of breast tissue, and if it dominates, breast lesions or tumors can form. Research tells us that isoflavones found in soy-foods actually bind to estrogen receptor sites, helping to inhibit the cellular reactions caused by circulating estrogen. It is for this reason that Japanese women, who eat plenty of soy and cabbage, which contains indoles, have much less breast disease.

Spirit/Mind Considerations

Benign breast disease can be a part of hormonally-related symptoms which also include anxiety, depression, tension, etc. The ability to recognize and treat symptoms that are caused by hormonal imbalances is vital to success. Understanding the physiological processes which can cause benign breast disease helps women to eat right, take the correct supplements and to effectively manage stress. Because so many women rely on caffeine drinks to get them through the day, the notion of stress management is more than pertinent. Caffeine consumption has been directly linked to fibrocystic disease, and yet, even women who suffer from breast problems have a hard time coping without it. Relaxation and the ability to get a good night's rest can help to provide the energy that caffeine artificially supplies.

Doctor's Notes

One of my patients, a 34-year-old female was diagnosed with fibrocystic disease of the breast. She had a more serious case with multiple cysts, some as large as the size of an egg. I put her on 800 to 1000 IU of vitamin E daily. She subsequently experienced a 50 percent reduction in her symptoms. I then placed her on a herbal combination which contained gotu kola and her symptoms were reduced by another 50 percent, resulting in an total 80 percent reduction. High doses of vitamin E (between 800 and 1,200 IU) per day are highly recommended for fibrocystic disease. In addition, butcher's broom works as a natural anti-inflammatory agent and also boosts circulation to breast tissue. Gotu kola is also useful in treating the symptoms of fibrocystic breast changes. Certain herbs help to modulate the hormonal fluctuations which cause breast tissue changes. These include chaste berry, black cohosh, and blue cohosh. I highly recommend consuming an increased amount of genistein through the use of soy products.

Endnotes

1. R.S. London, et al., "The effect of vitamin E on mammary dysplasia: A double-blind study," Obste Gyn, 1085, 65: 104-06.
2. N. Pashby et al., "A clinical trial of evening primrose oil in mastalgia," Bri Jour Surg, 1981, 68: 801-24.
3. Wei, "Antioxidant and antipromotional effects of the soybean isoflavone genistein," Proceedings of the Society for Experimental Biology and Medicine, 1995, 208: 124. and Wilcox G., et al., "Estrogenic effects of plant foods in postmenopausal women," Bri Med Jour, 1990, 301:905-6.
4. John R. Lee, MD., Natural Progesterone: The Multiple Roles of a Remarkable Hormone, revised. (BLL Publishing, Sebastopol, California: 1993), 4. See also U.S. Barzel, "Estrogens in the prevention and treatment of postmenopausal osteoporosis: a review," Am Jour Med, 1988, 85: 847-850 and D.R. Felson, Y. Zhang, and M.T. Hannan, et al., "The effect of postmenopausal estrogen therapy on bone density in elderly women." New England Journal of Medicine, (1993), 329: 1141-1146.
5. P. Band, et al., "Treatment of benign breast disease with vitamin A,"

Prev Med, 1984, 13: 549-54.

6. E.M. Duker, et al., "Effects of extracts from Cimicifuga racemosa on gonadotropin release in menopausal women and ovariectomized rats," Planta Medica, 1991, 57(5): 420-24.

7. D. Zhy, "Dong quai," Amer Jour Clin Med, 1987, 15(3-4): 1987.

8. E. Speroni and E. Minghetti, "Neuropharmacological activity of extracts from Passiflora incarnata," Planta Medica, 1988, 54(6): 488-91.

9. Mark Pederson, Nutritional Herbology, (Wendell Whitman, Warsaw, In: 1995), 145.

10. C. H. Costello, E.V. Lynn, "Estrogenic substances from plants: Glycyrrhiza," Jour Amer Pharm Soc, 1950, 39: 177-80.

11. P. H. List, et al., Hagers Hanbuch der Pharmazeutischen Praxis, vols. 2-5, Springer-Verlag, Berlin.

12. Rebecca Flynn, M.S. Your Guide to Standardized Herbal Products, (One World Press, Prescott, AZ: 1995), 67-69.

13. John R. Lee, MD, Natural Progesterone: The Multiple Roles of a Remarkable Hormone, revised, (BLL Publishing, Sebastopol, California: 1993).

FIBROMYALGIA

Fibromyalgia is one of the most common disorders seen by rheumatologists and yet it is probably one of the least familiar, least understood conditions today. Victims of this disorder—mainly women—are often unaware that they are suffering from a specific ailment. Fibromyalgia belongs to a family of disorders characterized by an overreaction to a normal stimulus and, until recently, was considered to be of a psychosomatic nature. Fibromyalgia is thought to be a by-product of Western lifestyle and is rarely seen in underdeveloped countries. It has also been linked to emotional trauma or depression. It is characterized by muscular aches that affect common points of the body and cause burning, stiffness, shooting pain or an overall throbbing sensation. It typically causes sleep disorders, characterized by an inability to fall into deep or restful sleep, the time when tissue healing and cell regeneration take place; hence, chronic fatigue results.

Symptoms

Fibromyalgia typically causes stiff or sore shoulders and pain in the hip, neck or back muscles. Fibromyalgia typically triggers pain in certain points such as the upper thigh, the knee joint, the base of the skull, the mid-back, the upper area of the buttocks, and to either side of the elbow. Pain can be throbbing, shooting or aching. Other primary symptoms are the inability to sleep well, persistent fatigue, and tenderness in the elbows and knees. If persistent muscle pain is accompanied by fever or weight loss, see your physician.

Secondary symptoms that can accompany fibromyalgia include depression, PMS, irritability, memory difficulties, skin problems, dizziness, lack of coordination, sleep disorders, anxiety, or chronic fatigue.

Causes

While the specific causes of this disorder are unknown, EEG tests reveal that victims manifest a specific type of disruption in their brain wave patterns while sleeping. This abnormality interrupts deep sleep with periods of wakefulness. Other possible causes include tension, viral infections, trauma, unusual exertion, thyroid disease (rare cases), immune dysfunction, brain chemistry, alteration, Epstein-Barr virus, mercury poisoning from amalgam dental fillings, anemia, parasites, underactive thyroid, or malabsorption of nutrients.

Anyone with fibromyalgia can experience a worsening of symptoms during periods of stress, overexertion, lack of sleep, trauma, extreme temperatures, infections or emotional crisis.

Conventional Therapies

Unfortunately, this disorder is easily misdiagnosed. As a result, doctors will routinely prescribe anti-inflammatory drugs such as naprosyn and motrin. These drugs are meant to treat inflammation and do not effectively treat afflictions that originate from muscular spasms. Frequently, tranquilizers and sleeping pills will be prescribed but this can further diminish the quality of sleep and cause dependence. On the whole, medical treatment is not particularly helpful to victims of fybromyalgia. If the disease is recognized and diagnosed correctly, the best medical therapy appears to focus on exercise and the use of antidepressants. For reasons not totally understood, low level doses of antidepressants such as amitriptyline (Endep, Elavil) and imipramine (Tofranil, Janimine) are effective in treating the sleep disturbances that accompany fibromyalgia. The use of these drugs should be discussed with your physician. Doctors often disagree on diagnostic terms to describe this particular disorder. It may be referred to as psychogenic rheumatism, fibrositis, non-articular rheumatism, or chronic muscle-contraction syndrome. If you suspect you have this disorder, see a rheumatologist who will be more familiar with effective treatment. Oral corticosteriods should not be used for this condition.

Dietary Guidelines

- Avoid red meats, fatty foods and acidic foods such as tomatoes and vinegar.
- White potatoes, green peppers and eggplant are not recommended.
- Drink plenty of fluids, especially fresh-squeezed vegetable and fruit juices. Carrot juice is highly recommended.
- Eat plenty of green leafy vegetables. Kelp and chlorophyll supplements are also recommended.
- Concentrate on raw foods (they contain plenty of enzymes) and eat small meals throughout the day.
- Limit or completely avoid foods that are high in hydrogenated or saturated fats, including shellfish.
- Eliminate caffeine and alcohol and greatly reduce sugar consumption.
- You also want to make sure you are not allergic to gluten or other foods.
- Keep the bowel functioning well by eating high-fiber foods or taking a fiber supplement.

Recommended Nutritional Supplements

PRIMARY NUTRIENTS

MALIC ACID Participates in the muscle cell metabolic processes that help muscles use glucose properly. This compound is part of the Krebs's cycle and is thought to reduce the severity of symptoms associated with fibromyalgia, especially when combined with magnesium.[1] *Suggested Dosage:* Take as directed with magnesium supplement.

MAGNESIUM Works to support muscle cell function and has a synergistic action when combined with malic acid. Tests have found that magnesium stores may be depleted in women with fibromyalgia.[2] Supplementation in test cases resulted in significant improvement. *Suggested Dosage:* 300 to 500 mg of magnesium daily. Use chelated products.

5-HYDROXY-TRYPTOPHAN Though tryptophan was previously removed from circulation, this new form of the amino acid is now available. Studies have found that supplementation with this compound significantly decreased symptoms of fibromyalgia.[3] *Suggested Dosage:* Take as directed.

PROTEOLYTIC ENZYMES Malabsorption of nutrients is common in fibromyalgia and these enzymes help to break down macronutrients from food for more efficient assimilation. They also act as natural anti-inflammatory agents and have been used with success in treating multiple types of rheumatic disorders.[4] *Suggested Dosage:* Take as directed with meals, upon arising and before retiring. Look for combination digestive enzymes.

GRAPE SEED OR PINE BARK EXTRACT A powerful antioxidant and natural anti-inflammatory compound that helps to inhibit the inflammatory response and scavenge for free radicals that cause muscle pain or damage.[5] *Suggested Dosage:* Take as directed. You may want to initially start with a higher dose to saturate cells and then taper down to less.

S-ADENOSYLMETHIONINE (SAM) Clinical studies confirmed the use of this compound reduces the type of pain that characterizes fibromyalgia. In recent studies, pain decreased in trigger points and mood was elevated as well.[6] *Suggested Dosage:* At this writing, this supplement is not available for purchase in the United States, although it is in Europe. Ask local suppliers when to expect its availability.

ESSENTIAL FATTY ACIDS These impressive natural anti-inflammatory agents inhibit prostaglandins that cause pain and swelling.[7] *Suggested Dosage:* Take as directed with meals. Look for combination products that contain fish oils as well as supplements containing flaxseed, evening primrose, borage, or black current oils. Take a vitamin E supplement whenever you take fish oil.

MANGANESE Like magnesium, tests suggest that anyone suffering from a disease that causes chronic inflammation or pain may be suffering from a manganese deficiency.[8] *Suggested Dosage:* Take as directed. It is also possible to use SOD (superoxide dimustase), a compound that is manganese rich.

COENZYME Q10 Clinical studies on compromised heart muscle have demonstrated that coenzyme Q10 helps to boost oxygen supplies to muscle tissue. Deficiencies of this enzyme have also been found in the muscle mitochondria of people with muscular dystrophy.[9] *Suggested Dosage:* Take as directed.

ALPHA LIPOIC ACID A powerful antioxidant agent that can potentiate the action of vitamin E, vitamin C and selenium in cells to protect them against free radical damage. Boosting the action of vitamin E and selenium may help decrease muscle pain.[10] *Suggested Dosage:* Take as directed.

GLUCOSAMINE/CHONDROITIN These two compounds can help to boost the production of collagen and exert a protective and regenerative effect on cartilage stores.[11] *Suggested Dosage:* Take as directed for extended periods of time to see results.

NERVINE HERBS Whether used singly or in combination, kava, passionflower, valerian root, hops, and skullcap are all herbs that can help to safely promote sleep. In addition, recent studies have found that St. John's wort can help to treat sleep disorders by promoting longer periods of deep sleep—the portion of the sleep cycle that is compromised in people with fibromyalgia.[12]

HERBAL COMBINATION This combination should include devil's claw, yucca, alfalfa leaves and seed, wild yam root, sarsaparilla root, kelp, white willow bark, cayenne, horsetail and chickweed. *Suggested Dosage:* Four to six capsules daily. For extreme cases it is best to use the maximum dosage of six capsules per day for a prolonged period of four to six months.

DEVIL'S CLAW: The analgesic and anti-inflammatory properties of this herb make it a favorite for rheumatic disorders.[13] It also boosts digestion, which may have a distinct bearing or fibromyalgia. Poor digestion or malabsorption usually results in greater putrefaction in the colon and, as a result, larger amounts of histamine are produced. Histamine triggers inflammation and could exacerbate rheumatic conditions. A second consequence of poor digestion may be the absorption of partially digested proteins called peptides into the bloodstream. Sometimes the body considers peptides to be a foreign substance (an antigen), and in response produces antibodies or larger amounts of histamine. Some people have found that when they improve the health of their digestive system, rheumatic symptoms disappear. YUCCA: Yucca has a similar action to that of devil's claw. It improves digestion, thereby reducing histamine production, so inflammation and pain may be alleviated.[14] The active constituents of yucca are called saponins. ALFALFA LEAVES AND SEEDS: People with fibromyalgia often suffer from malabsorption of nutrients. An impaired digestive system can cause malnutrition by starving the body of much needed macro- and micronutrients. If allowed to become chronic, serious and debilitating diseases can be the consequence. Alfalfa leaves and seeds provide a rich nutrient source to help the body to return to a healthy state.[15] WILD YAM ROOT: The antirheumatic property of this herb is primarily thought to be attributed to its cortisone precursor, diosgenin.[16] As diosgenin is converted to cortisone, anti-inflammatory activity results and a reduction of pain may be noticed. Also, wild yam root is a mild diuretic that helps to gently cleanse the body of toxins and waste. SARSAPARILLA ROOT: Sarsaparilla is officially recognized in Germany and the United Kingdom for its antirheumatic, anti-inflammatory, and diuretic properties.[17] Its activity is thought to be due to its saponin content. Historically, this herb has been used to treat gout and rheumatism and is classified as a tonic and blood purifier. KELP: Kelp, like alfalfa, is a dense source of nutrients, par-

ticularly trace elements that can improve the body's nutrition. It also provides mucilage in the form of algin, a substance soothing to the gastrointestinal tract. WHITE WILLOW BARK: White willow bark has been used for over a thousand years to relieve pain. Salicin, aspirin's forerunner, was discovered to be white willow's active constituent. Apart from its ability to assist with pain, salicin reduces inflammation. Unlike aspirin, however, it will not thin the blood or irritate the stomach. CAYENNE: Cayenne stimulates circulation and makes other herbs more effective. It can also help to improve digestion. Cayenne's "hot" principle, capsaicin, is a noted analgesic. HORSETAIL (SHAVEGRASS): While horsetail contributes to this formula as a mild diuretic, its main action is to strengthen and regenerate connective tissues. Connective tissue, found abundantly in joints, is destroyed by inflammation. Silica is vital in regenerating connective tissue and keeping it strong, and horsetail is one of the richest known sources of silica. CHICKWEED: Chickweed supports the overall cleansing of the body by providing a mild laxative effect. The effect from this herb is so gentle that most people will not be aware of the action.

SECONDARY NUTRIENTS

VITAMIN E: Improves overall circulation. A deficiency of vitamin E has been linked to muscular aches and cramping. *Suggested Dosage:* 400 to 800 IU per day.

MELATONIN: May help to promote better sleep rhythms by helping the body readjust its sleep parameters. *Suggested Dosage:* Start off with a smaller-than-suggested dose and see how you respond.

GINKGO: Promotes better muscle cell oxygenation when under periods of stress. *Suggested Dosage:* Take as directed using standardized or guaranteed potency products.

CAPSAICIN OINTMENTS: Can help relieve pain and boost circulation to tender muscle trigger points. Suggested Usage: Use as directed taking care not to apply cream close to any mucus membranes (mouth, eyes, etc.) An initial burning and reddening may occur but will diminish with use.

CALCIUM/MAGNESIUM: Both these minerals are crucial for proper muscle contraction and nerve function. They should be taken as a supplement daily. A calcium deficiency can actually cause muscle cramping. Good sources of dietary calcium are yogurt, skim milk, and low-fat cheeses. In the case of fibromyalgia, calcium/magnesium supplements may be more effective. Magnesium increase the body's absorption of calcium. Taking a calcium/magnesium supplement at bedtime may help reduce pain and promote sleep. *Suggested Dosage:* Take as directed using gluconate or citrate forms.

Home Care Suggestions

◆ Regular low-impact exercise can go a long way to strengthen muscle tone and discourage the spasms that create aches. Walking, low-impact aerobics, swimming, etc. are all recommended. Regular exercise also helps to promote better sleep. Make sure to warm up and stretch before beginning any exercise. Taking a hot shower or bath before exercising has been suggested by some professionals.

◆ Stretching exercises characteristic of yoga are recommended for their pain-relieving results. Yoga can also promote overall relaxation and promote better sleep. Stretching all muscle groups while lying in bed is a great way to relax before sleeping and upon rising.

◆ Chiropractic manipulations may also offer some relief.

◆ Physical therapy, including electrical muscle stimulation, should also be investigated for its potential benefits.

◆ Have a professional massage on a regular basis. The regular manipulation of muscle groups can help alleviate pain and improve tone. Massaging muscles can also help remove the lactic acid which cause muscles to feel sore after exercising.

◆ Use padded shoe soles if you have to stand for long periods of time.

◆ If you must sit at a desk while working, make sure your chair offers the proper back support.

◆ If this problem seems to significantly improve while on vacation, stress and tension may be significant causal factors and should be addressed.

◆ Sleep in roomy pajamas and do not weigh your body down with heavy blankets.

Other Supportive Therapies

HYDROTHERAPY: Using warm whirlpool baths can help with pain and facilitate muscle relaxation.

MASSAGE: Using oil of thyme, eucalyptus and lavender can help alleviate stiffness and pain.

ACUPUNCTURE: Specific treatment can address pain.

CHIROPRACTIC AND OSTEOPATHY: Helps to increase joint and muscle flexibility which, in turn, helps to reverse fibrotic changes in the musculo-skeletal system.

MEDITATION: Helps to diffuse stress and tension.

HOMEOPATHY: Rhus tox. 6, Arnica 6 and Bryonia 6 to build stamina.

MAGNET MATTRESS OR PADS: While there is no scientific data to support the use of these magnets, there is enough anecdotal evidence to warrant their investigation. Some people with fibromyalgia have found these pads to be extremely beneficial in controlling nighttime pain and promoting sound sleep.

Scientific Facts-at-a-Glance

People with fibromyalgia find that their symptoms are worse in cold or humid weather. In addition over 70 percent of people with this disease also suffer from depression. Anxiety and headaches are also common and almost all victims cannot get into a deep sleep where healing and tissue regeneration takes place. Some people have found that sleeping on magnet-embedded mattresses can be very helpful. While the exact scientific mechanisms of how the electromagnetic field affects this disease remains unknown, for those that cannot find relief through supplementation or exercise, these mattresses may be prove to be very helpful.

Spirit/Mind Considerations

Fibromyalgia can create a feeling of true discouragement and frustration in its victims. It is absolutely vital to find a physician who is familiar with this disorder. Some women with this disease have become even more troubled when their doctor suggests that it may be a psychosomatic illness. If you feel you are suffering from this particular ailment and it has not been recognized by your doctor, bring it to his or her attention. Fibromyalgia is a very real disease that is not fully understood. A variety of nervine herbs and supplements can help to promote better sleep and nourish muscle tissue. In addition, the notion of unresolved emotional stress or trauma may play a role in perpetrating this disease. Because so many women who suffer from fibromyalgia are also depressed, the mind/body connection must be addressed. Counseling may be helpful in combination with meditation or other techniques designed to bring about feelings of tranquility.

Prevention

◆ Keeping fit through regular exercise and eating a diet high in calcium and magnesium is recommended. In addition, staying at an ideal weight puts less strain on muscle groups.

◆ Employing a daily relaxation regimen can also help muscles from tensing up and causing stress-induced pain.

◆ Learn to express your feelings. Do not keep them internalized.

◆ Keep your digestive system working well by eating right and using digestive enzymes and nutrient supplements.

Doctor's Notes

While we still have much to learn about fibromyalgia we do know that inflammation and pain are involved at a muscular level. The herbs suggested above are intended to alleviate the symptoms of inflammation and pain, as well as provide a rich nutrient base to help the body's healing process. Because malabsorption is such a problem in many people suffering from this syndrome, boosting the assimilation of nutrients is vital. Proper nourishment of muscle cells plays a profound role in the development and course of this disease. Use a good multivitamin and mineral supplement along with the other nutrients suggested. It is also important to learn how to channel stress or unresolved emotional issues.

Additional Resources

USA Fibromyalgia Association
Phone: (614) 851 9177
Fax: (614) 851 9277

National Fibromyalgia Association
P.O. Box 500
Salem, OR 97302

Reversing Fibromyalgia
by Dr. Joe M. Elrod
Woodland Publishing
Lindon, Utah
(800) 777-2665

Endnotes

1. G. Abraham, "Management of fibromyalgia: Rationale for the use of magnesium and malic acid," Jour Nutri Med, 1992, 3: 49-59.

2. J. Eisinger, et al., "Donees actuelles sure les fibromyalgies:magneisum et transaminases," Lyons Mediterranee Med, 1988, 24: 11585-86.

3. I. Caruso, et al., "Double-blind study of 5-Hydroxytroptophan versus placebo in the treatment of primary fibromyalgia syndrome," Jour Int Med Res, 1990, 18(3): 201-09.

4. I. Horger, "Enzyme therapy in multiple rheumatic diseases," Therapiewoche, 1983, 33: 3948-57.

5. B. Schwitters and J. Masquelier, OPC in Practice: Bioflavonols and Their Application, (Alpha Omega, Rome: 1993).

6. P. Di Benedetto, et al., "Clinical evaluation of SAM versus transcutaneous nerve stimulation in primary fibromyalgia," Curr Ther Res, 1993, 53: 222-229.

7. Michael T. Murray, Encyclopedia of Nutritional Supplements, (Prima Publishing, Rocklin, Ca: 1996), 247-48

8. C. Paswuier, et al., "Manganese-containing superoxide dismustase deficiency in polymorphonuclear leukocytes of adults with rheumatoid arthritis," Inflammation, 1984, 8: 27-32.

9. K. Folkers, et al., "Two successful double-blind trials with coenzyme Q10 on muscular dystrophies and neurogenic atrophies," Biochem Biophys Acta, 1995, 1271: 281-86.

10. R. Van, et al., "Selenium deficiency in total parenteral nutrition," Amer Jour Clin Nutri, 1979, 32: 2076-85.

11. I. Setnikar, "Antireactive Properties of 'chondoprotective' drugs," Int-Jour-Tissue-React,1992, 14 (5): 253-61.

12. H. Schultz, and M, Jobert, "Effects of hypericum extract on the sleep EEG in older volunteers," Journal of Geriatric Psychiatry and Neurology, 1994, 7: S39-43.

13. L.R. Brady, et al., Pharmacognosy, 8th ed. Lea and Gebiger, Philadelphia: 1981, 480.

14. R. Bingham, et al., "Yucca plant saponins in the management of arthritis," Jour Applied Nutrition, 1975, 27: 45-50.

15. M.R. Malinow, et al., "Effect of alfalfa saponins on intestinal cholesterol absorption in rats," Amer Jour Clini Nutri, 1977, 30: 2061-67.

16. H.W. Feller, The Eclectic Materia Medica, Pharmacology and Therapeutics, Eclectic Medical Publications, Portland Oregon: 1983, first published in 1922.

17. Kiangsu Institute of Modern Medicine, Encyclopedia of Chinese Drugs, 2 vols. 1977, Shanghai, People's Republic of China.

GALLBLADDER DISEASE

SEE "GALLSTONES"

GALLSTONES

As many as 20 percent of the American population over 40 years old suffers from gallstones. Approximately 20 million people have gallstones, with at least one million new cases diagnosed each year. Gallstones can vary in size from smaller than a pea to as large as an egg. Often the presence of gallstones can go unnoticed.

If a gallstone becomes stuck within a bile duct, severe pain usually results. The gallbladder collects bile, a cholesterol rich fluid which comes from the liver. Bile is secreted when fatty substances are digested. Gallstones occur when cholesterol crystallizes and combines with the bile due to a chemical impairment.

There can be between one and 10 stones, which vary in size present, in the gallbladder. Gallstones are composed principally of cholesterol but may also contain bile pigment and chalk. Women who are over 40, obese and have had children are more likely to suffer from gallbladder disorders. Gallstones are rarely found in primitive cultures which strongly suggests that Western eating habits certainly have a great bearing on this condition. Gallbladder disease involves inflammation which, if left untreated, can be a very serious condition.

Symptoms

Gallstones

Interestingly, between one-third and one-half of people with gallstones have no symptoms. When the stones get stuck in the bile duct, though, unpleasant symptoms may appear, including a severe pain in the upper right section of the abdomen or between the shoulder blades. The pain can build to a peak and then fade over a period of hours and has been described as an intense, gnawing ache. It may be accompanied by bloating, nausea, and vomiting.

A gallstone attack may occur after a meal high in fatty or fried foods. Drinking alcohol has also been related to gallstone attacks. If the symptoms subside, the stone may have fallen back into the gallbladder or forced into the intestines.

Gallbladder Inflammation

Gallbladder inflammation is puncuated by fever, nausea,vomiting, and/or pain in the upper right abdominal area.

Causes

The high incidence of gallstones and gallbladder disease in the United States is thought to be directly related to

Western dietary habits. The older one gets, the chances for developing gallstones increase and women are far more susceptible to this disorder than men. Possible causes of both gallstones and gallbladder inflammation include elevated levels of cholesterol in the blood, food allergies, hormonal factors (pregnacy increases the risk of gallstones), prolonged periods of fasting, using birth control pills, rapid weight loss diets, overexposure to the sun (especially if you have fair skin), and a diet high in hydrogenated and saturated fats.

Conventional Therapies

Doctors who suspect gallstones will take a blood sample or offer a cholecystogram (a type of x-ray taken after ingesting a certain pill which enhances the visibility of the gallbladder). An ultrasound scan which detects up to 95 percent of gallstones or a CAT scan may also be recommended to detect gallstones that have not shown up in previous tests.

Standard treatment for gallstones usually involves surgically removing the gallbladder. New laser surgery techniques may be an option. This process of removing the gallbladder involves only a small incision and recovery is rapid. A new treatment called lithotripsy is also available in which stones are fractured by an external machine. Another technique uses a tube, inserted in the gallbladder, and a strong solution to dissolves the cholesterol. The value and safety of both of these methods is still being evaluated. Drug therapy may be suggested to dissolve small gallstones. This treatment is slow and is only effective with certain types of gallstones.

Removing the gallbladder surgically is 100 percent effective in resolving the problem of gallstones or gallbladder disease but is not without risk. Prevention, which is usually not stressed, should receive more emphasis.

Dietary Guidelines

◆ Eat a low-fat diet high in raw foods. Emphasize yogurt, broiled fish, beets, carrots, apples, lemons, oranges, grapes, celery, garlic, onions, tomatoes, dates, melons and fiber-rich foods.
◆ Fiber is thought to help prevent the formation of gallstones by stimulating bile flow from the liver and by preventing bile reabsorption.
◆ Avoid fried foods, fatty foods, animal fat, margarine, commercial oils, chocolate and coffee. Minimize your consumption of sugar and refined carbohydrates.
◆ If you need to lose weight, learn to push away from the table before feeling uncomfortably full. Beet juice is good for its ability to act as a liver cleanser.
◆ During a bout with inflammation, drink apple and green juices and avoid solid food.

Recommended Nutritional Supplements

PRIMARY NUTRIENTS

VITAMIN C Supplementation with ascorbic acid may be beneficial by actually reducing the formation of gallstones.[1]

Vitamin C deficiencies have been linked to gallstone formation. *Suggested Dosage:* 1,000 to 3,000 mg per day in divided doses with meals.

VITAMIN E Clinical studies suggest that vitamin E supplementation may prevent gallstone formation.[2] This vitamin also helps to scavenge for free radicals created by ingesting rancid fats. *Suggested Dosage:* 400 to 800 IU daily.

VITAMIN D Studies have found that vitamin D may not be properly absorbed if the gallbladder is impaired. *Suggested Dosage:* 400 IU per day.

LECITHIN Some research suggests that low levels of lecithin in the bile may cause gallstones. Lecithin also helps to emulsify fats which is important to proper cholesterol digestion. Lecithin, a dietary source of choline, may increase the capacity of the bile to solubilize cholesterol.[3] *Suggested Dosage:* 1,000 mg with each of three meals.

DIGESTIVE ENZYMES Helps to boost the digestion of foods which can be a problem if the gallbladder is impaired.[4] Use HCL or hydrochloric acid supplements with these enzymes if you suspect that you suffer from deficiency. Refer to the proper section of this book for more information. *Suggested Dosage:* Take as directed 30 minutes prior to eating.

ESSENTIAL FATTY ACIDS Observational studies indicate that supplying these acids can facilitate better cholesterol control and lipid metabolism which are both intrinsically linked to the formation of gallstones.[5] *Suggested Dosage:* Take as directed using a blend of oils such as evening primrose, borage, flaxseed, etc. Keep refrigerated.

PEPPERMINT OIL Several studies suggest that this essential oil may actually dissolve gallstones. Its terpene content also promotes the release of cholecystokinin which can keep gallstone blockage from occurring.[6] *Suggested Dosage:* Take as directed.

TAURINE This amino acid also affects bile. Taurine-supplemented diets increased the secretion and solubility of bile acids in both test groups.[7] *Suggested Dosage:* Take as directed on an empty stomach with fruit juice.

FIBER SUPPLEMENTS Psyllium, pectin, and guar gum can decrease cholesterol levels and keep the bile acid pool active which discourages disease and stone formation. The highest incidence of gallstones if found in animals receiving the lowest fiber diets.[8] *Suggested Dosage:* Take as directed using powdered formulas designed to be mixed with liquid just before retiring and in the morning.

CURCUMIN Studies have supported the use of this compound to increase the solubility of the bile.[9] *Suggested Dosage:* Take as directed.

HERBAL COMBINATION This combination should include dandelion root, milk thistle seeds, burdock root, peppermint leaves, artichoke and kelp. *Suggested Dosage:* Two to four capsules daily. For chronic conditions it is best to use maximum dosage of four capsules per day for a prolonged period of two to three months or until symptoms are gone. May be used every day.

DANDELION ROOT: Dandelion has been used to treat liver and gallbladder obstructions, improve overall liver function, and promote bile production. Dandelion is a mild laxative and diuretic.[10] Clinical use of dandelion is officially recognized in Britain, France, and Germany. MILK THISTLE SEEDS: Fortifying the liver is important when dealing with gallbladder disease or gallstones. In addition, the silymarin content of this herb can significantly reduce bile cholesterol concentration and saturation.[11] BURDOCK ROOT: Burdock root promotes bile production and secretion, but perhaps its best contribution to this formula is its ability to promote perspiration, reducing the load on the liver to process and neutralize toxins. The inulin content of this herb also contributes to better blood sugar control.[12] PEPPERMINT LEAVES: Peppermint leaves are indicated in conditions where sluggish bile flow may be present. Peppermint also supports the other herbs contained in this blend by stimulating circulation and acting as a catalyst to increase overall effectiveness. Its carminative and antigas properties help it to counteract some of the gastrointestinal tract irritation caused by dandelion, milk thistle, and burdock. It also contains terpenes which act to dissolve stones.[13] ARTICHOKE: Although commonly recognized as a table food, artichoke has been used historically to treat various conditions such as jaundice, dyspepsia and decreased liver function. Studies have shown it to be a more effective cholesterol-lowering agent than prescription drugs.[14] It should be taken to help facilitate the digestion of fats by anyone with gallbladder problems. KELP: While it has been reported that kelp can help with gallstones, its primary function in this formula is to provide a rich supply of trace nutrients as well as algin which is soothing and mildly laxative to the gastrointestinal tract.

SECONDARY NUTRIENTS

CATECHIN: This flavonoid has significant liver boosting properties which can help to support gallbladder function. *Suggested Dosage:* Take as directed only. Use under a doctor's supervision.

ALFALFA: Acts as a natural liver cleanser. *Suggested Dosage:* Take as directed using high-quality, pure products with no fillers.

BARBERRY ROOT BARK: Stimulates bile flow and helps to relieve liver congestion. *Suggested Dosage:* Take as directed using standardized products.

QUEEN OF THE MEADOW: Has a long history of use for gallbladder disorders. *Suggested Dosage:* Take as directed using guaranteed potency products.

Home Care Suggestions

◆ Drinking at least six to eight glasses of water per day is very important in helping maintain the proper water content of bile from which gallstones are formed.
◆ Do not overeat.

Other Supportive Therapies

AROMATHERAPY: Essential oil of Scot's pine can be helpful if pain is present.

ACUPUNCTURE: Helps the body to manage a healing crisis and can help stimulate liver and gallbladder function.

Scientific Facts-at-a-Glance

There is new evidence that slow transit time (the time it takes for food to digest and be eliminated as waste) may explain why some women who are not overweight suffer from gallbladder disease.[15] This suggests the value of increasing fiber to decrease transit time, especially in women with a history of gallbladder disease in their families. There is also new molecular evidence that bacteria actually colonize cholesterol gallstones.[16]

Prevention

◆ Gallstones are thought to be much easier to prevent than to treat. Reducing your risk factors for the formation of gallstones is of primary importance.
◆ Eat a diet low in fats and especially low in cholesterol. Avoid animal and saturated fats, sugar, and fried foods. Minimize your consumption of animal protein. Vegetable proteins such as soy are actually believed to prevent the formation of gallstones.
◆ Emphasize the following foods: fresh fruits and vegetables, fiber (oat bran, flaxseed, guar gum, pectin etc.) eating fiber regularly is believed to help prevent gallstones from forming.
◆ Do not become obese, which increases your risk for gallstones. Even slightly overweight people have twice the risk of developing gallstones. Lose weight safely and slowly. Losing weight too quickly can actually increase the risk of developing gallstones.
◆ Eat a diet high in fiber to prevent constipation.

Doctor's Notes

If you will notice, many of the herbs listed have the ability to make the bile more soluble which discourages the formation of stones. This is the only traditional herbal formula to incorporate dandelion, milk thistle, artichoke and peppermint—a very powerful and effective combination. Improvement in liver function is often noted by the amelioration of other conditions such as psoriasis. It is also important to keep in mind that a deficiency of hydrochloric acid may also predispose one to gallstones or gallbladder disease.[17] The practice of taking three tablespoons to a pint of olive oil with lemon juice before retiring in order to promote passage of stones in the stool, has been used with some success, although it is a therapy which can aggravate inflammation due to its high-fat content and should only be done under the care of a doctor.

Additional Resources

Gallstone Hotline: (800) 253-7888

Endnotes

1. E. Ginter, and L. Milus, "Reduction of gallstone formation by ascorbic acid in hamsters," Experientia, 1977, 33(6):716-7. See also M. Praza, et al., "Prevention of cholelithiasis with ascorbic acid: Experimental study in hamsters," Rev Gastroenterol Mex, 1979, 44(4):159-62.

2. T. Saito T and H. Tanimura, "The preventive effect of vitamin E on gallstone formation: A study of the biliary lipids in patients with gallstones," Arch Jpn Chir, 1987, 56(3):276-88.

3. G.L. Duff GL, et al., Amer Jour Medicine, 1951, 11:92.

4. W.M. Capper, et al., "Gallstones, gastric secretion, and flatulent dyspepsia," Lancet, 1967, 1:413-15.

5. R.A. Sturdevant, et al., "Increased prevalence of cholelithiasis in men ingesting a serum-cholesterol-lowering diet," New Engl Jour Med, 1973, 288(1):24-27.

6. D. Giachetti, et al., "Pharmacological activity of essential oils on Oddi's sphincter produced by morphine," Planta Medica, 1988, 54: 389-92.

7. W.Y. Wang and K.Y. Liaw KY, "Effect of a taurine-supplemented diet on conjugated bile acids in biliary surgical patients," JPEN J Parenter Enteral Nutr, 1991, 15(3):294-7.

8. B.L. Cohen, et al., "The effect of alfalfa-corn diets on cholesterol metabolism and gallstones in prairie dogs," Lipids, Mr. 1990, 25(3): 143-48.

9. C. Ramprasad, and M. Sirsi M, "Curcuma longa and bile secretion - Quantitative changes in the bile constituents induced by sodium curcuminate," Jour Sci Indust Res, 1957, 16C:108-10.

10. K. Bohm, "Choleretic action of some medicinal plants," Arzneimittel-Forsch, 1959, 9: 376-78.

11. G. Nassauto, R. Lemmolo, et al., "Effect of silibinin on biliary lipid composition: Experimental and clinical study," Jour Hepatol, 1991,12:290-5.

12. A.A. Silver, et al., "The effect of the ingestion of burdock root on normal and diabetic individuals: A preliminary report," Ann Intern Med, 1931, 5: 274-84.

13. D. Giachetti, et al., "Pharmacological activity of essential oils on Oddi's sphincter produced by morphine," Planta Medica, 1988, 54: 389-92.

14. A. Lietti, "Choleretic and cholesterol lowering properties of two artichoke extracts," Fitoterapia, 1977, 48(4): 153-58.

15. Heaton, "An explanation for gallstones in normal weight women: slow intestinal transit," Lancet, 1993, 341(8836): 8-10.

16. Swidsinski, et al., "Molecular genetic evidence of bacterial colonization of cholesterol gallstones," Gastroenterology, 1995, 108(3): 860-64.

17. W.M. Capper, et al., "Gallstones, gastric secretion, and flatulent dyspepsia," Lancet, 1967, 1:413-15.

GINGIVITIS

SEE "PERIDONTAL DISEASE"

GLAUCOMA

Unfortunately, glaucoma is one of the most prevalent eye disorders in people who are over the age of 60. It is responsible for 15 percent of all blindness in the United States, afflicting approximately 2 million people, and is the second leading cause of blindness. Glaucoma is a condition in which fluid pressure in the eye becomes high enough to cause damage. Small internal blood vessels can become compressed or obstructed in the optic nerve, resulting in nerve fiber destruction which can lead to partial or total blindness. Chronic open-angle glaucoma is the most common form of the disease and usually begins after the age of 40. A blockage of fluid in the eye gradually increases the pressure over a period of years. Acute closed-angle glaucoma refers to the sudden obstruction of fluid with a sudden rise in pressure. Congenital glaucoma results from structural abnormalities within the eye.

Symptoms

Chronic glaucoma can often progress without any symptoms due to the very slow loss of peripheral vision. Unfortunately, it is usually only after the disease is in its later stages, when irreversible damage has occurred, that vision loss becomes obvious. Possible symptoms include a severe dull ache or throbbing pain in the eye or above the eye, eye discomfort (which is usually worse in the morning), blurred or foggy vision, tunnel vision, inability to adjust to darkness, loss of peripheral vision, the perception of rainbow rings around lights, nausea or vomiting, a red, bloodshot appearance to the eyes, dilated pupils, hazy cornea.

Acute closed-angle glaucoma is considered a medical emergency and requires immediate medical attention. Go to an emergency facility if you feel sudden eye pain, blurred vision, halos around lights, and nausea or vomiting.

The only way that glaucoma can be detected in its early stages is with regular eye examinations. Applanation tonometry, which measures eye pressure, is used to detect the presence of the disease; visual field testing and gonioscopy, which measures the drainage angle in the eye, can also be performed along with applanation tonometry to detect glaucoma. See an ophthalmologist regularly.

Causes

Acute closed angle glaucoma typically runs in families. Other possible causes of glaucoma are injury to the eye, a dislocation of the lens, adhesions that grow between the iris and the cornea, diseases such as uveitis, malnutrition and stress, and impaired collagen metabolism.

There is some speculation that exposure to allergens, both airborne or environmental, can cause a rise in intraocular pressure, which could cause glaucoma-like symptoms. Certain drugs can hasten the onset of glaucoma. People with the following signs are also at a higher risk for developing glaucoma: anyone who has a family history of the disease, the severely nearsighted, those with cataracts, diabetics, anyone over 65, anyone taking certain blood pressure medication or cortisone. Also, black people have a higher incidence of glaucoma than Caucasians.

Conventional Therapies

If caught early enough, glaucoma can be controlled through medication and surgery, and blindness can be avoided. Normal vision can be restored if glaucoma has not progressed too far. Chronic glaucoma is commonly controlled with eye drops which reduce eye pressure. Timoptic (timolol maleate) reduces fluid formation and pilocarpine decreases the size of the pupil thus increasing fluid outflow. Propine (dipivefrin) is considered a cornerstone drug in the treatment of glaucoma. Careful monitoring of the eyes must be done during treatment to ensure its effectiveness. If pressure is still too high, other types of eye drops may be used. In persistent cases, tablets or capsules such as diamox (acetazolamide) may be prescribed which are generally taken as life long medications. If drug therapy fails, laser surgery or regular surgery may be necessary to enlarge the drainage area or to create an artificial channel in which the fluid can drain. Laser surgery involves aiming a beam at the iris and making a tiny hole to relieve pressure. Acute glaucoma is considered a medical emergency and requires immediate treatment. In this case, osmotic eye drops, oral medication and intravenous fluids may be administered to reduce eye pressure. Surgery will probably be recommended to prevent a reoccurrence of the problem. This procedure is called an iridectomy and involves making a small incision in the area around the iris so the fluid can drain. Medications may be recommended following the surgery.

Dietary Guidelines

- Eat a diet high in whole grains and fresh fruits and vegetables and low in animal and saturated fats.
- Avoid coffee, alcohol, nicotine, and all caffeine. Also, eat sugar and salt very sparingly.
- Try not to drink large amounts of fluid at once.

Recommended Nutritional Supplements

Avoid any eye drops that dilate the pupils, including certain herbs such as ephedra or belladonna, and do not take licorice.

PRIMARY NUTRIENTS

ALPHA LIPOIC ACID This antioxidant helps to raise and sustain glutathione levels, which work to protect the eye from free radical damage and strengthens the integrity of eye membrane tissue. Taking glutathione orally may not be as effective as boosting it through alpha lipoic supplementation.[1] It also has the distinct ability to raise and boost the action of vitamin C and vitamin E. *Suggested Dosage:* Take as directed.

VITAMIN E WITH SELENIUM The antioxidant properties of this duo are impressive and are also potentiated by taking lipoic acid. These nutrients provide the eye with additional protection from cellular damage.[2] *Suggested Dosage:* Take as directed.

VITAMIN B1 (NIACIN) Clinical studies have shown that thiamine supplementation did improve the condition of the eyes in chronic open-angle glaucoma.[3] *Suggested Dosage:* Take as directed.

VITAMIN A Following supplementation with vitamin A, the intraocular pressures of several patients with glaucoma dropped to normal, and they were able to discontinue their medications after a few months.[4] What this study suggests is that a vitamin A deficiency may contribute to this disease. *Suggested Dosage:* Take 50,000 IU per day. If you are pregnant, do not exceed 10,000IU per day.

VITAMIN C WITH BIOFLAVONOIDS It helps to lower intraocular pressure, which becomes elevated when glaucoma is present. High doses of vitamin C have proven their ability to lower pressure in the inner eye and have even resulted in more improvement than was seen with drug therapies for glaucoma (pilocarpine and acetazolamide).[5] *Suggested Dosage:* 10,000 to 20,000 mg per day in divided doses. Use buffered or esterized products to avoid stomach upset or diarrhea.

RUTIN (A BIOFLAVONOID) After 4 or more weeks of administration of rutin, 17 out of 26 patients with uncomplicated primary glaucoma demonstrated a 15 percent or greater reduction in intraocular pressure and responded better to other treatments.[7] *Suggested Dosage:* 20 mg three times daily.

CHROMIUM Studies have found that people with certain chromium levels are prone to lower intraocular pressure, suggesting that a dietary chromium deficiency may contribute to the development of the disease.[8] *Suggested Dosage:* Take as directed using GTF products.

MAGNESIUM Magnesium supplementation improved the peripheral circulation and visual field in test patients with glaucoma.[9] *Suggested Dosage:* 200 mg per day in divided doses.

ESSENTIAL FATTY ACIDS Help normalize membrane tissue in the eye and boosts cellular repair. *Suggested Dosage:* Take as directed using flaxseed, evening primrose or borage oil.

LECITHIN This nutrient which contains choline helps to nourish the membranes of the eye. It also works to conserve folic acid.[10] *Suggested Dosage:* Take as directed using granules or capsulized products.

FORSKOLIN A derivative of the coleus plant which has had some positive effects in treating glaucoma topically in some university studies and should be investigated.[11] *Suggested Dosage:* Take as directed using standardized products.

GINKGO BILOBA Studies have shown some improvement with gingko therapy in glaucoma patients which is probably due to its ability to boost circulation and oxygenation of eye tissue.[12] *Suggested Dosage:* Take as directed using standardized guaranteed potency products.

HERBAL COMBINATION This combination should include bilberry and blueberry. *Suggested Dosage:* Take as directed.

BILBERRY: This herb contains powerful flavonoid compounds called anthocyanosides, which are impressive antioxidants which improve the circulation of micro capillaries in the eye. It has been used to treat several retinopathies and has shown its ability to reduce permeability, hemorrhage and enlarge the visual field.[13]
BLUEBERRY LEAVES: This herb also contains anthocyanosides which can boost capillary integrity and protect against free radical damage in the eye. European practitioners use blueberry leaves extensively as treatments for eye diseases.[14]

SECONDARY NUTRIENTS

PYCNOGENOL (GRAPE SEED OR PINE BARK EXTRACT): The proanthocyanidin content of this compound acts as a powerful antioxidant to help protect the eye. *Suggested Dosage:* Take as directed.
VITAMIN B-COMPLEX: These vitamins can be given in injection form and may be helpful if glaucoma is stress related. *Suggested Dosage:* Take as directed using sublingual or injection form.
ZINC: Works to repair tissue and helps boost the action of vitamin A. *Suggested Dosage:* Take 50 mg per day using gluconate or lozenges.

Home Care Suggestions

◆ Avoid excessive or prolonged stress to the eye, such as watching too much television, reading, or doing minute work that puts extra strain on the eyes.
◆ Corticosteroids should not be used by anyone suffering from glaucoma due to their adverse effect on collagen structures within the eye. Cortisone also interferes with the fluid flow of the eye and can actually increase pressure.
◆ Avoid taking decongestants or antihistamines which can narrow eye-drainage canals and increase intraocular pressure.
◆ If taking eye drops for glaucoma, take them regularly and don't miss any doses. The best way to apply eye drops is to lay down, pull down your lower eyelid and place a drop of fluid in and then press against the tear duct in the corner of your eye with your finger.
◆ Regular exercise, especially cycling appears to also help reduce pressure within the eye. Glaucoma self-tests can be administered at home with a self-tonometer and should be done so with the consent of your doctor.

Other Supportive Therapies

HYDROTHERAPY: Home hydrotherapy treatments, which consist of putting hot and cold towels over the eyes, can be beneficial.
HOMEOPATHY: Continual treatments with belladonna have been used to treat the early symptoms of glaucoma. Gelsemium and alumina are also used.
YOGA: Certain exercises can help to relax the eye.

Scientific Facts-at-a-Glance

Several new procedures are available for glaucoma and include excimer laser-filtration surgery and subconjunctival injections of mitomycin. If you suffer from glaucoma, discuss this option with your doctor. New studies also strongly suggest that ALA (alpha lipoic acid) significantly boosts the presence of ascorbate, glutathione and other protective enzymatic compounds in the eye exerting a protective effect.[16] In essence, ALA was able to restore not only glutathione but ascorbate reductase as well in the eye lens of laboratory test animals.

Spirit/Mind Considerations

Anyone who has glaucoma is faced with compromised or lost vision. Fortunately, today there are many options for the visually impaired and taking advantage of those options is vital. If you find that you must rely or certain people or services in order to function, then do so graciously. Adapting our lifestyles to various biological changes that we may experience is what ensures continued quality of life. The resource addresses listed in this section offer valuable information and support. Use them.

Moreover, learning to manage stress with recuperative time is also very important when dealing with glaucoma. Meditation, yoga, visualization are all beneficial and can neutralize the damaging effects of stress.

Prevention

◆ Guard your eyes against flying objects, and wear protective goggles when involved in carpentry, metalwork, playing sports, chopping wood, etc.
◆ Avoid prolonged allergic irritation of the eyes.
◆ Make sure reading and work areas are well lighted.
◆ Use glasses if needed and update your prescription periodically.
◆ Take breaks from tedious eye work (computer entry, typing, lab work). Toning down the brightness of computer screen images is also less stressful on the eyes.
◆ Try not to work in direct sunlight, wear sunglasses if sun is bright or glare severe; however, try not to become dependent on tinted glasses by overusing them.
◆ See the eye doctor for a yearly, routine eye exam once a year, especially after age 40 for early detection of glaucoma.
◆ Avoid eye injury or eye strain.
◆ Placing herbal tea bags that have been steeped in an herb tea such as eyebright and then cooled on each eye can help relieve stress and relax the eye.

Doctor's Notes

One thing that must be addressed is the possibility that food allergies may be causing chronic simple glaucoma. Studies have found that certain individuals can experience an immediate rise in intraocular pressure after ingesting certain foods.[15]

Additional Resources

National Eye Institute
Building 31 Rm. 6A32
31 Center Drive, MSC 2510
Bethesda, MD 20892-2510
301-496-5248

Foundation for Glaucoma Research
490 Post St. Suite 830
San Francisco, CA 94102
415-986-3162

Endnotes

1. Han D. Tritschler, et al., "Alpha-lipoic acid increases intracellular glutathione in human T-lymphocyte Jurkat cell line," Biochem Biophys Res Commun, 1195, 207: 258-264.

2. M. Podda, et al., "Alpha-lipoic acid supplementation prevents symptoms of vitamin E deficiency," Biochem Biophys Res Commun, 1994, 204: 98-104.

3. E. Asregadoo, "Blood levels of thiamin and ascorbic acid in chronic open-angle glaucoma," Ann Ophthalmol, 1979, 11(7):1095-1100.

4. G. Todd, Nutrition, Health and Disease, (The Donning Co., Norfolk, Virginia: 1985).

5. Michael T. Murray, Encyclopedia of Nutritional Supplements, (Prima Publishing, Rocklin, CA: 1996), 452.

6. S. Evans, "Ophthalmic nutrition and prevention of eye disorder and blindness," Nutr Metab 1977, 21 (suppl 1): 268-72.

7. F. Stocker, "New ways of influencing the intraocular pressure," New York State Jour Med, 1949, 49:58-63.

8. B. Lane, "Diet and the glaucomas," abstract, Jour Amer Coll Nutr, 1991, 10(5):536.

9. A.Z. Gaspar, et al., "The influence of magnesium on visual field and peripheral vasospasm in glaucoma," Opthalmologica, 1995, 209: 11-13.

10. G Varela-Mreiras, et al., "Effect of chronic choline deficiency on liver folate content and distribution," Jour Nutr Biochem, 1992, 3: 519-22.

11. B. Meyer, et al., "The effects of forskolin eye drops on intraocular pressure," So Afr Med Jour, 1987, 71(9):570-1.

12. H. Merte and W. Merkle, "Long term treatment with Ginkgo biloba extract of circulatory disturbances of the retina and optic nerve," Klin Monatsbl Augenheilkd, 1980, 177(5):577-83 (in German).

13. L. Caselli, "Clinical and electroretinographic study on activity of anthocyanosides," Arch med int, 1985, 37: 29-35.

14. B. Bever, and G. Zahnd, "Plants with oral hypoglycemic action," Quar Jour Crude Drug Res, 1979, 17: 139-96.

15. L. Raymond, "Allergy and chronic simple glaucoma," Ann Allergy, 1964, 22:146-50.

16. I. Maitra, et al., "Alpha-lipoic acid prevents buthionine sulfoximine-induced cataract formation in newborn rats," Free Radical Biology and Medicine, 1995, 18: 823-829.

GOUT

Gout was traditionally thought of as a disease of the affluent who dined on fatty meats, wines and rich dairy products. It is an arthritis-like metabolic disorder which results from an increased concentration of uric acid which is formed from eating certain foods. This uric acid becomes crystallized and is deposited in joints, tendons, the kidneys and other tissues, causing inflammation, swelling and damage. Uric acid forms as a by-product of certain foods.

Gout has been referred to as a disease of the rich, alluding to its connection with the consumption of meats and wine. Today gout is a disease that primarily affects adult men over the age of 30. In women, gout occurs only after menopause. Approximately three adults in 1,000 suffer from gout. Once an initial attack of gout is experienced, subsequent episodes are common; however, a small percentage never experience a second attack.

Individuals that suffer from gout are typically obese, prone to high blood pressure and diabetes and may have a history of cardiovascular disease.

Symptoms

An attack of gout can be characterized by intense joint pain that resembles a dislocation. The first joint of the big toe is affected in 90 percent of people who suffer from gout. Gouty joints are swollen and red. Other symptoms of the disorder are fever and chills.

Attacks of gout commonly occur at night. They can be aggravated by overeating, drinking alcohol, trauma to the body and certain drugs and surgical procedures. An untreated attack of gout will not usually last longer that a week.

Other common sites of gout are the ankle, heel, knee and wrist. The shoulder, back or the hip are rarely affected by gout. Victims of chronic gout may also increase their risk for the development of uric acid kidney stones.

Causes

Gout is a diet-related condition. It is also linked to obesity, stress, enzyme defects, chemotherapy (causes cellular destruction which releases large amounts of uric acid), cancer, chronic anemia, kidney dysfunction, psoriasis, cytotoxic drugs, diuretics used to treat high blood pressure, heart failure (may impair the ability of the kidney to excrete uric acid).

It is possible to live with elevated levels of uric acid and never have an attack of gout.

Conventional Therapies

Gout needs to be controlled to avoid the risk of kidney disease. Traditionally, the medical profession places more emphasis on drug treatment rather than dietary modifications. Some physicians believe that changes in the diet are not effective and the gout can only be controlled through drug preparations.

Other individuals strongly support the idea that gout, like gallstones, is a diet-related disorder. A diagnosis for gout may involve the drawing out of fluid from a painful joint and testing it for the presence of uric acid. This is not considered a completely conclusive test.

An old, traditional approach for the treatment of gout is the administration of colchicine an anti-inflammatory drug, which can have some unpleasant side effects. This drug dates back to the time of Hippocrates. This particular medicine is aimed at reducing inflammation rather than decreasing uric acid levels. Allupurinol (zyloprim, lopurin) is also a common drug used to treat gout and works by inhibiting the enzyme that produces uric acid. Other drugs used to treat gout are probenecid (benemid) and sulfinpyrazone (anturane). Anti-inflammatory drugs, such as Naprosyn, Motrin, Advil, Nuprin, Feldene, Clinoril and Indocin, are also routinely prescribed for pain. Indocin is recommended for its effectiveness in treating gout. A corticosteroid injection is sometimes administered into the joint to relieve severe inflammation and pain.

Dietary Guidelines

◆ Dietary modification is a preferable approach to gout than simply addressing its symptoms with drugs.
◆ A low purine diet is essential in treating and preventing gout. Purine foods to avoid are anchovies, meat gravies and broths, all organ meats, mincemeat, luncheon meats, meat, asparagus, herring, sardines, mussels, and mushrooms.
◆ Avoid eating white flour and sugar also.
◆ Additional foods to limit are dried beans, cauliflower, fish, lentils, oatmeal, peas, poultry, spinach, yeast products, and saturated fats.
◆ Do not consume alcohol as it can increase the production of uric acid and significantly inhibit its elimination from the kidneys.
◆ Foods to emphasize are raw fruits and vegetables, fresh juices, (carrot, celery, and parsley), grains, vegetable broths, seeds and nuts and high-fiber foods, including complex carbohydrates.
◆ Drink large amounts of fluid (water) to keep the urine diluted and facilitate the excretion of uric acid through the kidneys. Becoming dehydrated can increase your chances of an attack of gout.
◆ Cherry juice helps to neutralize uric acid. Cherries, hawthorn berries, blueberries and strawberries have shown through studies to be effective agents in lowering levels of uric acid and in preventing collagen destruction.
◆ Eating large amounts of cherries regularly is highly recommended if you are prone to gout.

Recommended Nutritional Supplements

Niacin supplements may precipitate an attack of gout as nicotinic acid competes with uric acid for excretion from the kidneys.[1]

PRIMARY NUTRIENTS

PYCNOGENOL (GRAPE SEED EXTRACT) The proanthocyanidins contained in this compound scavenge for free radicals and work as natural anti-inflammatory agents.[2] *Suggested Dosage:* Take as directed.

VITAMIN C WITH BIOFLAVONOIDS May lower serum uric acid levels by increasing renal excretion. Taking megadoses of this vitamin is not recommended as it may actually increase uric acid levels.[3] *Suggested Dosage:* Take 3,000 mg in three divided doses.

FOLIC ACID Important in facilitating nucleoprotein breakdown and inhibits the production of the enzyme responsible for the production of uric acid.[4] Folic acid plays an intrinsic role in the conversion of amino acids from protein foods. *Suggested Dosage:* Take 200 mg per day.

VITAMIN E WITH SELENIUM Vitamin E and selenium help to keep the production of leukotrienes down which cause joint inflammation. It also acts to scavenge free radicals by potentiating the action of vitamin E and vitamin C.[5] *Suggested Dosage:* Take each supplement as directed together.

GLUCOSAMINE/CHONDROITIN Contains special compounds which fight inflammation and help to protect joint cartilage. *Suggested Dosage:* Take as directed.[6]

CMO A fatty acid which has anti-inflammatory capabilities and has been successfully used to treat inflammatory joint conditions.[7] *Suggested Dosage:* Take as directed.

OMEGA-3 AND OMEGA-6 FATTY ACIDS Eicosapentaenoic acid in fish oil helps to inhibit the production of the inflammatory agents released in gout.[8] In addition, the fatty acids found in flaxseed and primrose oil also fight inflammation and inhibit prostaglandin production which aggravates inflammation. *Suggested Dosage:* Take as directed.

TURMERIC AND BOSWELLA Two herbs with significant anti-inflammatory capabilities. Boswella contains an acid which has shown its ability to control arthritis in a number of animal studies. Among its actions are the ability to inhibit inflammation through interfering with inflammatory mediators, improve circulation to affected joint tissues, and prevent a drop in glycosaminoglycan levels.[9] The curcumin content of tumeric can also treat stiffness and joint pain and is especially effective when combined with boswella.[10] *Suggested Dosage:* Take as directed.

BLACK CHERRY AND CELERY SEED Both of these botanicals have the ability to reduce inflammation and can help to neutralize the harmful effects of uric acid. *Suggested Dosage:* Take as directed.

HERBAL COMBINATION Also recommended is an herbal combination containing devil's claw, yucca, alfalfa leaf and seed, wild yam root, sarsaparilla root, kelp, white willow bark, cayenne, horsetail and chickweed. *Suggested Dosage:*

Four to six capsules daily. For extreme cases it is best to use maximum dosage of six capsules per day for a prolonged period of four to six months.

DEVIL'S CLAW: This herb has an extensive history of use as an anti-inflammatory, analgesic and digestive stimulant. It has gained official recognition as an antirheumatic and digestive agent in many European countries, including France, Germany, Belgium, and Britain.[11] Improper digestion of protein causes gout due to uric acid buildup. Undigested proteins can also form peptides which can trigger an inappropriate immune response resulting in arthritic symptoms.
YUCCA: Yucca has a similar action to that of devil's claw. It improves digestion, thereby reducing histamine production, and, as a result, inflammation and pain may be alleviated. The constituents of yucca which are bioactive are saponins.[12]
ALFALFA LEAVES AND SEEDS: As mentioned previously, gout may be a result of poor digestion. An impaired digestive system can cause malnutrition by starving the body of much needed macro- and micronutrients. If allowed to become chronic, serious and debilitating diseases can be the consequence. Alfalfa leaves and seeds provide a rich nutrient source to help the body to return to a healthy state.[13] WILD YAM ROOT: Other common names for wild yam root include rheumatism root and colic root, suggesting its use as an antirheumatic and digestive aid. Its antirheumatic property is primarily thought to be attributed to its cortisone precursor diosgenin. As diosgenin is converted to cortisone, anti-inflammatory activity results, and the patient may notice a reduction of pain.[14] SARSAPARILLA ROOT: Sarsaparilla which is used as a food flavoring in the United States, is officially recognized in Germany and the United Kingdom for its antirheumatic, anti-inflammatory, and diuretic properties. Its activity is thought to be due to its saponin content. Historically, this herb has been used to treat gout and rheumatism and is classified as a tonic and blood purifier.[15]
KELP: Kelp, like alfalfa, is a dense source of nutrients, particularly trace elements which can improve the body's nutrition. It also provides mucilage in the form of algin which soothes the gastrointestinal tract. WHITE WILLOW BARK: White willow bark has been used for over a thousand years to relieve pain. Salicin, aspirin's forerunner, was discovered to be white willow's active constituent. Apart from its ability to assist with pain, salicin reduces inflammation, but unlike aspirin it will not thin the blood or irritate the stomach.
CAYENNE: Cayenne stimulates circulation and makes the other herbs more effective. Cayenne can help to improve digestion. Cayenne's hot principle, capsaicin, is also a noted analgesic and can be applied in topical ointment form.
HORSETAIL (SHAVEGRASS): While horsetail contributes to this formula as a mild diuretic, its main action is to strengthen and regenerate connective tissues. Connective tissue (found abundantly in joints) is destroyed by inflammation. Silica is vital in regenerating connective tissue and keeping it strong, and horsetail is one of the richest known sources of silica.

SECONDARY NUTRIENTS

GERMANIUM: Works to help control swelling and pain. Suggested Dosage: Take as directed. Do not exceed recommended dosages.

BROMELAIN: An enzyme found in the pineapple plant which functions as an effective anti-inflammatory. Suggested Dosage: Take as directed using chewable tablets. Eating plenty of fresh pineapple is also a good idea.
ALANINE, ASPARTIC ACID, AND GLYCINE: These amino acids have been known to reduce levels of uric acid. Suggested Dosage: Take as directed on an empty stomach with fruit juice.
TEA TREE OIL: Can be used externally by massaging it into the affected joints. Suggested Dosage: Use as directed.

Home Care Suggestions

- Keep the painful joint elevated. If the pain is severe use an ice pack. Iced gel packs used for physical therapy that stay soft are recommended.
- To keep the weight of bed sheets off of the affected joint, use a box or make a frame to keep the joint uncovered when sheets or blankets are pulled up.
- Try to achieve an optimal weight through a nutritious diet with a regular exercise program.
- If losing weight, do not do it too rapidly as uric acid levels may rise dramatically and result in an attack of gout.
- A charcoal poultice made from activated powdered charcoal and water may provide some pain relief.

Other Supportive Therapies

MASSAGE: Oils of peppermint, lavender, and geranium may be massaged into the affected joints. Try to self-mobilize the toe by gently pulling it and moving it around.
ACUPRESSURE: Massage of specific points relating to the feet can be helpful.
CHIROPRACTIC AND OSTEOPATHY: Both provide foot flexibility maneuvers to help alleviate uric acid deposits.

Scientific Facts-at-a-Glance

New studies have found that beer has a higher purine content than wine or other alcoholic drinks and that it may be a significant determining factor in predicting gout. Beer increases purine-nucleated metabolism in the liver, which increases uric acid production. One study found that the major dietary difference of 61 men with gout versus a control group was that 41 percent of them drank more than twelve cans of beer a day.[16]

Spirit/Mind Considerations

Gout is one of many conditions which demands that we reevaluate our eating habits and have the fortitude to make the necessary changes. We frequently want our doctors to hand us a magic pill that will be able to take care of our unpleasant symptoms without changing our bad habits. Gout typically results from overeating rich, fatty foods that are high in meat protein. Moreover, men who drink beer are particularly prone to gout. If we truly value our bodies as the entities which house our spirits, we need to pay more attention to their needs and give them the respect they require.

Often, the human body tries to signal us with certain symptoms, which in essence, act as a warning that we are abusing it through what we choose to consume.

All of us could do better; however, those of us with gout or other diseases linked to dietary choices or lifestyle habits need to bite the bullet and make the changes. Even if we are not able to eliminate everything from our "forbidden" list of foods, we can certainly improve considerably.

Prevention

- ◆ Drink at least 5 to 8 glasses of water per day to make sure waste products such as uric acid can be excreted easier by the kidneys.
- ◆ Protect your joints from injury. Joints that have been traumatized seem more susceptible to gout.
- ◆ Don't overuse diuretics. The abuse of these agents can impair the kidney's ability to excrete uric acid.
- ◆ Avoid a diet high in meat, alcohol and rich foods.
- ◆ If you are taking high blood pressure medication, you are at higher risk for developing gout. Watch your diet carefully, reduce salt, exercise and stay away from culprit foods and alcohols related to gout.
- ◆ Eat cherries and other dark red or blue berries on a regular basis.
- ◆ Do not consume large quantities of protein or take an excess of protein supplements.

Doctor's Notes

Gout is a problem which involves the improper metabolism of certain foods (especially red meat) which causes the formation of uric acid. This acid can deposit itself into joints, causing swelling and inflammation. The best way to approach gout is to adjust the diet and use supplements which help to lower or neutralize uric acid and work to alleviate joint inflammation.

A 47-year old male patient of mine had suffered with gout all his life. He was willing to alter his diet by significantly reducing the amount of animal protein he consumes. As a result, he has experienced a dramatic drop in the number of gout attacks. I also put him on a combination of black cherry extract and celery seed. Consequently, his uric acid level fell into the normal range. He has gone for over four months without an attack, which is the longest gout-free interval he has experienced in the past two years. As mentioned earlier, I believe that simple dietary changes combined with the help of certain herbs and nutrients can control gout without harsh drugs.

Endnotes

1. C. Pfeiffer, Elemental Nutrients, (Keats Publishing, New Canaan, Conn: 1975), 121.
2. Melvyn Werbach and Michael Murray, Botanical Influences on Illness: A Source book of Clinical Research, (Third Line Press, Tarzana, CA: 1994), 27-28.
3. H. Stein, et al., "Ascorbic acid-induced uricosuria: A consequence of megavitamin therapy. Ann Intern Med, 1976, 84(4):385-8.
4. H. Kalckar, and H. Klenow, "Milk xanthopterin osicase and pteroyl-glutamic acid," Jour Biol Chem, 1948, 172: 349-50.
5. V.E. Kagan, et al., "Dihydrolipoic acid: A Universal antioxidant both in the membrane and in the aqueous phase," Biochem Pharmacol, 1992, 44: 1637-49.
6. I. Setnikar, "Antireactive Properties of 'chondoprotective' drugs," Int-Jour-Tissue-React,1992, 14 (5): 253-61.
7. H. Deihl, "Cetyl myristoleate isolated from Swiss albino mice: an apparent protective agent against adjuvant arthritis," Journal of Pharmaceutical Sciences, 1994, vol. 83 (3): 296-299.
8. T. Stammers, et al., "Fish oil in osteoarthritis," Letter, Lancet, 1989, 2: 503.
9. G.Singh, et al., "Pharmacology of an extract of salai guggal ex-Boswellia serrata, a new non-steroidal anti-inflammatory agent." Agents Action, 1986, (18): 407-12.
10. R. Kulkarni, et al., "Treatment of osteoarthritis with a herbomineral formulation: a double-blind, placebo-controlled, crossover study," Jour Ethnopharmacol, 1991, 33(1-2): 91-95.
11. L.R. Brady, et al., Pharmacognosy, 8th ed. Lea and Gebiger, Philadelphia: 1981, 480.
12. R. Bingham, et al., "Yucca plant saponins in the management of arthritis," Jour Applied Nutrition, 1975, 27: 45-50.
13. M.R. Malinow, et al., "Effect of alfalfa saponins on intestinal cholesterol absorption in rats," Amer Jour Clini Nutri, 1977, 30: 2061-67.
14. H.W. Feller, The Eclectic Materia Medica, Pharmacology and Therapeutics, Eclectic Medical Publications, Portland Oregon: 1983, first published in 1922.
15. Kiangsu Institute of Modern Medicine, Encyclopedia of Chinese Drugs, 2 vols. 1977, Shanghia, People's Republic of China.
16. T. Gibson, et al., "A controlled study of diet in patients with gout," Ann Rheum Dis, 1983, 42(2): 123-27.

HALITOSIS

See "Bad Breath"

HEADACHES

See "Migraine Headaches"

HEART ATTACK

A heart attack refers to the sudden death of part of the heart muscle due to oxygen deprivation. An estimated one million heart attacks occur in the United States each year and one-third of these are fatal. Heart attacks are considered the single most common cause of death in developed countries of the world. Men are more susceptible to heart attacks than women.

If you have had a heart attack you have an increased risk of having another unless significant lifestyle changes are implemented. Many heart attack victims have a history of angina, which usually indicates the presence of coronary artery disease. Because heart disease occurs far less frequently in primitive societies, Western lifestyle must be addressed as the first and foremost contributing factor to heart-related disorders and deaths.

Symptoms

The pain of an heart attack usually comes on suddenly and ranges from a tight ache to an intense, crushing pain. It is persistent and does not decrease with rest. Heart attack pain can be characterized by a feeling of central chest pressure, squeezing or tightness, chest pain which radiates down the left arm, chest pain which may radiate into the jaw area and through the back, or pain in the upper abdomen which may be mistaken for indigestion or heartburn.

Other symptoms include shortness of breath, cold clammy skin, nausea, vomiting, diarrhea, anxiety, or loss of consciousness.

Long term complications of a heart attack include mitral valve damage and a weakened heart, which may require surgical repair.

If the attack is severe enough, heart failure can result after the heart has gone into an arrhythmia (referred to as ventricular fibrillation). Moreover, 20 percent of heart attacks are painless and usually occur in elderly people or diabetics.

If you or someone else is experiencing any of the above symptoms call an ambulance immediately and have them take some aspirin. Any type of chest pain requires immediate medical evaluation. The use of electrical defibrillation and clot-dissolving drugs can save lives if administered quickly enough. Most heart attack deaths occur before the victim ever reaches the hospital.

Causes

A heart attack results when blood supply to heart muscle is interrupted by a blockage of some kind causing the death of heart tissue.

Atherosclerosis of the coronary arteries is the most common cause of a heart attack. This buildup of fatty deposits develops on the inner lining of the arteries, and restrict blood flow and encourage the formation of clots, all of which can result in the sudden blockage of blood flow to the heart.

Risk factors which increase your chances of having a heart attack are a familial history of heart disease, cigarette smoking, high blood pressure, obesity, high blood cholesterol, physical inactivity, and coronary artery disease.

Factors which are thought to trigger a heart attack include an emotional crisis, a heavy meal, physical overexertion or heavy lifting.

Conventional Therapies

While doctors cannot cure the damage which results from a heart attack, advances in cardiac care and drug therapy can save lives. Cardiac arrests and arrythmias are easier to treat than heart failure. An ECG will be taken immediately to assess the severity of the heart blockage. A blood sample will be tested for the presence of a certain enzyme which is released into the bloodstream from damaged heart muscle. Emergency coronary artery angiography may be administered if surgery is being considered.

Standard medical procedures to treat a heart attack include administering pain killers and oxygen therapy. Diuretic drugs may be given to treat heart failure which can lead to fluid accumulation in the lungs.

Intravenous fluids will be given to prevent shock and antiarrhythmic drugs may be administered to control heart arrhythmias. Beta-blocker drugs are given in some cases to prevent further damage to heart muscle. In cases where the victim of a heart attack arrives at a hospital within three to six hours of the attack, thrombolytic drugs that dissolve blood clots can be given and significantly increase the chances of survival. Tissue plasminogen activator (TPA) is used to dissolve clots and is considered the best treatment for a heart attack. Streptokinase is another clot dissolver, which is not considered as effective as TPA.

Blood thinners will be given to prevent the formation of another clot until an angiogram can be done. Following this test an angioplasty, which widens the narrowed coronary arteries, or by-pass surgery may be indicated.

An angioplasty involves inserting a thin flexible tube into an artery located in the arm or leg and guiding it into the affected coronary artery in which a small balloon is inflated, which usually eliminates the clot obstruction.

Coronary by-pass surgery may be required to remove the blocked section of the artery and reconnect or reroute arterial blood flow by grafting in healthy vessels.

Dietary Guidelines

◆ Learn to eat plenty of raw fresh vegetables and fruits. Incorporate a diet which is high in fiber and low in animal fats and refined sugars.

◆ Add whole grains, almonds, plenty of fresh fruits and vegetables, all kinds of legumes, white skinless turkey or chicken meat, or fish to your diet.

◆ Avoid caffeine, red meats, and refined carbohydrates such as white sugar and white flour which can cause wide fluctuations in blood sugar that strain the heart.

◆ Minimize your intake of dairy products. Use low-fat varieties. Homogenized dairy products contain xanthine oxidasean, an enzyme which is believed to cause artery damage which could lead to arteriosclerosis.

◆ Avoid palm oil, coconut oil, peanut oil, cottonseed oil, crisco and butter. Only use margarine which is made from safflower or sunflower oils (hydrogenation, the process in which liquid oils are made into solid sticks, poses considerable health risks).

◆ Olive oil and canola oil are also good unsaturated oils that contain essential fatty acids. Olive oil is monounsaturated oil and should be added to the diet along with polyunsaturated oils.

◆ Decrease or eliminate salt and salty foods from your diet.

◆ Add plenty of raw onion and garlic to your diet. Both of these decrease the risk of blood clots.

◆ Pectin, which is found in fresh fruits and vegetables and can also be purchased as a supplement, can help to inhibit cholesterol buildup.

◆ Drinking barley water is a traditional old fashioned tonic considered to have valuable health benefits.

◆ Do not use alcohol.

◆ Taking two teaspoons of wheat germ oil daily is also recommended for any heart-related disorder.

Recommended Nutritional Supplements

PRIMARY NUTRIENTS

GARLIC AND ONION Both of these extracts have successfully treated both hypertension and high cholesterol or blood lipids which are directly linked to causing and exacerbating chronic heart disease.[1] *Suggested Dosage:* Take 2 to 3 capsules with each meal.

COENZYME Q10 Helps to strengthen and oxygenate heart muscle and contributes to metabolic processes. Studies have conclusively proven its significant benefit in treating both cardiovascular disease and hypertension.[2] *Suggested Dosage:* Take 100 mg daily. For established serious cases of CHD, take 300 to 400 mg daily.

ESSENTIAL FATTY ACIDS Both of these fatty acids which are found in fish oils and oils like flaxseed can decrease blood pressure and blood lipids. The fact that Eskimo cultures have diets high in saturated fats but have low cardiovascu-

lar disease is attributed to the effect of coldwater fish consumption.[3] *Suggested Dosage:* Take as directed a blend of fish oil or flaxseed oil with borage or evening primrose. Keep refrigerated. If you use fish oil, take a vitamin E supplement.

VITAMIN E Works to scavenge for free radicals and helps to protect against heart disease and stroke by also reducing LDL cholesterol. Low levels of this vitamin are considered a primary predictor of heart disease.[4] *Suggested Dosage:* If you are at low risk for these disorders, take 100 IU per day. If you are at high risk, take 400 to 800 IU per day.

VITAMIN C WITH BIOFLAVONOIDS These compounds act as free radical scavengers in the arteries and heart muscle and also have been shown to lower blood pressure in clinical tests. Supplementation may actually reduce blood pressure.[5] Incidence of heart attack may also be inversely correlated to bioflavonoid consumption. *Suggested Dosage:* 1,000 to 3,000 mg per day.

CALCIUM This mineral is very important in maintaining or normalizing blood pressure and ensuring proper heart muscle function. Supplementation can actually modify hypertension in some people.[6] *Suggested Dosage:* 1,000 mg of citrate variety per day.

MAGNESIUM The proper balance of minerals like magnesium is vital for regulating blood pressure and for nourishing heart muscle.[7] *Suggested Dosage:* 400 to 800 mg per day. Use chelated products.

SELENIUM Keeping selenium levels in the body high may be directly linked to blood pressure levels. Studies have found a direct correlation and because many American diets are selenium deficient, supplementation may be vital.[8] *Suggested Dosage:* Take as directed.

POTASSIUM The ratio of sodium to potassium is considered a profound determiner of blood pressure. Supplementation may be of value.[9] In addition, potassium is considered an electrolyte which helps regulate heart contraction. *Suggested Dosage:* Take only as directed.

NICOTINIC ACID A compound contained in niacin, this substance has the ability to substantially lower blood cholesterol and triglyceride levels.[10] *Suggested Dosage:* Take as directed.

HAWTHORN The proanthocyanidins found in this herb actually inhibit angiotensin-converting enzymes in much the same way as some prescription high blood pressure medications.[11] Anyone who has had a heart attack should go on a lifetime protocol of hawthorn therapy. *Suggested Dosage:* Take as directed. Combining with rosemary can also be helpful.

FIBER SUPPLEMENT Boosting fiber intake can be one of the single most effective treatments of hypertension and can also significantly lower blood cholesterol levels.[12] *Suggested*

Dosage: Take first thing in the morning and before going to bed. Use products that can be mixed in liquid.

FOLIC ACID AND VITAMIN B6 Very recent data suggests that taking more than RDA recommended requirements of these two vitamins can prevent heart disease. *Suggested Dosage:* Take as directed. You should, however, consult your doctor before increasing your dosage.

POLYUNSATURATED LECITHIN Can help with the proper emulsifying of fats in the blood stream. Animal studies indicate that lecithin facilitates the breakdown and elimination of cholesterol. *Suggested Dosage:* Take as directed.

SP PHOSPHATADITYL CHOLINE Helps reduce fat and triglyceride levels in the blood. *Suggested Dosage:* Take as directed.

HERBAL COMBINATION This combination should include hawthorn berries, motherwort, rosemary leaves, cayenne, kelp, wood betony, and shepherd's purse. *Suggested Dosage:* Four to six capsules daily.

HAWTHORN BERRY: Next to digitalis, hawthorn is probably the most recognized herb for positively affecting the heart. As demonstrated by scientific studies, hawthorn supports metabolic processes in the heart, dilates coronary vessels, reduces peripheral resistance and lowers blood pressure, reduces tendency for angina attacks, and strengthens damaged or weakened heart muscles.[13] MOTHERWORT: The use of motherwort as a cardiotonic spans centuries. Its other common names such as heart heal and heart wort are more indicative of its heart benefits than the name "motherwort." Motherwort is especially beneficial in cases of nervous heart conditions which can cause, among other things, palpitation or abnormally rapid or fluttering heart beats.[14] ROSEMARY LEAVES: A powerful antioxidant herb which supports the integrity of the veins, rosemary has also exhibited cardiotonic capacity which helps with normal heart function. It also causes mild perspiration, releasing toxins from the body and improving health.[15] CAYENNE: Cayenne supports and improves circulation. Cayenne is considered an herb activator that increases the effectiveness of other herbs. It stimulates digestion and promotes perspiration. Cayenne has been shown to reduce blood pressure, especially in conjunction with garlic. KELP: Kelp is a powerhouse of micronutrients that assist with various metabolic processes. Kelp has been considered a blood vessel cleanser and a treatment for atherosclerosis.[16] WOOD BETONY: Wood betony is carminative, diuretic, and nervine, which all support a healthy cardiovascular system. SHEPHERD'S PURSE: Shepherd's purse is a common weed that grows all over the United States. It is diuretic and has an ability to regulate blood pressure and heart action.

SECONDARY NUTRIENTS

L-CARNITINE: Helps to sustain cardiac muscle and is involved in caloric conversion of macronutrients to muscle. A deficiency of carnitine has been linked with heart disease. *Suggested Dosage:* Take as directed on an empty stomach with fruit juice.

GINKGO: This herb works to boost circulation and can help protect heart muscle by enhancing oxygenation. When combined with garlic, it contributes to lowered cholesterol levels. *Suggested Dosage:* Take as directed using standardized products.

POTASSIUM: Potassium helps to keep heart muscle in proper contraction and rhythm. A lack of potassium can cause abnormal heart beats. *Suggested Dosage:* Take with your doctor's approval as directed.

VITAMIN B-COMPLEX: These vitamins are necessary for healthy heart function. *Suggested Dosage:* Take as directed.

PROTEOLYTIC ENZYMES: Help to enhance the breakdown of fibrin, which decreases the risk of developing a blood clot. *Suggested Dosage:* Take 30 minutes before everymeal, in between meals and before going to bed. Look for supplements which contain pancreatin and papain.

Home Care Suggestions

◆ After you have sufficiently recovered, incorporate a sensible daily exercise regimen such as walking for fifteen minutes a day. (Begin this only after you have received your doctor's approval).

◆ Watch out for overprotective family members who may have a tendency to inhibit your participation in exercise. Discouraging much-needed exercise in heart disease patients can do more harm than good. Make sure your spouse or family member is well-educated on the benefits of exercise for the recovering heart patient.

◆ Eat a diet high in fiber, fresh fruits and vegetables, legumes, whole grains, and use low fat dairy products and skinless white meats and fish.

◆ Avoid sexual intercourse for four to five weeks following a heart attack.

◆ Do not smoke.

Other Supportive Therapies

ACUPUNCTURE: Can help to stimulate muscle flexibility and build strength after an attack.

HOMEOPATHY: Arnica 6c and the biochemic tissue salt kali mur 6x are traditionally used.

MASSAGE: Massage greatly enhances muscle tone and flexibility while promoting relaxation.

MEDITATION: Helps to diffuse the damaging effects of stress.

Scientific Facts-at-a-Glance

More and more clinical data is emerging which supports the idea that certain supplements, when taken in larger dosages than normally indicated, can help to significantly cut the risk of heart disease. Recently, an evening news broadcast announced that vitamin B6 and folic acid, if taken in greater-than-RDA doses, could dramatically reduce the risk of a heart attack for women in particular. What this says, in essence, is that larger than normal dosages of certain nutrients can have a very beneficial effect on the human body. In addition, receiving those nutrients from dietary sources alone is not always possible. Therapeutic doses of nutrients like these along with others such as vitamin E, vitamin C, garlic, etc., can achieve marvelous results, and supports the notion that supplementation should be considered absolutely essential for the maintenance of health and the treatment of disease.

Spirit/Mind Considerations

Make relaxation techniques an integral part of your life. Reduce and manage stress—stress can actually elevate blood cholesterol and clotting. Excessive adrenal stimulation, which can occur in periods of prolonged stress, not only increases the chance of arterial spasms and heart attacks but can decrease your chance of surviving a heart attack as well. Use biofeedback, music therapy, yoga, self hypnosis, etc., to control stress. Evaluate your emotional status. If you are resentful, fearful, or angry, get rid of these toxic reactions to the events of life and learn to mellow out. Make the pursuit of joy and serenity a daily goal. The power of prayer and meditation should not be minimized to this end.

Prevention

- Don't smoke. Nicotine constricts arteries, impairs circulation and raises blood pressure. It also reduces that capacity of the blood to carry oxygen and increases the risk of blood clot formation. Smoking is a great contributor to coronary heart disease and the incidence of heart attacks.
- Exercise daily, incorporating 30 minutes of aerobic exercise into your daily routine five days per week. Exercise has a multitude of physical as well as emotional benefits. It improves the efficiency of the heart, reduces cholesterol levels and the chance of blood clot formation and improves circulation in the heart muscle itself. Brisk walking is considered an excellent aerobic exercise.
- The best way to prevent a heart attack or heart disease is to build good habits of eating, exercise and relaxation which can protect coronary arteries from damage.
- Keep serum cholesterol levels low. High-serum cholesterol is the most important predictor of a heart attack. Use of cholesterol reducing drugs should come only as a last resort. Atherosclerosis can be stopped and even reversed without the use of drugs if dietary changes are implemented.
- Maintain an optimal weight. Obesity increases the risk of heart disease, high blood pressure, diabetes, and a number of other diseases.
- Keep your blood pressure normal—high blood pressure can significantly increase circulatory demands on the heart and may accelerate the development of coronary artery disease.

Doctor's Notes

Nutrient deficiencies can predispose us to cardiovascular disease or heart attack. We know that deficiencies in vitamin E and the B vitamins (vitamin B6, vitamin B12, and folic

acid) are associated with an increased risk of coronary artery disease. What this tells us is that what we eat and the supplements we take have a direct impact on our heart and vascular system. Many heart problems dramatically improve when dietary changes are made. Moreover, supplements like hawthorn have marvelous therapeutic actions to strengthen and protect the heart. Having a first heart attack should serve as a wake up call. If you are smart, you can end up healthier than you were before the attack occurred. If you don't heed the warning, it's only a matter of time before you have another attack. Something as simple as cutting saturated fat intake coupled with mild exercise can work wonders. If you smoke, stop. For women who are struggling with the issue of estrogen-replacement therapy and may be inclined to use it to lower their risk of cardiovascular disease, taking indole-3-carbinol and genistein may actually work in the same way as estrogen does to protect the heart. Clinical studies are finding that the indoles and isoflavones work as phytoestrogens and may eliminate the need for synthetic estrogen replacement therapy in some post-hysterectomy or post-menopausal women.

Additional Resources

American Heart Association
7272 Greenville Ave.
Dallas, Tx 75231
214-373-6300

Endnotes

1. D. Louria, et al., "Onion extract in treatment of hypertension and hyperlipidemia: A preliminary communication," Curr Ther Res, 1985, 37(1):127-31.
2. T.Yamagami, et al., "Bioenergetics in clinical medicine: Studies on coenzyme Q-10 and essential hypertension," Res Commun Chem Pathol Pharmacol, 1975, 11:273.
3. P. Singer, "Blood pressure-lowering effect of w-3 polyunsaturated fatty acids in clinical studies," in A.P. Simopoulos et al., eds."Health effects of w-3 polyunsaturated fatty acids in seafoods," World Rev Nutr Diet, 1991, 66:329-48.
4. K.F. Gey, et al., "Inverse correlation between plasma vitamin E and mortality from ischemic heart disease in cross-cultural epidemiology," Amer Jour Clin Nutri, 1991, 53: 326S_ 334S.
5. O. Osilesi. et al., "Blood pressure and plasma lipids during ascorbic acid supplementation in borderline hypertensive and normotensive adults," Nutr Res, 1991, 11:405-12. See also D. Brown, Quarterly Review Of Natural Medicine, Spring 1994
6. D. McCarron, et al., "Dietary calcium and blood pressure: Modifying factors in specific populations. Am J Clin Nutr, 1991, 54:215S-19S.
7. T. Moore, "The role of dietary electrolytes in hypertension," J Am Coll Nutr, 1989, 8: Suppl S:68S-80S.
8. J. Salonen, et al., "Blood pressure, dietary fats, and antioxidants," Am Jour Clin Nutr, 1988, 48:1226-32.
9. A. Sianin, et al., "Controlled trial of long term oral potassium supplements in patients with mild hypertension," Bri Med Jour, 1987, 294:1453-56.
10. J.R. DiPalma and W.S. Thayer, "The use of niacin as a drug," Ann Rev Nutr, 1991, 11: 169-87.
11. S. Uchida, et al., "Inhibitory effects of condensed tannins on angiotensin converting enzyme," Jap Jour Pharmacol, 1987. 43:242-5.
12. P. Little, et al., "A controlled trial of a low sodium, low fat, high fiber

diet in treated hypertensive patients: the efficacy of multiple dietary intervention," Postgraduate Medical Journal, 1990, 66(778): 616-21. F.L. Shinnick, et al., "Dose response to a dietary oat bran fraction in cholesterol-fed rats," Jour Nutri. 1990, 120(6): 561-68.

13. R. Blesken, "Crataegus in cardiology," Fortsc Med, 1992, 110(15): 290-92. See also D. Brown, Quarterly Review Of Natural Medicine, Spring 1994.

14. F. Arustamova, "Hypotensive effect of leonaurus cardiaca on animals in experimental chronic hypertension," Uzvestuta Akad Nauk Arm SSR Biol Nauki, 1963, 16(7): 47-52.

15. A. Boido, et al., "N-substituted derivatives of rosmaricine," Stu Sass Sez 2, 1975, 53(5-6): 383-93.

16. P. Searle, et al., "Study of a cardiotonic fraction from an extract of the seaweed undaria pinnatifida," Procee West Pharmacol Soc, 1981, 24: 63-65.

HEARTBURN

Even with the glut of antacids on our pharmacy shelves, new studies suggest that more people than ever may be suffering from persistent heartburn. Up to 21 million Americans are estimated heartburn victims, many of whom claim that the products they use often fail them. Heartburn, also called gastroesophageal reflux, is a burning sensation that originates from the stomach but may be experienced in the chest region. The feeling may travel from the breastbone to the throat. It is caused when hydrochloric acid backs up from the stomach into the esophagus. Occasional heartburn is no cause for alarm; however, anyone who suffers from it two days a week or more may have a more serious problem such as gastroesophageal reflux disease.

Symptoms

Heartburn is characterized by a burning pain or sensation that moves from the upper stomach area to the throat; a sour taste in the mouth; bloating; difficulty swallowing; belching; choking; coughing; hoarseness; chest pain; an uncomfortable feeling of fullness; headache; and nausea.

Ignoring persistent heartburn can lead to lesions on the esophagus, asthma, laryngitis, and even cancer. If heartburn is accompanied by the vomiting of black or bloody material or passing tar-like stool or chest pain that radiates to the back, difficulty swallowing, shortness of breath, or dizziness, see your doctor immediately. These symptoms may indicate the presence of ulcers, an obstruction of the esophagus or a heart attack.

Causes

Heartburn occurs when there is too much pressure on the stomach or when the sphincter muscle which separates the esophagus from the stomach does not completely close. If you experience heartburn on a regular basis, see your doctor. Repeated episodes of heartburn can damage the esophagus or cause ulcers.

Factors that may cause heartburn include excessive consumption of fried, fatty, spicy, rich or acidic foods; consumption of alcohol; smoking; excess aspirin or ibuprofen consumption; caffeine; obesity; enzyme deficiency; hiatal hernia; stomach ulcers; gallbladder disorders; allergies; stress; heart problems; pregnancy; and various drugs (anticonvulsants, antidepressants, birth control pills, estrogenic drugs, sedatives like Valium, and some antihistamines).

Chronic constipation can contribute to heartburn because straining during bowel movements puts added pressure on the abdomen, causing reflux. Recurring heartburn may also indicate the presence of esophagitis, a condition where the lower segment of the esophagus does not completely close off from the stomach. Lying down in a certain position or bending over after meal can also result in heartburn.

Conventional Therapies

Your doctor will have to determine if your symptoms are the result of stomach acid or not. An upper gastrointestinal x-ray may be required if the presence of an ulcer or hiatal hernia is suspected. Medications that decrease the secretion of acid may be prescribed and antacids will be recommended. While an antacid may provide relief, it does not treat the cause of the problem. It is important to select antacids that do not contain potentially dangerous compounds like aluminum or sodium. Calcium carbonate products include Tums, Chooz, Titralac and Alka-Mints. Magnesium salts are found in Milk of Magnesia products, and aluminum mixtures include Gaviscon, Gelusil, Mylanta, Maalox, Riopan, Di-Gel and Aludrox. New over-the-counter products that suppress stomach acid production rather than treat it after-the-fact are called H2 blockers and include Pepsid AC, Zantac and Tagamet. These must be taken prior to eating to be effective. Prescription-strength H2 blockers are also available. Surgery is warranted only in severe cases in which the upper part of the stomach and esophagus is stretched and warped, increasing pressure on the lower sphincter muscle.

Dietary Guidelines

◆ Avoid milk. Contrary to past beliefs, drinking milk to calm heartburn is not a good idea. Milk has only a transient neutralizing effect on gastric acidity followed by an actual rise in acid secretion.[1] Drinking water will actually neutralize acid more than milk will.

◆ Also stay away from culprit foods like fried foods, fatty foods, citrus fruits, coffee, alcohol, spicy foods, chocolate, tomato-based foods, and onions (although if cooked thoroughly they are considerably less likely to cause trouble).

◆ Certain varieties of onions such as the walla and maui are milder. Rich dairy products and carbonated beverages can also cause heartburn.

◆ Soda pop can cause bloating and put pressure on the abdominal sphincter.

◆ Eating buttered popcorn can also be a problem for some individuals.

◆ Eating fruits with a high enzyme content such as fresh papaya and fresh pineapple helps to boost digestion.

Recommended Nutritional Supplements

PRIMARY NUTRIENTS

PROTEOLYTIC DIGESTIVE ENZYMES These enzymes can facilitate better digestion and breakdown of macronutrients and should include pancreatin and papain.[2] *Suggested Dosage:* Take as directed 30 minutes prior to eating.

GINGER An excellent herb for heartburn due to is ability to absorb excess stomach acid. Can be taken in capsule form. Studies have found that ginger can prevent the formation of ulcers even in the presence of compounds like aspirin.[3] *Suggested Dosage:* Take as directed.

PAPAYA AND BROMELAIN This duo has the ability to treat a number of gastrointestinal disorders. Bromelain can remain active in either low or high pH environments.[4] *Suggested Dosage:* Take as directed 30 minutes prior to eating.

FENNEL AND CATNIP Both work as anti-inflammatory agents for the stomach and help to control gas and bloating. *Suggested Dosage:* Take as directed using standardized products.

SLIPPERY ELM This herb has a very high mucilage content which enables it to protect and soothe the mucus membranes of the gastrointestinal tract. *Suggested Dosage:* Take as directed. Capsulized products are good, however making a paste may afford better protection when swallowed.

HERBAL COMBINATION This combination should include papaya leaves, peppermint leaves, fennel seeds, ginger root, gentian root, and Irish moss. *Suggested Dosage:* Two to three capsules daily. Best if taken during a meal. Do not use if you are pregnant or lactating.

PAPAYA LEAVES: Papaya leaves are a rich source of an enzyme called papain. Papain is ideal for people with pancreatic insufficiency because it is a protein-digesting enzyme that functions similar to the body's pepsin and pancreatic protease enzymes. Papain also contains small amounts of lipase (a fat-digesting enzyme) and amylase (a carbohydrate-digesting enzyme). Papain can also help digest foods which may cause allergic reactions. PEPPERMINT LEAVES: Peppermint leaves contribute to this formula in several ways. If nervous disorders are the cause of heartburn, peppermint helps by calming the nerves and relaxing the muscles of the gastrointestinal tract. Peppermint can also help to calm a spastic intestine and cramping stomach.[6] Peppermint increases bile production and secretion which helps to prevent heartburn and gas. Great Britain, France, Belgium, Germany, Switzerland, and Russia are among the many countries that officially recognize and accept peppermint's remarkable influence on digestion. FENNEL SEEDS: The aromatic oils of fennel are believed to be responsible for its powerful effect on the digestive system. Fennel calms the stomach and soothes stressed spastic muscles of the gastrointestinal tract. It can relieve colic, treat heartburn and reduce flatulence.[7] Fennel reduces the need for laxatives and prevents the gripping discomfort often associated with their use. GINGER ROOT: No herb is better at supporting good digestion than ginger. The Japanese use it to clean and freshen the palate, stimulate saliva secretion, and improve digestion. Ginger can soothe and settle the stomach. Ginger also normalizes the action of the intestinal muscle and can protect the mucus membranes of the stomach from acid damage.[8] GENTIAN ROOT: Gentian is a very popular European bitter used to treat and prevent digestive disorders. Applications for gentian include indigestion, heartburn, vomiting, low bile and saliva secretion, and dyspepsia.[9] Gentian is officially recognized in Germany, France,

Belgium and the United Kingdom. IRISH MOSS: Irish moss is employed in this formula for its soothing demulcent properties. It contains mucilage which coats the gastrointestinal tract and improves the integrity of the lining. It serves to protect the stomach from excess acid damage.[10] For this reason, it is very beneficial for heartburn and gastritis.

SECONDARY NUTRIENTS

VITAMIN B12: Needed for good digestion and assimilation. *Suggested Dosage:* Take sublingual products at 200 mcg with each meal per day.

ANGELICA ROOT (DONG QUAI): Helps to relieve gas and other stomach ailments. *Suggested Dosage:* Take as directed using standardized products.

ACIDOPHILUS: Replaces friendly flora in the bowel which decreases gas and bloating. *Suggested Dosage:* Take as directed on an empty stomach using guaranteed bacterial count products with bifidobacteria that are milk-free. Be sure to check expiration date.

APPLE CIDER VINEGAR AND WATER: This mixture seems to counteract heartburn. *Suggested Dosage:* One teaspoon to a half glass of water sipped slowly.

ACTIVATED CHARCOAL: Helps to absorb excess acid in the stomach and neutralize its effects. *Suggested Dosage:* Take as directed.

ALGIN: A gel derived from algae that exerts a protective and healing effect on the mucus membranes of the stomach. *Suggested Dosage:* Take as directed.

Home Care Suggestions

◆ Over-the-counter antacids can be effective but can contain undesirable ingredients.

◆ Try to avoid products that contain sodium or aluminum. Riopan is low in sodium. Antacids such as Maalox, Mylanta or Gelusil may provide relief but should be used with caution by people who suffer from heart disease or high blood pressure. Tums are recommended because they contain calcium carbonate. Milk of Magnesia is also free of aluminum and sodium. There is some speculation that using antacids on a regular basis can actually encourage further stomach acid secretion. The continued use of antacids may also result in a depletion of calcium.

◆ Do not use sodium bicarbonate (baking soda) as a home remedy. It contains sodium and if misused can upset the acid/alkaline balance of the body and cause a potentially dangerous condition.

◆ While drinking milk can sometimes help to relieve the symptoms of heartburn, dairy products increase the stomach's production of hydrochloric acid.

◆ Don't smoke. Nicotine adversely affects the tone of the esophageal sphincter muscle and can directly contribute to heartburn.

◆ Loosen constrictive clothing or tight belts.

◆ Learn to eat slowly, chew thoroughly and relax during mealtime.

◆ Calcium carbonate can function as an antacid and can be purchased as a powder. It is also contained in Tums.

◆ Review other medications that you are taking to see if they are the cause of your heartburn. Certain high blood pressure drugs (calcium channel blockers) can cause stomach acid to back up into the esophagus. Birth control pills, antihistamines, and certain tranquilizers like Valium can also promote heartburn.

Other Supportive Therapies

AROMATHERAPY AND REFLEXOLOGY: Both of these therapies help in treating indigestion.

HOMEOPATHY: Arsenicum alb. 6c and Argentum nit. 6c can reduce pain and excess gas.

Scientific Facts-at-a-Glance

New studies have found that compared to the general public, nearly twice as many adults with chronic heartburn also suffer from asthmatic symptoms. Apparently, regurgitated stomach acid can end up in the lungs, especially in people with acid reflux disease. In addition, consuming chocolate, coffee and caffeine acts to relax the lower sphincter muscle of the esophagus and allows acid to back up.

Spirit/Mind Considerations

Heartburn, like a number of other physical conditions, can be brought on by anxiety and stress. It is important that during and after eating the mind is relaxed and tension alleviated. A case of "nerves" can result in adrenaline surges, causing poor digestion and excess stomach acid. Do not eat on the run and try to make mealtime a pleasant experience. Avoid topics of conversation that may cause intense emotional reactions. Make the eating environment tranquil and relaxing. Eating slower is part of gaining control of life.

Prevention

◆ Do not lay down after a meal, especially on your right side. Laying on the right side after eating can also produce uncomfortable bloating.

◆ Take a leisurely walk after dinner. This movement helps to facilitate better digestion.

◆ Do not consume large quantities of liquid with your meals as digestion may become impaired. Some professionals believe that drinking small amounts of water throughout your meal can help neutralize stomach acids.

◆ Don't smoke.

◆ Eat slowly, taking small bites and chew your food thoroughly. Gulping food can place stress on the stomach and impair digestion.

◆ Do not eat while on the run or in situations of high stress. Make meal time a time to relax your body and mind.

◆ Avoid rich, fatty, fried foods, carbonated drinks, and extremely spicy foods. Most fast food is high in fat. Fat slows the emptying of the stomach.

◆ Do not use caffeine or alcohol.

◆ At the first sign of heartburn, drink a glass of water.

- Do not overuse aspirin and ibuprofen as they can promote the production of excess stomach acid.
- Elevating the head of the bed may help to prevent the backflow of acid from the stomach into the esophagus.
- Don't wear clothing that is too constricting while eating.
- Don't eat too close to bedtime.
- Avoid constipation by eating plenty of fiber and drinking lots of water. Frequent straining during difficult bowel movements can place pressure on the stomach and increase the risk of heartburn.

Doctor's Notes

A patient I recently treated suffered from chronic heartburn, especially in the evening after retiring to bed. I had him raise the head of his bed four to six inches on blocks of wood to use gravity to his advantage. He also took slippery elm bark with digestive enzymes and within two weeks was relatively symptom-free. He found that fennel and catnip were also effective.

Consumption of antibiotics, alcohol, caffeine, rich foods, age and stress are all major contributing factors to digestive health. Digestive disorders can lead to many illnesses and in advanced cases the illnesses can be quite serious. The herbal formula listed contains herbs that improve all digestive functions and work in many different ways. No prescription or over-the-counter medicine will improve digestion and then maintain function as well as this herbal blend.

Endnotes

1. A. Ippoliti, et al., "The effect of various forms of milk on gastric-acid secretion," Ann Intern Med, 1976, 84:286-89.
2. W.M. Capper, et al.,. "Gallstones, gastric secretion, and flatulent dyspepsia," Lancet, 1967, 1:413-15.
3. M.A. Al Yahya, et al., "Gastroprotective activity of ginger in albino rats," Amer Jour Chin Med, 1989, 17: 51-56.
4. S. Taussig, et al., "Bromelain, a proteolytic enzyme and its clinical application, A review," Hiroshima, Jour Med Sci, 1975, 24: 185-93.
5. M. Messer, C.M. Anderson and L. Hubbard, "Studies on the mechanism of destruction of the toxic action of wheat gluten in celiac disease by crude papain," Gut, 1964, 5: 2950303.
6. R. Leicester and R. Hunt, "Peppermint oil to reduce colonic spasm during endoscopy," Lancet, 1982, II, 989.
7. Mark Pederson, Nutritional Herbology, Wendall Whitman Co., Warsaw, Indiana: 1995, 90.
8. M.A. Al Yahya, et al., "Gastroprotective activity of ginger in albino rats," Amer Jour Chin Med, 1989, 17: 51-56.
9. H. Glatzel and K. Hackenberg, "Roentgenological studies of the effect of bitters on digestive organs," Planta Medica, 1967, 15(3): 223-32.
10. W. Szturma, "Method for treating gastrointestinal ulcers with extract of herb cetaria," US Patent 4150123, issued April 17, 1979.

HEART DISEASE

SEE "CORONARY HEART DISEASE"

HEMORRHOIDS

As many as half of all Americans over the age of fifty deal with hemorrhoids. Like gallstones and constipation, many health experts believe this condition reflects Western eating habits and lifestyles. A hemorrhoid is a varicose vein that develops in the rectum or the anus. Internal hemorrhoids may be located near the beginning of the anal canal or close to the anal opening. When hemorrhoids protrude outside the anal opening, they are referred to as "prolapsed" hemorrhoids. This disorder is very common and may begin when a person is in his or her early twenties, but usually does not become obvious until the thirties. Approximately 50 percent of people over age fifty have hemorrhoidal symptoms. Up to one-third of the total population of the United States have hemorrhoids to some extent. While hemorrhoids are painful, they are rarely dangerous.

Symptoms

Hemorrhoids commonly cause rectal bleeding, pain and discomfort, inflammation, throbbing (especially during a bowel movement), mucus discharge, itching, formation of a tender lump and difficulty sitting. If a clot forms in the vein of a prolapsed hemorrhoid, intense pain can result. If hemorrhoidal bleeding is prolonged, iron deficiency anemia can occur.

If you find blood in the stool, or experience a change in bowel habits, see your doctor immediately. Other causes of rectal bleeding are anal fissures, intestinal disorders, and colon cancer.

Causes

The effects of gravity impose continual stress on the delicate vessels that supply blood to the anus. In addition, abdominal pressure of any kind can aggravate the pressure placed on these veins. Hemorrhoids can be the result of pregnancy (due to added weight and pressure on the rectum), childbirth, a congenital weakness in the veins of the anus, repeated straining during attempts to move hard feces, the repeated use of laxatives, prolonged coughing, violent sneezing, physical exertion, lifting the wrong way, standing or sitting for long periods of time, or a complication of liver disease

Conventional Therapies

Most hemorrhoids can be taken care of with proper home care; however, medical treatment is available if necessary.

Physical probing is usually done to determine the extent of the condition. In a proctoscopy, the rectum is viewed and examined for the possible presence of cancer. A barium enema and a sigmoidoscopy may be recommended if cancer is suspected.

In mild cases, hemorrhoids are traditionally treated with high-fiber diets, increased liquids and rectal suppositories. Rectal pads and creams that contain corticosteroid drugs reduce swelling and inflammation.

If these measures prove unsuccessful, a hemorrhoidectomy may be recommended. A new laser technique developed in Europe is now available in the United States. This procedure does not require hospitalization or general anesthesia and should be investigated as an option, although it is important to remember that many cases of hemorrhoids, when cared for properly, will resolve themselves. Monopolar direct current therapy is a painless treatment using a galvanic current source to shrink tissue.

Dietary Guidelines

- Like so many other disorders, many cases of hemorrhoids could be controlled by eating a diet low in refined, processed foods and high in whole grains, raw fruits and vegetables.
- Eat a high-fiber diet (oat bran, whole grains, dried prunes, dates, raw fruits and vegetables and beans). Individuals who do not get enough bulk fiber in their diets tend to strain during bowel movements due to the formation of small and hard feces.
- Avoid refined white flour, white sugar, and the empty calories found in high-fat junk foods.
- In addition, coffee, caffeine and alcohol are discouraged.
- Avoid salt; it can cause hemorrhoidal tissue to swell more due to the retention of fluid.
- Drink six to eight glasses of water per day to avoid constipation and the formation of hard stool.

Recommended Nutritional Supplements

PRIMARY NUTRIENTS

FIBER SUPPLEMENT These are natural bulking agents that can significantly reduce constipation and straining during bowel movements. They are less irritating to the bowel than whole wheat or cellulose products. Bulk-forming fiber supplements are considered a first-line therapy for hemorrhoids.[1] *Suggested Dosage:* Take as directed on an empty stomach before retiring and first thing in the morning. Look for powders that can be mixed with liquid.

BIOFLAVONOIDS Rutin (a bioflavonoid) is a component of vitamin C that acts to combat fragile capillaries. Bioflavonoids are very beneficial for any venous condition where weakness is involved. They help to strengthen the integrity of vein walls and increase the muscular tone of the veins.[2] *Suggested Dosage:* 500 to 1,000 mg per day.

GRAPE SEED OR PINE BARK EXTRACT The proanthocyanidins in these compounds work to calm inflammation while fortifying blood vessel strength.[3] *Suggested Dosage:* Take as directed.

BROMELAIN An enzyme from the pineapple plant that helps to prevent the formation of fibrin, a substance that surrounds varicose veins in the rectum or anus. Bromelain also has significant anti-inflammatory actions.[4] *Suggested Dosage:* Take as directed. Chewable tablets are available.

VITAMIN E Promotes tissue healing and helps control bleeding. *Suggested Dosage:* 600 IU per day.

VITAMIN A WITH BETA-CAROTENE Helps facilitate the healing of mucous membranes and damaged tissue. *Suggested Dosage:* 10,000 IU of vitamin A and 25,000 IU of beta-carotene.

HORSE CHESTNUT Horse chestnut seeds have a long folk history of use in the treatment of varicose veins and hemorrhoids. The active component works as a natural astringent to shrink swollen membranes.[5] *Suggested Dosage:* 300 to 500 mg three times daily.

BILBERRY This herb is well-known for its ability to boost the strength of blood vessels. It may even help to prevent or treat hemorrhoids and varicose veins associated with pregnancy.[6] *Suggested Dosage:* Take as directed. Use standardized products with guaranteed anthocyanoside content.

BUTCHER'S BROOM This herb has a long history of treating venous disorders and contains compounds that act as vasoconstrictors and anti-inflammatory agents.[7] *Suggested Dosage:* 100 to 200 mg three times daily.

HERBAL COMBINATION This combination should include witch hazel leaves, mullein leaves, cranesbill, slippery elm bark, plantain, butternut root bark, goldenseal root, peppermint leaves and aloe vera gel. *Suggested Dosage:* Two to four capsules daily. May be used every day.

WITCH HAZEL LEAVES: Witch hazel has quite a historical reputation for treating venous inflammation. It is still used today in over-the-counter medications to treat hemorrhoids. Witch hazel has a powerful astringent effect which reduces the size and itching associated with.[8] It also helps to maintain the integrity of the mucosal lining, important because mucus helps stools leave the body with greater ease. Witch hazel has also been used to treat phlebitis and varicose veins. It also promotes wound healing. MULLEIN LEAVES: Contain three to four times the amount of mucilage found in other mucilaginous herbs. Mucilage soothes the gastrointestinal tract and softens stools. Mullein leaves also contain astringent properties and cleanse the body by decreasing bowel transit time.[9] CRANESBILL: Cranesbill has earned the respect of herbalists for its powerful astringent properties. It has been used to treat hemorrhoids and periodontal disease characterized by inflammation.[10] SLIPPERY ELM BARK: Slippery elm is appropriately titled for its very significant mucilage content. It helps to heal and restore the mucus membranes of the gastrointestinal tract. Slippery elm, like other mucilage-containing herbs, soothes and heals tissue. It will reduce inflammation and heal sores.[11] PLANTAIN: Plantain contains two important healing compounds: mucilage and allantoin. Allantoin has been extensively used to promote wound healing. It is effective internally and externally for ulcers, lacerations, hemorrhoids, and periodontal conditions.[12] The *British Herbal Pharmacopeia* recommends plantain and witch hazel be used together to treat hemorrhoids. Plantain's diuretic action also promotes internal health. PEPPERMINT LEAVES: The only direct effect peppermint has on hemorrhoids is as a mild pain reliever. But peppermint improves digestion by increasing bile production and secretion; it also reduces gas, belching and flatulence, and settles a spastic colon and stomach.[13] Peppermint is also considered an activator, increasing the effectiveness of the astringent herbs. BUTTERNUT ROOT BARK: Butternut root bark is a mild laxative. With the assistance of peppermint, butternut will not cause the painful gripping associated with many laxatives. It softens the stool and relieves pressure from the hemorrhoids. Butternut root bark supports liver function.[14] GOLDENSEAL ROOT: Goldenseal is another astringent herb. It was employed by Russians during World War II to stop the bleeding in wounded soldiers due to its ability to constrict peripheral blood vessels.[15] Goldenseal also has a mild laxative effect. ALOE VERA GEL: Aloe vera gel is extremely soothing and healing to the gastrointestinal tract.[16] It promotes the growth of the healthy bacterial flora that are so crucial to proper gastrointestinal tract function. Aloe gel can also prevent the itching associated with hemorrhoids and has anti-inflammatory properties. BUTCHER'S BROOM: This herb has a long history in the treatment of hemorrhoids. It contains compounds that act as vasoconstrictors to help shrink hemorrhoidal tissue. Can be used both externally and internally.[17]

SECONDARY NUTRIENTS

ZINC: Helps to decrease the inflammation associated with hemorrhoids. *Suggested Dosage:* 30 mg per day using gluconate or picolinate products.

VITAMIN K: Recommended if hemorrhoidal bleeding is present. This vitamin can be found in alfalfa, kale and other dark green leafy vegetables. Chlorophyll is rich in vitamin K. *Suggested Dosage:* Use liquid fat-soluble chlorophyll supplements as directed to receive this vitamin.

ZINC OXIDE CREAM: This inexpensive over-the-counter ointment is also good for pain and swelling. Zinc oxide powder is also available. These preparations also help to toughen the skin over the hemorrhoid, which lessens the risk for additional irritation. *Suggested Usage:* Apply as directed.

VITAMIN A, D, OR E OINTMENTS: Good for pain and lubrication. *Suggested Usage:* Apply as directed.

ALOE VERA GEL: Can be used topically. Soothes and cools the area and promotes healing. *Suggested Usage:* Apply as directed.

GOTU KOLA (*Centella Asiatica*): Helps to heal and strengthen blood vessels. *Suggested Dosage:* Use as directed. A poultice can also be made from this herb and applied topically.

Home Care Suggestions

♦ When applying any ointment, cream or preparation to the anal area, make sure the surface has been cleaned and dried before application. Bacteria can become trapped under creams and ointments and cause additional inflammation.

♦ Exercise regularly to keep your bowels active. Brisk walks, low impact aerobics, yoga or dance classes are all excellent ways to exercise.

♦ Using witch hazel on hemorrhoids is a traditional treatment. Witch hazel is an astringent that constricts blood vessels and is an ingredient found in Tucks, Preparation H and other hemorrhoidal treatments. It can be purchased in a bottle and applied with cotton. Soaking a piece of cotton in witch hazel and leaving it on the anal opening overnight may provide additional relief.

♦ Keep the anal area clean but do not use abrasive toilet paper. Use a premoistened wipe then pat dry with toilet paper. Scented or colored toilet paper may cause additional irritation. If using toilet paper, moisten it first with witch hazel.

♦ Using petroleum jelly on the anal area can help to reduce pain. A cotton ball works nicely.

♦ Avoid topical anesthetic preparations that contain benzocaine. These may numb the area temporarily but can also cause more irritation. Preparation H, made from a combination of yeast culture and shark liver extract, is considered an effective ointment.

♦ An ice pack applied to the anal area may decrease swelling and pain. A product called Anurex is a type of ice pack specifically designed to reduce the swelling and pain of hemorrhoids.

♦ Sitting on a doughnut pillow (can be purchased at any pharmacy) can greatly help relieve pressure on anal tissue and provide some relief from pain.

♦ Try not to postpone bowel movements when you feel the urge. Constipation can result from this practice and may initiate difficult bowel movements. Sitting on the toilet for long periods of time may also aggravate hemorrhoids.

Other Supportive Therapies

HYDROTHERAPY: A warm sitz bath in which the temperature is between 100 to 105 degrees Fahrenheit can help with pain and swelling. Ice packs are also helpful.

AROMATHERAPY: Essential oils such as cypress, juniper, or peppermint can be applied directly or mixed into a warm bath to ease pain.

HOMEOPATHY: T. ratanhia 6c, Hamamelis 6c, Sepia 6c, and Sulfur 6c are traditionally used. Hamamelis or peony suppositories are also recommended. Aloe, Aesculus, and Pulsatilla are other possible homeopathic preparations.

YOGA: Lie with the legs at a 45 degree angle to a wall for three minutes every day. This can help to strengthen tissue and stimulate circulation.

Scientific Facts-at-a-Glance

The fact that hemorrhoids are rarely found in Third World countries strongly reiterates the profound health impact of a low-fiber diet has on the human body. One very interesting fact is that post-operative hemorrhoid patients who receive fiber have shorter hospital stays and do not have as much pain as other patients. A high-fiber diet seems to boost recovery and decrease side effects usually associated with the surgery.[18]

Prevention

- Eat a diet high in fiber to avoid hemorrhoids.
- Don't stand or sit for long periods of time.
- Engage in regular exercise.
- Do not become constipated. (Use herbal laxatives if you need to rather than commercial preparations.)
- Keep weight normal.
- Lift heavy objects correctly.

Additional Resources

UCLA Health Services/Hemmorhoids
(310) 825-4073

Endnotes

1. D. Burkitt, "Fiber as a protective against gastrointestinal diseases," Amer Jour of Gastroenterol, 1984, 79: 249-52.
2. M. Gabor, "Pharmacologic effects of flavonoids on blood vessels," Angiologica, 1972, 9: 355-74.
3. B. Schwitters and J. Masquelier, OPC in Practice: Bioflavonols and Their Application, (Alpha Omega, Rome: 1993).
4. H. Ako and P. Matsura, "Isolation of a fibrinolysis enzyme activator from commercial bromelain," Arch Int Pharmacodyn, 1981, 254: 157-67.
5. G. Hitzenberger, "The therapeutic effectiveness of chestnut extract," Wien Med Wochenschr, 1989, 139(17):385-9.
6. G. Grismond, "Treatment of pregnancy-induced phlebopathies," Minerva Gynecol, 1981, 33:221-30.
7. G. Marcelon, et al., "Effects of Ruscus aculeatus on isolated anaine cutaneous veins," Gen Pharmacol, 1983, 14: 103.
8. H. Felter, The Eclecta Materia Medica, Pharmacology and Therapeutics, (Eclectic Medical Publications, Portland Oregon: 1983).
9. V. Vogel, American Indian Medicine, (Ballentine Books, New York: 1970).
10. H. Smith, Ethnobotany of the Meskwaki Indians, Bulletin of the Public Museum, vol 1v, 2: Milwaukee, 1928.
11. Mark Pederson, Nutritional Herbology, (Wendell Whitman Co., Warsaw, Indiana: 1987), 160.
12. Ellingwood, American Materia Medica, Therapeutics and Pharmacognosy, (Eclectic Medical Publications, Portland: 1983).
13. R. Leicester and R. Hunt, "Peppermint oil to reduce colonic spasm during endoscopy," Lancet, 1982, II, 989.
14. J.D. Gunn, Domestic Physician or Home Book of Health, (Moore, Wilstach, Keys, Cincinnati: 1971).
15. Daniel B. Mowrey, The Scientific Validation of Herbal Medicine, (Keats Publishing New Canaan, CT: 1986), 147-48.
16. R. Davis, et al., "Aloe vera and wound healing," Jour Amer Pod Med Asso, 1987, 77: 165-69.
17. G. Marcelon, et al., "Effects of Ruscus aculeatus on isolated anaine cutaneous veins," Gen Pharmacol, 1983, 14: 103.
18. C. Johnson, et al., "Laxatives after hemorrhoidectomy," Diseases of the Colon and Rectum, 1987, 10: 780-81.

HIGH BLOOD PRESSURE/ HIGH CHOLESTEROL

High blood pressure and high cholesterol levels can lead to other debilitating and even deadly conditions. They should be taken seriously. High blood pressure is considered one of the major medical problems of modern times.

Technically speaking, hypertension refers to a condition where too much pressure is exerted on the arteries when the blood is pumped by the heart. A person with high blood pressure, the heart has to pump the blood through the circulatory system with greater force, resulting in added strain on the entire cardiovascular system.

Blood pressure can vary in each individual. When measuring blood pressure, both the systolic and diastolic pressure is read. Systolic pressure refers to the highest pressure which occurs when the heart contracts. Diastolic pressure is the pressure at the moment when the heart relaxes. Systolic pressure will therefore be higher than diastolic. A reading of 120 over 70 refers to a systolic pressure of 120 over a diastolic reading of 70.

There are two types of high blood pressure: essential hypertension, which results for no apparent reason, and secondary hypertension, a complication of another condition.

Essential hypertension comprises 92 percent of all diagnosed cases of high blood pressure. High blood pressure is extremely common in North America. Approximately one in ten Americans (60 million) suffers from hypertension. The incidence of high blood pressure dramatically rises with age and is twice as high among black Americans. Men are more affected than women. Of the many risk factors related to heart attack, high blood pressure remains the most accurate indicator of potential victims of cardiovascular disease after the age of 65. A normal blood pressure reading is 120 over 80. Acceptable blood pressure readings can vary from 110 over 70 to 140 over 90.

High cholesterol refers to blood serum cholesterol readings. Remember that you should always take more than one reading on two different occasions. If you are free of coronary artery disease, a desirable reading in total cholesterol is seen as less than 200 mg per 100 ml of blood. Borderline readings range from 200 to 239. If you fall into this area, dietary changes and the use of certain supplements may be enough. Anything over 240 is considered high and may prompt your doctor to advise using cholesterol lowering drugs.

The ratio of LDL (bad cholesterol) to HDL (good cholesterol) is even more important than total amounts. High-risk LDL counts are over 160, borderline is from 130 to 159 and desirable levels are less than 130. If you have coronary artery disease, you should keep your LDL levels down to less than 100 mg per decaliter of blood. Now, keep in mind that even if your total cholesterol count is acceptable, if you lack in HDL, you may need some dietary adjustments. HDL readings less than 35 mg per decaliter of blood are considered risky.

Symptoms

Hypertension

A person can be suffering from hypertension and not have any noticeable symptoms until the disease is quite advanced. Symptoms of advanced hypertension include dizziness, headache, rapid pulse, sweating, visual disturbances, and frequent nosebleeds.

Anyone suffering from high blood pressure should be under a doctor's care. Because high blood pressure is often asymptomatic, it should be monitored every six months to a year. High blood pressure is a serious condition which should not be taken lightly. Prolonged high blood pressure can result in heart disease, kidney damage, stroke and atherosclerosis. Untreated high blood pressure can significantly reduce life expectancy.

High Cholesterol

High cholesterol levels rarely cause any discernible symptoms until damage from plaque accumulations is significant. Plaque deposits can eventually block carotid arteries, cause impotence, heart attack or stroke.

Causes

The exact cause of essential hypertension remains somewhat of a mystery. Factors that do contribute to it are genetic predisposition, obesity, diet, high blood cholesterol, cigarette smoking, alcohol consumption, stress, the excessive use of stimulants, drug abuse and high sodium intake.

The incidence of essential hypertension increases with age and is higher among blacks. Secondary hypertension can be the result of arteriosclerosis, atherosclerosis, congestive heart failure, kidney disease, diabetes, hormonal disorders, taking birth control pills, pregnancy, and exposure to heavy metals such as lead and cadmium. Genetic research suggests that two specific genes may identify children who will develop high blood pressure later in their lives.

Conventional Therapies

While blood pressure-reducing drugs are effective and may be necessary, it is also true that many cases of high blood pressure can be controlled through changes in diet and lifestyle. The fact that blood pressure-reducing drugs are so widely prescribed supports the fact that changes in lifestyle and diet are not considered as effective or realistic. High blood pressure is generally treated with either diuretic drugs or beta-adrenergic drugs. Hypotensive drugs, which include vasodilators and reserpine alkaloids, are also used. Your doctor will have to choose from diuretics, beta-blockers, alpha-blockers, calcium blockers, vasodilators, or alpha-simulators. Angiotensin-converting enzymes are currently considered a good treatment with the lowest incidence of side-effects, and are known as Capoten, Prinivil, Zestril or Vasotec. Using diuretics and other high blood pressure medication can cause hypotension (or very low blood pressure). This condition is seen in elderly people and medication levels should be checked if fainting, headaches, or weakness results. Several drugs are available which lower cholesterol levels and include cholestyramine, nicotinic acid, gemfibrozil, probucol, statins and even aspirin. These drugs all have serious side effects that should be taken into account before usage. Ideally, diet and exercise can be of more value than drug therapy.

Dietary Guidelines

- Make sure you are not drinking soft water. Emphasize a low-fat, high-fiber diet. Eat plenty of oat bran, pectin fruits, vegetables (such as bananas, apples and melons), broccoli, cabbage, green leafy vegetables, peas, prunes, beets, carrots, and spinach. The incidence of high blood pressure is considerably lower in vegetarians.
- Reduce salt intake in the diet which can promote the retention of fluids and increase blood pressure. Look for the symbol "na" or the word "sodium" in products. Watch for hidden salts.
- Avoid ingesting monosodium glutamate (Accent), some canned vegetables and soups, ibuprofen medications, diet sodas, meat tenderizers, most sugar substitutes soy sauce and softened water. Many salt substitutes still contain up to 50 percent sodium chloride. Check your ingredient label.
- Avoid smoked or aged cheeses and meats, chocolate, animal fats, gravies, broths, and processed foods.
- Avoid using Nutri-Sweet which contains phenylalanine.
- Do not consume caffeine. Caffeine can temporarily elevate blood pressure.
- Watch your intake of white sugar. Some studies have shown that ingesting white sugar can increase sodium retention and can also stimulate adrenaline production which can cause blood vessel constriction.
- Garlic has been shown to be effective in not only lowering high blood pressure but in decreasing cholesterol and triglyceride levels in the blood. Garlic may be eaten fresh, in cooked foods, or taken in capsule form. Because most people do not receive therapeutic levels of garlic from their diets, odorless capsules are recommended. Onion has some of the same benefits as garlic.
- Eating celery has a beneficial effect on high blood pressure. Studies have suggested that routinely eating celery can help to bring blood pressure down. Celery oil and celery seed have been used for generations by folk healers and Chinese physicians in the treatment of high blood pressure.
- Use olive and flaxseed oil and watch out for hydrogenated fats (margarines). Coldwater fish and lean white meats are also recommended.

Recommended Nutritional Supplements

PRIMARY NUTRIENTS

GARLIC OR ONION Both of these extracts have successfully treated hypertension and high cholesterol/blood lipids.[1]

Suggested Dosage: Take two to three capsules with each meal.

COENZYME Q10 Helps to strengthen and oxygenate heart muscle and contributes to metabolic processes. Studies have conclusively proven its significant benefit in treating both cardiovascular disease and hypertension.[2] *Suggested Dosage:* Take as directed.

ESSENTIAL FATTY ACIDS Fatty acids, found in fish oils and oils like flaxseed, can contribute to decreased blood pressure and blood lipids. The fact that Eskimo cultures eat diets high in saturated fats but have low cardiovascular disease is attributed to the effect of coldwater fish consumption.[3] *Suggested Dosage:* Take as directed a blend of fish oil or flaxseed oil with oils like borage or evening primrose. Keep refrigerated. If you use fish oil, take a vitamin E supplement.

VITAMIN E Works to scavenge for free radicals and helps to protect against heart disease and stroke by also reducing LDL cholesterol. Low levels of this vitamin are considered a primary indicator of heart disease.[4] *Suggested Dosage:* If you are at low risk for these disorders, take 100 IU per day. If you are at high risk, take 400 to 800 IU per day.

VITAMIN C WITH BIOFLAVONOIDS These compounds act as free radical scavengers in the arteries and heart muscle and also have been shown to lower blood pressure in clinical tests. Supplementation may actually reduce blood pressure.[5] *Suggested Dosage:* 1,000 to 3,000 mg per day.

CALCIUM This mineral is very important in maintaining or normalizing blood pressure. Supplementation can actually modify hypertension in some people.[6] *Suggested Dosage:* 1,000 mg per day of citrate variety.

MAGNESIUM The proper balance of minerals like magnesium is vital when treating hypertension.[7] *Suggested Dosage:* 400 to 800 mg per day. Use chelated products.

SELENIUM Keeping selenium levels in the body high may be directly linked to blood pressure levels. Because many American diets are selenium deficient, supplementation may be vital.[8] *Suggested Dosage:* Take as directed.

POTASSIUM The ratio of sodium to potassium is considered a profound determiner of blood pressure. Supplementation may be of value.[9] *Suggested Dosage:* Take only as directed.

NICOTINC ACID A compound contained in niacin, this substance has the ability to substantially lower blood cholesterol and triglyceride levels.[10] *Suggested Dosage:* Take as directed.

HAWTHORN The proanthocyanidins found in this herb actually inhibit angiotensin-converting enzymes in much the same way as some prescription high blood pressure medications.[11] *Suggested Dosage:* Take as directed. Combining with rosemary can also be helpful.

FIBER SUPPLEMENT Boosting fiber intake can be one of the single most effective treatments of hypertension and can also significantly lower blood cholesterol levels.[12] *Suggested Dosage:* Take first thing in the morning and before going to bed. Use products that can be mixed in liquid.

CHITOSAN A form of fiber that absorbs dietary fat in the gut and can also inhibit LDL cholesterol (bad cholesterol) while boosting desirable HDL cholesterol levels. One study in the *American Journal of Clinical Nutrition* found that chitosan acted as effectively in controlling blood serum cholesterol levels as cholestryramine, a cholesterol-lowering drug with very undesirable side effects.[13] *Suggested Dosage:* Take as directed. Five to seven capsules with a lipid-containing meal is typical. Don't use unless you eat fats and do not take fat-soluble vitamins at the same time. Drink lots of water.

HERBAL COMBINATION This herbal combination should include garlic, valerian root, black cohosh root, cayenne, kelp, blessed thistle and parsley leaves. *Suggested Dosage:* Four to eight capsules daily. After an adequate reduction of blood pressure is achieved, slowly reduce dosage while maintaining the effect. Do not use this formula if your are pregnant or nursing.

GARLIC: Clinical tests have proven the ability of garlic to decrease blood pressure and to lower triglycerides, cholesterol and lipoproteins found in the blood.[14] Garlic also contains compounds which inhibit platelet aggregation, helping to prevent stroke. Strokes are often related to high blood pressure. VALERIAN ROOT: Valerian root is particularly beneficial for stress-induced hypertension. Valerian will calm and relax an anxious person.[15] Valerian has the ability to reduce arrhythmia (irregular heart beats), and dilate blood vessels. The actives include valepotriates and valeric acid. BLACK COHOSH ROOT: Compounds like actein have been isolated from black cohosh and have been demonstrated to lower blood pressure in some animals. Herbalists have known for years that black cohosh can calm the cardiovascular system. In addition, its diuretic and diaphoretic effects help to expel excess fluids from the body and assist in keeping the blood healthier and blood pressure lower.[16] CAYENNE: Cayenne or capsicum has been used extensively and successfully with garlic in affecting a lower blood pressure. Cayenne is considered to be a blood pressure normalizer or adaptogen. It raises blood pressure that is too low and lowers blood pressure that is too high. Cayenne also serves to stimulate sluggish circulation and makes the other herbs of this formula work faster and better. It can also help to lower blood triglycerides associated with high cholesterol levels.[17] KELP: Kelp is a storehouse of nutrients which assist in maintaining various metabolic processes of the body and provides improved nutrition. Kelp has been employed in Japanese medicine to keep blood pressure under control. It can help to stimulate the production to bile acids which works to control cholesterol levels.[18] Kelp also provides soluble fiber in the form of algin, improving gastrointestinal tract health and mildly stimulating bowel function. BLESSED THISTLE: Blessed thistle is considered a tonic herb which helps to improve general health. It enhances digestion by

correcting liver and gallbladder disorders. It is also diuretic and promotes perspiration. PARSLEY LEAVES: Parsley is used extensively in Europe as a diuretic and antispasm medicine. It is considered to be one of the more nutritious herbs. Apiole is a chemical constituent of parsley that helps to dilate blood vessels, which aids in reducing high blood pressure.[19]

SECONDARY NUTRIENTS

VITAMIN D: Some studies have suggested that levels of this vitamin correlate with blood pressure. *Suggested Dosage:* Take as directed.

ZINC: Supplementation has actually reversed high blood pressure which was artificially induced in laboratory animals. *Suggested Dosage:* Take 15 to 30 mg per day. Use picolinate products.

LECITHIN: This compound contains choline which works to increase bile solubility and lower cholesterol levels. *Suggested Dosage:* Take as directed in either capsule or granulated form.

CHROMIUM: Studies have conclusively shown that chromium supplementation does indeed lower elevated blood cholesterol and triglyceride levels. *Suggested Dosage:* 200 mcg per day. Use GTF forms.

GINGER: Studies have found that ginger can reduce cholesterol levels by inhibiting its absorption. *Suggested Dosage:* Take as directed before meals. Fresh ginger can be used.

Home Care Suggestions

♦ Buy a blood pressure monitor so that you can chart your daily readings and evaluate drug therapy.

♦ If you are overweight, choose a gradual weight reduction and exercise plan. Stay away from weight lifting or isometric exercises, which can actually raise blood pressure. Try low-impact aerobics, such as walking, etc. While reaching an optimal weight is no guarantee that hypertension will disappear, thinner people are much less prone to high blood pressure and the diseases which cause it.

♦ Reduce or eliminate salt. It can cause fluid retention which can raise the water content of the blood thus contributing to high blood pressure.

♦ Stop smoking. A definite link exists between smoking and coronary artery disease which can also cause high blood pressure. Giving up smoking can decrease your risk for high blood pressure by half. In addition, smokers often have higher concentrations of lead and cadmium in their systems than non-smokers.

♦ Don't take antihistamines without consulting your doctor.

♦ Learn to relax and fight stress. Use breathing techniques, yoga, exercise, music, etc. to inhibit tension. When you feel tense, stop and use visualization techniques to achieve tranquility. Slow down if your pace of living has become too stressful.

♦ Get a pet or set up a fish aquarium. Stroking a pet and watching an aquarium are both activities which can help reduce stress and consequently lower blood pressure.

◆ Don't drink alcohol. Even moderate amounts of alcohol can produce an immediate rise in blood pressure and increased adrenalinee secretion. The continual consumption of alcohol is considered a significant predictor of hypertension.

Other Supportive Therapies

MEDITATION: Helps to diffuse stress which is known to raise both blood pressure and blood triglycerides.

AROMATHERAPY: Oils of lemon, lavender, sage or marjoram can be used in conjunction with massage to treat hypertension.

ACUPUNCTURE: Stimulating points on the wrist, head, knee, and back are beneficial.

Scientific Facts-at-a-Glance

Ironically, in some individuals, reducing salt intake actually caused their blood pressure to rise. What this study suggests is that there are many parameters involved in the effect of sodium on blood pressure. It is obviously contingent on other factors or mineral ratios and cannot be looked at as a singular effect. Reducing dietary salt may increase blood pressure.[20] While moderate salt restriction may be beneficial, eliminating all salt may not be necessary. You can test yourself for a salt sensitivity by eliminating all salt and then seeing if your diastolic pressure falls below 90.

The same complex dietary relationships can be seen in the effect of saturated fat on cholesterol. If Eskimo diets are high in saturated fat but low in blood cholesterol counts, another factor comes into play here. The consumption of essential fatty acids may well help to negate the type of cholesterol-raising effect we see from the saturated fats we consume every day in the United States.

Spirit/Mind Considerations

While high blood pressure effects every cultural strata to some extent, there is some conjecture that certain types of personalities seem more prone to the disorder. The type A personality, which is usually typified by perfectionism, ambition, high levels of motivation and standards of achievement, is thought to be more susceptible to stress-related high blood pressure. Some studies advocate that people who are always in a rush have a tendency to look at their watches often, have trouble sleeping and don't find time to relax, need to monitor their blood pressure and take steps to counteract stress. Regular exercise, music therapy, breathing techniques, yoga, etc. can greatly help in reducing tension.

Several physicians believe high blood pressure is a physiological condition which cannot result from anxiety or tension alone. Their approach to the value of relaxation and stress reduction therapy on the disease is skeptical at best. However there is plenty of data to show that during meditation or visualization, blood pressure can drop significantly. Clearly, science does support the notion that stress can indeed, raise blood cholesterol which predisposes us to hypertension and cardiovascular disease.

Prevention

◆ Keep stress levels down or learn to manage stress through meditation, relaxation, exercise, etc.
◆ Use olive and flaxseed oils.
◆ Eat plenty of fish.
◆ Try to drink water that has not been softened. Softened water often has higher concentrations of lead due to the acidity of the water. Exposure to lead and cadmium can cause elevated levels of blood pressure. In these areas, bottled drinking water is recommended.
◆ Keep your diet low in hydrogenated and saturated fats, and salt and high in fiber and fresh fruits and vegetables.
◆ Keep your weight down. Obesity directly contributes to the development of high blood pressure.
◆ Do not smoke. Smoking is directly linked with the development of coronary artery disease.
◆ Do not consume alcohol.

Doctor's Notes

High blood pressure is considered a primary killer in the United States and is closely linked to coronary artery disease. In addition, high cholesterol counts are predictors of both hypertension and cardiovascular disease.

High blood pressure is not as easy to diagnose as it may seem. To illustrate, some people will experience temporary elevation in blood pressure merely because of the anxiety generated when being diagnosed. Also, there is still some controversy over what is considered to be high blood pressure.

Lifestyle changes can help to alleviate symptoms. It is best to cut out tobacco, alcohol and caffeine and to exercise according to the advice of a health care professional. Weight reduction, improving diet and exercise are the most effective tools in treating both high blood pressure and high cholesterol. It is important to realize that one must be willing to make these changes or all the herbal treatments in the world will not be effective.

Taking calcium, magnesium and potassium in the proper amount is crucial to treating both of these disorders. Herbs that significantly boost circulation include capsicum. When combined with B-vitamins, especially niacin, the diameter of the arteries can actually increase, which reduces blood pressure. High cholesterol, like hypertension, can be a complex problem. Remember that the count is not as important as the ratio of LDL cholesterol to HDL cholesterol.

People under stress oxidize cholesterol differently because the stress causes the release of chemicals like epinephrine and cortisol. These stress hormones can cause abnormal oxidative processes which increase the chance of cholesterol adhesion to artery walls. In addition, they cause the release of a certain amino acid which also impairs cholesterol metabolism. Unquestionably, stress contributes to plaque formation and obstruction. Learning to deal with stress is so important in controlling both high blood pressure and high cholesterol.

Taking adequate B-vitamins with extra B6, B12 and folic acid is highly recommended. In addition, vitamin E also helps to reduce the oxidation which can damage artery walls and interfere with the proper use of cholesterol. Reduce your dietary consumption of cholesterol containing foods which always come from animal sources and are found in saturated fat. Increase your use of olive and flaxseed oil and add tofu dishes to your menu. Use garlic liberally and learn to consistently take a fiber supplement every day. It is important to keep in mind that people who are likely to suffer from high cholesterol do not necessarily eat too much cholesterol. Their bodies have tendency to produce too much cholesterol in the liver. For this reason, herbs that improve liver function and boost the production of bile acids are also helpful. Milk thistle and tumeric are good.

Additional Resources

American Heart Association
7272 Greenville Ave.
Dallas, TX 75231
214-373-6300

Endnotes

1. D. Louria, et al., "Onion extract in treatment of hypertension and hyperlipidemia: A preliminary communication," Curr Ther Res, 1985, 37(1):127-31.

2. T.Yamagami, et al., "Bioenergetics in clinical medicine: Studies on coenzyme Q-10 and essential hypertension," Res Commun Chem Pathol Pharmacol, 1975, 11:273.

3. P. Singer, "Blood pressure-lowering effect of w-3 polyunsaturated fatty acids in clinical studies," in A.P. Simopoulos et al., eds. "Health effects of W-3 polyunsaturated fatty acids in seafoods," World Rev Nutr Diet, 1991, 66:329-48.

4. K.F. Gey, et al., "Inverse correlation between plasma vitamin E and mortality from ischemic heart disease in cross-cultural epidemiology," Amer Jour Clin Nutri, 1991, 53: 326S_ 334S.

5. O. Osilesi. et al., "Blood pressure and plasma lipids during ascorbic acid supplementation in borderline hypertensive and normotensive adults," Nutr Res, 1991, 11:405-12.

6. D. McCarron, et al., "Dietary calcium and blood pressure: Modifying factors in specific populations. Am J Clin Nutr, 1991, 54:215S-19S.

7. T. Moore, "The role of dietary electrolytes in hypertension," J Am Coll Nutr, 1989, 8: Suppl S:68S-80S.

8. J. Salonen, et al., "Blood pressure, dietary fats, and antioxidants," Am Jour Clin Nutr, 1988, 48:1226-32.

9. A. Sianin, et al., "Controlled trial of long term oral potassium supplements in patients with mild hypertension," Bri Med Jour, 1987, 294:1453-56.

10. J.R. DiPalma and W.S. Thayer, "The use of niacin as a drug," Ann Rev Nutr, 1991, 11: 169-87.

11. S. Uchida, et al., "Inhibitory effects of condensed tannins on angiotensin converting enzyme," Jap Jour Pharmacol, 1987. 43:242-5.

12. P. Little, et al., "A controlled trial of a low sodium, low-fat, high-fiber diet in treated hypertensive patients: the efficacy of multiple dietary intervention," Postgraduate Medical Journal, 1990, 66(778): 616-21. F.L. Shinnick, et al., "Dose response to a dietary oat bran fraction in cholesterol-fed rats," Jour Nutri. 1990, 120(6): 561-68.

13. George Vahouny, et al., "Comparative effects of chitosan and cholestryramine on lymphatic absorption of lipids in the rat," Amer Jour Clinical Nutri, 1983, 38(2): 278-84.

14. B.H. Lau, et al., "Allium sativum (garlic) and atherosclerosis; A review," Nutri Res, 1983, (3): 119-128.

15. T. Mennini, et al., "In vitro study on the interaction of extracts and pure compounds from Valeriana officinalis roots with GABA. Benzodiazepine, and barbiturate receptors in rat brain," Fitoterapia, 1993, 54(4): 291-300.

16. J. Young, American Journal of Medical Sciences. 9, 310, 1831, P.S. Benoit, H.H.S. Fong, G.H. Svoboda and N.R. Farnsworth. "Biologic and phytochemical evaluation of plants: XIV. Anti-inflammatory evaluation of 163 species of plant," Lloydia, 1976, 39(2-3), 160-61.

17. T. Kawada, et al., "Effects of capsaicin on lipid metabolism in rats fed a high-fat diet," Jour Nutri, 1986, 116: 1272-78.

18. N. Iritani and J. Nogi, "Effect of spinach and wakame on cholesterol turnover in the rat," Atherosclerosis, 1972, 15: 87-92.

19. V. Petkov, "Plants with hypotensive, antiatheromatous and coronarodilatating action," Amer Jour Chin Med, 1979, 7(3): 197-236.

20. M. Brent Egan, Director of the hypertension program, Medical College of Wisconsin in Milwaukee, reported in The Los Angeles Times, March 19, 1990.

HYPERTENSION

SEE "HIGH BLOOD PRESSURE"

HYPOGLYCEMIA

Glucose (blood sugar) is the energy source for the body. Hypoglycemia is a glucose metabolism disorder where the pathology is the opposite of diabetes. Diabetes is a condition of too much glucose in the blood because too little insulin is being produced by the pancreas. Hypoglycemia is a condition of too little glucose in the blood often as a result of the pancreas producing too much insulin. A diabetic who injects too much insulin can cause a state of hypoglycemia. At one time it was believed that hypoglycemia did not occur except in diabetics who overdosed on insulin. When glucose is used up too rapidly or when the pancreas produces an excess of insulin which results in an abnormally low level of blood sugar, hypoglycemia can result.

Legitimate cases of hypoglycemia are extremely rare and usually occur in people suffering from diabetes mellitus. Functional hypoglycemia, on the other hand, is a relatively new classification that refers to a form of hypoglycemia directly related to dietary habits rather than physiological abnormalities. This type of hypoglycemia has been the subject of ongoing debate. While some doctors accept it as a valid disorder, others deny its existence. More and more evidence points to the existence of blood glucose disorders of this type, which are difficult to diagnose yet certainly exist in some sensitive individuals.

It is important to know that two kinds of hypoglycemia exist. The first is called reactive hypoglycemia, which refers to people who experience symptoms 30 minutes to one hour after eating a meal high that is high in sugar. The other is called simple hypoglycemia which occurs hours after fasting or may not occur for four to six hours after eating. Reactive hypoglycemia is considered more severe and troublesome.

Symptoms

Hypoglycemia commonly causes dizziness, fatigue, irritability, mood swings, anxiety, sweating, cold sweats, weakness, fainting, tremors, strong sensation of hunger, food cravings, eye pain, visual disturbances, palpitations, insomnia, mental disturbances, and swollen feet.

In severe cases of hypoglycemia experienced by diabetics a coma is possible.

A large number of people who suffer from the symptoms of hypoglycemia have reduced thyroid function and should see a physician. Also, persistent symptoms of hypoglycemia may indicate the presence of a serious disorder and should not be ignored.

Causes

True hypoglycemia can be a complication of people suffering from insulin-dependent diabetes, from ingesting large amounts of alcohol, or from a insulinoma, which is an insulin producing tumor of the pancreas. Other glandular disorders such as thyroid abnormalities or glandular tumors may also cause hypoglycemia. Functional hypoglycemia can also result from inherited tendencies and dietary factors. People with certain metabolic types that very quickly digest carbohydrates can also become hypoglycemic.

Conventional Therapies

A five-hour glucose tolerance test (GTT) can be administered where a large amount of sugar water is consumed and subsequent blood tests are taken at certain intervals to determine glucose levels.

Hypoglycemia that does not have a specific physiological cause is considered by some physicians as a pseudo disease. Some critics of the glucose tolerance test point out that giving the body such high levels of glucose may result in false readings.

If your physician determines that low blood sugar exists, diet changes where protein is stressed and carbohydrates are minimized will be recommended. There is some controversy surrounding this approach. Some health care professionals believe that complex carbohydrates should be stressed and protein kept to a minimum.

In addition, some physicians will suggest eating a piece of candy when symptoms of hypoglycemia begin. Critics of this approach point out that by quickly raising the blood glucose level with refined, quickly assimilated sugars, blood sugar may drop down even lower to compensate, perpetrating a vicious cycle.

Dietary Guidelines

- ◆ Designing the right kind of diet is vital to controlling hypoglycemia. It is important to eat complex carbohydrates which are assimilated slower in combination with the proper ratio of protein and good fats.
- ◆ Avoid the following foods altogether: sugars, refined and processed foods, white flour, soda pop, salt, caffeine, alcohol, extremely sweet fruits, dried fruits and fruit juices (which if consumed, should always be diluted with water), noodles, gravy, white rice and corn.
- ◆ Pre-sweetened cold cereals can cause a rapid rise in blood sugar and can precipitate the over-secretion of insulin.
- ◆ Alcohol can also induce a dramatic drop in blood sugar. Eating sugar and consuming alcohol aggravates the cycle of hypoglycemia.
- ◆ Emphasize fresh fruits and vegetables, sprouts, brown rice, seeds, grains, nuts, cottage cheese, lean meats, fish, high-fiber foods such as oat bran, popcorn and other whole grains. Eat several small meals a day to prevent the onset of low blood sugar.

◆ Carry nuts and high-protein snacks with you. Make sure to eat enough protein and add good fats like olive oil to meals to keep sugar from entering the bloodstream too rapidly.

◆ Something as simple as eating a piece of cheese before going to bed can help prevent nighttime episodes. (Mozzarella cheese, which is made partly from skim milk, is recommended.)

Recommended Nutritional Supplements

PRIMARY NUTRIENTS

CHROMIUM Supplementation can be very helpful in reducing glucose-induced insulin secretion and in helping to normalize blood sugar levels. Adequate supplies of chromium are necessary for proper insulin secretion and glucose metabolism. Also, studies have found that supplementation with chromium can help reverse hypoglycemia.[1] *Suggested Dosage:* 200 mcg per day. Use GTF varieties.

VITAMIN B3 (NIACIN) Studies with patients suffering from hypoglycemia related to alcoholism have found that niacin supplementation significantly alleviated its symptoms.[2] *Suggested Dosage:* 100 mg per day.

MAGNESIUM This mineral may reduce glucose-induced insulin secretion. Studies have found that low levels of magnesium can actually initiate hypoglycemic responses by overstimulating insulin secretion.[3] *Suggested Dosage:* 500 to 700 mg per day.

ZINC A zinc deficiency has been linked to hypoglycemia. This mineral contributes to the proper metabolism of insulin and is involved in every aspect of insulin utilization.[5] *Suggested Dosage:* Take 50 mg per day.

FIBER SUPPLEMENT Increasing fiber in the digestive tract can substantially slow the infusion of glucose into the blood which helps to modify insulin reaction and prevent hypoglycemic symptoms from occurring. Studies conclusively show that increasing dietary fiber improves glucose metabolism.[6] *Suggested Dosage:* Take as directed using powdered forms which can be mixed with liquid. Take first thing in the morning or before going to bed. Look for psyllium-based products.

OMEGA-6 FATTY ACIDS These acids can actually serve to inhibit excess insulin secretion even in the presence of glucose. Linoleic acid found in oils like flaxseed can be very valuable.[7] *Suggested Dosage:* Take as directed using blends containing flaxseed, evening primrose or borage oils. Keep refrigerated.

HERBAL COMBINATION This herbal combination includes licorice root, gotu kola, Siberian ginseng, ginger root, and kelp. *Suggested Dosage:* Four to six capsules daily.

LICORICE ROOT: For people in acute hypoglycemic conditions, licorice root can stimulate adrenal hormone production as a response to provide quick energy.[8] This will allow the person to function until food can be consumed. A hypoglycemic condition can be the result of a dysfunctional digestive system. Poor digestion may not allow the required nutrients to be absorbed creating a condition much like that produced by fasting. Licorice root will improve digestion by stimulating the secretion of a soothing mucus in the gastrointestinal tract. Licorice also has the ability to modulate and increase the effectiveness of the other herbs in this formula. (Do not use licorice if you have hypertension or kidney disease and no one should use this herb for extended periods of time.) GOTU KOLA: Gotu kola is said to be able to improve energy stores. It has a tonic and an adaptogenic effect on the central nervous system which relies heavily on proper brain function. Gotu kola is a mental stimulant, a stress reducer and memory enhancer.[9] Clinical studies in Europe confirm gotu kola's ability to stimulate circulation. Increased circulation can deliver more nutrients to the various tissues of the body, even when those nutrients are in short supply in the blood. Of course, in a hypoglycemic state, glucose would be in short supply. SIBERIAN GINSENG: Siberian ginseng is called an adaptogen which refers to an innocuous substance that normalizes systems of the body irrespective of the pathology. A common example used to support ginseng's claimed adaptogenic effects is its clinically documented ability to normalize blood sugar levels.[10] Ginseng will bring the blood sugar level to normal whether it is high or low. Ginseng has a similar effect on blood pressure and the central nervous system. Stress and anxiety may have a significant influence on hypoglycemic states. Ginseng has a well documented ability to fight the effects of stress. GINGER ROOT: Ginger root's applications in this formula are to improve digestion and stomach and bowel function. Ginger will settle nervous stomachs.[11] Ginger improves circulation which will help make other herbs of this formula more effective. KELP: Kelp provides many trace elements which are involved in various metabolic processes. Some trace elements like chromium are vital to carbohydrate metabolism. Kelp provides a soothing soluble dietary fiber called algin, which improves gastrointestinal function.

SECONDARY NUTRIENTS

L-CARNITINE, CYSTEINE, GLUTAMINE AND METHIONINE: These amino acids help to normalize glucose metabolism. *Suggested Dosage:* Take as directed on an empty stomach with fruit juice.

MANGANESE: Low levels of this trace mineral have been found in people with hypoglycemia. *Suggested Dosage:* Take as directed.

VITAMIN C WITH BIOFLAVONOIDS: Helps to boost proper adrenal function. *Suggested Dosage:* 3,000 to 5,000 mg per day.

GLUCOMANNAN: This herb helps with carbohydrate metabolism which helps to normalize insulin response. *Suggested Dosage:* Take as directed, using standardized products.

ACIDOPHILUS: Helps to ensure proper digestion which is integral to keeping blood sugar levels normal and to enhance nutrient assimilation. *Suggested Dosage:* Take as directed using bifidobacteria-containing products that are not milk-based. Check expiration date.

Home Care Suggestions

◆ Lose weight if you need to. The relationship of fat stores to the metabolism of sugar has been firmly established.
◆ Exercise is extremely beneficial in helping the body regulate sugar metabolism.
◆ If you are an insulin-dependent diabetic, always carry sugar lumps with you and take them at the first sign of a hypoglycemic reaction.
◆ Taking injections of B-vitamins has produced some good results in keeping the pancreas from over secreting insulin when certain foods are ingested.

Other Supportive Therapies

AROMATHERAPY: Massage with orange blossom, and lemon and rosemary can help to treat the pancreas and can facilitate relaxation.
ACUPUNCTURE: Stimulation of key areas can help to normalize adrenal function.

Scientific Facts-at-a-Glance

More and more evidence is suggesting that people who are sensitive to glucose may also gain weight easily and find it difficult to shed. We are just beginning to understand why fat is deposited into adipose tissue. Too much insulin fills up glucose stores quickly which results in the surplus being stored as fat. For this reason, the rapid absorption of carbohydrates and high release of insulin promotes obesity. Consequently, hypoglycemics need to emphasize protein foods and even good fats in order to feel satisfied and to keep blood sugar levels even, thereby making it easier to shed those pounds. Using fiber and herbs like glucomannan (an inabsorbable carbohydrate that can absorb 50 to 200 times its weight in water) can help to promote weight loss and is specifically suited for the hypoglycemic.[12]

Spirit/Mind Considerations

It is a well-established fact that abrupt drops in blood glucose levels can cause dramatic mood swings, irritability, combativeness and depression. Low blood sugar can result in feeling of confusion, impatience and the inability to cope. The brain is highly dependent on glucose as an energy source. Several studies indicate that psychiatric patients have a higher incidence of low blood sugar. In addition, hypoglycemia can be a significant contributing factor to depression. Learning to understand what foods trigger low blood sugar and how it affects mental function is vital.

Prevention

◆ Good dietary habits combined with regular exercise are once again the formula to help prevent not only low blood sugar but several other common diseases of our age.
◆ Eating small meals several times of day may be preferable to two or three large meals which can shoot the blood sugar level up.
◆ Keep yourself at an ideal weight.
◆ Do not consume alcohol.
◆ Do not consume an excess of white sugar products, candy, cakes, sugared cereals, desserts, etc. Reach for the fruit instead.

Doctor's Notes

Hypoglycemia can be a problem that initiates a variety of symptoms which are often mistaken for other disorders. Hypoglycemia usually occurs after eating a meal high in simple sugars and involves an excessive insulin response, which drives blood sugar so low that symptoms result.

The simplest way of controlling hypoglycemia is to adapt your eating habits by eating the right kinds of foods every two to three hours. These foods should contain protein or complex carbohydrates. Be aware, however, that some people metabolize even complex carbohydrates too quickly and may need to concentrate on protein snacks only. One-fourth cup of low-fat cottage cheese and a few nuts such as almonds or peanuts are recommended. In non-diabetic individuals, hypoglycemia can easily be misdiagnosed for other conditions such as panic or anxiety attacks. Today, even though more doctors and patients are aware of the possibility of hypoglycemia, it is often overlooked due to its wide array of possible symptoms which mimic a variety of disorders. Fasting or going without food for a few hours can result in inadequate blood sugar which can generate a state of hypoglycemia. Consuming something sweet like orange juice or a candy bar can quickly solve the problem. Severe hypoglycemia is potentially a serious condition sometimes resulting in a coma or death. One of my favorite blends is called SP35 and includes licorice root, gotu kola, Siberian ginseng, ginger root and kelp. By taking this two or three times a day blood sugar can stabilize itself if diet is altered.

Additional Resources

American Diabetes Association
Two Park Avenue
New York, NY 10016
(212) 683-7444

Endnotes

1. R.A. Anderson, et al., "Effects of supplemental chromium on patients with symptoms of reactive hypoglycemia," Metabolism, 1987, 36(4):351-55. See also R. Anderson et al., "Chromium supplementation of humans with hypoglycemia," Fed Proc, 1984, 43:471.
2. A. Shansky, "Vitamin B3 in the alleviation of hypoglycemia," Drug Cosmetic Industry, 1981, 129(4):68.
3. D. Curry. et al., "Magnesium modulation of gluco-induced insulin secretion by the perfused rat pancreas," Endocrinology, 1977, 101:203.
4. W.M. Capper, et al., "Gallstones, gastric secretion, and flatulent dyspepsia," Lancet, 1967, 1:413-15.

5. M.W. Tadros, "Protective effects of trace elements," Ind Jour Exp Biol, 1982, 20: 93-94.

6. J.G. Pastors et al., "Psyllium fiber reduces rise in post prandial glucose and in insulin concentration in patients with non insulin dependant diabetes," Amer Jour Clin Nutr, 1991, 53:1431-5.

7. D. Gugliano and R. Torella, "Prostaglandin E1 inhibits glucose-induced insulin secretion in man," Prostaglandins Med, 1979, 48:302.

8. D. Armanini, et al., "Affinity of licorice derivatives for mineralocorticoid and glucocorticoid receptors," Clin Endocri, 1983, 19: 609-12.

9. A.S. Ramaswamy, et al., "Pharmacological studies on Centella Asiatica," Jour Res Indi Med, 1070. 4: 160-175.

10. N.R. Farnsworth, et al., "Siberian ginseng: Current status as an adaptogen," Econ Med Plant Res, 1985, 1: 156-215.

11. Y. Yamahara, et al., "Gastrointestinal motility enhancing effect and its active constituents," Chem Phar Bull, 1990, 38: 430-31.

12. D. Walsh, et al., "Effect of glucomannan on obese patients: A clinical study," Inter Jour Obes, 1984, 8(4): 289-93.

IMPOTENCE

Impotence refers to the inability to achieve or to maintain a penile erection. It can also refer to premature ejaculation or the inability to ejaculate.

Impotence is the most common sexual disorder among males and will probably affect most men at some time in their lives. It is estimated that more than 30 million American men are chronically impotent. By the age of 75, 55 percent of men suffer from impotence. Aging effects impotence due to lowered levels of testosterone and decreased circulation from plaque deposits in penile arteries. At one time, impotence was considered an emotional disorder. Recently, however, physicians have to come to accept that well over half of all cases of impotence have a physiological cause.

Symptoms

Impotence is characterized by the inability to achieve or maintain an erection adequate enough for normal sexual intercourse. It may be an isolated incident, a chronic disorder or may come in spells and then recur.

Causes

Impotence can result from diabetes mellitus, peripheral vascular disease, Parkinson's disease, liver or kidney disease, stroke, hypothyroidism, pelvic trauma, epilepsy, atherosclerosis, multiple sclerosis, Alzheimer's disease, lower back problems, hormonal diseases, neurological disorders, alcoholism and spinal cord damage.

Impotence can be the result of psychological factors such as stress, performance anxiety, fatigue, boredom, anxiety, guilt, depression, marital discord and age.

Over 200 drugs can cause impotence and include antipsychotics, antidepressants, some tranquilizers such as Valium, antihypertensives and diuretics. Some over-the-counter antihistamines and decongestants have also been linked to incidence of temporary impotence.

Conventional Therapies

Medical doctors take this disorder more seriously today and will check if both psychological and physical factors involved. Your doctor will order certain tests to rule out the possibility of a physical cause. A test to determine if there is adequate blood flow to the penis may be performed. It is referred to as a aultasonography which is a non-invasive method of measuring blood flow to the penis. The health of the spinal cord will also be assessed. A history will be taken and a blood glucose test may be ordered to eliminate the possibility of diabetes. In addition, a testosterone level test should be performed. Certain medications may be stopped or dosages adjusted. If depression is a factor, it is usually treated with antidepressants and counseling.

Testosterone shots may be prescribed. Thyroxine is another name for a testosterone medication that can be effective in some cases. Determining and administering the best levels of testosterone is difficult. A testosterone patch is currently being developed and will be used for men who experience sexual dysfunction as the result of a physiological disorder. A urologist may need to be consulted if the problem is severe; you can discuss surgical options available. If blood insufficiency to the penis is the cause of the impotence, a surgical procedure to unblock the arteries involved may be necessary. Special vacuum devices can be surgically implanted; these draw blood into the penis. Penile implants are surgically implanted prosthetic devices which facilitate an erection. NOTE: A new drug, Viagra, is now available and has shown impressive results. Consult with your doctor.

Dietary Guidelines

- ◆ Losing weight, exercising and eating a low-fat, high-fiber diet can help to improve circulation and counteract impotence that is caused by reduced blood flow.
- ◆ Avoid alcohol and tobacco and limit animal fats and high-sugar foods.

Recommended Nutritional Supplements

PRIMARY NUTRIENTS

GINKGO BILOBA Studies have found that the glycosides contained in this herb may be effective in cases of impotence which are due to insufficient blood supply. Ginkgo can boost vascular oxygenation of tissue.[1] *Suggested Dosage:* Take as directed using standardized products.

VITAMIN E Boosts circulation and helps to strengthen reproductive organs by effectively scavenging for free radicals. Because it helps to prevent arteriosclerosis, it is also beneficial as a preventative nutrient for impotence.[2] Taking alpha lipoic acid can help to boost the function of vitamin E in the body. *Suggested Dosage:* 400 to 800 IU per day.

VITAMIN C WITH BIOFLAVONOIDS Helps maintain proper circulation and keeps the arteries clean while it strengthens the collagen content of veins.[3] It is also known as the anti-stress vitamin. *Suggested Dosage:* 3,000–5,000 mg per day.

ZINC Important in maintaining healthy reproductive organs and contributes to normal prostate gland function. Zinc is involved in virtually every aspect of male reproduction. Zinc works to keep testosterone levels up.[4] *Suggested Dosage:* 50 mg per day. Use picolinate or gluconate varieties.

GRAPE SEED OR PINE BARK EXTRACT An impressive antioxidant which can help to keep arteries clear. The proanthocyanidin content of this compound scavenges for free radicals which also helps to prevent arterial damage to veins in the penis.[5] *Suggested Dosage:* Take as directed.

YOHIMBE BARK This herb is also sold under brand names which include Dayto, Yocon and Yohimex. These are prescription forms of the herb which should not be used by anyone with high blood pressure. Yohimbe is a bark that contains alpha-adrenergic blocker compounds which has been used for both psychological and physically-induced impotence and is the only drug currently approved by the FDA for erectile dysfunction.[6] *Suggested Dosage:* Use as directed only on an occasional basis not exceeding 20 to 30 mg per day. This substance can cause significant side effects.

POTENCY WOOD This herb, also called *muira puama*, has been used effectively in South America to restore libido and treat erectile dysfunction.[7] *Suggested Dosage:* Take as directed.

HERBAL COMBINATION This combination should include damiana leaves, Siberian ginseng, saw palmetto berries, kelp, sarsaparilla root and buckthorn bark. *Suggested Dosage:* Three to six capsules daily. For chronic conditions it is best to use maximum dosage of six capsules per day for a prolonged period of two to three months. When adequate results have been achieved, cut dosage to three capsules daily.

DAMIANA LEAVES: Damiana's reputation began when it was discovered that native Mexican Indians used it for nervous and sexual debility and for mild constipation. Germany's Commission E (the regulatory body that oversees phytomedicines) has published an official monograph on damiana suggesting it to be used as an aphrodisiac and for prophylaxis as well as a treatment for sexual disorders.[8] Damiana seems to be particularly effective when combined with saw palmetto berries. SIBERIAN GINSENG: Siberian ginseng, like damiana, has been popular for centuries as an aphrodisiac, not because it stimulates sexual desire, but because it improves the health of the reproductive system. Thus, people who feel reproductively and sexually revitalized will experience greater sexual performance and satisfaction. Frequently, stress is a major cause of infertility and sexual dysfunction. Siberian ginseng has a clinically supported reputation as a stress fighter. It helps the body to cope with stress and maintain proper function. It has also been able to raise the sperm count of certain animals.[9] SAW PALMETTO BERRIES: The saw palmetto berry has been popular among the American Indians of the South for treatment of urinary disorders. While the product has been listed in the National Formulary, it has become very popular in Europe as a treatment for benign prostate hypertrophy (BPH).[10] In South America, it is used in combination with other herbs by women who find it to be more effective than prescription drugs for painful menstruation and pelvic congestion. Saw palmetto seems to exert a hormone balancing effect irrespective of gender. KELP: Kelp performs three major functions in the herbal formula. First, it provides organic iodine for proper function of the thyroid gland. A dysfunctional thyroid gland can cause weakness, general malaise and obesity. These conditions can contribute to lack of sexual desire and function. Second, it provides trace elements so often lacking in the American diet. Trace elements are co-factors in many metabolic processes of the body which can contribute to overall health. Third, it provides mucilage which helps to soothe the gastrointestinal tract and maintain its proper function.[11] SARSAPARILLA ROOT: Sarsaparilla has a reputation as a fighter of syphillis and other venereal diseases. It also contains hormone precursors which help the body to maintain proper hormonal balance.[12] Sarsaparilla root is a diuretic as well as a reputed blood purifier helping to maintain general health. BUCKTHORN BARK: Buckthorn bark is included in this formula as an extremely mild laxative. Its effect is so subtle it may not be obvious. Stress and sexual debility may result in constipation. This could exacerbate lower abdominal pelvic congestion and compromise a sense of well being.

SECONDARY NUTRIENTS

L-TYROSINE: An amino acid which may help to boost reproductive function. *Suggested Dosage:* Take as directed on an empty stomach with fruit juice.

VITAMIN A: A natural antioxidant which also boosts the immune system and can help strengthen tissue. *Suggested Dosage:* Take as directed. Do not take over 25,000 IU per day.

B-VITAMINS: These vitamins play an important role in proper hormone synthesis and reproductive health. *Suggested Dosage:* Take as directed.

GINKGO, BUTCHER'S BROOM, CAYENNE AND BILBERRY: These herbs can boost circulation to the penis. *Suggested Dosage:* Take as directed using standardized products.

Home Care Suggestions

- Home impotence tests are used to determine whether impotence is psychologically caused or has an organic source. These are set up prior to sleeping and determine if any erections occur during sleep. If there are no erections while sleeping, there may be a mechanical or organic cause present. Contact a urologist if this is the case. If you discover that erections do occur during sleep but you still experience impotence when awake, then the problem has a psychological basis and an appropriate counselor may be consulted.
- Discuss your problem openly with your partner. Express your feelings, especially if you have negative feelings toward your partner.
- There is some speculation that exercising right before sex directs blood away from the penis and may hinder achieving an erection.
- Use relaxation techniques such as yoga, biofeedback, etc. to counteract the negative effects of stress and tension.
- Do not become preoccupied with the physical aspects of an erection. Relax and do not set your expectations unrealistically high.

Other Supportive Therapies

HYDROTHERAPY: Taking baths in cold water, sitz baths, or cold water frictions is a traditional therapy for impotence.

ACUPUNCTURE: This therapy can help to stimulate circulation to the penis and can also facilitate relaxation.

MEDITATION: Learning to de-stress is invaluable for both physical and psychologically caused impotence.

Scientific Facts-at-a-Glance

Atherosclerosis of the main artery than runs through the penis is the primary cause of impotence in over 50 percent of men that are over the age of 50. This strongly suggests that keeping cholesterol levels low could significantly prevent the buildup of plaque in this particular artery.

Spirit/Mind Consideration

If the causes of impotence are psychological in nature, sex counseling or psychotherapy may be helpful, although it is vital that you choose a therapist that has good credentials and is respected in his or her field. Traditional methods of psychotherapy have not enjoyed a great deal of success in treating impotence. A sex therapist may be more qualified in this area. If alcoholism is a factor, it will have to be treated appropriately.

Prevention

- The Boston University School of Medicine has recently found that a man's overall health is the key predictor of impotence. Men who suffered from high blood pressure, heart disease or diabetes were one to four times more likely to become completely impotent later in their lives. Having a low level of HDL (good cholesterol) was also linked to eventually becoming impotent.
- Try to maintain an active, healthy and regular sex life. It is thought that testosterone levels stay higher when sex is more frequent.
- Try not to become obsessed with sexual performance. Performance anxiety can lead to psychological impotence.
- Do not drink alcohol. Impotence among men in their late forties and early fifties is associated with the excessive consumption of alcohol than with any other single factor.
- Don't smoke. Smoking impairs circulation and contributes to hardening of the arteries which can effect erections.
- Learn to relax and to counteract stress and fatigue with exercise and relaxation techniques such as yoga, music therapy, etc.
- Eat a diet low in fat and high in fiber. Cholesterol deposits can effect the arteries that supply blood to the penis also.

Doctor's Notes

There are so many possible causes for impotence. If a man is experiencing impotence during attempted sexual intercourse (but has normal erections during the night or early morning) then a psychological cause may be at the center of the problem. If this is the case, I find it beneficial to treat the patient for depression with St. John's wort, kava kava and valerian root.

If someone has completely lost the ability to have an erection altogether, it is wise to consult with a urologist. I like to use *Ginkgo biloba* due to its effects on the neurological and cardiovascular system. Using relaxation techniques such as mediation is also good.

One of the most common causes of impotence is the misuse of drugs, both the prescription and illegal variety. Narcotics, antihypertensive drugs, antianxiety medication, and antidepressant medication can all cause impotence. If you suspect a drug is at fault, tell your doctor.

Yohimbe has proven itself to be useful in men who know that the cause of their impotence is organic rather than emotional, but yohimbe can cause side effects such as anxiety, depression, increased heart rate or blood pressure. I like the yohimbe product from Neutraceuticals. If you decide to use yohimbe on a regular basis, monitor your blood pressure and heart rate. Using yohimbe on an occasional basis can be done very safely if precautions are taken. Although the ancient Mayans used damiana leaves as an aphrodisiac, this formula is not considered a magical solution to sexual dysfunction. Herbs designed to boost circulation may also be very helpful; these include cayenne, ginkgo, bilberry and butcher's broom.

Remember that any psychological cause of impotence, such as stress, should be addressed before any treatment is incorporated. Also, keep in mind that blood pressure pills, the use of narcotic drugs and alcohol can all lead to impotence.

Endnotes

1. R. Sikora, et al., Ginkgo biloba extract in the therapy of erectile dysfunction," Jour Urol, 1989, 141: 188A.

2. E.B. Rimm, et al., "Vitamin E consumption and the risk of coronary heart disease in men," New Eng Jour Med, 1993, 328: 1450-56.

3. J.A. Simon, "Vitamin C and cardiovascular disease: A review," Jour Amer Coll Nutr, 1992, 11: 107-125.

4. A. Netter et al., "Effect of zinc administration on plasma testosterone, dihydrotestosterone and sperm count," Arch Androl, 1981, 7: 69-73.

5. M.T. Meunier, et al., "Free radical scavenger activity of procyanidolic oligomers and anthocyanosides with respect to superoxide anion and lipid peroxidation," Plant Med Phytotherapy, 1989, 4: 267-74.

6. J. Susset, et al., "Effect of yohimbine hydrochloride on erectile impotence" a double- blind study," Jour Urol, 1989, 141(6): 1360-63.

7. J. Wayneberg, "Aphrodisiacs: Contribution to the clinical validation of the traditional use of ptychopetalum guyanna," Presented at the First International Congress of Ethnopharmacology, Strasbourg, France, June 5-9, 1990.

8. R. Roys, The Ethnobotany of the Maya, (Middle America Research Series, Tulane University, New Orleans, La: 1931), 265

9. N. Farnsworth, "Siberian ginseng: Current status as an adaptogen," Econ Med Plants, 1985, 1: 156-215.

10. B. Del Valio, "The use of a new drug in the treatment of chronic prostatitis," Minerva Urol, 1972, 26: 81-94.

11. N. Iritani and J. Nogi, "Effect of spinach and wakame on cholesterol turnover in the rat," Atherosclerosis, 1972, 15: 87-92.

12. Kiangsu Institute of Modern Medicine, Encyclopedia of Chinese Drugs, 1977 Shanghai, People's Republic of China.

INFERTILITY

Infertility refers to the inability to conceive after a year or more of normal sexual intercourse. It may also refer to the inability to carry a pregnancy to full term. Infertility is an increasingly common problem among American couples. As many as one in six couples will have to seek the aid of an infertility specialist. Roughly 30 percent of infertility cases are due to factors that affect the male; another 30 percent are due to female problems, and the remaining 40 percent are caused by a combination of the two. Male infertility usually involves low sperm count or structural abnormality. For women, a failure to ovulate or tubal obstruction are common causes of infertility.

The inability to conceive can be a heartbreaking and frustrating experience. Fortunately, several medical and natural treatment options exist which have good success rates in treating infertility.

Symptoms

As mentioned, a failure to conceive after one year or more during periods of normal sexual intercourse constitutes infertility. You should consult an Ob/Gyn if you have any of the following situations:

♦ You or your partner have had a venereal disease (especially chlamydia, which can cause fallopian tube damage in women and ductal scarring in men).

♦ Your menstrual periods are irregular or abnormally scant.

♦ You have a history of endometriosis, pelvic infections, abdominal or urinary tract surgery, mumps, measles, excessively high fevers, polycystic ovary disease, exposure to toxic chemicals such as lead, or significant exposure to radiation.

♦ You can find no evidence that ovulation is occurring (taking temperature, using standard ovulation kits, etc.), and you have symptoms of too much testosterone in your system (ie., hair growth on your chest, upper lip, or chin).

Causes

A hormonal imbalance is the most common cause of infertility. Other possible causes are chlamydia or other venereal diseases, pelvic inflammatory disease, an allergic reaction to sperm, endometriosis, obstruction of the fallopian tubes due to cysts or scar tissue, physical injury to reproductive organs, cervical mucus, chromosomal abnormalities, congenital defects or deformities, and/or eating disorders.

Low sperm count in male semen can be due to varicocele (a varicose vein in the scrotum), prostate infections, mumps, alcohol use, certain prescription drugs, nicotine, illness or fatigue, impotence, malnutrition, high or prolonged fever, radiation, and/or testicular mumps or cancer.

Diets that are deficient in certain vitamins and minerals have also been linked to infertility. Some health care experts believe that escalating rates of infertility are due to our widespread consumption of refined and processed foods, the effects of pollution and toxins and hormonally treated cattle, poultry and pork.

Conventional Therapies

Approximately half of all couples who seek professional infertility treatment will achieve conception. Your physician will take a complete history and evaluation of both physical and psychological factors which may be related to infertility. Separate interviews of both partners are sometimes conducted where sexual habits are discussed. If the problem is physical, you will be referred to a fertility clinic where the first lab test is usually a sperm count. If sperm production is normal (at least 60 million sperm per milliliter of ejaculate), the female reproductive system will be examined. A sample of the cervical mucous and a biopsy of the uterine lining will be taken and tested to see if ovulation is occurring. You may be asked to keep a chart of morning temperatures with a basal thermometer to also confirm ovulation (which is usually marked by a rise in temperature of one to two degrees). A post-coital semen test may also be ordered. If ovulation is absent, a fertility drug such as Clomid may be advised. In addition, the fallopian tubes may be tested with a hysterosalpingography to check for any obstruction. A laparoscopy, which involves inserting a scope through the abdominal wall, may be ordered if the presence of adhesions, scar tissue, fibroid tumors, endometriosis, a tipped uterus, cysts or tumors is suspected. In some cases, surgical correction can take place at the same time. In cases involving low sperm count, artificial insemination with the male semen may be successful. If sperm count is low because of an endocrine imbalance, drugs such as slomiphene or gonadotropin may be prescribed.

Artificial insemination with donor sperm is also a possibility and should be done only if both partners agree. Surrogate pregnancy is another option that should be explored only if attitudes permit and all legalities are discussed. In vitro fertilization (test tube baby) where an egg and sperm meet inside of test tube with subsequent implantation into the woman's uterus is another possibility. In vitro fertilization is expensive ($6,000 or more for each attempt). Research in Great Britain confirms that in vitro fertilization success rates decline with age. The study found that conception and live birth rates fell 20 percent and 14 percent respectively in women over the age of 40 who had attempted five in vitro cycles. In contrast, more that 50 percent of women between the ages of 20 and 34 conceived after five cycles. Sometimes adopting a baby seems to increase chances for conception for reasons that are not totally understood.

Dietary Guidelines

- ◆ Limit animal fats, white sugar, refined flour and junk foods.
- ◆ Eat plenty of soybean-based foods like tofu that have isoflavones which have desirable estrogenic actions.
- ◆ Eat plenty of whole grains and raw fruits and vegetables.
- ◆ Avoid caffeine. Some recent studies have linked caffeine consumption with infertility—give up coffee, cola beverages and chocolate. The same is true for alcohol which can reduce sperm count and actually inhibit fertilized egg implantation in the uterine lining. Make sure you are getting enough B-vitamins through protein-rich foods. Look to fish, lean meats, nuts, legumes and low-fat dairy products.

Recommended Nutritional Supplements

PRIMARY NUTRIENTS

FOLIC ACID Studies have strongly suggested that a folate deficiency can contribute to infertility for both sexes.[1] Folic acid is also crucial to the normal development of the fetus and may depend, to some extent, on prepregnancy levels. *Suggested Dosage:* Take as directed.

VITAMIN E AND SELENIUM Vitamin E has the ability to contribute to hormone normalization although its exact mechanism is not fully understood. Selenium levels have also been linked to sperm counts in men and lack of ovulation in women.[2] *Suggested Dosage:* 400 to 800 IU of vitamin E per day and 200 to 400 mcg of selenium per day. Taking lipoic acid can help boost the action of both of these nutrients.

VITAMIN B6 Women with irregular periods have found that this vitamin can help to restore normal cycles. In addition some studies have shown that this vitamin contributes to normal pituitary gland secretions that are involved in reproductive processes.[3] *Suggested Dosage:* Take as directed. Do not take over 250 mg per day.

VITAMIN C WITH BIOFLAVONOIDS Some European studies suggest that bioflavonoids may help women prone to miscarriages to sustain the pregnancy. Bioflavonoids in conjunction with vitamin C can also help to strengthen blood vessels and prevent free radical damage to sperm.[5] *Suggested Dosage:* 3,000 to 5,000 mg per day. Men who smoke need to make sure they are taking this supplement.

IRON Studies have found women who are iron-depleted can become infertile. These tests suggest that supplementation may restore ovulation and result in conception.[7] Because women can be anemic and not know it, their iron levels should be tested. *Suggested Dosage:* Take 35 mg with a vitamin C supplement for better absorption.

ISOFLAVONES These compounds are found in soy-based foods and have very beneficial effects on deranged estrogenic hormones. Genistein is one of the best for female problems.[8] *Suggested Dosage:* Take as directed. Look for genistein content.

EVENING PRIMROSE OIL The essential fatty acids found in this oil help to normalize female hormones and have been used to treat hormonally induced female disorders like PMS.[9] *Suggested Dosage:* Take as directed and keep refrigerated.

L-ARGININE This amino acid has the ability to raise sperm count in infertile men.[10] *Suggested Dosage:* Take as directed on an empty stomach with fruit juice.

HERBAL COMBINATION This combination should include damiana leaves, Siberian ginseng root, saw palmetto berries, kelp, sarsaparilla root and buckthorn bark. *Suggested Dosage:* Three to six capsules daily. Use a maximum dosage of six capsules per day for a period of two to three months.

DAMIANA LEAVES: Damiana's reputation began when it was discovered that native Mexican Indians used it for nervous and sexual debility and for mild constipation.[11] Germany's Commission E (the regulatory body that oversees phytomedicines) has published an official monograph on damiana suggesting it to be used as an aphrodisiac and for prophylaxis, as well as a treatment for sexual disorders. Damiana seems to be particularly effective when combined with saw palmetto berries. SIBERIAN GINSENG: Siberian ginseng, like damiana, has been popular for centuries as an aphrodisiac. It has probably enjoyed this reputation not because it stimulates sexual desire, but because it improves the health of the reproductive systems of the body. Stress, quite often, is a major cause of infertility and sexual dysfunction. Siberian ginseng has a clinically supported reputation as a stress fighter. It helps the body to cope with stress and maintain proper function.[12] KELP: Kelp performs three major functions in the herbal formula. First, it provides organic iodine for proper function of the thyroid gland. A dysfunctional thyroid gland can cause weakness, general malaise, and obesity. These conditions can contribute to lack of sexual desire and function. Second, kelp provides trace elements so often lacking in the American diet. Trace elements are cofactors in many metabolic processes of the body which can contribute to overall health.[13] Third, kelp provides mucilage which helps to soothe the gastrointestinal tract and maintain its proper function.[14] SARSAPARILLA ROOT: Sarsaparilla has a reputation as a fighter of syphilis and other venereal diseases. It also contains hormone precursors which help the body to maintain proper hormonal function.[15] Sarsaparilla root is a diuretic as well as a reputed blood purifier helping to maintain general health. BUCKTHORN BARK: Buckthorn bark is included in this formula as an extremely mild laxative. Its effect is so subtle it may not be obvious. This could exacerbate lower abdominal pelvic congestion and compromise a sense of well being.

SECONDARY NUTRIENTS

DONG QUAI AND LICORICE ROOT: Both of these herbs have estrogenic action and can help to boost estrogen in women who may have a hormonal deficiency. *Suggested Dosage:* Take as directed using standardized products. Do not use combinations containing licorice for over two weeks at a time or if you have hypertension or kidney disease.

CRUCIFEROUS SUPPLEMENTS (INDOLES): These compounds help to protect breast and reproductive organ tissue from the effects of deleterious estrogen. *Suggested Dosage:* Take as directed.

PANTOTHENIC ACID: Can help to restore reproductive health in both sexes. *Suggested Dosage:* Take as directed.

Home Care Suggestions

- Home ovulation kits such as Ovu-Stick can be purchased to determine the most optimal time for conception to take place. The test is simple and is done by using a chemically-treated stick which is placed in a urine sample. A positive result indicates that ovulation will occur within twelve to thirty-six hours.
- Men can take a cold bath 30 minutes before intercourse. There is some speculation that cold water not only increases sperm count but also makes them more active.
- Do not use commercial vaginal douches. Douching can disturb the natural pH balance of the vagina which may impair or actually kill sperm.
- Usually couples under the age of thirty are advised to try to achieve conception for a year before consulting a fertility specialist. Fertility does decrease with age. Often women in their thirties and forties do not regularly ovulate, which significantly reduces the probability of conception.
- Avoid extreme exercise, and the repeated use of **hot** saunas which can induce changes in normal ovulation. Exercising for more than an hour per day is not recommended.
- Men should not take hot showers, baths, or saunas which may reduce sperm count. In addition stay away from electric blankets and occupational exposure to high temperatures.
- Use a vaginal lubricant that won't disturb the natural acid/alkaline balance of the vagina. Egg white has been suggested as being the least disruptive to normal sperm motility. Use the egg white after it has reached room temperature just prior to intercourse on fertile days.
- If your are thin, gain enough weight to put you close or at your ideal weight. Stored body fat can actually produce estrogen.
- Women should remain lying down and even prop their feet up for at least twenty minutes after intercourse.
- Men should not take any steroids. They can adversely affect the pituitary gland or damage the testicles.
- Men should avoid tight underwear or athletic supporters which may also decrease sperm count.
- Abstain for at least two days prior to ovulation or fertile days to increase sperm count.
- Don't smoke.
- Some medications can actually decrease sperm count or impair motility. Tagamet, certain antibiotics and antiseizure preparations are among these drugs. Get off any over-the-counter or prescription drugs that aren't necessary.

Other Supportive Therapies

AUTOGENIC TRAINING: This therapy may be useful if infertility is stress-related in origin.

MEDITATION: Relieving stress and learning to relax is very important when trying to conceive.

Scientific Facts-at-a-Glance

A recent article in *Time* magazine addressed the troubling fact that statistics published in the *British Medical Journal* found that men born after 1970 had a sperm count 25 percent lower than those born before 1959. Other studies have found the same trend among the French and Danish, who have experienced a decline in sperm by nearly 50 percent over the last fifty years. In addition, the rate of testicular cancer has also escalated over the same time period. Male infertility was considered somewhat rare thirty years ago. Today the Fertility Research Center in New York finds that 40 percent of their patients have a fertility problem. The reasons for this dramatic change have been attributed to stress, pollution, smoking and drugs. New evidence strongly supports the notion that chemical toxins in our environment, including DDT and PCBs, are responsible. Some industrial chemicals that enter water and soil can actually cause the feminization of male organs. These substances are called environmental estrogens. Dr. Neils Skakkebaek, a Danish endocrinologist, published a startling report in which he found that the average male sperm count has fallen from 113 million per ml in 1938 to 66 million ml in 1990.[16]

Spirit/Mind Considerations

While it is not completely understood, the ability to relax seems unquestionably connected to increasing your chances of conception. Often it is best to concentrate on passion and forget about mechanics or temperature charts. Going on a cruise or other restful type of vacation is recommended. Regular meditation can be very useful. A prescribed sexual regimen to achieve fertility can also result in a lack of interest in sex, which can become more of a chore than anything else. Women are sometimes impatient with men, who are perceived as uncooperative or resistant. Some men can mistakingly view infertility as a sign that they lack virility.

Prevention

- ◆ Eat right; dietary habits when you are sixteen can affect health in your twenties.
- ◆ Use a strong multivitamin and mineral supplement.
- ◆ Use olive and flaxseed oil.
- ◆ Do not use drugs, alcohol or tobacco.
- ◆ Do not over-exercise.
- ◆ Do not use steroid drugs.
- ◆ If you have difficult or heavy periods, get checked for hormonal imbalances or the presence of cysts.
- ◆ Try to limit or avoid eating hormonally treated meats.

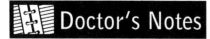 Doctor's Notes

The herbal formula suggested is excellent for both men and women afflicted with infertility, impotence and other hormone imbalance-related conditions. It does more than treat symptoms—it attacks the root of the problem and returns the body to normal function. Its mode of action is both pharmacological and nutritive. Although the ancient Mayans used damiana leaves as an aphrodisiac (damiana maintains some of the same popularity today), this formula is not a magic potion of alluring aphrodisiacal properties or consequences. However, this formula is a serious remedy that will revitalize reproductive and sexual function. It may also be used prophylactically to maintain good reproductive and sexual function and prevent degeneration of the same. It is also important to realize that studies tell us that being too underweight or overweight can contribute to infertility. Ovulation seems to be affected in both situations.

Additional Resources

The Society for Assisted Reproductive Technology
Birmingham, Alabama
(205) 978-5000

Footnote References

1. D. Dawson and A. Sawers, "Infertility and folate deficiency," Case Reports, Br Jour Obstet Gynaecol, 1982, 89:678-80.

2. G.N. Schrauzer, "Benefits of natural selenium," Anabolism, 1988, 7(4): 5.

3. G.S. Kidd, "The effects of pyridoxine on pituitary hormone secretion in amenorrhea-galactorrhea syndrome," Jour Clin Endocrin Metab, 1982, 54(4): 872-75.

4. Y. Kumamoto et al., "Clinical efficacy of mecobalamin in treatment of oligozoospermia: Results of double-blind comparative clinical study," Acta Urol Jpn, 1988, 34:1109-32.

5. C. Fraga, et al., "Ascorbic acid protect against endogenous oxidative DNA damage to sperm," Proc Natl Acad Sci, 1991, 88(24): 11003-6. See also E. Dawson, et al., "Effect of vitamin C supplementation on sperm quality of heavy smokers," Faser Jour, 1991, 5(4):A915.

6. A.S. Prasad, "Zinc in growth and development and spectrum of human zinc deficiency," Jour Amer Coll Nutr, 1988, 7(5):377-84.

7. D. Rushton, et al., "Ferritin and fertility," Letter, Lancet, 1991, 337:1554.

8. H. Wei, "Antioxidant and antipromotional effects of the soybean isoflavone genistein," Proceedings of the Society for Experimental Biology and Medicine, 1995, 208: 124.

9. D. Horrobin, "The role of essential fatty acids and prostaglandins in the premenstrual syndrome," Jour Repro Med, 1983, 28(7): 465-68.

10. J. Pryor et al., "Controlled clinical trial of arginine for infertile men with oligospermia," Bri Jour Urol, 1978, 50:47-50.

11. R. Roys, The Ethnobotany of the Maya, (Middle America Research Series, Tulane University, New Orleans, La: 1931), 265

12. N. Farnsworth, "Siberian ginseng: Current status as an adaptogen," Econ Med Plants, 1985, 1: 156-215.

13. B. Del Valio, "The use of a new drug in the treatment of chronic prostatitis," Minerva Urol, 1972, 26: 81-94.

14. N. Iritani and J. Nogi, "Effect of spinach and wakame on cholesterol turnover in the rat," Atherosclerosis, 1972, 15: 87-92.

15. Kiangsu Institute of Modern Medicine, Encyclopedia of Chinese Drugs, 1977 Shanghai, People's Republic of China.

16. Michael D. Lemonick, "What's Wrong with our Sperm?" Time Magazine, March 18, 1996, 147(12).

INFLAMMATORY BOWEL DISEASE (IBD)

SEE "COLITIS"

INSECT BITES

While we all agree insect bites are annoying, they can vary in their seriousness from mild to potentially fatal. Some insect bites carry disease, such as the tick responsible for Lyme disease. Minor insect bites are usually simple to treat. Insect bites and stings are a common occurrence during the summer months and can result from mosquitoes, lice, midges, gnats, horseflies or houseflies, sand flies, fleas, bedbugs, bees, spiders ticks and mites.

Symptoms

Physical symptoms of minor insect bites include pain, redness, swelling, itching, and burning. If multiple stings have occurred, muscle cramps, headaches, fever, drowsiness, weakness or unconsciousness can occur. Any insect bite that causes weakness, difficult breathing, wheezing, abdominal pain, fainting, hives or a skin rash should receive immediate medical attention.

SPIDER BITES

Spider bites can be dangerous for children or elderly people. There are three varieties of poisonous spiders found in the United States. They are the black widow, the brown recluse, and the tarantula.

Physical symptoms from a black widow bite include abdominal cramps, a hard abdomen, difficulty breathing, grunting, nausea, vomiting, headache, sweating, twitching, shaking, and tingling sensations in the hand. (Symptoms from a brown recluse spider, identified by the violin pattern on their backs, cause significant pain and local reactions, but are not as dangerous as the black widow spider).

First Aid for Spider Bites

Put an ice pack or cold compress on the bite and seek medical attention as soon as possible. CAUTION: The bite of a black widow or brown recluse spider requires immediate medical attention.

BEE STINGS

The sting of bumblebees, wasps, hornets, fire ants and yellow jackets can cause an allergic reaction in five out of 1,000 people. This reaction can be life threatening and requires immediate medical treatment.

First Aid for Simple Bee Stings

Remove the stinger with a clean sharp blade that you scrape against the skin. Using a pair of tweezers can squeeze a venom sac located at the end of the stinger and cause more pain and inflammation. Wash the area with soap and water.

Dietary Guidelines

Eating a lot of onions and garlic in your diet can make you repugnant to flying bugs (not to mention people as well). Large doses of vitamin C have been used to treat a bite by a venomous insect such as the brown recluse spider. Some studies have suggested that people who eat diets that are high in thiamine or vitamin B1 are not as attractive to insects possible due to a body odor given off in perspiration which cannot be detected by humans. Taking a thiamine supplement up to three times a day when camping is recommended, or one 100 mg tablet before going outside.

Recommended Nutritional Supplements

PRIMARY NUTRIENTS

Internal

QUERCETIN AND HESPERIDIN The powerful antioxidant and anti-inflammatory action of these bioflavonoids helps to calm swelling and redness and modulates the release of histamine which causes pain.[1] *Suggested Dosage:* Take as directed.

VITAMIN C WITH BIOFLAVONOIDS Helps to minimize inflammation and to detoxify affected tissue. *Suggested Dosage:* 6,000 to 12,000 mg daily in three equal divided doses.

External

VITAMIN C, ALOE GEL, MYRRH AND WINTERGREEN Rub a paste of these ingredients on the bite area to control inflammation and pain.

PABA AND ALCOHOL This mixture has had good results as a topical treatment and has been particularly successful with large and persistent mosquito bites.

OIL OF LAVENDER AND EUCALYPTUS Help to repel insects and calm inflammation after a bite.

OIL OF OREGANO Apply to the bite to control itching.

OIL OF ST. JOHN'S WORT Helps to promote tissue healing.

HERBAL COMBINATION This combination should contain burdock root, gotu kola, yellow dock, dandelion root, milk thistle seeds, Irish moss, red clover blossoms, kelp, cayenne, and sarsaparilla. *Suggested Dosage:* Two to six capsules daily.

BURDOCK ROOT: Burdock promotes liver function and increases bile flow, which in turn cleanses the blood and reduces toxin production in the gastrointestinal tract. In addition, burdock root is a mild laxative and diuretic which action further cleanses toxins from the body.[2] GOTU KOLA:

This herb has the ability to boost skin tissue healing and can decrease possible scarring.[3] YELLOW DOCK: Yellow dock root is a reputed blood purifier. Its laxative effect is well documented and supports the body's detoxifying ability.[4] DANDELION ROOT: This herb can strengthen the liver, improve bile formation, regulate the bowels, purify the blood, and tonify the skin.[5] IRISH MOSS: The contribution of Irish moss is very simple. It provides a demulcent and soothing source of mucilage. RED CLOVER BLOSSOM: Red clover helps to purify the blood and is used in Britain for any kind of skin disorder or injury.[6] MILK THISTLE: This marvelous herb cleanses, strengthens, and protects the liver and its functions which plays a major role anytime the body deals with poisons or allergic reactions.[7] KELP: Kelp serves a similar function as Irish moss, but kelp is thought to be a blood purifier with the ability to alleviate skin problems, burns, and insect bites.[8] CAYENNE: Cayenne is a stimulant that helps to make all the other herbs function better. Such herbs are referred to as activators. SARSAPARILLA ROOT: Sarsaparilla possesses diuretic and diaphoretic actions, which cleanse the body of toxins.[9]

SECONDARY NUTRIENTS

COMFREY: Mix dry comfrey powder with aloe vera juice to promote healing and reduce swelling.

PAPAYA: Contains papain an enzyme which is also found in some meat tenderizers. Applying papaya to an insect bite promotes healing and reduces inflammation.

ELECAMPANE: This herb is considered a natural insect repellent when used externally.

Home Care Suggestions

- Toothpaste applied to the bite can help to cool burning, stop pain and decrease inflammation.
- Rubbing meat tenderizer on an insect bite can reduce pain. A paste can be made with meat tenderizer and water.
- Lotions such as Alpha Keri and Skin-so-Soft (an Avon product) have been reported to repel bugs. Vick's Vaporub seems to have the same effect.
- Lindane and crotamiton, both prescription drugs, can kill mites and alleviate itching.
- Taking antihistamines or Benadryl can help to lessen allergic symptoms that sometimes accompany insect bites.
- Calamine lotion helps with itching.
- A charcoal paste can be applied to bites to help draw out poisons and reduce inflammation.
- Insect repellents such as Deet or Off (which contain N-diethyltoluamide) can repel mosquitos and ticks. Some allergic reactions to this substance have been reported; it should be used with caution on children. Insect repellents containing R-11 have been banned by the EPA as being potentially hazardous to humans. Don't use any insect repellent on broken skin.
- Apply distilled witch hazel to inflamed area for a soothing effect.
- Apply a slice of fresh onion on insect stings for pain relief.
- Rubbing meat tenderizer on an insect bite can reduce pain.
- Topical steroid creams can be used for itching if not used for prolonged periods of time. Use an antibiotic cream if it looks as though the bite has become infected.
- Applying wet clay or making a mudpack and applying it to the bite can also help with pain and swelling.
- After removing the stinger, apply honey to the bite area.

Other Supportive Therapies

HOMEOPATHY: Ledum 6C is used to prevent and treat insect stings.

Scientific Facts-at-a-Glance

There is some speculation that if you eat sugar, your skin will actually emit a sweet "essence" which quickly attracts insects. It is thought that mosquitos in particular can pick up the smell of glucose. It is fascinating to watch who mosquitos seem to pick on out of a group of people. Perhaps blood sugar levels have something to do with their preferences. Another interesting observation is that wearing hair spray or certain colognes or perfumes can actually attract flying insects.

Prevention

- Hanging dried tomato leaves in each room of the house has been a traditional way to repel insects of all kinds.
- Wear light-colored clothing that does not have brightly colored patterns.
- Avoid wearing perfumes, sweet smelling soaps, lotions, or hair sprays, suntan oil or metallic jewelry.
- Don't eat sweet, drippy foods, such as watermelon or ice cream outside.
- If attacked by a swarm of insects, lie down and cover your head.
- Don't wear sandals or loose fitting, short sleeved clothing. Tuck your pants inside of your shoes.
- Take garlic and vitamin B1 supplements before going out.
- Avoid alcoholic drinks that cause the skin to flush and blood vessels to dilate; this can attract mosquitos and flies.
- Black widows like to nest in dark woodpiles. Exercise caution when going into these kinds of areas. Spray woodpiles regularly for spiders.

Endnotes

1. M. Farrandiz and M. Alcarez, "Anti-inflammatory activity and inhibition of arachidonic acid metabolism by flavonoids," Agents Action, 1991, 32: 283-87.

2. F. Ellingwood, American Materia Medica, Therapeutics and Pharmacognosy, (Eclectic Medical Publications, Portland: 1983).

3. T. Chakrabarty, et al., "Centella asiatica in the treatment of leprosy," Sci Culture, 1976, 42: 573.

4. J.P. Bosse, et al., " Clinical study of a new antikeloid drug," Ann

Plastic Surgery, 1979, 3: 13-21.

5. H.W. Felter, The Eclectic Materia Medica: Pharmacology and Therapeutics, (Eclectic Medical Publications, Portland: 1983).

6. K. Bohm, "Choleretic action of some medicinal plants," Arzneimittel-Forsch, 1959, 9: 376-78.

7. G. Weber and K. Galle, "The liver, a therapeutic target in dermatoses," Med Welt, 1983, 34: 108-111.

8. D. Brown, Quarterly Review Of Natural Medicine, Spring 1994, 17.

9. F. Thurman, "The treatment of psoriasis with sarsaparilla compound," New Eng Jour Med, 1942, 227: 128-33.

INSOMNIA

This particular problem plagues thousands of people and in many cases, the exact cause of this disorder remains a mystery. Insomnia simply refers to having trouble falling asleep or staying asleep. It is a very common problem with an incidence of one in three adults in the United States, or approximately 120 million Americans. Sleep requirements vary in each individual and can range from four to ten hours per night. Generally speaking, the older one gets, the less sleep is required. Often an individual who thinks they are suffering from insomnia is getting more sleep than they think. Sleeping pills or hypnotics are among the most widely prescribed drugs in this country.

Symptoms

People who suffer from insomnia generally complain of tossing and turning, short intervals of sleep, the inability to get comfortable, getting up several times a night, a generally frustrated feeling and hearing voices or repetitive melodies in their mind.

The lack of sleep may result in daytime fatigue, irritability, impatience, the inability to concentrate, malaise, headaches and lack of energy. If a particular physical problem is keeping you awake, such as chest pain, shortness of breath, heart palpitations, etc., consult your doctor as soon as possible.

Causes

The most common cause of insomnia is anxiety, which results from worrying about a problem. Other possible causes of insomnia include caffeine consumption, malnutrition, sleep apnea, indigestion, low blood glucose, some over-the-counter and prescription drugs, lack of exercise, pain, a feeling of restlessness in the legs, overwork, the misuse of hypnotic drugs, emotional trauma and fibromyalgia.

Withdrawing from certain drugs such as hypnotics, antidepressants, tranquilizers, illicit drugs or alcohol can also result in the inability to sleep. Poor sleeping routines such as sleeping late or excess napping are also considered contributory factors.

Conventional Therapies

Your doctor will want to check for a physical or psychological cause and then treat it accordingly. In cases of persistent insomnia, which has no apparent cause, an EEG may be recommended to access brain wave patterns during periods of rest. If your physician determines that you have a sleeping disorder (such as sleep apnea), you may be referred to a specialist.

Most cases of insomnia are treated with sedative-hypnotic drugs such as the barbiturates (Seconal, Nembutal, Tuinal) and the benzodiazepines (Valium, Librium). Prescription sleeping pills induce an unnatural sleep which is not necessarily restful. Consequently, the use of hypnotics may leave you feeling more tired than before, which may prompt an increased dosage of the drug. This cycle of disturbed sleep with continual drug treatment is referred to as "drug-dependent insomnia" and is thought to plague a significant number of Americans. Any type of sedative-hypnotic can create a psychological and physical dependency in its users.

Sleeping pills are not a cure for insomnia. On the contrary, they can actually worsen the condition and create an aggravated sense of fatigue upon arising. Insomnia is often treated as a disease by physicians, when in fact, it may be more a result of poor sleeping habits. Relaxation techniques such as bio-feedback and self-hypnosis are much more preferable to drug therapy. Several herbs and other natural compounds can promote sleep without dangerous side effects.

Dietary Guidelines

- ◆ Low blood glucose levels at night have been associated with insomnia and may require a small pre-bedtime snack to be stabilized. A plain baked potato or piece of bread eaten 30 minutes prior to retiring may be helpful.
- ◆ Foods high in tryptophan have a calming effect on the brain. These include bananas, turkey, figs, tuna, dates, yogurt and milk.
- ◆ Avoid eating spicy foods, chocolate, smoked meats, sauerkraut and tomatoes too close to bedtime. There is some speculation that these foods stimulate a release of norepinephrine, a brain chemical stimulant
- ◆ A folk remedy for insomnia is to drink a mixture of two teaspoons of cider vinegar, one teaspoon of honey to a cup of warm water.
- ◆ A traditional nightcap for insomnia used in Spain is made by mixing two tablespoons of honey and the juice of one lemon in a glass of buttermilk.

Recommended Nutritional Supplements

PRIMARY NUTRIENTS

5-HYDROXY-TRYPTOPHAN This new product is a form of the amino acid tryptophan which was taken off the market several years ago due to an isolated incident where a batch of product was contaminated. Tryptophan has proven its ability to increase total sleep time and prevent sleep interruptions.[1] *Suggested Dosage:* Take as directed on an empty stomach with fruit juice. If you find that you feel nauseated, then take it with food.

CALCIUM/MAGNESIUM These two minerals work to calm the central nervous system and to relax muscle tissue respectively. Magnesium's effect on muscles is well documented.[2] *Suggested Dosage:* Take 1,500 mg of calcium and 1,000 of magnesium. Use chelated products such as calcium citrate and magnesium gluconate. It may be more effective to take 500 mg of the magnesium in the evening.

MELATONIN This hormone is intrinsically involved in promoting sleep and has proven its ability to initiate and sustain sleep in test subjects. A lack of melatonin may be the underlying cause of insomnia in some people.[3] *Suggested Dosage:* 1 to 3 mg is the common dosage. Start with a very small dose and monitor your reaction.

HERBAL COMBINATION This herbal combination includes valerian root, hops, skullcap, passionflower, dandelion root, chamomile, marshmallow root and hawthorn berries. *Suggested Dosage:* Two to four capsules daily. This formula should not be used when driving or operating heavy equipment or with conditions of low blood pressure.

VALERIAN ROOT: Valerian root has significant therapeutic value as demonstrated by many scientific, clinical and pharmacological studies. Compounds found in this herb interact with brain receptor sites to promote sleep.[4] There are literally dozens of pharmaceutical and tea preparations throughout Europe which employ its tranquilizing benefits. One should not confuse valerian with the popular drug Valium; they are not related in any way. HOPS: Hops has a sedative effect which has been well-documented. Even the people collecting hops for beer production were known to become abnormally sleepy while working. Hops has a calming effect on the nervous system that helps with insomnia and restlessness, particularly when associated with anxiety.[5] SKULLCAP: Skullcap brings even more sedative action to this herbal formula. This plant has proven itself useful for sleep disorders, nervous conditions, tremors, and spasms. Skullcap is officially recognized in Europe as a sedative.[6] PASSIONFLOWER: This herb is widely used in Europe as a sedative and to treat common nervous conditions including nervous headaches and restlessness.[7] It is officially recognized in Britain, Belgium, France and Germany and has been listed in the *National Formulary* of the United States. DANDELION ROOT: Dandelion root plays a supportive role in this formula, even though it has no sedative or antianxiety action. It does have a mild laxative effect that helps cleanse the body and return it to a more normal state of health.[8] Quite often, conditions of anxiety and pain cause digestive disorders that interfere with sleep. CHAMOMILE: This herb has been the subject of a tremendous amount of chemical, scientific, and pharmacological research. Chamomile supports the overall sedative properties of this formula, is a natural anti-inflammatory and provides a carminative action that is settling to the gastrointestinal tract.[9] MARSHMALLOW: Marshmallow is accepted in Britain, Belgium, France and Germany as an emollient and demulcent. Its demulcent properties provide soothing activity for the gastrointestinal tract, improving digestion.[10] Marshmallow root does not have any sedative action, but also plays a supporting role in this herbal formula. HAWTHORN BERRIES: While its cardiotonic benefits may improve overall feeling of well-being, it has two lesser known properties. Hawthorn berries have been used as a mild tranquilizer as well as an antispasmodic. Their ability to lower blood pressure may be indirectly involved.[11] Interestingly, hawthorn berries have been incorporated in many European natural sedative formulas.

SECONDARY NUTRIENTS

KAVA: This herb has long been used in the South Pacific to calm and tranquilize. *Suggested Dosage:* Take as directed using standardized or guaranteed potency products.

VITAMIN B-COMPLEX: Necessary to nourish the central nervous system and promote rest. *Suggested Dosage:* Take as directed.

FOLIC ACID: Helps to calm restless leg syndrome which can cause insomnia. *Suggested Dosage:* Take as directed.

SUANZAORENTANG: A Chinese herbal combination designed to promote sleep. *Suggested Dosage:* Take as directed.

Home Care Suggestions

◆ Exercise regularly; it helps body to relax at night. Exercise earlier in the day and not too close to bedtime. Twenty to thirty minutes of aerobic exercise at least three days a week is recommended.

◆ An outside stroll prior to bed is recommended.

◆ Go to bed at the same time every night to establish a sleeping/waking routine for the body.

◆ Try to keep the bedroom as tranquil as possible, making it a place exclusively for sleep rather than other activities. Keep noise low and if necessary purchase curtains that effectively block out light.

◆ Purchase a white noise machine that emits a sound that masks other sounds and can help lull a person to sleep. A fish aquarium filter, a fan or a humidifier can produce the same effect.

◆ Make sure your bedroom is not too hot and is well ventilated.

◆ Some people sleep better with an electric blanket or hot water bottle.

◆ Try switching to pure cotton or linen sheets. Often the fabric that comes in contact with our skin can cause a subconscious annoyance.

◆ Make sure your pillow is not too high or puffy. Feather pillows that compress or special pillows designed to support your neck may be more comfortable.

◆ Avoid drinking alcohol, especially in the evening. Alcohol can temporarily induce sleep but a drink before bedtime can actually cause you to wake up during the middle of the night.

◆ Don't use nicotine. Smokers have more difficulty going to sleep.

◆ Don't eat a large meal prior to bedtime. Not only can this result in insomnia, it can cause nightmares as well.

◆ Eliminate any over-the-counter or prescription drugs you do not need to take. Barbiturates and benzodiazepines can actively interfere with the sleep cycle.

◆ Never sleep in what you wore during the day. Use a light pajama or nightgown that is not too constricting or heavy

◆ Get in bed and do breathing exercises while gently stretching your limbs. Listening to a stress-reducing tape which plays the sound of rain falling or ocean waves may also be helpful.

◆ Relax and unwind before you go to bed by reading, watching TV, listening to music, taking a bath, etc.

◆ Try some aromatherapy. The smell of lavender is recommended for its ability to relax the body.

◆ A bedtime snack is often helpful. The traditional home remedy of drinking a warm glass of milk has a scientific basis. Milk contains L-tryptophan which does help to induce sleep.

◆ If you can't sleep, get up and stay up reading, etc., until you feel sleepy.

◆ Yoga has been an effective meditative technique for combating insomnia.

Other Supportive Therapies

RELAXATION THERAPIES: Mediation and yoga can initiate relaxation and free your mind from anxiety.

AROMATHERAPY: A warm bath scented with a few drops of essential oils, such as meadowsweet and orange blossom, will soothe and relax the body and mind. Herbal baths can be quite relaxing and can be made by filling a muslin bag with herbs or with lavender and attaching it to the faucet so that hot water runs through it as the tub fills.

MASSAGE: Hot oil massages can do more to relax a tense body than perhaps any other therapy.

HOMEOPATHY: Aconite is used for insomnia caused by fear, arnica if you are overtired, and coffee for the racing mind. Phosphorus is also prescribed for nightmares and nux vomica for insomnia caused by alcohol consumption.

Scientific Facts-at-a-Glance

The Chinese herbal combination "Suanzaorentang" has been tested in double blind studies and may help to not only treat insomnia but actually improve daytime performance and alertness as well. Unlike the prescription drug Diazepam, it did not result in feelings of irritability, depression, or anxiety the next day. To the contrary, this combination of five herbs actually promoted a sense of well-being after its use.[12]

Spirit/Mind Considerations

Frequently, people who cannot sleep are plagued with a number of anxieties or emotional concerns that have not been resolved. They are known to "stew" over their problems and cannot let them go in order to relax and tranquilize their mind in preparation for sleep. Spiritual issues can also come into play as some people believe that prayer before bed can prompt feelings of peace and contentment. Insomnia can also be symptomatic of a psychiatric illness or an emotional problem. People who suffer from anxiety disorders and depression often have difficulty sleeping. The typical pattern in these instances is to awaken very early in the morning and not be able to resume sleeping. Manic-depressives usually sleep much less than normal and schizophrenics often pace at night. Victims of dementia may become afraid of the dark and act confused and restless at night. Make peace with those who you resent and cultivate an attitude of gratitude and faith.

Prevention

- Learn to relax and relieve stress before bedtime.
- Establish a routine with set sleeping and waking hours.
- Make your bedtime environment as soothing and comfortable as possible.
- Exercise regularly.
- Avoid ingesting caffeine, nicotine or alcohol.
- Avoid the use of over-the-counter and prescription drugs to induce sleep. These can end up promoting insomnia and are often counter-productive.
- Don't sleep in too late. Taking daytime naps may actually help you sleep better at night although it is generally recommended that sleeping during the day be avoided.

Doctor's Notes

Insomnia is a very common malady. Technically, it can be defined as terminal insomnia, beginning insomnia, or a combination of both. Unquestionably, stress leads to insomnia. One of the most important things I've done for my patients is to encourage them to reduce the effects of stress. Meditation exercises are good as are various yoga exercises. Mild to moderate exercise reduces insomnia, but vigorous exercise can actually aggravate it.

One should not dwell on an occasional bout with insomnia or it may become a chronic occurrence. We all have periods of time when we find it difficult to sleep. The harder you try to sleep, the less successful you will be. Get in the habit of telling yourself that you will be able to go to sleep. Incorporate a nightly routine that prepares you for bed. I have found that it is pointless to try to force yourself to sleep. If sleep doesn't come easily, pick up a book or do something constructive until you feel tired.

Remember that sleep medication can become habit-forming. Magnesium supplementation can help to relax the mind and body. 5-hydroxy-tryptophan can raise serotonin levels and allow people with insomnia to sleep. Melatonin should not be used for extended periods of time. It works better if used only occasionally. Valerian root in singular herb form or as part of a combination is also effective. Kava kava is also recommended. A good old-fashioned cup of chamomile tea before bed is still considered an effective means of combating insomnia.

Endnotes

1. E. Hartman, "L-tryptophan, a rational hypnotic with clinical potential," Amer Jour Psychi, 134: 366-70.

2. D. Shaw, "Management of fatigue: a physiologic approach," Amer Jour Med Sci, 1962, 243: 758-69.

3. S.P. James, et al, "Melatonin administration in insomnia," Neuropsychopharm, 1990, 3: 19-23.

4. T. Mennini, et al., "In vitro study on the interaction of extracts and pure compounds from Valeriana officinalis roots with GABA. Benzodiazepine, and barbiturate receptors in rat brain," Fitoterapia, 1993, 54(4): 291-300.

5. M. T. Murray, The Healing Power or Herbs, 2nd ed. Prima Publishing, Rocklin, Ca: 1992), 371.

6. K.L. Reichelt, et al., "Gluten, milk proteins and autism: Dietary intervention effects on behavior and peptide secretion," Jour Appl Nutr, 1990, 42(1):1-11.

7. N. Sopranzi, et al., "Biological and electroencephalographic parameters in rats in relation to Passiflora incarnata," Clin Ter, 1990, 132(5): 329-33.

8. J. K. Bohm, "Choleretic action of some medicinal plants," Arzneimittel-Forsch, 1959, 9: 376-78.

9. L. R. Della, et al., "Evaluation of the anti-inflammatory activity of chamomile preparations," Planta Med, 1990, 56:657-8.

10. "Marshmallow," The Lawrence Review of Natural Products: Facts and Comparisons, 1991, St. Louis.

11. S. Uchida, et al. "Inhibitory effects of condensed tannins on angiotensin converting enzyme," Jap Jour Pharmacol, 1987. 43:242-5.

12. M. Chen, and M Hsieh, "Clinical trial of Suanzaorentang in the treatment of insomnia," Clin Ther, 1985, 7(3): 224-27.

KIDNEY STONES

Kidney stones have plagued humans for thousands of years. Today, over 10 percent of all males and 5 percent of females will suffer from a kidney stone sometime during their lifetime. Approximately 6 percent of the entire United States population develops kidney stones. The incidence of kidney stones seems to be increasing and, like other Western diseases such as gallstones, gout, etc., may be directly linked with Western diet and lifestyle.

Kidney stones occur when either calcium oxalate, phosphates or uric acid crystallize into stones. Seventy percent of all kidney stones are calcium oxalate based. Usually, all three of these compounds are in solution form due to normal pH levels and the presence of other compounds. When there is a disruption of the chemical balance, stones can form and lodge anywhere within the urinary tract. Small stones that are present in the kidney will often cause no symptoms until they start to pass down into the ureter.

Once you have had a kidney stone, you are at somewhat of a higher risk of getting another. Approximately 60 percent of patients treated for a stone will develop another within seven years. Interestingly, there are more kidney stones reported during the summer months. This may imply that due to increased sweating, the urine can become more concentrated.

Symptoms

Kidney stones typically cause intermittent upper back pain (acute and sharp) that can radiate to the lower abdomen and groin area. Kidney stone pain almost always occurs on one side of the body at a time and is the type of pain that causes "doubling up." The following symptoms may also occur: chills, vomiting, fever, frequent urination which can contain pus or blood, and impaired urination with poor flow rate or dribbling.

Contact a physician immediately if you are experiencing any type of unexplained intense pain or the presence of blood in the urine. If you have passed a stone, save it for laboratory analysis. The most serious complication of not treating an obstructive kidney stone is infection which can lead to kidney damage.

Causes

Various factors can cause the formation of kidney stones:

- an excess of vitamin D
- Cushing's syndrome
- degenerative bone disease
- hyperparathyroidism
- cystinuria
- sarcoidosis
- gout
- kidney disease
- deformities of the kidney
- ingesting aluminum salts
- excessive intake of milk and alkali (antacids)
- prolonged immobility
- an excess of vitamin C
- anticancer drugs
- high-protein diets
- high alcohol consumption
- exposure to certain heavy metals such as cadmium
- genetic predisposition

Conventional Therapies

There is really no satisfactory medical treatment for kidney stones that do not flush out on their own. If stones are being caused by other medical conditions, certain drugs can be prescribed to help prevent the formation of future stones. Recent advances in ultrasonic and shock wave therapy offer better treatment options. Surgery should be considered only as a last resort.

It is vital that the type of kidney stone that you have is diagnosed in order to design an effective treatment based on the stone's composition. Urine will be examined, as it may contain the presence of stone crystals. Approximately 90 percent of urinary tract kidney stones will show up on an x-ray. The use of intravenous or retrograde pyelography (IVP) can confirm the site of the stone. This test can also indicate any obstruction of the tract above the stone which can be monitored by ultrasound scanning. A chemical analysis of the blood and urine may be required if another physical condition is thought to have caused the stone.

The usual treatment for a small kidney stone is bed rest accompanied by the use of narcotic analgesics. Increased fluid intake is encouraged. The majority of stones that are less than 0.2 inch in diameter can be passed without too much difficulty. In the case of a larger stone, surgical treatment may be indicated to prevent kidney damage. Surgery should only be done as a last resort. Surgery to remove kidney stones is invasive and causes considerable trauma to the area affected. Stones that are located in the bladder and the lower ureter can be crushed and removed using a cystoscopy. The extra corporeal shock-wave lithotritor can actually disintegrate stones using a focused shock wave. This method is continually being improved and is preferable to surgery.

Dietary Guidelines

- Drinking large amounts of cranberry or cherry juice has long been considered a folk remedy for kidney stones. Cherry juice contains bioflavonoids which can help reduce inflammation and heal damaged tissue. Most physicians, however, believe that in order to make the urine acid enough, unrealistic quantities of these juices would have to be consumed. The majority of the scientific community sees cranberry and cherry juice as just other ways to increase fluid intake, which is seen as desirable.
- Drink plenty of fluids every day—at least six to eight glasses of water. Keeping the body well hydrated is one of the most effective ways of avoiding kidney stones.

- Drink the juice from a freshly squeezed lemon in water first thing in the morning and at night.
- Calcium-based kidney stones (which make up the majority of kidney stones) can be the result of dietary patterns characterized by low-fiber and high intake of alcohol, fat, animal protein, sugar and salt. Several studies indicate that vegetarians, as a whole, have a decreased risk of developing kidney stones. Because calcium-rich foods can create stones, reduce the amount of milk, butter, cheese and other dairy products that you consume.
- Eat whole grains exclusively. Research has indicated that increasing fiber intake can lower the calcium content of urine.
- Avoid white sugar and refined carbohydrates; after ingesting sugar, a rise in urinary calcium can occur.
- Limit dairy products and try to avoid those fortified with vitamin D—it is thought to contribute to the formation of stones.
- Avoid foods that are high in oxalate, namely cocoa, black tea, beet leaves, spinach, parsley, celery, grapes, blueberries, strawberries, summer squash and nuts.
- Watch your protein intake (meats, cheeses, poultry and fish). Eating too much protein can increase the presence of urinary calcium, phosphate and uric acid.
- Cut your daily salt intake. Cutting down on salt helps to decrease the concentration of urinary calcium. Watch for hidden sources of salt or sodium such as ketchup, mustard, pickled foods, smoked meats, chips, pops and pretzels.

Recommended Nutritional Supplements

PRIMARY NUTRIENTS

MAGNESIUM AND VITAMIN B6 Magnesium increases the solubility of calcium and helps to reduce the urinary oxalate that often comprises kidney stones.[1] Lab tests with animals have shown that a magnesium deficient diet produces kidney stones. Magnesium supplemented with vitamin B6 has been shown to be effective in preventing the recurrence of kidney stones.[2] This combination has had dramatic results in curtailing the incidence of kidney stone recurrence, with a success rate in some studies as high as 90 percent. *Suggested Dosage:* 200 mg twice daily of magnesium and 50 mg of B6. Use chelated forms of magnesium.

POTASSIUM This mineral actually inhibits the chemical process that leads to kidney stone formation. In addition, eating potassium-rich foods can actually reverse the hypercalciuria which can be caused by high meat consumption.[3] *Suggested Dosage:* Use as directed.

L-GLUTAMIC ACID This compound has been found to be very low or even absent in the urine of people who have trouble with kidney stones.[4] *Suggested Dosage:* Take as directed on an empty stomach with fruit juice.

GLYCOSAMINOGLYCANS These compounds are found in supplements like glucosamine and in some cartilage products. They are powerful inhibitors of the aggregation process that causes calcium oxalate to harden into stones.[5] *Suggested Dosage:* Take as directed.

VITAMIN A A deficiency of this vitamin has been linked to the formation of kidney stones. Apparently, a lack of vitamin A causes the excretion of compounds in the urine which promote crystallization.[6] Interestingly, this reaction is made worse if you eat dairy products and lack vitamin A.[7] *Suggested Dosage:* 10,000 to 25,000 IU daily. If you are pregnant, do not exceed 10,000 IU.

CRANBERRY Clinical studies have found that cranberry not only helps to prevent bladder infections, but may also inhibit the formation of calcium oxalate kidney stones in the urine.[8] *Suggested Dosage:* Take as directed using standardized products.

PROTEOLYTIC ENZYMES Because improper digestion of protein may contribute to the formation of kidney stones, adding enzymes can help to prevent undigested peptides from initiating chemical reactions which affect uric acid and urine content. *Suggested Dosage:* Take as directed, making sure to look for papain and pancreatin containing products.

HERBAL COMBINATION This combination includes parsley, uva ursi, cleavers, juniper berries and kelp. *Suggested Dosage:* Take 3-6 capsules per day with a large glass of water.

PARSLEY: Parsley is used in Germany not only as a diuretic, but also to provide irrigation in treating kidney stones. It has an historical record of kidney stone application.[9] The main constituents of parsley which initiate its antikidney stone action are myristicin and apiole. Parsley also provides a carminative action. UVA URSI: Uva ursi is one of the best researched diuretics obtained from the plant kingdom. Its urinary tract applications extend far beyond diuresis, urethritis, cystitis, and other urinary inflammatory diseases.[10] It contains arbutin, a compound which is converted to hydroquinone in the body, producing antiseptic properties for the urinary tract. CLEAVERS: Cleavers is considered by some herbalists to be one of the best herbs for kidney and bladder troubles. It is especially good for cases of kidney stones and water retention.[11] It is beneficial for painful urination, and also provides a mild laxative effect, further cleansing the body and returning it to a more normal state of health. JUNIPER BERRIES: Juniper berries are an important weapon against urinary tract disorders and water retention. Juniper is particularly effective at expelling the uric acid associated with stone formation in the kidneys.[12] KELP: Kelp exhibits only mild diuretic activity, but its real application to this blend is its ability to replace trace elements that are lost through urination.[13] Trace element imbalances and loss are a major problem with extended diuretic use.

SECONDARY NUTRIENTS

VITAMIN K: Vitamin K plays a significant role in the synthesis of urinary proteins that are necessary to keep calcium oxalate from crystallizing. Vitamin K is found in green leafy vegetables and fat-soluble liquid chlorophyll. *Suggested Dosage:* Take as directed.

CITRATE: This compound is found in potassium citrate or sodium citrate. A low level of citrate has been found in various people who suffer from kidney stones. A decreased level of citrate can be the result of chronic diarrhea, urinary tract infections or acidosis. Citrate supplementation is thought to be of significant value in preventing kidney stones. *Suggested Dosage:* Take as directed.

VITAMIN E, SELENIUM AND ALPHA LIPOIC ACID: A powerful antioxidant trio that can scavenge for free radicals in the kidney. *Suggested Dosage:* Take each supplement as directed making sure to get 400 IU of vitamin E.

ZINC: Can help to discourage the formation of crystals in the urine which can solidify into stones. *Suggested Dosage:* Take 50 mg per day.

ALOE VERA: This herb can reduce the growth rate of urinary calcium. It can be used to prevent as well as reduce the size of an existing stone. Take in juice form. *Suggested Dosage:* Take as directed. Aloe vera has a distinct laxative action and may cause some gripping. Take with ginger to minimize this effect.

KHELLA: Used by the ancient Egyptians for the treatment of kidney stones. It works by relaxing the ureter and allowing the stone to pass. *Suggested Dosage:* Take as directed.

GRAVEL AND STONE ROOT: These herbs have a long history of use for kidney stones. *Suggested Dosage:* Take as directed using standardized products.

Home Care Suggestions

◆ At the first sign of a kidney stone, drink large quantities of water to help flush out the stone.

◆ Analgesics can help if the pain is not severe.

Other Supportive Therapies

HOMEOPATHY: Magnesia phos and Calcarea are used to treat kidney stones.

ACUPUNCTURE: Can help to relieve pain and stimulate better kidney function.

Scientific Facts-at-a-Glance

Drinking hard water may have its advantages. In an American study, there was a negative correlation between the hospital incidence of kidney stones and local water hardness.[14] Some people believe that if your water is high in calcium, however, it should be filtered out.

Prevention

◆ There is a sizable consensus that the majority of kidney stones can be prevented through dietary changes.

◆ Increase your daily fluid intake; drink six to eight glasses of pure water every day. If you have a hard water supply, drink bottled water that is lower in mineral content. Magnesium is a mineral that should be ingested and calcium avoided.

◆ Increase dietary fiber, complex carbohydrates and green leafy vegetables.

◆ Avoid excess sugar, salt, simple carbohydrates, animal fats and meats.

◆ Make sure you supplement your diet with adequate doses of magnesium and vitamin B6.

◆ Limit your intake of dairy products, especially those that have been fortified with vitamin D.

◆ Limit your intake of animal protein. Uric acid kidney stones can form from a diet high in purines.

◆ Keep yourself at an ideal weight. Excess weight may lead to an insensitivity to insulin which can cause hypercalciuria, a condition that increases your risk for stone formation.

◆ Do not use calcium-based stomach medications or antacids such as Tums, and avoid aluminum compounds.

◆ Keep yourself active. Exercise regularly. Prolonged inactivity can cause calcium levels in the blood to rise. Exercising helps to pull calcium out of the bloodstream and back into the bones.

◆ CAUTION: Ascorbate can be metabolized to oxalate; therefore, megadoses of vitamin C may increase urinary oxalate levels and contribute to kidney stone formation in predisposed individuals. It is also important to not take more than 200 IU of vitamin D per day.

Doctor's Notes

Kidney stones can cause excruciating pain that feels like it will last forever. Anyone who has experienced an episode will want to do everything in their power to prevent another one. Unfortunately, if you have had one occurence, you are prone to have more. Like so many of the diseases we have discussed, kidney stones seem to be linked to Western eating habits. Countries which had very low rates of kidney stones in the past are now experiencing a rise in incidence due to their change from whole, raw foods to the refined, sugary and animal protein foods typical of our culture. Drinking pure cranberry juice on a daily basis is one of the best things you can do to prevent stones. Decreasing animal protein foods and boosting raw vegetable and fruit intake are also very beneficial. If you are waiting for a stone to pass, you can urinate through a piece of gauze to trap it. It can be taken to your doctor for chemical analysis. I believe that the inadequate digestion of proteins is a little addressed factor in the formation of kidney stones. Boosting your ability to digest protein by taking proteolytic enzymes is highly recommended.

Additional Resources

American Kidney Fund
6110 Executive Blvd, Suite 1010
Rockville, MD 20852
(800) 638-8299

Endnotes

1. J. Lindberg, et al., "Effect of magnesium citrate and magnesium oxide on the crystallization of calcium salts in urine: changes pro-

duced by food-magnesium interaction," Jour Urol, 1990, 143(2):248-51.

2. D. Gibbs, "The action of pyridoxine in primary hyperoxaluria," Clin Sci, 1970, 38:277-86.

3. K. Kaneko, et al., "Urinary calcium and calcium balance in young women affected by high protein diet of soy protein isolate and adding sulfur-containing amino acids and/or potassium," Jour Nutr Sci Vitaminol (Tokyo), 1990, 36(2):105-16.

4. M. Mcgeown, "The urinary excretion of amino acids in calculus patients," Clin Sci, 1959, 18:185.

5. Y. Michacci, et al., "Urinary excretion of glycosaminoglycans in normal and stone forming subjects," Kidney Int, 1989, 36(6):1022-8.

6. H. Bichler, et al., "Influence of vitamin A deficiency on the excretion of uromucoid and other substance in the urine of rats," Clin Nephrol 1983, 20:32-39.

7. S. Gershoff and R. McGandy, "The effects of vitamin A-deficient diets containing lactose in producing bladder calculi and tumors in rats," Am Jour Clin Nutr, 1981, 34:483.

8. H. Hirayama, et al., "Effect of desmodium styracifolium-triterpenoid on calcium oxalate renal stones," Bri Jour Urol, 1993, 71(2):143-7.

9. Mark Pederson, Nutritional Herbology, (Wendell Whitman, Warsaw, IN: 1995), 131-32.

10. A. Leung, Encyclopedia of Common Natural Ingredients Used in Foods, Drugs, and Cosmetics, (John Wiley and Sons, New York: 1980), 316-17.

11. H.W. Felter, The Eclectic Materia Medica, Pharmacology and Therapeutics, (Eclectic Medical Publishers, Portland, Oregon: 1992), 83.

12. E. Racz-Kotilla and G. Racz, Farmacia, 1971, 19:165.

13. N. Iritani and J. Nogi, "Effect of spinach and wakame on cholesterol turnover in the rat," Atherosclerosis, 1972, 15: 87-92.

14. R. Seirakowski, "Stone incidence as related to water hardness in different geographical regions in the United States," Urol Res, 1979, 7: 157-60.

LUPUS

Lupus is an autoimmune disease of unknown origin that can affect a variety of organs. Basically, it is a chronic inflammatory condition that occurs when the body's immune system attacks itself. The term *lupus* means "wolf" and refers to the rash that sometimes accompanies the disease which gives the face a wolf-like appearance. There are two type of lupus: systemic lupus erythematosus (SLE), affecting the organs and joints; and discoid lupus (DLE), a less serious skin disease. Lupus may go into spontaneous remission, but in severe cases it can be fatal. Lupus generally affects young women more than any other segment of the population. The kidneys are particularly susceptible to the inflammation brought on by lupus. Approximately 50 percent of people with systemic lupus develop nephritis. Drug-related lupus is usually mild and subsides when use of the offending drug is discontinued.

Symptoms

In systemic lupus, symptoms can mimic arthritis in the beginning with joint pain and swelling. In addition the following may be present:

- sun sensitivity
- fatigue
- chills
- weight loss
- abdominal pain
- enlarged lymph nodes
- malaise
- low grade fever
- anorexia
- diarrhea
- anemia
- mouth sores

NOTE: In more advanced cases the brain, kidneys and heart may become involved. If the central nervous system is affected, amnesia, irritability, depression, psychosis or seizures may result.

Causes

The causes of systemic lupus are not conclusively known. There is some speculation that a viral infection has caused the immune system to develop inappropriate antibodies which attack organs and tissues. Other factors related to the onset of lupus are streptococcal bacteria, pregnancy and genetic predisposition. Discoid lupus can be triggered by ultraviolet rays, fatigue, childbirth, infection, chemicals, stress and some drugs such as hydralazine for high blood pressure or procainamide for irregular heartbeat. Other factors which are thought to contribute to the development of lupus are:

- pollution
- food additives
- faulty genes
- vaccines
- undigested proteins
- hydrochloric acid deficiency

Conventional Therapies

An accurate diagnosis of lupus is difficult. Lupus is considered an incurable disease, therefore medical treatment involves symptomatic therapy and treatment designed to inhibit immune function, which is always accompanied by serious side-effects. Lupus, like other autoimmune diseases, has a high probability for long remissions. A false positive blood test for syphilis can occur with lupus and should be considered a possible first marker of the disease. According to some criteria, four of the following eight symptoms must be present before a diagnosis can be made:

1. arthritis
2. butterfly rash on the cheeks
3. sun sensitivity
4. low white blood cell count, low platelet count or the presence of hemolytic anemia
5. mouth sores
6. abnormal cells in the urine
7. the presence of a specific antibody in the blood
8. seizures or psychosis

In the initial stages of lupus, anti-inflammatory drugs are usually prescribed. Some antimalarial medications are effective in treating the sun-sensitivity and skin rashes associated with lupus. Corticosteroids are routinely prescribed for lupus and can have serious side-effects. Other drugs used are immunosuppressants, and antirheumatics. The value of radiation therapy is still in the experimental stage and involves giving low doses of radiation to the lymph nodes to suppress immune reaction. In the same way, anti-cancer drugs may be used to treat lupus. Physical therapy and plasmapheresis, a type of blood therapy, may also be suggested. CAUTION: Always inform any medical workers that you have lupus before you are treated for any disorder or given any immunization.

Dietary Guidelines

- Eat a diet comprised of mild foods that is high in raw vegetables and fruit juices.
- Drink several glasses of pure water a day.
- Keep your protein consumption low and emphasize complex carbohydrates, fresh fruits and vegetables.
- Garlic, asparagus, brown rice, fish, oatmeal fresh pineapple, and whole grains are recommended.
- Avoid all dairy products.
- Avoid eating alfalfa sprouts which contains canavain, a compound that may cause some problems in people suffering from lupus.[1]
- Don't eat nightshade vegetables, including potatoes, peppers, eggplant and tomatoes.
- The benefit of drinking several glasses of carrot juice is promoted by some victims of lupus.
- Make sure to find out if you are suffering from a hydrochloric acid deficiency, a symptom rarely addressed by physicians.

Recommended Nutritional Supplements

PRIMARY NUTRIENTS

ESSENTIAL FATTY ACIDS The role of both omega-3 and omega-6 fatty acids is vitally important in any immune disease. These acids inhibit the formation and action of prostaglandins that initiate the inflammatory response so typical of diseases like lupus. Using fish oils in combination with oils like flaxseed or evening primrose can affect the severity of lupus.[2] *Suggested Dosage:* Take as directed using fish oils and flaxseed or evening primrose. Take with vitamin E and keep refrigerated.

PROTEOLYTIC ENZYMES These digestive enzymes work to breakdown the peptides found in protein foods. Undigested protein deposits in tissue are suspected as one of the causes of autoimmune diseases.[3] *Suggested Dosage:* Take as directed prior to meals and between meals. Look for blends containing papain and pancreatin.

PANTOTHENIC ACID Extended therapy with this nutrient has been effective in treating the symptoms of lupus.[4] *Suggested Dosage:* Tests subjects took six grams daily and tapered to two grams. This is a megadose and should be done only under the supervision of your doctor. Taking vitamin E with pantothenic acid has been found to be more effective. Calcium pantothenate is the form generally used.

VITAMIN A WITH BETA-CAROTENE This combination helps to boost immunity and promotes the regeneration of tissue. Beta-carotene has been used in clinical studies to treat lupus.[5] In addition, a lack of vitamin A actually increases the production of certain antibodies associated with lupus in laboratory animals.[6] *Suggested Dosage:* Take 25,000 IU of vitamin A and 25,000 IU of beta-carotene daily. CAUTION: If you are pregnant, do not take over 10,000 IU of vitamin A.

VITAMIN E WITH SELENIUM Various studies strongly suggest that this combination is intrinsically involved in autoimmune response. Levels of glutathione-peroxidase in the skin are directly impacted by these two nutrients.[7] In addition, topical application of vitamin E oil directly on skin lesions may be helpful.[8] *Suggested Dosage:* Take 400 to 800 IU of vitamin E and selenium as directed.

GLUCOSAMINE SULFATE/CHONDROITIN SULFATE Help to promote cartilage and collagen repair. This prevents joint inflammation that occurs from the arthritic component of lupus.[9] *Suggested Dosage:* Take as directed.

CMO This is a fatty acid derivative that is fairly new and has great potential for treating inflammatory joint disorders.[10] *Suggested Dosage:* Take as directed.

GRAPE SEED OR PINE BARK EXTRACT The powerful antioxidant actions of the proanthocyanidins found in this compound help to quiet inflammation, especially in joints.[11]

Suggested Dosage: Take as directed with higher initial doses for two weeks to achieve cellular saturation, and then taper down.

TRIPTERYGIUM WILFORDI An herbal compound that has been used in 26 cases of discoid lupus with significant success.[12] *Suggested Dosage:* Take as directed using guaranteed potency or standardized products.

L-CYSTEINE, L-METHIONINE, L-LYSINE This trio of amino acids helps to keep the skin healthy and promotes tissue repair. *Suggested Dosage:* Take as directed on an empty stomach with fruit juice.

HERBAL COMBINATION This combination should contain devil's claw, yucca, alfalfa, wild yam root, sarsaparilla root, kelp, white willow bark, cayenne, and horsetail. *Suggested Dosage:* Four to six capsules daily. For extreme cases it is best to use maximum dosage of six capsules per day for a prolonged period of four to six months.

DEVIL'S CLAW: This herb has a long history of use in Europe for inflammatory disorders.[13] It also stimulates digestion and helps to prevent the presence of undigested proteins called peptides which can trigger an inappropriate immune response. Sometimes the body considers peptides to be a foreign substance (antigen) and in response antibodies or larger amounts of histamine are produced. YUCCA: Yucca has a similar action to that of devil's claw. It improves digestion, thereby reducing histamine production. As a result, inflammation and pain may be alleviated. The bioactive constituents of yucca are saponins.[14] ALFALFA LEAVES AND SEEDS: As mentioned earlier, autoimmune diseases characterized by unwanted inflammatory responses may be a result of poor digestion. In addition, an impaired digestive system can cause malnutrition by starving the body of much needed macro and micronutrients. Alfalfa leaves and seeds provide a rich nutrient source to help the body to return to a healthy state.[15] WILD YAM ROOT: Other common names for wild yam root include rheumatism root and colic root, suggesting its use as an anti-inflammatory and digestive aid. Its antirheumatic property is primarily thought to be attributed to its cortisone precursor diosgenin. As diosgenin is converted to cortisone, anti-inflammatory activity results, and the patient may notice a reduction of pain.[16] SARSAPARILLA ROOT: Sarsaparilla is officially recognized in Germany and the United Kingdom for its antirheumatic, anti-inflammatory, and diuretic properties. Its activity is thought to be due to its saponin content. Historically, this herb has been used to treat gout and rheumatism and is classified as a tonic and blood purifier.[17] KELP: Kelp, like alfalfa, is a dense source of nutrients, particularly trace elements that can improve the body's nutrition. It also provides mucilage in the form of algin, a compound that soothes the gastrointestinal tract. WHITE WILLOW BARK: White willow bark has been used for over a thousand years to relieve pain. Salicin, aspirin's forerunner, was discovered to be white willow's active constituent. Apart from its ability to assist with pain, salicin reduces inflammation. Unlike aspirin, however, it will not thin the blood or irritate the stomach. CAYENNE: Cayenne, also known as capsicum, stimulates circulation and makes other herbs more effective. Cayenne can help to improve digestion. Cayenne's "hot" principle, capsaicin, is also a noted analgesic and can be applied in topical ointment form. HORSETAIL (SHAVEGRASS): While horsetail contributes to this formula as a mild diuretic. Its main action is to strengthen and regenerate connective tissues. Connective tissue (found in joints) is destroyed by the inflammation caused by lupus. Silica, abundantly contained in this herb, is vital in regenerating connective tissue and keeping it strong.

SECONDARY NUTRIENTS

VITAMIN B12: Supplementation or injections of this vitamin have shown some promise for people with lupus. *Suggested Dosage:* 1,000 mg intramuscularly twice weekly or use sublingual products.

DHEA: This hormone helps to modulate and normalize the inflammatory response. *Suggested Dosage:* Take as directed although this supplement is not recommended for anyone who has had or has hormonally related cancer.

GOTU KOLA: Research demonstrates that gotu kola is effective in the treatment of various skin disorders associated with cellulitis and lupus. It also possesses wound healing activity and has been shown to decrease scarring. *Suggested Dosage:* Take as directed using guaranteed potency or standardized products.

ZINC: Helps to boost tissue repair and nourishes the immune system. *Suggested Dosage:* Take 50 mg per day. Use gluconate or picolinate products.

GARLIC: Helps to fortify immunity and fights secondary infection. *Suggested Dosage:* Take two tablets with each meal.

CHINESE HERBAL BLEND: A special autoimmune formula is offered by Seven Forest Company. This blend is also good for multiple sclerosis, lupus, rheumatoid arthritis, ulcerative colitis, myasthenia gravis and scleroderma.

Home Care Suggestions

- Minimize your exposure to environments where viral infections would be more likely to exist such as classrooms, nurseries, etc.
- Avoid using birth control pills. They have been linked with lupus flair-ups.
- Keep a positive mental attitude. Use visualization therapy or hypnotherapy to help facilitate a better chance for remission.
- Avoid exposure to strong sunlight or ultraviolet light. Use strong sunscreens and protective hats and clothing if necessary.
- Exercise regularly. Swimming is particularly good if arthritis exists.
- Use regular message therapy to help with joint aches and toxin removal.
- Seek medical treatment for any infection, no matter how minor.
- Find a physician with a positive attitude.

Other Supportive Therapies

MEDITATION AND YOGA: Help to facilitate true relaxation and stress relief.

MASSAGE WITH ESSENTIAL OILS: Can help to ease painful joints and stimulate circulation.

ACUPUNCTURE: Specific trigger points help to control the pain associated with lupus.

Scientific Facts-at-a-Glance

Recent studies have found that the ability to metabolize sulfur in the body may be impaired in people with lupus. This suggests that sulfur-containing foods may cause a problem and that sulfur levels may not be normal.[18] In addition, sensitivities to certain chemicals and foods may be much more pronounced in individuals with lupus. In some studies people with lupus also had a much higher incidence of hives, conjunctivitis, and other allergy-induced disorders. When certain foods were eliminated and supplements were taken, remissions occurred.[19]

Spirit/Mind Considerations

Because of the nature of the disease, lupus can cause a great deal of mental stress and anxiety in its victims. When the disease is active, mental and physical support should be available. There are lupus support groups and foundations that can be of great value in promoting self-help. If systemic lupus has attacked the central nervous system, symptoms can resemble those of various abnormal psychological disorders. Excessive irritability, deep depression and psychotic behavior are not uncommon in these instances.

Prevention

◆ Take proteolytic enzymes with meals.
◆ Do not give your baby high-protein foods too early.
◆ As with any autoimmune disease, it is recommended to keep the immune system healthy through proper diet, rest and exercise.
◆ Avoid exposure to chemical agents, pollutants, drugs, and other toxins that can impair immune function.

Doctor's Notes

As I continue to practice medicine, I am more and more convinced that undigested proteins can initiate a serious dysfunction of the immune system, causing autoimmune diseases like lupus. If protein molecules are not properly broken down and assimilated, they can circulate in the bloodstream, deposit in joints and organs, and may eventually stimulate an abnormal immune response. In such cases, the immune system actually turns against the body instead of against legitimate invaders.

Additional Resources

Lupus Foundation of America
Box RD 4 Research Place, Suite 180
Rockville, MD 20850-3226
(800) 558-0121

Endnotes

1. R. Malonow, et al., "Systemic lupus erythematosus-like syndrome in monkeys fed alfalfa sprouts: Role of a non-protein amino acid," Science, 1982, 216:415-17.
2. N. Alexander, et al., "The type of dietary fat affects the severity of autoimmune disease in NZB/NZW mice," Am J Pathol, 1987, 127(1): 106-21.
3. K. Ransberger, "Enzyme treatment of immune complex diseases," Arth Rheum, 1986, 8: 16-19. See also "Enzyme therapy in multiple sclerosis," Der Kassenarzt, 1986, 41: 42-45.
4. A. Welsh "Lupus erythematosus: Treatment by combined use of massive amounts of pantothenic acid and vitamin E," Arch Dermatol Syphil, 1954, 70:181-98. See also L. Goldman, Preliminary and Short Report: "Intensive pantheol therapy for lupus erythematosus," J Invest Dermatol, 1950, 15:291.
5. P. Newbold, "Beta-carotene in the treatment of discoid lupus erythematosus," Bri Jour Dermatol, 1976, 95:100-101.
6. M. Gershwin, et al., "Nutritional factors and autoimmunity: Dietary vitamin A deprivation induces a selective increase in IgM autoantibodies and hypergammaglobulinemia in New Zealand Black mice," Jour Immunology 1984, 133(1):222-26.
7 M. Block, "Vitamin E in the treatment of diseases of the skin," Clin Med, 1953, January, 31-34.
8. S. Ayres S, "Is vitamin E involved in the autoimmune mechanism?" Cutis, 1978, 21:321-25.
9. I. Setnikar, "Antireactive Properties of 'chondoprotective' drugs," Int-Jour-Tissue-React,1992, 14 (5): 253-61.
10. H. Deihl, "Cetyl myristoleate isolated from Swiss albino mice: an apparent protective agent against adjuvant arthritis," Journal of Pharmaceutical Sciences, 1994, vol. 83 (3): 296-299.
11. M.T. Meunier, et al., "Free radical scavenger activity of procyanidolic oligomers and anthocyanosides with respect to superoxide anion and lipid peroxidation," Plant Med Phytotherapy, 1989, 4: 267-74.
12. Q. Wanzhang et al., "Clinical observations on Tripterygium wilfordi in treatment of 26 cases of discoid erythematosus," Jour Trad Chin Med, 1983, 3(2):131-2.
13. L.R. Brady, et al., Pharmacognosy, 8th ed. (Lea and Gebiger, Philadelphia: 1981): 480.
14. R. Bingham, et al., "Yucca plant saponins in the management of arthritis," Jour Applied Nutrition, 1975, 27: 45-50.
15. M.R. Malinow, et al., "Effect of alfalfa saponins on intestinal cholesterol absorption in rats," Amer Jour Clini Nutri, 1977, 30: 2061-67.
16. H.W. Feller, The Eclectic Materia Medica, Pharmacology and Therapeutics (Eclectic Medical Publications, Portland Oregon): 1983, first published in 1922.
17. Kiangsu Institute of Modern Medicine, Encyclopedia of Chinese Drugs, 2 vols. 1977, Shanghi, People's Republic of China.
18. M. Diumenjo, "Allergic manifestations of systemic lupus erythematosus," Aller Immunopathol, 1985, 13(4): 323-26.
19. H. Cook and C. Reading, "Dietary intervention in systemic lupus erythematosus: 4 cases of clinical remission and reversal of abnormal pathology," Int Clin, Nutr Rev, 1985, 5(4): 166-67.

MENINGITIS

Meningitis is a contagious disease characterized by an inflammation of the meninges, membranes that cover the brain and spinal cord. Victims of meningitis are generally under the age of thirty. There are two types of meningitis: viral and bacterial. Viral meningitis is a relatively mild disease that is far more common than the bacterial form and tends to occur in outbreaks during the winter months. It usually clears up within two weeks. Bacterial meningitis, on the other hand, can be life threatening and requires immediate medical attention. It affects between 9,000 and 12,000 people in the United States annually. Meningococcal meningitis is the most common form of bacterially caused meningitis and can occur in small epidemics. Approximately 2,000 to 5,000 cases are reported annually in the United States, with 70 percent of victims under the age of five. Bacterial meningitis can be cured with prompt medical treatment and usually takes two weeks under a doctor's care.

Symptoms

Symptoms of bacterial meningitis include the following:

- fever
- severe headache
- stiff neck
- nausea
- vomiting
- sensitivity to light
- red rash
- the fontanelle (soft spot) on a baby may become raised and tight

Viral meningitis causes milder symptoms and can be mistaken for influenza. The symptoms of bacterial meningitis can develop suddenly, sometimes over a period of just a few hours and are followed by drowsiness and, in some cases, a loss of consciousness. In 50 percent of these cases, a red, blotchy rash appears. CAUTION: Any headache accompanied by vomiting, fever, drowsiness, a shrill cry or a stiff neck should receive immediate medical attention. In an infant who has meningitis, the soft spot on the top of the head may feel tight to the touch. Meningitis is a potentially fatal disease that requires prompt medical treatment. Some of the potential consequences of failing to diagnose and treat bacterial meningitis properly and in time are impaired learning, mental retardation, paralysis, blindness, deafness, and even death.

Causes

The organisms responsible for meningitis usually come from an infectious source elsewhere in the body and reach the meninges through the bloodstream. Some of these viruses are the same ones that cause polio and measles.

Bacteria such as meningococcus, pneumococcus, streptococcus and tuberculosis can also cause the disease. Meningitis can also be a complication of a skull fracture, or can occur when cavities in the skull become infected from the presence of an ear or sinus infection. In rare instances, cryptococcus, a fungus spread in pigeon droppings, can also cause the disease.

Conventional Therapies

Meningitis is a disease that requires immediate medical attention. A lumbar puncture or spinal tap will be performed to examine a small sample of cerebrospinal fluid for the presence of certain microbes. A number of blood tests will also be performed. If viral meningitis is present, generally no medical treatment is required. Bacterial meningitis will be treated with large doses of intravenous antibiotics and usually requires hospitalization. New cephalosporin antibiotics enable physicians to successfully treat the majority of meningitis cases if caught early enough. Anyone who has come into close contact with a person who suffers from the meningococcus variety should receive prophylactic antibiotics such as rifampin for two days.

Dietary Guidelines

- First of all, take a good acidophilus supplement and eat live culture yogurt to replace the friendly bacteria which are readily destroyed by antibiotic therapy.
- Encourage a dramatic increase in fluids using water, fresh citrus juices, vegetable juices, broths and herbal teas. Increasing fluid helps to control fever, prevent dehydration and eliminate toxins.
- Eat raw foods extensively. Cut up carrots, broccoli, cucumbers, cauliflower, green peppers, bananas, apples, and oranges.
- Avoid caffeine, alcohol, nicotine, fatty foods, etc.

Recommended Nutritional Supplements

PRIMARY NUTRIENTS

LACTOBACILLUS ACIDOPHILUS Supplementing friendly bacteria is important to counteract its destruction by antibiotics and to afford the immune system added fortification.[1] Tests have found that acidophilus caused a 50 percent inhibition in the growth of 27 different strains of bacteria.[2] *Suggested Dosage:* Take as directed on an empty stomach first thing in the morning and before retiring. Look for nonmilk products with bifidobacteria that have guaranteed bacteria count. Check the expiration date.

VITAMIN A There is no question that this vitamin boosts immunity and facilitates better tissue repair, especially during times of infection. Moreover, a lack of this vitamin can predispose us to infection.[3] *Suggested Dosage:* 25,000 IU for duration of infection. CAUTION: If you are pregnant, do not take over 10,000 IU per day.

VITAMIN C WITH BIOFLAVONOIDS Ascorbic acid combined with flavonoids like quercitin can stimulate the immune system to better fight infection by enhancing phagocyte activity.[4] *Suggested Dosage:* 10,000 mg per day divided into three doses with meals.

ZINC Zinc is absolutely vital to proper immune function. During periods of infection it can help fight some strains of bacteria that even antibiotics may fail to treat.[5] *Suggested Dosage:* 100 mg per day. Do not take more than 100 mg daily of zinc.

ESSENTIAL FATTY ACIDS Fish oils, evening primrose and flaxseed oil are rich in certain acid compounds that have antibacterial properties. Studies have referred to these actions as antibiotic-like.[6] *Suggested Dosage:* Take as directed, using blends that contain both the omega-3 and omega-6 acids. Keep refrigerated.

CHINESE MUSHROOMS Shitake, reishi, or maitake varieties have the distinct ability to rev up immune defenses by enhancing T-cell activity.[7] *Suggested Dosage:* Take as directed using standardized products.

ASTRAGALUS This Chinese herb has impressive immuno-stimulatory properties, especially in cases of viral infection.[8] *Suggested Dosage:* Take as directed using guaranteed potency or standardized products.

HERBAL COMBINATION This combination should contain echinacea, goldenseal root, myrrh gum, garlic, licorice root, blue vervain, butternut root bark, and kelp. *Suggested Dosage:* Six to twelve capsules daily. Should not be used for more than three weeks at a time.

ECHINACEA: This herb has a long history and impressive credentials in fighting pathogenic conditions like meningitis. In Germany it is widely used to treat infections of the head, nose and throat. Echinacea exerts a bactericidal effect against infectious organisms while stimulating the immune response by improving phagocytic activity.[9] GOLDENSEAL ROOT: Goldenseal root is recognized by many herbalists for its ability to strengthen the mucus linings of the body, making it harder for pathogens to penetrate. Two of its active compounds, hydrastine and berberine, have demonstrated effectiveness in treating ulcers and various bacterial and viral infections, especially those of the respiratory tract.[10] MYRRH GUM: Myrrh gum stimulates phagocyte activity and reduces inflammation of the mucus secreting mucosa.[11] Myrrh gum also acts as an antiseptic and anti-inflammatory. Myrrh gum is officially recognized in Britain, France, and Germany for its medicinal value. GARLIC: Garlic is another herb that can be considered a tonic. It is a powerful warrior against infections of various types and origins and is considered a natural bactericide. Garlic can increase the number of leukocytes (white blood cells) that help fight infections.[12] In addition, garlic increases perspiration, which further cleanses the body. LICORICE ROOT: Licorice root contributes in several important ways to this formula. It stimulates secretion of the hormone aldosterone from the adrenal cortex. This can produce a higher energy level, which is usually needed when combating infections like meningitis. Licorice has antiviral and antibacterial properties.[13] Long-term consumption of licorice is not recommended as it may cause weakness, electrolyte imbalances, water retention and hypertension. BLUE VERVAIN: Blue vervain has the ability to break the cycle of chronically occurring infections. It has been used for colds and flu and has an ability to reduce fever. BUTTERNUT ROOT BARK: Butternut is a laxative that does not produce the sometimes painful gripping associated with other laxatives. Butternut improves liver function and stimulates bile production and flow. KELP: Kelp's function in this formula is to provide needed trace elements important in many metabolic processes in the body. These nutrients may further support the healing process and return the body to normal function. Kelp contains a soluble fiber called algin which is soothing to the gastrointestinal tract and improves bowel function.

SECONDARY NUTRIENTS

VITAMIN B6: Helps to boost tissue repair and regeneration during periods of infection and fever. *Suggested Dosage:* Take 100 to 150 mg divided up with meals per day.

MAGNESIUM: The ability of the body to cope with infection may be profoundly determined by magnesium intake and availability. *Suggested Dosage:* Take as directed, using chelated products.

ST. JOHN'S WORT: This herb is useful if the infection is viral. The hypericum compounds of St. John's wort have the ability to stop viral replication. If your meningitis is virally-caused, this is an excellent herb to use. *Suggested Dosage:* Take 800 mg per day in two divided doses.

ISATIS (BAN LAN GEN): A Chinese herb that has immunostimulatory properties. *Suggested Dosage:* Take as directed.

VITAMIN E: Supplementation increases phagocyte action and stimulates the body to better immune response. *Suggested Dosage:* Take 800 IU daily.

BEE PROPOLIS: This resinous substance has distinct antibacterial properties. *Suggested Dosage:* Take as directed using local products with guaranteed potency.

PAU D'ARCO: This herb, along with cat's claw, has the ability to fight both viral and bacterial invaders. *Suggested Dosage:* Take as directed using standardized products. Pau d'arco teas are also very good.

DIMETHYLGLYCINE: This odd-sounding compound helps the body deal with infection and boosts immunity and cellular function. *Suggested Dosage:* Take as directed.

GRAPEFRUIT SEED EXTRACT: The anthocyanidins found in this compound help to reduce inflammation and are also good for fever. *Suggested Dosage:* Take as directed.

Home Care Suggestions

- Get adequate rest in a dimly lit room.
- Use cool ginger baths to reduce fever.

Other Supportive Therapies

MASSAGE: Helps to stimulate circulation which supports immune function.

Scientific Facts-at-a-Glance

One of the most interesting theories concerning meningitis is that it may stem from faulty waste elimination in the bowel. If antigens and putrefied toxins from undesirable bacteria are harbored in the colon, their presence may trigger infections like meningitis.[14] Ironically, it may be our previous misuse of antibiotics for other infections which can add to this bowel toxicity by killing friendly flora. Moreover, people who have taken antibiotics needlessly contribute to the creation of new antibiotic-resistant bacteria which are not eliminated by existing antibiotics. For this reason, new and more powerful antibiotic compounds must be continually created in order to keep up. The notion of one day facing an infectious organism that exsisting antibiotics cannot contain is not far fetched. For this reason, it is important to keep our immune systems strong. It is important to understand, however, that with an infection like meningitis, antibiotic therapy is absolutely essential and is often life saving.

Prevention

- ◆ It is advisable to avoid becoming constipated by eating a diet high in fiber, drinking plenty of water and exercising regularly.
- ◆ In some cases, vaccination may be of some value in controlling an outbreak of certain strains of bacterial meningitis.
- ◆ Taking antibiotics is recommended if you come in contact with anyone suffering from the disease. In some cases this is more effective than vaccination. The meningitis vaccination has met with limited success due to the variety of organisms which can produce the disease.

Doctor's Notes

The herbal formula suggested includes compounds that address four areas: fighting viral and bacterial infections, enhancing and supporting the immune response, reducing fevers, and cleansing the body. This formula is good for infections of varying types and origins.

Endnotes

1. G. Zoppi, et al., "Oral bacteriotherapy in clinical practice, the use of different preparations in the treatment of acute diarrhea," Euro Jour Ped, 1982, 139: 22-24.
2. K. Shahani, et al., Cult Dai Pro Jour, 1977, 12: 8-11.
3. A. Sommer, et al., "Increased risk of respiratory disease and diarrhea in children with pre-existing mild vitamin A deficiency," Amer Jour Clin Nutr, 1984, 40: 1090-95.
4. R. Anderson, "The immunostimulatory, anti-inflammatory and anti-allergenic properties of ascorbate," Adv Nutr Res, 1984, 6: 19-45.
5. F. Willmott, et al., Lancet, 1983, 1: 1053.
6. U. Das, "Antibiotic-like action of essential fatty acids," Letter, Cana Med Asso Jour, 1985, 132(12): 1350.
7. T. Aoki et al., "Low natural killer syndrome: clinical and immunologic features," Nat Immunol Cell Growth Regu, 1987, 6(3): 116-28.
8. Y. Yang, "Effect of astragalus membranaceous on natural killer cell activity and induction with Coxsackie B viral myocarditis," Clin Med Jour, 1990, 103(4): 304-7.
9. R. Bauer and H. Wagner, "Echinacea species as potential immunostimulatory drugs," Econ Med Plant Res, 1991, 5: 253-321.
10. D. Sun, et al., "Berberine sulfate blocks adherence of streptococcus pyogenes to epithelial cells, fobronectin and hexadecane," Antimivrob Agents Chemo, 1988, 32: 1370-74.
11. Encyclopedia of Chinese Drugs, 1977, Shanghai Scientific and Technical Publications, People's Republic of China.
12. H.P. Koch, "Garlicin, Fact or Fiction," Phytother Res, 1993, 7: 278-80.
13. Melvyn R. Werbach and Michael T. Murray, Botanical Influences on Illness (Third Line Press, Tarzana, Ca: 1994).
14. J. Finne, et al., "Antigenic similarities between brain components and bacteria causing meningitis," Lancet, 1983, II: 355-57.

MENOPAUSE

Today, as the baby boomers head into middle age, record numbers of women are facing what has managed to remain a physiological enigma for many: menopause. The next two decades will see over 40 million American women entering their 40s and early 50s. By the year 2000, it is estimated that 17 million women will be over the age of 50. By the year 2020, 60 million women will be experiencing or will have passed through menopause. Most of those women will live out at least twenty-five post-menopausal years.

Menopause is a medical term referring to the cessation of ovulation and menstrual periods. It is also referred to as "change of life." A woman can experience her last period sometime between the ages of 40 and 50, although in some cases, menopause can happen as late as age 60. The average age for menopause is 51. The years leading up to menopause are characterized by disruptions in the menstrual cycle and in the nature of the periods themselves. It is important to remember that many women experience menopause with little or even no discomfort. A woman is considered post-menopausal when she is past 45 and has had no periods for six months.

Symptoms

Half of all women experience some symptoms associated with menopause and 25 percent of women consider the symptoms distressing. Symptoms may include hot flashes, flushed face, vaginal dryness, sweating, palpitations, irregular periods, joint pains, headaches, weight gain, beginnings of osteoporosis, depression, anxiety, irritability, lack of concentration, mood swings, sleep disorders, lack of confidence, increased emotional sensitivity, crying for no apparent reason, forgetfulness, or social withdrawal.

The mood changes that accompany menopause are not all necessarily negative. For example, an increase in energy and motivation may result from the hormonal changes typical of menopause. Both the physical and psychological symptoms of menopause can last from a few months up to five years. The average length of menopausal symptoms is a year to two years. Caution: Bleeding between periods, or prolonged or excessive menstrual bleeding may indicate the presence of a uterine tumor. Bleeding after menopause is not normal and should be investigated by a doctor as soon as possible.

Causes

Menopause occurs because the production of estrogen and progesterone in the ovaries greatly decreases. Without the presence of sufficient estrogen, the uterine lining that is shed during menstruation cannot form. This change can occur quite suddenly and can initiate a variety of physical and emotional symptoms. Contrary to some popular notions, the loss of estrogen experienced during menopause does not redistribute fat, contribute to a loss of muscle tone or cause wrinkles to appear.

Conventional Therapies

Hormone replacement therapy is the usual treatment for menopausal symptoms. These hormones may be a combination of progesterone and estrogen or estrogen alone. These hormones can be taken in tablet form, vaginal creams, or as surgically placed implant patches. In addition, tranquilizers, antidepressants and sleeping pills are also routinely prescribed for emotional and psychological disturbances typical of menopause. A recent evaluation of hormone replacement therapy has concluded that the value of estrogen outweighs its possible risks. Estrogen therapy is thought to help slow osteoporosis, and actually reduce a woman's risk for heart attack. Recent studies indicate that the death rate from heart disease among women who take post-menopausal estrogen is significantly lower. Hormone replacement therapy should be discussed thoroughly with your doctor. Not all health care professionals approve of hormone therapy. It certainly has some potentially serious side effects, including ovarian cancer, breast cancer and even autoimmune disorders like lupus. Herbal phytoestrogens or plant estrogens are much safer and may offer a viable alternative to drug therapy.

Dietary Guidelines

- Eat a diet high in raw foods and low in red meats, sugar and dairy products.
- Emphasize the following foods: whole grains, sesame seeds, sunflower seeds, almonds, fresh vegetables and fruits, garlic, beans and whole grain pastas.
- Try to add soybean-based foods which have natural estrogenic properties like tofu.
- Other phytoestrogenic foods include flaxseed oil, dates and pomegranates.
- Avoid the following foods: rich dairy products, sugar, fatty greasy foods, red meats, coffee, tea, alcohol and nicotine.
- Avoid alcohol and caffeine as they can aggravate hot flashes.
- Eating frequent light meals is preferable to three heavy ones. Doing this seems to discourage hot flashes.

Recommended Nutritional Supplements

PRIMARY NUTRIENTS

VITAMIN E Tests with vitamin E dramatically support its use for hot flashes and other menopausal symptoms. In some tests, it worked better than barbiturates to calm anxiety, hot flashes, etc.[1] *Suggested Dosage:* 800 to 1,000 IU daily.

WILD YAM We are beginning to understand now that boosting progesterone levels rather than estrogen may be of much more value for menopause and other hormonally-related female problems. The diosgenin content of this herb is a progesterone precursor which can help minimize menopausal symptoms safely by its absorption through the skin.[2] Wild yam is used in cream or topical form.

EVENING PRIMROSE OIL This oil contributes to estrogen production and works as a sedative and diuretic to help stop hot flashes. It also has antiprostaglandin properties that inhibit deranged hormonal activity and inflammatory response.[3] *Suggested Dosage:* Take as directed using high quality sources that need to be refrigerated. Using fish or flaxseed oil with this supplement is also recommended.

GAMMA-ORYZANOL This compound is extracted from rice bran and can help to modulate hot flashes and other menopausal symptoms.[4] *Suggested Dosage:* 20 mg daily.

PHYTOESTROGENS While certain foods like tofu and other soybean based foods should be eaten, supplements that contain isoflavones like genistein can also be purchased. They have been shown to protect tissue from bad estrogen and to contribute to balancing hormones.[5] *Suggested Dosage:* Take as directed, looking specifically for isoflavone supplements with genistein content.

VITAMIN C WITH BIOFLAVONOIDS Clinical studies involving 94 menopausal women found that using vitamin C with hesperidin (a bioflavonoid) relieved symptoms in 50 percent.[6] Leg cramps, bruising, and hot flashes significantly decreased. Certain bioflavonoids actually resemble estradiol in their structure.[7] *Suggested Dosage:* Take as directed.

CALCIUM AND MAGNESIUM These minerals help calm the central nervous system. They also afford bone protection—important because after menopause the risk of osteoporosis increases for some women.[8] *Suggested Dosage:* 2,000 mg of calcium and 1,000 mg of magnesium daily. Use calcium citrate lactate or gluconate and chelated magnesium.

VITAMIN D Many postmenopausal women have impaired synthesis of vitamin D which inhibits the absorption of calcium.[9] *Suggested Dosage:* Take as directed.

5-HYDROXY-TRYPTOPHAN Studies have found that low blood levels of tryptophan and estrogen were found in women who suffered from depression during menopause.[10] Moreover, this supplement may also help promote more restful sleep which can be impaired during menopause. *Suggested Dosage:* Take as directed.

HERBAL COMBINATION This combination should include black cohosh root, dong quai, passionflower, red raspberry leaves, fenugreek seeds, licorice root, chamomile, black haw bark, saw palmetto berries, wild yam root, kelp and butternut root bark. *Suggested Dosage:* Four to six capsules daily. For chronic conditions and imbalances maximum dosage of six capsules per day should be taken for several months or until normal function is restored. Best if used daily throughout the month. This formula should not be taken by pregnant or lactating women.

BLACK COHOSH ROOT: Black cohosh has been proven to be such an effective remedy for menopausal disorders and premenstrual complaints that it has received official recognition in Britain and Germany. Studies have shown black cohosh root to have endocrine activity with the ability to mimic estrogen.[11] Antispasmodic and diuretic actions are other properties which contribute to the herb's usefulness in this formula. DONG QUAI: There is no other herb used more widely in Chinese medicine for treatment of gynecological ailments than dong quai. Dong quai helps to relieve the unpleasant symptoms associated with menopause.[12] Dong quai is said to have analgesic properties but this is probably due, in part, to its antispasmodic effect. It also boosts elimination. PASSIONFLOWER: Many women experience anxiety prior to and during menses, and discomforts such as hot flashes when adjusting to menopause. Passionflower contributes a sedative action for anxiety and relieves spasms and cramps.[13] It has an overall calming effect. RED RASPBERRY LEAVES: Red raspberry leaves have long been used for various female afflictions during pregnancy and child birth in addition to those associated with menses. More specifically it strengthens and tones the uterus, stops hemorrhages, decreases excess and increases deficient menstrual flow, and relieves painful menstruation by relaxing the smooth muscles.[14] FENUGREEK SEEDS: Although fenugreek seed has been used to assist proper menstruation and promote lactation, its main role in this formula stems from its other properties. Fenugreek is a tonic, mild diuretic, and a source for mucilage which provides soothing demulcent properties. LICORICE ROOT: Licorice root is incorporated into about one-third of all Chinese herbal formulas and a majority of the formulas dealing with female reproductive problems. This is an indication that the herb has tremendous versatility. Indeed, licorice supports the effects of all the other herbs in this formula. Licorice not only contains hormonal precursors but stimulates the production of estrogen.[15] This has been shown to decrease the symptoms associated with hormone fluctuation. CHAMOMILE: Aside from chamomile's carminative and tonic properties, this herb has gained world recognition for its anodyne (pain relieving), antispasmodic, and antianxiety properties. Chamomile has demonstrated its worth in many clinical studies and is officially monographed in Britain, Belgium, France, and Germany. BLACK HAW BARK: Another name for black haw bark is cramp bark, suggesting the reason for its inclusion in this formula. Historical and folkloric use, as well as scientific evidence, have proven this bark to be effective against muscle spasms and menstrual dysfunction. It is especially good for the inconsistent estrus cycles typical of perimenopausal women.[16] SAW PALMETTO BERRIES: Saw palmetto berries have been used by American Indians for hundreds of years. Today this herb has been scientifically and clinically proven effective for male and female genitourinary problems. One study has shown it to be many times more effective than prescription anti-inflammatory medication in the treatment of pelvic congestion associated with menstrual dysfunction.[17] WILD YAM ROOT: Wild yam root contains the steroidal saponins botogenin and diosgenin. These are precursors to cortisone and other hormones like progesterone, which play a vital role in menopause. Wild yam has antispasmodic effects and is soothing to the nerves.[18] KELP: Kelp provides important trace elements that are often missing or deficient in Western diets. Trace elements assist with many metabolic processes in the body and a lack may lead to various problems. Kelp contains algin which provides soothing benefits to the gastrointestinal tract. BUTTERNUT ROOT BARK: Butternut is a soothing laxative that helps to restore general health and a sense of well-being. Its laxative effect in this formula may be too gentle for it to be obvious.

SECONDARY NUTRIENTS

VITAMIN B-COMPLEX: Helps to fight depression and stress and boosts circulation. *Suggested Dosage:* Take as directed. Use sublingual products if possible.

VITAMIN B6: Specifically treats water retention and helps to fight emotional or mental disorders that can occur during menopause. *Suggested Dosage:* 150 mg per day in three equal divided doses.

CHASTE TREE: This herb helps to normalize hormonal function and balance. Some university studies indicate that chaste tree appears to stimulate the pituitary gland to secrete hormones which can help produce estrogen and progesterone. *Suggested Dosage:* Take as directed using guaranteed potency or standardized products.

GOTU KOLA, GINKGO AND ST. JOHN'S WORT: These herbs help to boost brain function and fight the anxiety and depression associated with menopause. *Suggested Dosage:* Take as directed using standardized products.

Home Care Suggestions

◆ The value of regular aerobic exercise in helping combat both the physical and psychological symptoms of menopause cannot be stressed enough. Regular exercise can increase the secretions of certain brain chemicals which can elevate moods and counteract depression. Walk , swim, climb stairs, join a spa—do whatever you can to involve yourself in some sort of exercise. Weight bearing exercises have been found to work especially well in preventing the onset of osteoporosis.

◆ Having regular sexual intercourse seems to discourage both vaginal dryness and hot flashes.

◆ Do not smoke. When combined with hormone replacement therapy it can cause an interaction that dramatically increases the risk of stroke, high blood pressure and heart disease.

◆ Use a vaginal lubricant (Lubifax, K-Y) for vaginal dryness and itching. Other preparations that might be helpful are unscented creams such as Albolene and Lubrin.

◆ For hot flashes, particularly at night, wear light cotton fabrics that have "breathability."

◆ Drink plenty of water to help with hot flashes.

◆ Carry of packet of premoistened towelettes with you to cool off your face. Small battery operated fans are also available.

◆ Use relaxation techniques such as yoga or breathing exercises to combat anxiety or nervousness.

◆ Discussing your menopause with an understanding partner goes a long way. Knowing that certain symptoms are perfectly normal and temporary can be extremely valuable.

◆ View menopause not as a tragic end to your youth and sexuality but rather as a natural transition.

Other Supportive Therapies

ACUPUNCTURE: Can help to alleviate emotional symptoms and treat hot flashes or back pain using points along the urinary bladder, governing vessel, kidney meridians and gallbladder.

YOGA: Postures designed to relax muscles and promote relaxation can be very helpful.

MEDITATION: Helps to calm the mind and fights anxiety and depression.

HOMEOPATHY: Several medications are used for specific symptoms of menopause and include Pulsatilla for moods, Belladonna for hot flashes, graphites for emotional problems, Bryonia for vaginal dryness, Cimicifuga for depression or anxiety, and Arnica for muscle or back aches.

Scientific Facts-at-a-Glance

One of the reasons why Japanese women do not seem to suffer with menopausal symptoms like American women is attributed to their consumption of phytoestrogenic foods. In a study where 25 postmenopausal women supplemented their diets with soya flour, red clover sprouts and linseeds, significant improvement in vaginal dryness was seen after only six weeks.[19] What this study implies is that American women need to increase their intake of soy-based foods or take isoflavone supplements. Using soy flour and learning to eat and cook with tofu is highly recommended.

Spirit/Mind Considerations

Menopause can be a time of either great contentment and optimism or it can be full of emotional problems, pessimism and feelings of deep frustration. Typical associations we may have unknowingly made with menopause may seem strangely frightening as "the passage" nears. The notion that menopause signals the advent of a matronly life bereft of youthful vigor, sexuality and productivity no longer applies. Knowing the "whys and wherefores" of this normal female physiological modification combined with applying nutritional strategies and exercise can make all the difference between a successful menopause and one filled with anxiety. Menopausal myths include:

◆ Menopause signals the end of sexuality.
◆ The hormonal chaos of menopause makes most women crazy.
◆ Weight gain is an inevitable consequence of menopause.
◆ Once menopause occurs, signs of aging (wrinkling, osteoporosis, etc.) always accelerate.
◆ Menopause signals the end of physical activity and fitness.

◆ Menopause is a marker of overall physical and mental decline.

The good news is that for many women, menopause signals the beginning of a new and exciting phase of life.

Prevention

◆ Exercising regularly, eating a good nutritious diet and leading a happy, full life can greatly help to minimize psychological and physical menopausal symptoms.
◆ Keep involved and active. Finding something that you love to do can help you through menopause. Walk with someone, try a new hobby, take a class, etc.
◆ Eat soy-based phytoestrogenic foods. Use soy flour and tofu.
◆ Take essential fatty acid supplements, including both omega-3 and omega-6 compounds.
◆ Emphasize raw fruits and vegetables, whole grains and low-fat dairy products, and reduce animal protein foods.
◆ Use olive oil and stay away from hydrogenated fats.

Doctor's Notes

Menopausal symptoms are rooted in hormonal dysfunction or imbalance. There are women who start having symptoms related to hormone fluctuation at menarche, the beginning of menstrual flow, right up to those who begin having symptoms only after menopause, the cessation of menstrual flow. There are also women who will live their entire lives without any symptoms related to hormone fluctuations. Then there are those who seem to be incessantly plagued by continually revolving symptoms surrounding hormone function and dysfunction. This formula is specially designed to help modulate and decrease or eliminate symptoms associated with hormone fluctuation and dysfunction. This formula incorporates other herbs that will allay symptoms of anxiety and pain.

Endnotes

1. B. Rubenstein, "Vitamin E diminishes the vasomotor symptoms of menopause," Abstract, Fed Proc, 1948, 7:106. See also R. Reitz R, Menopause: A Positive Approach (Penguin Books, New York: 1979).
2. John R. Lee, M.D., Natural Progesterone: The Multiple Roles of a Remarkable Hormone, revised (BLL Publishing, Sebastopol, California: 1993). See also U.S. Barzel, "Estrogens in the Prevention and Treatment of Postmenopausal Osteoporosis: A Review," Amer Jour Med, (1988), 85: 847-850. and D.R. Felson, et al., "The Effect of Postmenopausal Estrogen Therapy on Bone Density in Elderly Women," The New England Journal of Medicine, 1993, 329: 1141-1146.
3. Michael T. Murray, Encyclopedia of Nutritional Supplements, (Prima Publishing, Rocklin, CA: 1996), 255-56.
4. M. Ishihara, "Effect of gamma oryzanol on serum lipid peroxide level and climacteric disturbances," Asi-Oceania Jour Obstet Gynaecol, 1984, 10(3):317. See also M. Ishihara et al., "Effect of gamma-oryzanol on serum lipid peroxide level of patients with climacteric disturbances," Jour Aichi Med Univ Assoc, 1983, 11(3): 278-85.
5. H. Wei, "Antioxidant and antipromotional effects of the soybean isoflavone genistein," Proceedings of the Society for Experimental Biology and Medicine, 1995, 208: 124. (Wilcox G., et al. "Estrogenic effects of plant foods in postmenopausal women," Bri Med Jour, 1990, 301:905-6.)
6. C. Smith, "Non-hormonal control of vaso-motor flushing in menopausal patients," Clin Med, 1964, 67(5): 193-95.
7. C. Clemetson, et al., "Capillary strength and the menstrual cycle," Ann NY Acad Sci, 1962, 93: 277-300.
8. M. Horowitz, et al., "Biochemical effects of calcium supplementation in postmenopausal osteoporosis," Euro Jour Clin Nutr, 1988, 42: 775-78.
9. C. Park, "Calcium metabolism," Jour Amer Coll Nutr, 1989, 8(s): 46S-53S.
10. J. Thomson, et al., "Relationship between nocturnal plasma estrogen concentration and free plasma tryptophan in perimenopausal women," Jour Endocrinol, 1977, (3):395-6.
11. E.M. Duker, et al., "Effects of extracts from Cimicifuga racemosa on gonadotropin release in menopausal women and ovariectomized rats," Planta Medica, 1991, 57(5): 420-24.
12. D. Zhy, "Dong quai," Amer Jour Clin Med, 1987, 15(3-4): 1987.
13. E. Speroni and E. Minghetti, "Neuropharmacological activity of extracts from Passiflora incarnata," Planta Medica, 1988, 54)6): 488-91.
14. Mark Pederson, Nutritional Herbology (Wendell Whitman, Warsaw, In: 1995), 145.
15. C.H. Costello, E.V. Lynn, "Estrogenic substances from plants: Glycyrrhiza," Jour Amer Pharm Soc, 1950, 39: 177-80.
16. P.H. List, et al., Hagers Hanbuch der Pharmazeutischen Praxis, vols. 2-5, Springer-Verlag, Berlin.
17. Rebecca Flynn, M.S. Your Guide to Standardized Herbal Products, (One World Press, Presscott, AZ: 1995), 67-69.
18. John R. Lee, M.D., Natural Progesterone: The Multiple Roles of a Remarkable Hormone, revised (BLL Publishing, Sebastopol, California: 1993).
19. G. Wilcox, "Estrogenic effects of plant foods in postmenopausal women," Brit Med Jour, 1990, 301: 905-06.

MENSTRUAL CRAMPS

Menstrual cramps were considered more psychosomatic than physical just a few decades ago. Today, however, they are recognized as a real problem for many women. The involvement of hormones called prostaglandins explains the presence of menstrual cramping. Most women experience menstrual cramps several times before they reach menopause. Menstrual cramps usually begin two to three years after the first period, once ovulation becomes established. Menstrual discomfort occurs in at least half of all adolescent females and is the leading cause of school absences. In some cases, cramping will decrease after the age of 25 or after childbirth. The existence of cramps has no relationship with the amount of flow. Approximately 10 percent of women have menstrual cramping severe enough to interfere with their daily routine.

Symptoms

Cramping can start up to 24 to 48 hours prior to the onset of a period and continue for up to a day or so. Most women who experience cramps find that they are worse during the first two days of the period. Menstrual cramps are characterized by pains in the lower abdomen or back that can come and go in a wave-like pattern, pain which can radiate down the thighs, dull, nagging lower back pain, and squeezing pain in back or lower abdomen.

Menstrual cramps typically begin shortly before the onset of a period and generally last for 12 hours. Cramps can be accompanied by nausea, vomiting and anxiety. Menstrual discomfort that begins at an early age should be mentioned to a physician.

If menstrual cramps are intense see your doctor to make sure that endometriosis or a pelvic infection is not present

Causes

Following ovulation, progesterone stimulates the uterus to produce prostaglandin, forcing muscle contraction in the uterus. This contraction, combined with the constricting of blood vessels that cut off blood supply to the uterine lining so that it will be shed monthly, can also cause discomfort. Excessive production of prostaglandins or a hypersensitivity to them may be responsible for severe cramps. Heredity does not seem to be a significant factor. Factors which have been linked to cramping include being overweight, having regular periods rather than irregular ones, or having a flow that lasts longer than three days.

Conventional Therapies

In most cases, the severity of cramps can be controlled, but they are rarely totally eliminated. Pain killers that are prostaglandin inhibitors will be recommended by your physician. Ibuprofen-based preparations are the most effective (Motrin, Rufen, Nuprin, Medipren, Advil). Nonsteroidal anti-inflammatory drugs (Naprosyn, Anaprox, Clinoril, Feldene) function in the same way; however, they require a prescription and are costly. Aspirin is considered an antiprostaglandin, although it is not as effective as ibuprofen. Acetaminophen-based products (Tylenol, Anacin-3, etc.) are not antiprostaglandins. As a result, they do not have a significant effect on the mechanism that causes menstrual cramps. In more severe cases, birth control pills are sometimes prescribed to suppress ovulation which, in turn, minimizes the intensity of menstrual cramps. Non-contraceptive hormones (that come with significant side effects) may also be prescribed.

CAUTION: Do not use oral contraceptives if you might be pregnant, if you have a history of stroke, if you have high blood pressure, if you have or have had liver, breast or reproductive organ cancer, or if you have blood clots. Using oral contraceptives is not recommended if you have irregular or scanty periods. There are a number of other physical disorders that may pose a health risk if taking oral contraceptives. Any existing condition should be discussed with your doctor.

Dietary Guidelines

- ◆ Emphasize fresh fruits/vegetables, chicken and fish.
- ◆ Eat soy-based foods like tofu or use soya flour.
- ◆ Avoid taking diuretics. They can deplete your body of essential minerals that help to control menstrual cramping.
- ◆ Avoid salt, caffeine, junk foods and refined sugars. Drink plenty of water and fruit juice.
- ◆ Do not drink alcoholic beverages; alcohol can increase water retention.

Recommended Nutritional Supplements

PRIMARY NUTRIENTS

ESSENTIAL FATTY ACIDS These are natural antiprostaglandin compounds that promote uterine relaxation and inhibit the response that initiates cramping and pain.[1] *Suggested Dosage:* Take as directed using multiblend oils.

CALCIUM AND MAGNESIUM Calcium helps to quiet the central nervous system and alleviate muscle cramping. It is also good for breast tenderness. Magnesium inhibits prostaglandins and has been shown to calm cramps by acting as a natural muscle relaxant.[2] *Suggested Dosage:* 1,500 mg of calcium and 1,000 of magnesium. Use calcium lactate, gluconate or citrate, and chelated magnesium. Take with vitamin B6 for better assimilation.

VITAMIN E Studies have shown that this vitamin actually acts as a natural analgesic in test cases with menstrual cramps.[3] *Suggested Dosage:* Take 400 IU per day throughout the month.

VITAMIN B-COMPLEX Helps to reduce premenstrual tension. In some instances, taking brewer's yeast has decreased the severity of menstrual discomfort, including depression. Some research suggests that menstruation may cause a functional deficiency of vitamin B6. *Suggested Dosage:* 150 mg per day.

VITAMIN B3 (NIACIN) In a recent study, 90 percent of 80 women with serious menstrual cramps who were treated with niacin found relief. It is thought that niacin acts as a natural vasodilator.[4] *Suggested Dosage:* 200 mg per day and every two to three hours during cramps. Expect flushing and some dizziness during intensive therapy.

VITAMIN C WITH BIOFLAVONOIDS Helps to strengthen blood vessels and capillary walls in the uterine system.[5] *Suggested Dosage:* Take as directed.

IRON Clinical studies found that women with cramps who were anemic experienced a complete disappearance of menstrual pain following iron supplementation.[6] *Suggested Dosage:* Take as directed.

HERBAL COMBINATION This combination should contain black cohosh, blue cohosh, dong quai, passionflower, red raspberry leaves, fenugreek seeds, licorice root, chamomile, black haw bark, saw palmetto berries, wild yam root, kelp and butternut root bark. *Suggested Dosage:* Four to six capsules daily. For chronic conditions and imbalances, a maximum dosage of six capsules per day should be taken for several months or until normal function is restored. Best if used daily throughout the month. CAUTION: Do not take these herbs if pregnant or lactating.

BLACK COHOSH ROOT: Black cohosh has been proven to be an effective remedy for painful menstrual cramps and has received official recognition in Britain and Germany. Studies have shown black cohosh root to have endocrine activity with the ability to mimic estrogen.[10] BLUE COHOSH: This herb was used so extensively by Native American women it also became known as squaw root. It is effective for menstrual cramps and other female disorders. It acts as a natural antispasmodic to help to relax uterine muscle. DONG QUAI: There is no other herb used more widely in Chinese medicine for treatment of gynecological ailments than dong quai. Dong quai relieves menstrual cramps, corrects irregular or retarded menstrual flow, and alleviates unpleasant symptoms associated with menopause. Dong quai is said to have analgesic properties but this is probably due, in part, to its antispasmodic effect.[11] As a side note, dong quai has been used to treat anemia, a condition that can result from excessive blood loss during menstruation. PASSIONFLOWER: Many women experience anxiety prior to and during menses, and discomforts such as hot flashes when adjusting to menopause. Passionflower contributes a sedative action for anxiety and relieves spasms and cramps.[13] It has an overall calming effect. RED RASPBERRY LEAVES: Red raspberry leaves have long been used for various female afflictions during pregnancy and child birth in addition to those associated with menses. More specifically it strengthens and tones the uterus, stops hemorrhages,

decreases excess and increases deficient menstrual flow, and relieves painful menstruation by relaxing the smooth muscles.[14] FENUGREEK SEEDS: Although fenugreek seed has been used to assist proper menstruation and promote lactation, its main role in this formula stems from its other properties. Fenugreek is a tonic, mild diuretic, and a source for mucilage which provides soothing demulcent properties. Like many other seeds, fenugreek is nutritious and restorative, strengthening those recovering from illness or imbalances. LICORICE ROOT: Licorice root is incorporated into about a third of all Chinese herbal formulas and a majority of the formulas dealing with female reproductive problems. This is an indication that it has tremendous versatility. Indeed, licorice supports the effects of all the other herbs of the formula. Licorice not only contains hormonal precursors but stimulates the production of estrogen.[15] This has been shown to decrease the symptoms associated with hormone fluctuation. CHAMOMILE: Aside from chamomile's carminative and tonic properties, this herb has gained world recognition for its anodyne (pain relieving), antispasmodic, and antianxiety properties. Chamomile has demonstrated its worth in many clinical studies and is officially monographed in Britain, Belgium, France, and Germany. BLACK HAW BARK OR CRAMP BARK: Historical and folkloric use as well as scientific evidence have proven this bark to be effective against muscle spasms and menstrual dysfunction, especially inconsistent estrus cycles and menstrual cramping.[16] SAW PALMETTO BERRIES: One study has shown this herb to be many times more effective than prescription anti-inflammatory medication in the treatment of pelvic congestion associated with menstrual dysfunction.[17] As an interesting side note, saw palmetto can prevent the growth of unwanted facial hair in women. WILD YAM ROOT: Wild yam root contains the steroidal saponins botogenin and diosgenin. These are precursors to cortisone and other hormones like progesterone.[18] Wild yam has antispasmodic effects and is soothing to the nerves. It is also diuretic and helps to eliminate painful urination. It is highly recommended for cramping. KELP: Kelp provides important trace elements which are often missing or deficient in Western diets. Trace elements assist with many metabolic processes in the body, without which may lead to various problems. Kelp contains algin which provides soothing benefits to the gastrointestinal tract. BUTTERNUT ROOT BARK: Butternut is a soothing laxative that helps to restore general health and a sense of well-being. Its laxative effect in this formula may be too gentle for it to be obvious.

SECONDARY NUTRIENTS

NERVINE HERBS (VALERIAN, KAVA, PASSIONFLOWER, SKULLCAP AND HOPS): These herbs can safely promote muscle relaxation and sleep during painful periods. *Suggested Dosage:* Take as directed. These herbs may be taken individually or in a combination.

MELATONIN: Also helps to initiate and sustain restful sleep. *Suggested Dosage:* Take as directed starting with smaller than suggested doses and see how you react.

LECITHIN: Helps with nerve transmissions. *Suggested Dosage:* Take as directed in granule or capsule form.

Home Care Suggestions

◆ Take ibuprofen immediately at the beginning of cramping and repeat according to drug directions. Waiting to use these medications until cramping is severe is less effective. Do not take this medication on an empty stomach. Be aware that misuse of this drug can cause stomach or liver damage.

◆ Take a good brisk walk and breathe deeply as you walk. Do not over exert yourself. Make it a pleasant walk and pace yourself. Walking can help reduce muscle tension and can help release brain chemicals which can actually elevate your mood.

◆ Use a hot water bottle or heating pad on the small of your back or on your abdomen. Taking a long, leisurely hot bath can also help with menstrual pain. Some women apply heat to the small of the back before they anticipate having cramps and find this minimizes menstrual discomfort.

◆ For some women, applying a soft ice pack to the abdomen helps to reduce pain.

◆ Drink plenty of hot herbal teas, such as raspberry leaf tea.

Other Supportive Therapies

YOGA: Engage your body in a number of stretches. A yoga routine can also be quite effective in minimizing pain. Yoga exercises that should be investigated are: shoulder stand, plow, fish, uddiyana, cobra, and posterior stretch.

REFLEXOLOGY OR ACUPRESSURE: These therapies help to relax muscles, dilate arteries and veins, and may offer some beneficial results. You can measure a hand width from the inner ankle and press for pain relief.

MASSAGE: Regular foot massages may help alleviate pain caused by uterine muscle contraction.

Scientific Facts-at-a-Glance

There has been some speculation that some menstrual cramps are aggravated by eating hormonally-treated meats and milk. The notion is that estrogenic compounds given to cattle, chickens or pigs enter the female body and cause an estrogen overload or dominance, characterized by several symptoms including menstrual cramps and hormonally-caused disorders.[18] In addition, we know that fat cells contribute to estrogen production so if a woman is overweight, she may find herself battling symptoms of an estrogen dominance, including difficult periods.

Spirit/Mind Considerations

The mood fluctuations associated with difficult periods can be quite dramatic. Feelings of frustration and depression are common in women who also suffer severe menstrual cramping. It is vital to recognize hormonally-induced mood disorders and combat them with serotonin-raising herbs and other supplements. Having to deal with debilitating pain on a monthly basis can be very discouraging.

Informing your family or spouse about your condition is also important. If you tense up under stress, it can make cramping even worse. Learn to meditate or relax with controlled breathing and try not to let stress build up during the month. Learn to diffuse it on a daily basis.

Prevention

◆ Limit your intake of animal protein and fats.
◆ Take isoflavone supplements or eat soy-based foods.
◆ Use essential fatty acids on a daily basis.
◆ Don't become overweight. Women who are overweight suffer more from menstrual cramping.
◆ Exercise regularly. Women who are physically fit have a lower incidence of menstrual cramps.
◆ Take a good vitamin and mineral supplement all month long. Prior to your period increase your intake of calcium and magnesium.

Doctor's Notes

I recently treated a sixteen-year-old white female who had suffered from severe menstrual cramps ever since she began her period. Physical exams had failed to turn up anything abnormal and she continued to miss school on a monthly basis due to the severity of the pain, which was accompanied by nausea. I put her on an herbal product that contained cramp bark: it made a world of difference, enabling her to function normally during her periods. The cramps are not completely gone but they are of the mild variety. Another good preventive treatment would be to take boswellia, devil's claw, turmeric or ginger a day or two before your anticipated period, or when it first begins. The more extensive herbal formula listed is specially designed to help modulate and decrease—or eliminate—symptoms associated with hormone fluctuation and dysfunction. This formula incorporates other herbs that will allay symptoms of anxiety and painful cramping. Most women with the above related conditions would greatly benefit from consistent use of this particular formula.

Endnotes

1. G.E. Abraham, "Primary dysmenorrhea," Clin Obstet, Gyn, 1978, 21(1): 139-45.

2. H. Fontana-Klaiber and B. Hogg, "Therapeutic effects of magnesium in dysmenorrhea," Schweiz Rundsch Med Prax, 1990, 79(16): 491-94.

3. E. Butler and E. McKnight, "Vitamin E in the treatment of primary dysmenorrhea," Lancet, 1955, 1: 844-47.

4. A. Hudgins, "Vitamins P, C, and niacin for dysmenorrhea therapy," West Jour Surg Gyn, 1954, 62: 610-11.

5. B. Cox and W Butterfield, "Vitamin C supplements and diabetic cutaneous capillary fragility," Bri Med Jour, 1975, 3: 205.

6. N. Shafer, "Iron in the treatment of dysmenorrhea: A Preliminary report," 1965, 7: 365-66.

7. G. Singh, "Pharmacology of an extract of salai guggal ex Bosewellis serrata, a new non-steroidal anti-inflammatory agent," Agents Action, 1986, 18: 407-12.

8. A. Mukhopadhyay, et al., "Anti-inflammatory and irritant activities

of curcumin analogues in rats," Agents Actions, 1982, 12: 508-15.

9. "New methods is pharmacognosy: chromatographic evaluation of commercial viburnum drugs," Deytsche Apot Zei, 1965, 105(40): 1371-72.

10. E.M. Duker, et al., "Effects of extracts from Cimicifuga racemosa on gonadotropin release in menopausal women and ovariectomized rats," Planta Medica, 1991, 57(5): 420-24.

11. D. Zhy, "Dong quai," Amer Jour Clin Med, 1987, 15(3-4): 1987.

12. E. Speroni and E. Minghetti, "Neuropharmacological activity of extracts from Passiflora incarnata," Planta Medica, 1988, 54)6): 488-91.

13. Mark Pederson, Nutritional Herbology, (Wendell Whitman, Warsaw, In: 1995), 145.

14. C.H. Costello, E.V. Lynn, "Estrogenic substances from plants: Glycyrrhiza," Jour Amer Pharm Soc, 1950, 39: 177-80.

15. P.H. List, et al., Hagers Hanbuch der Pharmazeutischen Praxis, vols. 2-5, Springer-Verlag, Berlin.

16. Rebecca Flynn, M.S., Your Guide to Standardized Herbal Products, (One World Press, Prescott, AZ: 1995), 67-69.

17. John R. Lee, M.D., Natural Progesterone: The Multiple Roles of a Remarkable Hormone, revised, (BLL Publishing, Sebastopol, California: 1993).

18. Orville Schell, Modern Meat: Antibiotics, Hormones and the Pharmaceutical Farm, (Random House, New York: 1984).

MIGRAINE HEADACHES

The word *migraine* is derived from the French and Greek languages, and means "half a head," referring to the fact that most migraines attack only one side of the head. Migraine headaches are surprisingly common and affect 15 to 20 percent of men and 25 to 30 percent of women. Migraines most frequently afflict people between the ages of 20 and 35. Seventy percent of migraine sufferers are women.

The nature of migraines can vary significantly with each individual. Migraines can last up to 18 hours and are debilitating and extremely painful. There is some speculation that unexplained recurring abdominal distress in some children can be an indicator that they may be susceptible to migraines later in life. In some individuals, migraines cease after age 40.

Symptoms

Typically, the initial stage of a migraine, called an aura, is characterized by a feeling of fatigue. In rare cases, a migraine begins with sensory disturbances, such as seeing sparks, flashes or geometric shapes. This sensation may be followed by nausea and vomiting, and occasionally diarrhea. Visual disturbances and a sensitivity to light are also common at this point. Some time after these symptoms, an intense, gripping headache will occur. The pain commonly begins on one side of the forehead and gradually spreads, causing the entire head to throb and ache. During this stage, it is common to have bloodshot eyes, pallor and a runny nose or weepy eyes. Other possible symptoms include numbness, tingling, dizziness, ear ringing and mental confusion.

The duration and frequency of migraines is unpredictable. "Cluster headaches" are characterized by several painful headaches per day which can persist for weeks. This type of headache is a variation of the migraine and commonly afflicts more men than women. Smoking and drinking are thought to be significant contributory factors. CAUTION: Any severe and persistent headache should be reported to your physician. If you are suffering from a migraine headache, do not drive or operate machinery.

Causes

Specific causes for migraine headaches remain unknown. The physical mechanism that causes a migraine involves an instability in the blood flow system. Basically, arterial constriction is followed by a rebound dilation, bringing on the headache.

More than half of people who suffer from migraines have a family history of the disease. Other possible contributing factors include alcohol consumption (especially red wine), nitrates, monosodium glutamate, emotional stress, hormonal changes, birth control pills, fatigue, exhaustion, chocolate, cheese or cured meats, barometric pressure changes, exposure to sun or glare, TMJ syndrome, lack of exercise, constipation, and environmental pollutants. Using nitroglycerine or the withdrawal from certain drugs such as caffeine and ergotamine may also precipitate a migraine headache.

Conventional Therapies

Migraines are usually treated with strong drug therapy that can significantly reduce pain, but the side effects of these drugs must be considered. Frequently, migraines are incorrectly treated by doctors who give out strong pain killers that are not considered effective against migraines. Ergotamine is the only preparation that has shown significant success in treating true migraines. Most doctors can diagnose migraines from a family history and physical examination. In some cases, a full neurological examination may be indicated to exclude the possibility of a brain tumor.

Taking aspirin plus an antiemetic drug is usually recommended for simple migraines. If this combination is not effective, ergotamine is usually prescribed. In the drug Cafergot, ergotamine is combined with caffeine. The effect of this drug is to stiffen blood vessels in the brain to avoid constriction and dilation. It can be taken in pill or suppository form when a migraine is first coming on. Inhalers or sublingual pills are also available and work faster. Some doctors will prescribe pain medications such as Darvon or Tylenol with codeine, but these are not effective treatment for a true migraine headache. Doctors also routinely prescribe Fiorinal for migraines; this is often ineffective and can become addictive. Imitrex, a relatively new drug, works on these headaches by boosting serotonin levels in the brain. It must be administered by injection and has significant side effects.

Dietary Guidelines

◆ Avoid chocolate, cheese, citrus fruits, shellfish and alcohol. These foods contain vasoactive amines, such as tyramine, that can cause brain vessels to constrict. (They are also common food allergens.) Some people who suffer from migraines are deficient in platelet enzymes that normally break down these amines. Other foods which contain these amines are avocados, bananas, cabbage, eggplant, pineapple, potatoes, canned fish, aged meat, yeast extracts, yogurt, canned figs, onions and peanut butter.

◆ Avoid aspartame (found in Nutra-Sweet). This particular chemical has been implicated in various studies as a migraine inducer.

◆ Eating several small meals may help inhibit blood sugar swings.

◆ Nitrates and monosodium glutamate are considered migraine inducers. Check ingredients of food items and in restaurants.

◆ Low blood sugar is also a possibility and has been found to be a factor in clinical studies.[1] For this reason, avoid excess carbohydrate consumption. Some migraine patients may develop headaches when hypoglycemic.

◆ There have been significant studies done which suggest that some migraines may be caused by food allergies.[2] Some foods most commonly found to induce migraine headaches in some people are dairy products, wheat, chocolate, eggs, oranges, tomatoes, rye and beef.

Recommended Nutritional Supplements

PRIMARY NUTRIENTS

GINKGO BILOBA AND FEVERFEW These herbs have impressive actions in oxygenating brain cells and serving as powerful antioxidant agents. Studies have found that feverfew works on the smooth muscle of the veins of the brain.[3] Ginkgo also boosts oxygenation and acts as a very effective free radical scavenger.[4] *Suggested Dosage:* 60 mg of a 24 percent extract of ginkgo taken two to three times a day. Take feverfew as directed. Use both of these supplements for at least four to six weeks before assessing their effectiveness.

CALCIUM AND MAGNESIUM Calcium helps to calm the central nervous system and can help to control pain. A lack of magnesium has been found in people who suffer from migraines, and it has been found that magnesium supplementation positively effects the vascular system of the brain.[5] *Suggested Dosage:* 2,000 mg of calcium and 1,000 mg of magnesium daily. Use calcium citrate, gluconate or lactate and chelated forms of magnesium.

VITAMIN B6 Tests have shown that some people who experience these headaches as a side effect of medications they must take can be helped by boosting their vitamin B6 levels.[6] *Suggested Dosage:* Take as directed.

LECITHIN Lecithin contains a compound called choline which is profoundly important to proper nerve cell activity. Tests found that blood levels of choline were low in people with cluster-type migraine headaches.[7] *Suggested Dosage:* Take as directed using capsules or granulated products.

OMEGA-3, OMEGA-6 FATTY ACIDS Tests conclude that even a severe migraine can be treated with omega-3 fatty acids.[8] The brain itself is composed of unsaturated fatty acids. *Suggested Dosage:* Take as directed using a combination of both omega-3 and omega-6 acids. Use flaxseed or fish oil and evening primrose or borage oils. Keep refrigerated.

NIACIN A natural vasodilator that has been traditionally used for migraine, niacin helps to increase blood flow to the brain. It is not recommended for cluster-type migraine headaches.[9] *Suggested Dosage:* Take as directed, although you can take this supplement every two to three hours during periods of pain. Expect flushing and some dizziness.

CAPSICUM Tests results indicate that intranasal capsaicin (the key compound in capsicum) may provide a new therapeutic option for the treatment of migraines.[10] *Suggested*

Dosage: This is a relatively new way to apply capsicum and should not be attempted unless supervised by a health care professional. Capsaicin can cause intense burning.

GINGER This carminative herb has relieved migraines in clinical tests.[11] *Suggested Dosage:* Take two capsules every two hours during headache. Look for guaranteed potency products.

HERBAL COMBINATION This combination should include white willow bark, blue vervain, feverfew leaves, rosemary leaves, skullcap and kelp. *Suggested Dosage:* Three to five capsules daily. May be used for extended periods. Do not use if you are pregnant or nursing.

WHITE WILLOW: This herb contains a substance called salicin that is believed by some to convert to salicylic acid (the key component of aspirin) in the body.[12] While they both help with pain, salicin does not thin the blood or irritate the stomach like aspirin does. BLUE VERVAIN: Blue vervain is recognized in Europe and elsewhere for its ability to reduce inflammation and pain.[13] It also helps to reduce muscle spasms. Blue vervain promotes perspiration, adding to the cleansing action of white willow. FEVERFEW: While this herb was undergoing a scientific study to confirm other actions, it was noted that some of the subjects found relief from migraine. It has since been clinically studied for migraine and shown to be very effective, especially in chronic conditions and in cases where other medications have failed.[14] It is believed that feverfew works on migraines by reducing inflammation in the areas where pain is generated. ROSEMARY LEAVES: Rosemary performs two major functions in this formula: it relieves painful spasms and assists in reducing pain associated with migraines.[15] Rosemary also improves liver function, promotes bile production, and assists digestion. SKULLCAP: Skullcap has gained recognition in many parts of the world. Its two main functions are the alleviation of nervous tension and sedation.[16] Tension headaches, or headaches caused by lack of sleep, are often helped by skullcap. KELP: Kelp's storehouse of micronutrients assist in many metabolic processes in the body. Kelp provides electrolytes that can help prevent edema. Edema and inflammation have both been associated with migraines. Kelp also contains algin, a mild laxative that soothes the gastrointestinal tract.[17]

SECONDARY NUTRIENTS

DL-PHENYLALANINE: This amino acid has the ability to decrease pain in some people. *Suggested Dosage:* Take as directed on an empty stomach with fruit juice. Do not use this amino acid if you have high blood pressure or are taking antidepressant drugs.

ST. JOHN'S WORT: This natural and effective serotonin raiser in the brain may help with migraine treatment and prevention. *Suggested Dosage:* 800 mg day of standardized .3 percent hypericum product.

5-HYDROXY-TRYPTOPHAN: This metabolite of tryptophan helps to raise brain amines like serotonin and may be intrinsically involved in what causes a migraine. *Suggested Dosage:* Take on an empty stomach with fruit juice as directed.

WINTERGREEN, PEPPERMINT AND CAPSICUM: Can help dispel headaches through their carminative and stimulant effects. *Suggested Dosage:* Take as directed. The wintergreen and peppermint can be used in essential oil form for aromatherapy or massage as well.

Home Care Suggestions

- ◆ Keep track of what you were doing or eating before a migraine to see if there is any connection between ingesting chocolate, cheese, etc.
- ◆ If your migraines seem related to taking birth control pills, notify your doctor. Changing the type of oral contraceptive may eliminate the headaches.
- ◆ At the very first indication that a migraine is coming on, take aspirin, apply a cold compress to your face and a soft ice bag to your head, and lie in a quiet dark room for two to three hours. Listen to music or try breathing or visualization exercises. Do not read during this time.
- ◆ A rather unusual, yet successful, treatment for migraines involves, at the first sign of a headache, placing your head under a bonnet-type hair dryer on the warm/hot setting. The use of heat to treat migraines has not been scientifically proven.
- ◆ Try getting a neck and head massage to see if this aggravates or alleviates your symptoms.

Other Supportive Therapies

CHIROPRACTIC MANIPULATION: There is some indication that while chiropractic treatments do not necessarily reduce the occupance of migraines, they may help with pain reduction during an attack.

RELAXATION AND BIOFEEDBACK: Several studies suggest that electrothermal biofeedback may reduce the frequency and severity of migraines and should be investigated.

TENS (TRANSCUTANEOUS ELECTRICAL STIMULATION): If TENS is appropriately administered, it has been found to significantly reduce migraines and other headaches which are the result of muscle tension.

ACUPUNCTURE: There is some evidence to suggest that acupuncture may reduce the frequency of migraine headaches and should be investigated as a possible treatment. After traditional acupuncture treatments, migraine victims can learn to use acupressure to stop the onset of a migraine. Several physicians recommend acupuncture for migraine treatment. It is an alternative which, unlike drugs, has no side effects and may prove valuable.

Scientific Facts-at-a-Glance

Taking too many analgesics (painkillers) is now considered a cause (often unrecognized) of chronic headaches. In several cases, when barbiturates, acetaminophen and narcotics were discontinued, headaches decreased dramatically. This particular phenomenon is referred to as "analgesic rebound" and may contribute to aggravating migraines. Caffeine withdrawal and the use of aspartame (Nutra-Sweet) have also been linked to migraines.[18]

Spirit/Mind Considerations

Migraine headaches can be related to mental illness. They have also been linked to perfectionist, type-A personalities who demand a great deal from themselves. Because tension is considered a primary contributing factor, "de-stressing" is essential. Using meditation or other relaxation techniques can be of tremendous value. People in the workplace who internalize job stress are prone to headaches of all kinds.

Prevention

- ◆ Avoid any "trigger" factors, such as culprit foods, loud noisy environments, bright lights, etc.
- ◆ For patients who suffer from severe and persistent migraines, certain drugs that are thought to prevent migraine headaches may be prescribed. Some of these are high blood pressure drugs, some antidepressants, nonsteroidal anti-inflammatories and some antihistamines. Any ongoing drug therapy has negative side effects which should be carefully evaluated.
- ◆ Some doctors recommend the use of steroid drugs to help prevent migraines. This approach is not recommended. The dangers of steroids outweigh any possible benefits.
- ◆ Taking aspirin every other day has also been found to help cut the incidence of migraine attacks in people who are susceptible to the headaches. Always check with your physician before initiating any kind of ongoing drug therapy. Do not give aspirin to anyone under the recommended age.
- ◆ Use biofeedback techniques regularly to learn to relax muscles and even to control blood vessels. Biofeedback has been found to be especially helpful for headache sufferers.
- ◆ Taking regular naps, keeping fit through exercise and avoiding unhealthy foods can help reduce both the physical and mental stress associated with migraines.
- ◆ Take time to relax every day through yoga, massage etc. people who operate under stress and tension for prolonged periods of time and then relax may be prone to experience a migraine. Learn to relax on a regular basis.

Doctor's Notes

There are two types of headaches: those that are brought on by tension and stress, and those caused by actual physical phenomena. A tension headache often starts with pains in the upper back, shoulders, or neck. Stress increases the incidence of these types of headaches. I remember treating a 42-year-old female who suffered from headaches, including both the tension type characterized by tight muscles in the neck and upper back, and a migraine headache. We treated her with boswellia and this alone reduced her tension headaches by 70 percent and her migraines by 80 to 90 percent. People who suffer from combination headaches need to get the tension headache under control, which will inevitably lessen the severity of the migraine. If my patient hadn't responded to this therapy, I would have put her on a muscle relaxant herb, either kava or valerian, and suggested regular massage therapy.

Stress-control techniques, such as meditation or deep breathing exercises, are also excellent and help control muscle tension and spasms. Calcium and magnesium and herbs such as kava kava and valerian are also good natural tranquilizers. Getting a massage on a regular basis can work wonders for headaches.

For simple migraines I like to use a feverfew product that has a guaranteed amount of active ingredient (in the range of .3 to .7 percent) once a day. You need to remember that often, this herb needs to be taken four to six weeks before effects will be noted. Patience and persistence is the key. *Ginkgo biloba*, used daily, or taking two to three capsules at the beginning of the headache, can help to cut it short or avoid it altogether. Using a combination of both ginkgo and feverfew can be very helpful. Acupuncture can be very helpful in treating migraines and preventing them by easing tension. Many people I have seen find that tightness in the shoulder and neck muscles can precipitate a migraine. At the first sign of tightness or tension, take magnesium in higher doses or use herbs (such as kava or valerian) that relax both muscles and the central nervous system.

Keep in mind that stress is a major cause of migraines. If you notice that you get more migraines on weekends, a change in weekly routine may be a triggering factor. Sleeping in on Saturday mornings can precipitate a headache. Try to maintain the same schedule and eating habits throughout the weekend. I've seen people who eat ice cream and chocolate on Friday night and then wake up every Saturday morning with a migraine. In the case of headaches, you must also realize that a treatment that works for one person may not work as well for another.

One unusual treatment is to generate static electricity which can stop the headache immediately. Rub some 40-gauge PVC pipe with a dust mitten, then pass the mitten over your head for five to fifteen minutes. While this therapy sounds a bit eccentric, it is worth trying. The same treatment can be used in treating swelling on the hand, ankle, etc.

Additional Resources

National Headache Foundation
5252 North Western Avenue
Chicago, IL 60625
(800) 843-2256

Endnotes

1. J. Pierce, "Insulin-induced hypoglycemia in migraine," JNNP, 1971, 34:154-56.

2 L. Mansfield, et al., "Food allergy and adult migraine: Double-blind and mediator confirmation of an allergic etiology," Ann Allergy, 1985, 55:126.

3. J. Murphy, et al., "Randomized double-blind placebo controlled trial of feverfew in migraine prevention," Lancet, II: 1988, 189-92. See also R. Barsby, et al., "Feverfew and vascular smooth muscle: Extracts form fresh and dried plants show opposing pharmacological profiles,

dependent upon sesquiterpene lactone content."

4. I. Hindmarch and Z. Subhan, "The psychopharmacological effects of Ginkgo biloba extract in normal healthy volunteers," Int Jour Clin Pharma, 1984, 4: 89-93.

5. G. Abraham and M. Lubran, "Serum and red cell magnesium levels in patients with premenstrual tension," Am J Clin Nutr 1981, 34:(11)2364-66. See also K. Weaver, "Magnesium and its role in vascular reactivity and coagulation," Contemp Nutr, 1987,12(3).

6. A. Bernstein, "Vitamin B6 in clinical neurology," Ann N Y Acad Sci, 585:250-60.

7. J. Belleroche, et al., "Red blood cell choline levels may be deficient in patients with cluster headache," and "Erythrocyte choline concentrations and cluster headache," Br Med J 1984, 288: 268-270.

8. C. Glueck et al., "Amelioration of severe migraine with omega-3 fatty acids: A double-blind, placebo-controlled clinical trial," Abstract, Am J Clin Nutr, 1986, 43:710.

9. M. Atkinson, "Migraine headache," Ann Int Med, 1944, 22: 990.

10. D. Marks, et al., "A double-blind placebo-controlled trial of intranasal capsaicin for cluster headache," Planta Medica, 1983, 59: 20-5.

11. T. Mustafa, "Ginger (Zingiber officinale) in migraine headache," Jour Ethnopharmacol 1990, 29(3): 267-73.

12. W. Thompson, Herbs That Heal, (Charles Scribner's Sons, New York: 1976), 81-82.

13. S. Sakai, "Pharmacological actions of vervena officinalis extracts," Gifu Ika Daug Kiyo, 1963, 11(1): 6-17.

14. E. Johnson, et al., "Efficacy of feverfew as prophylactic treatment of migraine," Brit Med, 1985, 291: 569-73.

15. A. Boido, et al., "N-substituted derivatives of rosmaricine," Studi Sassar, 1975, 53(5-6): 383-93.

16. B. Kurnakov, "Pharmacology of skullcap," Farm Toksik, 1957, 20(6): 79-80.

17. G. Binding, About Kelp, (Thorson's Pub, Wellingborough, England: 1974).

18. R. Lipton, "Aspartame as a dietary trigger of headaches," Headache, 1989, 29: 90-92.

MONONUCLEOSIS

Infectious mononucleosis (also known as "the kissing disease") is an acute viral disease. It affects the respiratory system and lymph glands and can be mistaken for influenza. Approximately 90 percent of the American population has been exposed to the Epstein-Barr virus (the cause of mononucleosis) by the time they reach the age of 21. Mononucleosis usually affects young adults and is rarely seen after the age of 35. Most cases occur between the ages of 15 and 17. The onset of the disease can be sudden or gradual and most victims recover with no complications. The illness usually lasts between one and four weeks, but it can persist for up to three months. Most victims recover without medications. Exactly how the disease spreads is not known. There is some evidence that anyone who has lowered immunity due to malnutrition, excessive fatigue or who has had recent surgery is more vulnerable to the disease.

Symptoms

Mononucleosis can cause flu-like symptoms, including sore throat, headache behind the eyes, fatigue, malaise, fever, muscle aches, swollen lymph glands in the neck, underarms or groin, depression, spleen enlargement, loss of appetite, a measle-like rash, yellowing of the skin, and/or a loss of taste for cigarettes.

In some cases of mononucleosis, mild liver damage develops. If the tonsils become swollen, breathing may become obstructed. If spleen enlargement is present, precautions should be taken during any activity to protect that area of the body from trauma. For months after recovering from mononucleosis, symptoms such as depression, lack of energy, and malaise may continue.

Infectious mononucleosis can be confused with acute leukemia because the two conditions share many of the same symptoms.

Causes

Mononucleosis is caused by the Epstein-Barr virus, a member of the herpes family. Epstein-Barr is also believed to cause chronic fatigue syndrome. Once in the body, the virus multiplies in the lymph system and causes the proliferation of white blood cells.

Conventional Therapies

Because mononucleosis is a viral infection, medical treatment is limited. The use of antibiotic therapy is of no value. Supportive treatments can help with complications but bed rest and good nutrition take precedence in most cases.

Diagnosis is made by testing the blood for an increase in certain lymphocytes and antibodies. Rest is prescribed for at least a month to allow the immune system to destroy the virus. In some cases in which inflammation is severe, corticosteroid drugs may be recommended. Mononucleosis is a viral disease and does not respond to antibiotics. Using steroids to treat the disease should be avoided unless specific conditions persist, such as chronic fever or tonsil swelling. If ampicillin is mistakenly prescribed, it may produce a rash and actually worsen symptoms.

Dietary Guidelines

- Eat a diet especially high in raw foods. Drink plenty of vegetable and fruit juices.
- Emphasize the following foods: citrus fruits, baked potatoes with the skin left on, vegetable broths, celery, parsley, onions, garlic, cabbage, baked squash, fish, turkey, and chicken, and whole grains.
- Avoid foods which are considered immune system depressants such as white sugar, white flour, caffeine, and high-fat/empty calorie junk foods.
- Protein supplements mixed into shakes may help combat fatigue, especially if the appetite is depressed.

Recommended Nutritional Supplements

PRIMARY NUTRIENTS

MULTIPLE VITAMIN/MINERAL SUPPLEMENT Take a good supplement daily which has a wide array of organic nutrients and is rapidly assimilated. *Suggested Dosage:* Take as directed.

VEGETABLE-BASED PROTEIN SUPPLEMENT Some evidence exists that rice protein may help to boost liver function and toxicity and treat abnormal gut permeability which may be compromised in some cases of Epstein-Barr infection.[1] *Suggested Dosage:* Look for quality vegetable-based products that taste good and mix easily in liquid.

VITAMIN A WITH BETA CAROTENE Enhances immune function and scavenges for damaging free radicals. Several clinical studies have found that this duo has the ability to boost immunological function.[2] Studies have found that taking a beta-carotene supplement is even better absorbed than food sources.[3] *Suggested Dosage:* Use up to 25,000 IU of vitamin A per day for two weeks after which reduce to 10,000 IU per day. If you are pregnant, do not exceed 10,000 IU daily.

GERMANIUM Clinicians have reported that between 20 and 50 percent of their patients who had Epstein-Barr and received germanium supplements experienced significant symptom relief.[5] *Suggested Dosage:* Take as directed. Use this supplement with your doctor's approval and only take recommended dosages.

MAGNESIUM AND ZINC After six weeks of magnesium supplementation, 32 people with Epstein-Barr experienced improved energy, better mood and less pain.[6] Zinc also helps to stimulate better immune function and can boost a suppressed appetite as well. *Suggested Dosage:* Take as directed.

HERBAL COMBINATION This combination should include St. John's wort, kava kava, Siberian ginseng, gotu kola, kelp, astragalus, shitake mushroom, reishi mushroom, schizandra, and licorice root. *Suggested Dosage:* Four to eight capsules daily. Botanicals have been employed by many cultures to support and improve immune function. This formula contains some of the best herbs known to build and strengthen the body's resistance to disease. It is ideal for sufferers of chronic immune deficiency and may be used daily.

ST. JOHN'S WORT: One of the most impressive properties of this herb is its ability to fight viral infections. Interestingly, people who suffer from viral conditions such as chronic fatigue syndrome, mononucleosis, herpes simplex, and AIDS are also often depressed. In these conditions, St. John's wort will provide mood elevation while it fights viral infection.[10] KAVA KAVA: Used by people throughout the South Pacific, where it is an important ceremonial drink. People who consume kava kava note a sense of well-being and happy contentment. After much clinical research, several European countries approved kava kava for the treatment of nervous anxiety and restlessness.[11] SIBERIAN GINSENG: Chronic stress can lead to illness by eroding immune function. Siberian ginseng has a clinically supported reputation as a stress fighter. It also improves energy levels, mental function and stamina—all often lacking in chronically ill people. In the past 10 years, research has demonstrated Siberian ginseng's ability to increase important T-lymphocytes of the helper variety. These lymphocytes are significantly reduced in HIV infections. Double blind studies have confirmed the ability of this herb to improve and normalize immune system actions.[12] GOTU KOLA: Ayurvedic doctors use gotu kola as a central nervous system tonic to improve mental stamina and enhance memory. Its application for mononucleosis is as a mental stimulant with antistress properties that also have a mild tranquilizing effect.[13] KELP: Kelp provides organic iodine which promotes healthy thyroid function. A dysfunctional thyroid has been associated with lethargy and general malaise. Kelp further provides trace elements that may be lacking in the diet. Thus, kelp may help to provide chemical balance to the body.[14] ASTRAGALUS: Astragalus is one of the most popular herbs in Chinese medicine where it is regarded as a tonic, energizer, and potent immune builder. Recent scientific studies have confirmed astragalus' benefit for immune function. Astragalus has been shown to increase phagocytosis and interferon production. This herb can stimulate the production of interferon and has been used for centuries by the Chinese to enhance immune function.[15] SHITAKE AND REISHI MUSHROOM: Shitake mushrooms have received considerable attention for their immune system-building abilities. This mushroom has been scientifically studied and shown to stimulate interferon production and increase helper T-lymphocytes. This mushroom contains powerful immunostimulating polysaccharides. LICORICE ROOT: Licorice root is one of the most used plants in Chinese medicine and is referred to as the "Great Adjunct" because it increases the effectiveness of other herbs. However, animal studies have shown licorice to enhance the production of interferon and macrophage (a large phagocyte) activity and inhibits herpes-type viruses.[17] Licorice should not be used by anyone with high blood pressure, kidney disease or who is taking digitalis.

SECONDARY NUTRIENTS

VITAMIN C WITH BIOFLAVONOIDS: Studies have shown that these supplements can enhance resistance to fatigue while boosting immunity.[18] *Suggested Dosage:* 1,000 mg with each of three meals.

GOLDENSEAL: Berberine and other alkaloids found in this herb can boost white cell activity and improve liver function.[19] *Suggested Dosage:* Take as directed, but do not use for more than one week consecutively.

ACIDOPHILUS: Replenishes friendly flora which can help to fight infections and restore vitality. *Suggested Dosage:* Take as directed using guaranteed bacterial count products with bifidobacteria. Check expiration date.

GARLIC: Garlic has proven itself as an effective antiviral agent which also serves to boost the immune system.[20] *Suggested Dosage:* Take two capsules with each of three meals.

MILK THISTLE (SILYMARIN): Several theories suggest that liver toxicity or malfunction is intrinsically linked to this disease as well as to chronic fatigue syndrome. This herb has the ability to stimulate liver tissue regeneration while detoxifying at the same time.[21] *Suggested Dosage:* Take as directed using standardized, guaranteed potency varieties.

PROTEOLYTIC ENZYMES: Improve the assimilation of nutrients and are recommended in cases where malabsorption is suspected as a possible contributor to mononucleosis. *Suggested Dosage:* Take before each meal as directed.

CARNITINE, TAURINE AND CYSTEINE: This trio of amino acids helps to support immune function. *Suggested Dosage:* Take as directed on an empty stomach with fruit juice.

DHEA: Low levels of this hormone have been linked to Epstein-Barr infections. As with any hormonal supplement, check with your doctor first. *Suggested Dosage:* Take as directed.

BLUE VERVAIN, SARSAPARILLA, GINSENG AND RED CLOVER BLEND: This blend helps to increase stamina and detoxify the blood. *Suggested Dosage:* Take as directed.

Home Care Suggestions

- ◆ Adequate rest and good nutrition are essential in the treatment of mononucleosis. While moderate activity is now recommended, taking naps and eating properly is stressed for heightened recovery.
- ◆ Be patient and realize that it takes a substantial amount of time to recover from mononucleosis. Use this time well—read, learn a new language through instructional tapes, and learn to relax while recuperating. Putting life on hold can have its advantages.

Scientific Facts-at-a-Glance

Studies on the Epstein-Barr virus suggest that mononucleosis as well as chronic fatigue syndrome are indicative of a seriously compromised immune system. Research has found that antibodies to the Epstein-Barr virus have also been found in people suffering from other diseases related to weakened immunity.[22] In this regard, it remains unknown whether this virus causes immune dysfunction or invades after the fact. If you suffer from this or any other related disease, strengthening your immune system is vital. Consider this a wake-up call that your immunity suffers either from poor nutrition, intense stress, lack of sleep or a combination of these factors. If you have mononucleosis, you may be predisposed to other more serious diseases, so take action.

Spirit/Mind Considerations

Stress is one of the major contributing factors to immune dysfunction. Adrenal exhaustion, which is common in people who do not relieve stress, is also linked to diseases like mononucleosis. Use whatever works for you, whether it be meditation, biofeedback, visualization or even counseling. Do not underestimate the impact of unresolved emotional stress on the immune system.

Prevention

- ◆ The best way to keep from getting mononucleosis is to keep from getting worn out. Eat right, exercise and get enough rest.
- ◆ A diet high in raw foods and low in fat and sugar has been proven to promote good health.
- ◆ Immunity can become impaired when the body is under physical and mental stress, making it easier to contract viral and bacterial infections.
- ◆ If you know someone who has this disease, do not use the same eating utensils, glasses, etc. While the disease is considered contagious, it is not as easily contracted as the common cold or influenza.

Doctor's Notes

Because this disease is caused by the Epstein-Barr virus, it must be treated with supplements and herbs that demonstrate significant antiviral properties. I have had good success with St. Johns wort, which actually interferes with the ability of viruses to replicate. The earlier you incorporate this therapy, the better. In other words, the severity and duration of mononucleosis can be dramatically altered by taking these agents early on. The same is true for echinacea. Don't wait. It's important to remember that mononucleosis is very difficult to recover from for most people, so herbs and supplements which contribute to stamina, detoxification and immune support are vital.

Endnotes

1. J.S. Bland, et al., "A medical food-supplemented detoxification program in the management of chronic health problems," Altern Therap, 1995, 1: 62-71.

2. A. Bendich, "Beta-carotene and immune response," Proc Nutr Soc, 1991, 50: 263-74.

3. E.D. Brown, et al., "Plasma carotenoids in normal men after a single ingestion of vegetables or purified beta-carotene," Amer Jour Clin Nutr, 1989, 49: 1258-65.

4. C.W. Lapp, "Chronic fatigue syndrome is a real disease," North Carolina Family Physician, 1992, 43(1): 6-11.

5. G.R. Fallona and S.A. Lavine, "The use of organic germanium in chronic Epstein-Barr virus syndrome: An example of interferon, modulation of herpes reactivation," Jour Orthomol Med, 1988, 3(1):29-31.

6. I.M. Cox et al "Red blood cell magnesium and chronic fatigue syndrome," Lancet, 1991,337:757-60.

7. A. Goldberg, CFIDS Chronicle, 1989 Summer/ Fall.

8. P.O. Behan, et al, "Effect of high doses of essential fatty acids on the post viral fatigue syndrome," Acta Neurol Scand, 1990 82(3):209-16.

9. J. Moz, "Effect of echinacin on phagocytosis and natural killer cells," Med Welt, 1983 34:1463-67.

10. G. Lavie, et al., "Hypericin as an inactivator of infectious viruses in blood components," Transfusion, 1995, 35: 392-400.

11. Rebecca Flynn, M.S., and Mark Roest, Your Guide to Standardized Herbal Products. (One World Press, Prescott Arizona: 1995: 52-58).

12. B. Bohn, et al., "Flow-cytometric studies with Eleutherococcus senticosus extract as an immunomodulatory agent," Arzneimittel-Forsch, 1987, 37: 1193-96.

13. A.S. Ramaswamy, et al., "Pharmacological studies on Centella asiatica, Jour Res India Med, 1970, 4: 160-75.

14 Daniel B. Mowrey, Ph.D. The Scientific Validation of Herbal Medicine, (Keats Publishing, Connecticut, 1986): 123.

15. H. Yunde et al "Effect of radix astragalus on the interferon system," "Chinese Medical Jour. 1981 94:35-40.

16. F. Fukucuoka, "Polysaccharide extract active against tumors," Chem Abstracts, 1971, 74:324-25.

17. N. Abe, et al., "Interferon induction by glycyrrhizin and glycyrrhetinic acid in mice," Micorb Immunol, 1982, 26: 353-359.

18. E. Cheraskin, et al., "Daily vitamin C consumption and fatigability," Jour Amer Geria Soc, 1976, 24: 136-37.

19. Y. Kumazawa, et al., "Activation of perotenil macrophages by berberine alkaloids in terms of induction of cytostatic activity," Int Jour Immunofarmocal, 1984 6: 587-92.

20. N.D. Weber, et al., "In vitro virucidal effects of Allium sativum (garlic) extract and compounds," Planta Medica, 1992, 58: 417-23.

21. H.A. Salmi and S. Sarna, "Effect of silymarin on chemical, functional, and morphologic alteration of the liver: A double-blind controlled study," Scand Jour Gastroent, 1982, 17: 417-21.

22. W. Henle and G.Henle, "Epstein-Barr virus specific serology in immunologically compromised individuals," Cancer Res, 1981, 44.

MOTION SICKNESS/NAUSEA

Motion sickness refers to a condition which is produced in some people when they travel by car, plane or boat. It is a phenomenon created by conflicting sensory input to the eyes and the brain when certain motion is present. It can affect adults as well as children and is created when rapid motion changes, irregular motions or rolling sensations are experienced by the inner ear and the eyes. Nausea can be caused by a number of factors but usually results from the presence of an intestinal bug, food poisoning, pregnancy or drug reactions and motion sickness.

Symptoms

Nausea or motion sickness in its mild form can cause stomach upsets, a headache or feeling of uneasiness. In more severe cases possible symptoms include excessive sweating, dizziness, cold clammy skin, pallor, anxiety, excess salivation, gagging, and vomiting.

Nausea and vomiting that do not stop after motion has stopped may indicate the presence of a variety of disorders, from food poisoning to appendicitis. Any time vomiting persists or is accompanied by fever, pain, diarrhea, or profuse sweating, a physician should be seen as soon as possible.

Causes

Motion sickness is caused by the effect of any prolonged movement or sense of motion on a specific organ located in the inner ear that controls balance. Motion sickness is a result of the eyes perceiving one sense of motion and the brain another. It is commonly experienced in cars, boats, airplanes, swings or amusement park rides. Factors contributing to motion sickness are anxiety or fear (such as a fear of flying or of water in the case of boat trips), certain fumes, crowded, stuffy environments, reading or doing anything that requires eye movement while traveling, a full stomach, certain food smells or bad smells such as dead fish or rotting garbage, and focusing on objects that are close by rather than far off.

Simple nausea can result from pregnancy, drug reactions, food poisoning, types of influenza, liver disease, gallbladder trouble, diarrhea, constipation and other gastrointestinal disorders.

Conventional Therapies

Various antiemetic drugs are prescribed to help control motion sickness. Scopolamine is routinely prescribed and is available in patch form (transdermal) which is worn behind the ear. It delivers steady, tiny doses of this drug through the skin. Longer acting antihistamines such as promethazine, hydroxyzine, or meclizine should be taken one day before starting to travel. Phenergan is a prescription cough medicine that is used for motion sickness, but it does cause drowsiness. Dramamine, Marezine, Bonine and Benedryl are over-the-counter antihistamines used for motion sickness. Simple nausea is treated with Emetrol or other carbohydrate preparations that can be purchased as over-the-counter drugs at your pharmacy.

Dietary Guidelines

◆ Fresh ginger can help to ease nausea and can be grated into water or steeped as a tea.

◆ Eating grated lemon, orange or lime peel is recommended for the nausea that accompanies motion sickness. The bitter nature of these peels seems to calm both nausea and feelings of dizziness.

◆ Eating olives or sucking on a lemon can help control salivation that normally occurs when nausea sets in.

◆ Eating frequently while traveling helps control motion sickness.

◆ One very tried and true combination is to alternate eating a fresh banana with something salty like a dry salted cracker. Avoid dairy products that can produce more stomach acid and contribute to further nausea.

Recommended Nutritional Supplements

PRIMARY NUTRIENTS

`GINGER` This herb can be taken as a capsule or a tea. Most people would admit that there is little worse than being subject to nausea and vomiting. Nutritional deficiencies such as a lack of vitamin B6 may contribute to the condition and pregnancy is notorious for causing nutrient depletion. Clinical studies on ginger have found it to be more effective than prescription medications.[1] *Suggested Dosage:* Take two capsules every three hours.

`VITAMIN B6 AND MAGNESIUM` Both of these nutrients can help with nausea that is related to pregnancy. *Suggested Dosage:* Take as directed by your doctor.

`HERBAL COMBINATION` This combination includes ginger root, cayenne, licorice root, and chamomile. *Suggested Dosage:* Two to six capsules. May be used every day to prevent or treat nausea. Use maximum dosage if necessary.

GINGER ROOT: Ginger is a strong carminative in that it settles the stomach. It improves digestion, reduces gas, tonifies the intestinal muscle, and stimulates the liver to bile secretion. The highly acclaimed and respected British medical journal *Lancet* published a study that found ginger root to be more effective than either dimenhydrinate (Dramamine) or placebo in fighting motion sickness. In another double-blind clinical study, ginger reduced the incident of postoperative nausea and vomiting after major surgery. Yet another trial confirmed that it reduced nausea in even the most severe cases of morning sickness (referred to as "hyperemesis gravidarum"), which can lead to hospitalization and may be fatal if untreated. CAYENNE: The British regard cayenne (or capsicum) highly. In fact, it is officially recognized in the

British Herbal Pharmacopeia as a treatment for colic, flatulence, and poor digestion. It will also prevent painful spasms of the stomach and intestines. LICORICE ROOT: Licorice root is a demulcent which works to soothe the gastrointestinal tract. It receives this reputation because it stimulates the secretion of mucus in the stomach and bowels. The mucus improves bowel function and protects the stomach and intestines. CHAMOMILE: Chamomile is extremely popular in Germany where it is considered a cure-all. For this formula it imparts a strong carminative action and relaxes the nerves. Chamomile calms muscle spasms of the stomach bowels and throughout the body.

SECONDARY NUTRIENTS

PROTEOLYTIC ENZYMES: Digestive enzymes can help boost digestion which is often impaired in pregnancy which helps prevent heartburn and indigestion and contributes to better nutrient assimilation for mother and child. *Suggested Dosage:* Take as directed 30 minutes before eating or with meals. Look for supplements with papain.

RED RASPBERRY LEAF TEA: Promotes uterine muscle health. This particular herb is well known for its use in pregnancy. It helps to decrease bleeding after delivery and is believed to shorten the duration of labor. *Suggested Dosage:* Take as directed.

PAPAYA, FENNEL, MINT, GINGER AND ALFALFA TEA: All of these are good for heartburn, nausea and indigestion. *Suggested Dosage:* Take as directed.

WILD CHERRY BARK OR WILD YAM: An herbal stomachic which treats a nervous stomach and can help reduce nausea and vomiting. *Suggested Dosage:* Take as directed.

BASIL TEA: Has a good reputation for easing severe cases of nausea and vomiting. *Suggested Dosage:* Take as directed.

PEPPERMINT: Can be taken in tincture drops while traveling. Peppermint helps prevent vomiting and is an antispasmodic. *Suggested Dosage:* Take as directed.

Home Care Suggestions

◆ Emetrol, an over-the-counter high-carbohydrate nausea preparation, is effective in alleviating nausea and vomiting. It is available at any pharmacy and should accompany you on your travels.

◆ Have someone give you a good neck and head massage. Trigger points located in the neck, between the shoulder blades and at the base of the head if stimulated with deep massage can alleviate feelings of queasiness and nausea.

◆ When traveling focus on objects that are far away or on the horizon rather than things that are close up.

◆ Do not attempt to read, put together puzzles or do anything that requires eye movement when traveling.

◆ Biofeedback techniques designed to condition the body's reflexes to motion stimuli can help train the body to go into a different mode when experiencing travel.

◆ Plug your nose if unpleasant smells are causing you to become nauseated. Closing your eyes and taking several deep breathes can help relax the stomach and decrease the anxiety that accompanies nausea.

◆ Smoking will actually intensify motion sickness.

Other Supportive Therapies

AROMATHERAPY: Add four drops of peppermint and giner essential oils to glycerine and rub on your chest. Drops can be sniffed from a handkerchief or an inhaler.

ACUPRESSURE: Exerting pressure using your thumb placed on the inside of either wrist approximately 1 inch up from bottom of hand can bring some relief. Massage firmly on this area for at least 60 seconds then repeat on other wrist. Commercial wristbands that accomplish this same effect can be purchased if you are going on a trip.

MASSAGE: A deep massage of the scalp, neck and shoulder muscles can sometimes ease feelings of nausea.

Scientific Facts-at-a-Glance

Doctors have routinely prescribed vitamin B6 for the nausea that accompanies morning sickness; however, clinical trials have found that many women continued to experience vomiting after supplementation. For this reason, using ginger in combination with prenatal vitamins or B-complex vitamins is highly recommended. New guidelines sent to doctors in medical journals now suggest the duo as a better approach to morning sickness. A 1992 article found in *Current Opinions in Obstetrics and Gynecology* highly recommends adding ginger to vitamin B6 for its remarkable antiemetic properties.

Spirit/Mind Considerations

Adrenaline surges can bring on waves of nausea. Most of us have experienced the stomach upset that can precede public speaking, performances or even spells of anger, which boost the release of stress hormones. Moreover, if you find yourself on a plane or ship and are experiencing nausea, anxiety will only serve to make it worse. Learning to take controlled deep breaths which are exhaled very slowly can help to calm the entire body and ease nausea. Remember that stress tightens muscles and prompts the stomach to do flip flops all by itself. Visualization and meditation can sometimes help us get through an episode of motions sickness or nausea if we don't have any ginger on hand. In addition, massaging the neck can also inhibit stomach spasms.

Prevention

◆ Don't read, crochet, do puzzles or move your head around to converse while riding in your car. All of these activities aggravate motions sickness with reading being the worst offender.

◆ Avoid eating heavy meals that have a high-fat content before traveling. Make sure to eat a light meal that is low in fat. Traveling on an empty stomach only increases motion sickness.

◆ If you would like a special meal during air travel you can call 24 hours prior to your flight and order a low fat, vegetarian, low sodium, kosher, or diabetic meal. If you need, bring your own snack foods on board like saltines, melba toast, candied ginger or bananas.

◆ Sit in the front seat of a car and make sure to crack your window for access to fresh air.

◆ Do not drink alcohol before or during travel.

◆ If you are on a boat, stay amidship and topside.

◆ Elevate small children who must sit in a back seat on a car seat or cushion so they will be able to focus on distant points.

◆ Don't sit in a seat on a bus or boat in which you will be traveling backwards. This sensation can cause significant motion sickness.

◆ Wear head phones and listen to soothing music. Controlled breathing exercises and relaxation techniques such as visualization, meditation, etc, can focus your mind. People who drive rarely get motion sickness because they are preoccupied with the mechanics of driving.

◆ Don't take drugs or vitamin pills on an empty stomach.

◆ Keep temperatures cool in your traveling environment. Overly warm or stuffy conditions can create feelings of nausea.

◆ Travel at night so that passing scenery is not visible. This approach works whether the setting is a car, airplane or boat.

◆ Being overly tired greatly increases your susceptibility to motion sickness and feelings of nausea. Get adequate rest before taking a trip.

Doctor's Notes

Most of us would readily affirm that there is little worse than being subject to motion sickness and nausea. Interestingly, it's usually not the driver of the car, bus, boat or airplane that experiences nausea, but the passengers. Motion sickness can hit without warning and puts us in some rather precarious positions. Frequently, relief only comes after one turns pale, and then green, and subsequently vomits.

Motion alone is not responsible for all the nausea that people experience, though. Stomach and digestive disorders, contaminated food, pregnancy, stomach flu, and other conditions have caused their fair share of nausea. Nutritional deficiencies such as a lack of vitamin B6 may contribute to the condition. Treating the condition can be quite simple, but preventing it may be a better choice. Safe and natural products have proven in clinical studies to be more effective than some prescription medications. This formula contains herbs that have been used for thousands of years to treat these types of disorders. No automobile glove box or medicine chest should be without ginger, considering its remarkable culinary and medicinal uses. Clinical trials back up its folk use of treating nausea and vomiting.

I can recall a 38-year-old female patient of mine who suffered from sporadic bouts with nausea. She used some medication but found that it made her feel drowsy. She decided to try ginger root and found that it could effectively control her nausea. Now, keep in mind that unexplained nausea warrants a trip to the doctor. If you find, however, that there are no underlying causes for the nausea, then ginger should work very well for you. It can also be used to treat the nausea typical of morning sickness or that which comes as a side effect of chemotherapy.

Endnotes

1. W. Fischer-Rasmussen, et al., "Ginger treatment of hyperemesis gravidarum," Eur Jour Gyn Repro Bil, 1990, 38: 19-24.

MULTIPLE SCLEROSIS

Multiple sclerosis (MS) is a progressive, degenerative disease of the central nervous system that usually affects people between the ages of 25 and 40. It is the most commonly acquired disease of the nervous system in young adults. The incidence of multiple sclerosis in temperate climates is approximately one in every 1,000 and more women than men suffer from MS. It can affect several areas of the nervous system by destroying the myelin sheaths that form a protective covering for the nerves. As a result of this destruction, an inflammatory response occurs. The severity of MS varies markedly with each individual. In some cases, the disease is characterized by mild relapses or exacerbations, followed by long symptom-free periods. Other victims of MS may experience a series of flare-ups that cause some permanent disability. Even in these cases, remission periods may be lengthy.

Symptoms

Symptoms can vary according to the location of the myelin sheath damage. Possible symptoms include slurred speech, staggering, a tendency to drop things, blurred or double vision, numbness, tingling, electrical sensations, dizziness and nausea, breathing difficulties, weakness, tremors, bladder and bowel problems, incontinence, impotence and paralysis.

Some victims of MS experience serious debilitating symptoms within the first year. Others may become gradually more disabled. Additional problems that victims of MS may have to deal with include painful muscle spasms, urinary tract infections, constipation, skin ulcers and mood swings which can vacillate from euphoria to depression. Only a limited number of people are crippled by MS.

Causes

The causes of MS remain unknown. Multiple sclerosis is thought to be an autoimmune disorder in which the body's immune system attacks myelin as if it were a foreign substance. There is some evidence to support that MS is more likely to occur after periods of stress or malnutrition. Once the disease is contracted and is in remission, the presence of other infections, emotional stress or trauma due to an injury can help to trigger an attack.

Multiple sclerosis is not hereditary, but a genetic predisposition does exist in those with the disease. Relatives of affected people are more likely to contract the disease. Environmental factors may also play a role. MS is five times more common in temperate zones than in tropical areas. In Japan, however, the disease is rare at any latitude. Possible reasons for the geographic distribution of the disease include diet, sun exposure and genetics. Mainstream medicine has been attempting to link MS with the presence of a virus such as the one which causes measles, but a substantial amount of research suggests that MS is probably a disorder of the immune system. The association between diet and MS has also been investigated. A diet rich in animal fat and dairy products and low in essential fatty acids has been strongly linked to the incidence of MS.

Conventional Therapies

Once a diagnosis is made, unfortunately, medical science has little to offer victims of this disease. Frequently, physicians approach the disease with a pessimistic attitude. Using corticosteriods can provide some symptomatic relief, however the side effects of these drugs are significant. A great deal of research promises the emergence of medications which may dramatically improve the prognosis of the disease. There is no single diagnostic test to confirm the presence of multiple sclerosis. When symptoms of MS are present, a spinal tap will usually be ordered, along with CAT scanning, brain wave tests and an MRI. Corticosteroid drugs such as Prednisone may be prescribed to alleviate acute symptoms during an attack. ACTH and cyclophosphamide may also be used to suppress immune reactions. Muscle relaxants may be prescribed for muscular stiffness or pain and occasionally surgery to relieve spasms may be advised. In some cases, antidepressants may be recommended. Physical therapy will be suggested to help strengthen muscles and promote better mobility.

Newer medical approaches to the disease include X-ray irradiation of the lymph glands and spleen, which have halted the progress of MS in a significant percentage of patients treated. Radiation therapy, however, can depress the immune system and increase susceptibility to infection. Discuss this treatment with your physician. The use of spinal injections of human fibroblast interferon is also under current investigation. The value of acupuncture, acupressure and chiropractic should be investigated for their potential in helping to control pain and promote mobility.

Dietary Guidelines

- Interestingly, Japan has an unusually low rate of MS, even in its temperate zones. Analysis of the Japanese diet reveals that the consumption of marine foods, seeds and fruit oil is high. These foods contain abundant polyunsaturated fatty acids, including omega-3 oils. As a result, there is some speculation that a deficiency of omega-3 oils may interfere with the proper formation of myelin.
- Victims of MS appear to suffer from a defect in their ability to absorb fatty acids. Eating saturated or hydrogenated fats further aggravates that deficiency.
- There is no question that the role of diet and nutrition in the treatment and prevention of MS is significant. Eat a diet low in saturated fats. Several studies support the fact that avoiding saturated fats for a prolonged period of time can retard the process of this disease and reduce the number of attacks.
- Do not eat over 10 grams of saturated fat per day and eat 40 grams of polyunsaturated oils per day. Oils that can be used sparingly are extra virgin olive oil, canola oil, safflower, soy and sunflower oils.

- Do not eat margarine, shortening, or hydrogenated oils. Take 1 tsp of cod liver oil daily. Taking black currant oil on a regular basis is also recommended. Evening primrose oil is also beneficial.
- Consume fish abundantly. Fish provides an excellent source of omega-3 oils. These oils are essential to normal nerve cell function and myelin sheathe production. Sardines are also a good source of omega-3 oils.
- Eat plenty of legumes, grains, vegetables and fruits. Increase the fiber content of your diet to avoid becoming constipated.
- Taking acidophilus culture and psyllium is recommended.
- Drink plenty of fresh vegetable and fruit juices. A mixture of carrot and green pepper is recommended.
- Avoid sugar, coffee, chocolate, salt, dairy products, meat, highly seasoned foods, processed foods, and caffeine, alcohol, nicotine and saturated fats.

Recommended Nutritional Supplements

PRIMARY NUTRIENTS

OMEGA-3 FATTY ACIDS These oils contain materials that are directly linked with the maintenance of nerve cells. The myelin is composed primarily of unsaturated lipid compounds. Studies using fish oil and linoleic oils strongly support the use of these fatty acids for MS for symptom control and maintenance of remission.[1] *Suggested Dosage:* Take products which contain both types of fatty acids and use pure oils that require refrigeration. Flaxseed oil at one tablespoon per day is recommended. If you use fish oil, take it with vitamin E.

LECITHIN This compound contains choline which works to ensure proper lipid metabolism which may be deranged in people with MS. Choline is required to transfer lipids from the liver.[2] *Suggested Dosage:* Take 1,200 mg with each of three meals per day.

NADH This form of niacin may be very effective in treating the symptoms of MS by lowering blood lipids and boosting circulation.[3] It works to increase energy and stamina as well. *Suggested Dosage:* Five to ten mg daily. You can even go up as high as 15 mg per day, for at least one or two months and evaluate the results.

VITAMIN E, SELENIUM AND LIPOIC ACID The strong antioxidant action of this trio is very beneficial for MS in protecting the cells of the nervous system from additional damage. Lipoic acid considerably boosts the action of vitamin E.[4] In addition, low soil content of selenium has been linked to the prevalence of MS. *Suggested Dosage:* Take 800 to 1,200 IU of vitamin E and selenium and lipoic acid as directed.

COENZYME Q10 Helps to oxygenate cells and supports the immune system.[5] *Suggested Dosage:* 90 mg per day.

PROTEOLYTIC ENZYMES These enzymes help to prevent the circulation of undigested protein molecules thought to stimulate autoimmune responses seen in diseases like MS.[6] *Suggested Dosage:* Take as directed using products with papain and pancreatin.

THIAMINE Clinical studies support the use of vitamin B1 injections for central nervous system diseases like MS to control pain.[7] *Suggested Dosage:* Consult your doctor about the use of injections on a regular basis. Sublingual products may also be tried.

VITAMIN B6 AND B12 Deficiencies of these vitamins have been linked to multiple sclerosis.[8] *Suggested Dosage:* Take as directed using sublingual products if possible.

CALCIUM AND MAGNESIUM A lack of calcium during adolescence has been linked with the later development of MS.[9] Studies using calcium/magnesium with vitamin D and cod liver oil found that the incidence of exacerbations decreased.[10] *Suggested Dosage:* 2,500 mg of calcium lactate, gluconate or citrate and 1,000 mg of magnesium (use chelated varieties).

D-PHENYLALANINE Using this amino acid to prevent MS symptoms has been successful in some clinical trials.[11] *Suggested Dosage:* Take as directed on an empty stomach with fruit juice. Do not use if you have high blood pressure or kidney disease or are on medications for hypertension or antidepressant drugs.

5-HYDROXY-TRYPTOPHAN A supplement of this compound helped to improve mood and the neurological symptoms associated with MS in case studies.[12] *Suggested Dosage:* Take as directed on an empty stomach with fruit juice.

HERBAL COMBINATION This herbal combination should include *Ginkgo biloba* and other antioxidant compounds. *Suggested Dosage:* Look for products with a 24 percent content of ginkgoflavoglycosides and take as directed.

GINKGO BILOBA: The ginkolide content of this herb has helped to inhibit outbreaks of multiple sclerosis in subjects with MS.[13] Padma 28 is a commercial product based on an ancient Tibetan (lamaistic) formula. It contains a mixture of 28 different herbs.[14]

SECONDARY NUTRIENTS

L-GLYCINE: Works to protect myelin coverings of the nerves. *Suggested Dosage:* Take 1,000 mg per day in two divided doses on an empty stomach with fruit juice.

DHEA: When DHEA levels fall below 180 ng/dL in men and 130 ng/dL in women, supplementation is advised. *Suggested Dosage:* Men should take 50 to 100 mg daily, and women 20 to 75 mg daily.

VITAMIN B-COMPLEX: Essential for tissue repair and the proper functioning of the immune system. A vitamin B deficiency can result in further nerve damage. *Suggested Dosage:* Take as directed.

COPPER: Deficiency is associated with defects in myelination in animal studies.[15] *Suggested Dosage:* Ask your doctor to test you for a copper deficiency.

ZINC: Important for normal immune function and healing. *Suggested Dosage:* Take as directed using no more than 100 mg per day. Use picolinate products.

Home Care Suggestions

◆ Portable electro-stimulator units have been used with some success in controlling pain and increasing mobility. These can be obtained through a physician or physical therapist. Acupuncturists also use these units.
◆ If you are under a physician's care who has a negative attitude and makes you feel depressed, get a new doctor immediately.
◆ Avoid emotional stress. Take time every day to relax. Breathing exercises can be quite valuable. Other meditative techniques, like music therapy, hypnotherapy and visualization, can help counteract tension.
◆ Regular exercise is recommended but avoid overexertion and fatigue. Swimming is particularly beneficial. Some exercises which can significantly increase body temperature are discouraged. In some cases, changes in body temperature can aggravate symptoms.
◆ Avoid extremely hot baths, hot tubs, showers, etc. Abrupt rises in temperature have been associated with triggering MS attacks.
◆ Regular massage is excellent for relieving pain and improving muscle tone.
◆ Be wary of questionable practitioners who claim to have a cure for multiple sclerosis.

Other Supportive Therapies

ACUPUNCTURE: Helps to limber up muscles and stimulate nerve function while controlling pain.

MEDITATION AND YOGA: Help to diffuse stress and keep muscles toned.

HYDROTHERAPY: Warm (not hot) baths can help relax muscles and manage stress.

CHIROPRACTIC AND OSTEOPATHY: Improves posture and helps to keep muscles toned.

HOMEOPATHY: Phosphorus, Agaricus, Kali phos., Magnesia phos. and Tarantula are all used for multiple sclerosis.

Scientific Facts-at-a-Glance

Food allergies and their possible link to MS are rarely discussed in patient/doctor conversations. Gluten and milk allergies have been linked to the development of MS and people suffering from MS often have intestinal derangement commonly seen in celiac disease.[16] While scientific studies are few, the notion of antibody production to certain foods could certainly contribute to any autoimmune disease. MS is considered by many experts to be one of several autoimmune diseases which occurs when the immune system begins to attack the body. In this case, the myelin sheaths of the nerves are targeted.

Spirit/Mind Considerations

Victims of MS can lead very productive lives with minimal limitation. If you have been diagnosed with MS, it is imperative to realize that a positive attitude toward the disease is invaluable. MS can be a very manageable disorder; it is important not to approach the condition with a negative or fatalistic attitude. Educating yourself and your family about MS is essential. Even after a particularly severe exacerbation, recovery can be dramatic. Learning to manage stress through meditation can be very helpful. The impact of stress or tension on exacerbations must be considered. It unquestionably predisposes individuals with MS to more episodes.

Prevention

◆ Avoiding a diet high in animal fats may help to prevent a susceptibility to the disease although there is no scientific evidence to support this.
◆ Do not start babies on gluten foods or cow's milk too early. Breast feed whenever possible.
◆ Use soy or flaxseed oil in cooking and avoid hydrogenated fats altogether.
◆ Take essential fatty acids daily.
◆ Use proteolytic enzymes with each meal.

Doctor's Notes

Compelling new research suggests that the herpes simplex virus no. 6 is associated with this disease. It has been discovered in the plaques that develop in the brain and central nervous system. While more research is warranted, using antiviral herbs may be of value. Echinacea, licorice root, cat's claw, pau d'arco, St. John's wort, garlic, astragalus and Chinese mushrooms have significant antiviral properties. In addition, the notion that MS may be one of several autoimmune diseases caused by food allergies or incomplete digestion must also be addressed. Food allergies to gluten and milk have been implicated, as have vaccines and hydrogenated fats. The fact that the Japanese have such a low incidence of this disease strongly suggests that eating certain types of fats and oils has a profound effect on the nervous system. If we get adequate supplies of essential fatty acids, we may be able to protect ourselves from diseases like MS. Using hydrogenated fats found in vegetable margerines is thought to be particularly harmful due to the creation of trans-fatty acids. There are many people with MS who manage to control their symptoms with natural supplementation rather than harsh drugs. Diet changes are extremely important as are using certain supplements on a daily basis.

Additional Resources

Multiple Sclerosis Foundation
6350 North Andrews Avenue
Fort Lauderdale, FL 33309
(800) 441-7055

Endnotes

1. W. Cendrowski, "Multiple sclerosis and Max-EPA," Bri Jour Clin Prac, 1986, 40:365-67. See also R. Dworkin, et al., "Linoleic acid and multiple sclerosis: A reanalysis of three double-blind trails," Neurology, 1984, 34:1441-45, and R. Dworkin, "Linoleic acid and multiple sclerosis," Lancet, 1981, 1:1153-4.
2. D. Canty and S. Zeisel, "Lecithin and choline in human health and disease," Nutr Rev, 1994, 52: 327-39.
3. J. DiPalma and W. Thayer, "The use of niacin as a drug," Ann Rev Nutr, 1991, 11: 169-87.
4. M. Podda, "Alpha lipoic acid supplementation prevents the symptoms of vitamin E deficiency," Biochem Biophy Res Comm, 1994, 204: 98-104.
5. B. Frei, et al., "Ubiquinol-10 is an effective lipid-soluble antioxidant at physiological concentrations," Proc Nat Acad, 1990, 87: 4879-4883.
6. K. Ransberger et al., "Enzyme therapy of immune complex diseases," Arth Rheum, 1986, 8: 16-19.
7. E. Stern, "The intraspinal injection of vitamin B1 for the relief of intractable pain, and for inflammatory and degenerative diseases of the central nervous system," Am Jour Surg, 1938, 34:495.
8. D. Mitchell and E. Schandl, Am Jour Clin Nutr, August, 1973, See also R. Ransohoff et al., "Vitamin B12 deficiency and multiple sclerosis," Letter, Lancet, 1990, 335:1285-86.
9. P. Goldberg, "Multiple sclerosis: Vitamin D and calcium as environmental determinants of prevalence," Int Jour Environ Stud, 1974, 6:19-27 and 121-29.
10. P. Goldberg, et al., "Multiple sclerosis: decrease relapse rate through dietary supplementation of calcium, magnesium and vitamin D," Med Hypoth, 1986, 21(2): 193-200.
11. A. Winter, "A new treatment for multiple sclerosis," Jour Neural Trans, 1975, 37:297-304.
12. M. Hyyppa, et al., "Effect of L-tryptophan treatment on central indole amine metabolism and short-lasting neurologic disturbances in multiple sclerosis," Jour Neural Tran, 1975, 37:297-304.
13. B. Brochet, et al., "Pilot study of Ginkgolide B, a PAF specific inhibitory in the treatment of acute outbreaks of multiple sclerosis," Rev Neurol, (Paris) 1992, 148(4):299-301.
14. T. Korwin-Piotrowska et al., "Experience of Padma 28 in multiple sclerosis," Phytother 1992, Res 6:133-6.
15. E. Underwood, Trace Elements in Human and Animal Nutrition, 4th Ed. (Academic Press, New York: 1971).
16. L. Lange and M. Shiner, "Small bowel abnormalities in multiple sclerosis," Lancet, 1976, II: 1319-22.

OBESITY

In 1996, the total number of prescriptions for the weight-loss drug "phen-fen" written in this country exceeded 18 million. Statistics suggest that as many as 30 percent of patients using phen-fen may have lesions on their heart valves caused by combining fenfluramine and phentermine. Those who thought they had finally found the ultimate weight loss panacea, find themselves back at square one again. So the question remains: Are there any safe substances that can effectively inhibit the appetite, supply energy, and boost caloric burning without compromising health? The answer is a definitive "yes."

Obesity refers to a weight condition which is defined as being 20 percent over the prescribed weight for a particular age, build or height. Estimates assessing the extent of obesity in the United States range from 10 percent to 50 percent of the overall population. The number of obese children in Western countries has dramatically increased, nearly doubling between the years of 1965 and 1980. One in every four American children is overweight. One in every five men and almost one in every three women is considered obese.

Simply stated, obesity is an excessive amount of body fat. It is important to remember that weight alone is not a good indicator of body fat composition. Obesity is a complex and frustrating problem which involves more than just overeating. Factors that influence obesity are genetics, cultural background, physical characteristics and social or economic status.

Symptoms

The most apparent sign of obesity is an increase in body weight due to a rise in the fat percentage of total mass. Secondary symptoms of obesity are increased foot problems, back problems, reduced physical endurance, labored breathing, and sleep difficulties (especially sleep apnea).

Complications of obesity include an increased risk for kidney disease, heart trouble, stroke, gallbladder disease, certain types of cancer, hemorrhoids, varicose veins, diabetes, high blood pressure, hormonally related disorders, problems in pregnancy, liver damage and psychological disorders.

Causes

Overeating and lack of exercise are considered the most common causes of obesity. We know that a diet that is low in fiber and high in refined carbohydrates and fat is believed to be one of the major factors responsible for the high rates of obesity found in Western cultures. Other possible causes are glandular malfunctions, genetic predisposition or defect, emotional relationship with eating, malnutrition and boredom. Clearly, as we age our bodies make less of calorie-burning hormones like DHEA and pyruvate.

Genetic abnormalities and even the presence of a certain virus have been linked with certain types of obesity.

Certainly food is not the only factor involved in all cases of obesity.

Experts at the University of Florida have concluded through their research that people who are extremely obese may be victims of Prader-Willi syndrome, which is caused by a defective gene that causes them to store fat abnormally. These people have to actually reduce food intake to below normal levels just to maintain their weight.

Conventional Therapies

Traditional medical treatment of obesity has proved to be rather frustrating for both patient and doctor. Using drugs or drastic surgical procedures has a poor success rate and comes with a number of negative side effects. Obesity is extremely difficult to successfully treat. Most physicians will suggest a diet that will usually lower caloric intake to 1,500 calories per day combined with 15 to 20 minutes of aerobic exercise at least three or four times a week. Gradual weight loss is recommended (one-half pound to one pound per week). Antiobesity drugs such as non-amphetamine appetite suppressants are prescribed by some physicians, but their use is discouraged due to their significant side effects. Drugs which are designed to increase the body's energy requirements are currently being tested. Wiring the teeth together to prohibit eating is another possible medical treatment for obesity. The treatment is uncomfortable and while it may produce results, they are usually temporary and have nothing to do with eating habit modification. In addition, wiring the jaw may promote tooth decay and mouth infections.

Surgical options are always accompanied with severe risks and side effects. Liposuction, one form of surgical weight loss, involves cutting an incision through which a vacuum tube is placed to literally suck out fat cells. The procedure is extremely traumatic to surrounding tissue and causes a considerable amount of bruising and pain. The possibility of developing a life-threatening blood clot from this procedure exists.

Colectomy, another type of fat-reduction surgery, reduces the area of the intestine through which food can be absorbed. It can also decrease appetite. This is considered a major surgical procedure and carries with it the risk of serious complications or death. The proper assimilation of vitamins and minerals is also impaired. The use of this particular surgery has declined due to its adverse effects.

Stomach stapling, a third type of fat-reduction surgery, reduces the size of the stomach to limit the amount of food which can be ingested at one time. This also is a major surgical procedure that carries with it serious complications or the risk of death. In several instances, the staples do not hold and the surgery has to be repeated. Eating disturbances, like involuntary regurgitation can result from this procedure. A significant percentage of people who use drastic surgical procedures to lose weight will eventually gain it back.

Dietary Guidelines

◆ Some studies indicate that when there is an inadequate intake of essential nutrients, fat is not burned efficiently, which may contribute to obesity. For this reason, supplementing the diet with a good multivitamin and mineral supplement is highly recommended.

- Research indicates that the amount of calories consumed is not as important as what comprises those calories.

- Eating a diet that is high in fiber, complex carbohydrates, fresh vegetables, fruits and low in fat is the winning combination. In addition, raising your caloric intake of nonfat foods seems to enhance weight loss rather than slow it.

- Cultures that routinely eat high-fiber diets have a very low incidence of obesity (and they probably don't count calories). High-fiber diets improve the excretion of fat in the feces, improve glucose tolerance, and provide a feeling of satisfaction and fullness. In addition, studies support that if we eat a diet that is nutritious, we will not experience food cravings.

- Sugar in the form of soda pop, candy, cookies, cakes, ice cream and pastries is responsible for much of childhood obesity. Salted snack foods such as potato chips and corn chips are as much as 40 percent fat. Making these foods unavailable to family members can go a long way to fight obesity. Many breakfast cereals are up to 60 percent sugar.

- Emphasize the following foods: lentils, beans, plain baked potatoes, baked squash, brown rice, whole grain breads (low-fat or no fat), whitefish, tuna, chicken, skim milk, low-fat cottage cheese, low-fat active culture yogurt, turkey, tofu, fresh fruits and vegetables and high protein lean foods.

- Avoid the following foods: high-fat dairy products (cheese, sour cream, ice cream, butter, whole milk), rich dressings, soda pop, mayonnaise, fried foods, red meats, gravies, custards, pastries, cakes, and peanut butter and junk foods.

- Do not eat too little. Any diet that is less than 1,200 calories is not effective as a means of weight loss. In addition, all diets should contain some percentage of desirable fat which can be ingested in the form of olive, flaxseed or safflower oil. Supplementing your diet with 1 to 2 teaspoons of these oils is thought to actually improve the burning of fat. Do not consume alcohol: all alcoholic beverages are high in calories.

- Fiber supplements can be taken in the form of guar gum, psyllium or glucomannan. Avoid artificial sweeteners. There is some evidence that artificial sweeteners can actually increase appetite and result in weight gain. Barley malt sweetener can be used instead of sugar. Omit all substances which are thought to be appetite stimulants such as salt, hot spices, coffee, tea, tobacco and sugar.

Recommended Nutritional Supplements

PRIMARY NUTRIENTS

FIBER SUPPLEMENT Adding a fiber supplement to your diet can help reduce blood sugar, control appetite and promote feelings of fullness. Study after study supports its efficacy in promoting weight loss.[1] *Suggested Dosage:* Take in the morning and at night using products designed to mix in liquid. Drink plenty of water.

5-HYDROXY-TRYPTOPHAN A twelve-week study in Rome using oral hydroxy-tryptophan (5-HTP) was administered without any dietary restriction and weight loss averaged 4 pounds per week. The drug is a serotonin precursor and can inhibit the desire to eat carbohydrates.[2] *Suggested Dosage:* Take as directed on an empty stomach with fruit juice.

CHROMIUM PICOLINATE This mineral increases the ability of body cells to utilize insulin which plays a vital role in appetite control, thermogenesis and the creation of muscle mass. Low levels of this nutrient have been discovered in obese individuals and supplementation has initiated weight loss.[3] *Suggested Dosage:* 300 to 600 mg per day.

OMEGA-6/OMEGA-3 FATTY ACIDS These compounds stimulate brown fat activity which is where calories are burned. Individuals who have repeated trouble losing weight can especially benefit from this effect.[4] *Suggested Dosage:* Take as directed, using flaxseed, evening primrose and fish oil blends. Take a vitamin E supplement whenever you take fish oil.

GLUCOMANNAN As a carbohydrate that cannot be absorbed, this compound can absorb 50 to 200 times its weight of water and acts as a good colon cleanse and fiber source.[5] *Suggested Dosage:* 3 grams daily.

GARCINIA CAMBOGIA (HCA) This compound interferes with the conversion of carbohydrates to fat and is an excellent supplement to any weight loss program.[6] *Suggested Dosage:* 500 mg three times daily with meals.

PROTEOLYTIC ENZYMES These help to break down macronutrients in the gut and promote better digestion. Laboratory tests using pancreatin resulted in unanticipated weight loss.[7] *Suggested Dosage:* Take as directed, looking for products which contain pancreatin and papain.

VITAMIN C WITH BIOFLAVONOIDS May theoretically reduce obesity by increasing cellular energy consumption through increasing sodium pump activity.[8] *Suggested Dosage:* Take 1,000 to 3,000 mg per day.

PYRUVATE This end product of sugar metabolism in the body has been proven in clinical studies to boost weight loss by 20 to 40 percent by increasing cellular respiration in the mitochondria.[9] *Suggested Dosage:* 6 to 8 grams per day with fruit juice.

EPHEDRA (MA HUANG) This thermogenic herb actually promotes the conversion of calories to heat.[10] Adding certain substance like aspirin to ephedra can potentiate its action even further.[11] *Suggested Dosage:* Take only as directed but do not take after 3 p.m. or insomnia may occur. Do not use if you have anxiety or panic disorder, heart disease, high blood pressure, glaucoma, or if you take an MAO inhibitor drug.

DHEA Studies using this hormone have found that it boosts the burning of fat.[12] *Suggested Dosage:* Take as directed. CAUTION: Should not be used by anyone who has had a hormonally-caused cancer or who has a family history of this type of cancer.

HERBAL COMBINATION This combination should include chickweed, celery seeds, psyllium seeds, horsetail, fennel seeds, Irish moss, kelp and white willow. *Suggested Dosage:* Six to ten capsules daily. Should be used daily.

CHICKWEED: Chickweed is considered by many herbalists to be one of the better appetite suppressant herbs. It also cleanses plaque from blood vessels and is able to break down and eliminate fatty substances from the body. Chickweed supports the cleansing action by stimulating the body's own system of elimination. CELERY SEED: Celery seed helps return the body to a positive energy state. In other words, the amount of energy consumed is equal to the amount of energy burned. Less energy will be converted to fat. It has insulin-like activity and is an excellent diuretic and diaphoretic (promotes perspiration).[13] This property will be of use in cleansing the body of toxins whether or not one chooses to fast. PSYLLIUM SEEDS: Psyllium seeds provide a bulking, water-soluble fiber that promotes bowel elimination and cleansing. Psyllium will absorb many times its weight in fluids causing appetite cessation while contributing very little in calories. It also reduces serum cholesterol and removes fatty substances from the body.[14] HORSETAIL: Horsetail is a mild diuretic and has traditionally been used in Europe as a main component of weight-loss diets. It stimulates the body's metabolism. In addition to this, horsetail contains silica which is essential in maintaining a stronger, healthier skeleton, which can be beneficial to obese individuals.[15] FENNEL SEEDS: Fennel seeds, like several other herbs of the formula, are mildly diuretic. Fennel has a strong carminative action which reduces flatulence and bloating. Like celery, fennel reduces spasm and may prove useful during and after exercise. Fennel helps the bowel to better adapt to the laxative effect produced by some of the other herbs. IRISH MOSS: Irish moss is an excellent mucilage-containing demulcent. The mucilage is similar to psyllium in that it absorbs large amounts of fluids and imparts a feeling of fullness. In this way it is an appetite suppressant. Irish moss is considered to be very nutritive. Overweight people quite often have nutrient imbalances that can be helped and possibly fully corrected by Irish moss. KELP: Obesity is quite often associated with the dysfunction of thyroid gland. Kelp, like Irish moss, is very nutritious. However, kelp's iodine content also helps to maintain normal function in the thyroid gland which is the main reason for its addition to this formula.[16] The thyroid gland regulates metabolism and controls the use of oxygen and heart rate. Kelp contains algin which is another soluble fiber and further adds mucilage and bulking to this formula. WHITE WILLOW: White willow has been included in several traditional weight loss formulas. It is an analgesic but when combined with other compounds like ephedra can boost thermogenesis.

SECONDARY NUTRIENTS

L-PHENYLALANINE: Works to suppress the appetite by working on brain amines. *Suggested Dosage:* Take as directed on an empty stomach with fruit juice. Do not use if you have high blood pressure or are taking antidepressant drugs.

L-TYROSINE: Raises serotonin and other brain neurotransmitters to help discourage eating. *Suggested Dosage:* Take as directed on an empty stomach with fruit juice.

LIPOIC ACID: Boosts cellular levels of glutathione and vitamin E to scavenge for free radicals created when fat is burned. *Suggested Dosage:* Take as directed.

CHITOSAN: A form of fiber made from ground shrimp shells, which can bind to fat in the stomach and prevent its absorption. *Suggested Dosage:* Use as directed. Usually five to seven capsules are required for an average meal. Do not use unless fat is being consumed and do not take with any fat-soluble vitamins or other supplements. You may experience a laxative effect.

CARNITINE AND METHIONINE: Helps to promote the creation of lean muscle mass while inhibiting hunger. *Suggested Dosage:* Take as directed on an empty stomach with fruit juice.

VITAMIN D: People with weight problems are often low in circulating levels of this vitamin. *Suggested Dosage:* Take as directed.

Home Care Suggestions

- Exercise regularly. Exercise is considered the best method to control weight. Begin slowly. Take a ten-to-fifteen minute walk three days a week and then slowly increase your distance and your pace. Light exercise right after eating is recommended and can help to burn calories that have just been consumed.
- Don't chew gum. Chewing gum can activate the flow of gastric juices and make you feel like eating.
- Eat only when you are truly hungry. Often thirst can be mistaken for hunger. Drink when you feel the urge to eat.
- Don't become constipated. Drink six to eight glasses of water per day.
- Keep all high calorie foods on high shelves or on the back selves of the refrigerator and low-calorie foods easily accessible.
- Eating too fast or improper chewing can also result in the consumption of more calories during a certain period of time. Eating a diet that is high in fiber can automatically increase chewing time and slow the eating process. People who eat too fast can often become hungry again soon after eating. Listen to calm, soothing music while you eat and chew slowly.
- Don't eat when you are depressed, lonely or angry.
- Avoid fad diets which can make your body feel as if it's starving and actually lower your metabolism; this slows the burning of fat stores.
- Do not use diuretics or laxatives to induce weight loss.

These can be potentially hazardous to your health and result in temporary weight loss only.

- Join a support group like Weight Watchers or Overeaters Anonymous, which both take a sensible and healthful approach to losing weight. Be wary of diet organizations that are costly or limit you to their own foods.
- Be patient. More permanent results will be obtained if weight loss is gradual. Remember that it takes time for the body to readjust to its new programmed weight set point.
- Do not eat when you are anxious, bored or frustrated. Find something else to do when you feel inclined to eat under these circumstances.
- Do not eat while reading or watching TV. As fun as this might be, it promotes inactivity and weight gain. If you have to eat during these activities, munch on raw veggies.
- Never nibble on food after the meal is over. Mothers are particularly susceptible to this. While they may eat sensibly during the meal, picking at leftovers while washing dishes can significantly contribute to weight gain.
- Do not use food as a reward.

Other Supportive Therapies

ACUPUNCTURE: Stimulating certain meridian points can help to suppress the appetite.

Scientific Facts-at-a-Glance

Once again, the notion that food allergies may play a role in obesity may seem far fetched but is worth investigating. Some very intriguing clinical studies have found that when people ate foods they were sensitive to, they gained weight and when they eliminated these foods, they lost weight. The interesting thing about these studies is that caloric intake remained the same in both instances, suggesting that many more factors are involved in weight control than we may have assumed.[17]

Spirit/Mind Considerations

Obesity carries with it a significant societal stigma and the pressure to be thin is enormous. Discrimination is routinely experienced by obese individuals. As a result, these people often adopt self-defeating and self-degrading attitudes. Low self esteem, depression and overeating may result.

Counseling can afford the obese person an opportunity to change attitudes, and improve self-esteem. Initial counseling prior to any weight loss program has been found to increase the rate of success. In addition, the value of meditation and visualization may be of great benefit in setting the mental and emotional stage for weight loss. It is also important to remember that if you are not getting enough carbohydrates on any weight loss diet, you may feel depressed and irritable. Try to find a plan that is suited to your tastes so that you will have a much greater chance of succeeding.

Prevention

- Weigh yourself regularly and record your weight on a chart. If you go up three pounds from your ideal weight, adjust your diet and exercise to lose those three pounds. It is easier to lose three pounds than to lose 20.
- Stay off the diet roller coaster of overeating and then crash dieting. Keep a consistent, healthy lifestyle centered around sensible eating and regular exercise.
- Keep your kitchen stocked with healthy low-fat, low sugar snacks.

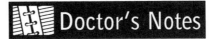 Doctor's Notes

Obesity is a common problem which is directly or indirectly responsible for many other health problems. Obesity has no single underlying cause. Sometimes it can be the result of disorders associated with psychogenic, genetic, thyroid and hypothalamic problems that can be complex and difficult to diagnose. Since obesity is a complex condition, an herbal formula designed to address several of the more common underlying causes is most appropriate. Any weight loss effort should include consulting a health care professional, exercise, and fat and calorie control for maximum and lasting benefits. A cleansing fast done under the care of a health care professional can help to expedite weight loss and stop food cravings.

Endnotes

1. K. Porikos, "Is fiber satiating? Effects of high-fiber preload on subsequent food intake of normal-weight and obese young men," Appetite, 1986, 7: 153-62.
2. M. Holder and G. Huether, "Role of pre-feedings, plasma amino acid ratios and brain serotonin levels in carbohydrate and protein selection," Physl Behav, 1990, 47:113-19.
3. L. Van Gaal, et al., "Exploratory study of co-enzyme Q-10 in obesity,", in K. Folkers and Y. Yamamura, Eds., Biomed and Clin Aspects of Coenzyme Q-10, vol. 4, (Amsterdam, Elsevier Science Publishers, 1984: 369-73).
4. R. Lowndes and R. Mansel, "The effects of evening primrose oil (Efamol) on serum lipid levels of normal and obese subjects," in D.F. Horrobin, ed., Clinical Uses of Essential Fatty Acid (Eden Press, Montreal: 1982), 37-52.
5. G. Reffo, et al., "Glucomannan in hypertensive outpatients," Curr Ther Res, 1988, 44(1):22-27.
6. J. Watson and J. Lowenstein, "Citrate and the conversion of carbohydrate into fat," Jour Biol Chem, 1970, 245:599.
7. D.H. Dean and R.N. Hiramoto, "Weight loss during pancreatin feeding of rats," Nutrition Reports International, 1984, 29: 167-72.
8. G. Naylor, et al., "A double-blind placebo-controlled trial of ascorbic acid in obesity," Nutr Health, 1985, 4:25-8.
9. R. Stanko, et al., "Body composition, energy utilization and nitrogen metabolism with a severely restricted diet supplemented with pyruvate," Amer Jour Clin Nut, 1992, 55: 771-75.
10. R. Pasquali, "A controlled trial using ephedrine in the treatment of obesity," Int Jour Obes, 1985, 9(2): 93-8.
11. T. Horton and C. Geissler, Aspirin potentiates the effect of

ephedrine on the thermogenic response to a meal in obese but not lean women," Int J Obes, 1991, 15(5):359-66. See also L. Bukowiecki, et al., "Ephedrine, a potential slimming drug, directly stimulates thermogenesis in brown adipocytes via B-adrenoreceptors," Inter Jour Obes, 1982, (6): 343-50, and L. Landsberg, et al., "Sympathoadrenal activity and obesity: physiological rational for the use of adrenergic thermogenic drugs," Inter Jour Obes, 1993, (17) suppl 1: s29-34.

12. G. Bush and D. Bush, New England Journal of Medicine, 1986, 315, 1519-24, W.D. Drucker et l., "Biologic activity of dehydroepiandrosterone sulfate (DHEA) in man," Journal of Clinical Endocrinology, 1972, 35: 48-54.

13. C. Best and D. Scott, "Possible sources of insulin," Jour of Met Res, 1923, 3:177-79.

14. G. Enzi, et al., "Effect of hydrophilic mucilage in the treatment of obese patients," Pharmatherapeutica, 1980, 2(7): 420-28.

15. P. List and L. Hoerhammer, Hagers Hanbuch der Pharmazeutischen Praxis, Vols. 2-5 (Springer-Verlag, Berlin).

16. H. Johnsons, "Composition of edible seaweeds," Proceedings of the Seventh International Seaweed Symposium, (Wiley and Sons, New York: 1972), 429-35.

17. T. Randolph, "Masked food allergy as a factor in the development and persistence of obesity," Abstract, Jour Lab Clin Med, 1947, 32: 1547.

OSTEOPOROSIS

Osteoporosis literally means "porous bones," and is considered a natural part of aging. Bones become brittle and easily fractured as a result of decreasing bone density. By age 70, it is estimated that the density of the skeleton has decreased by approximately one-third.

For hormonal reasons, osteoporosis is much more common in women than men. Twenty-five percent of all postmenopausal women have the disorder. Bones that are affected by osteoporosis can become thin and porous, which makes them vulnerable to fractures. The most common sites of bone loss are in the spine, hips and ribs. Osteoporosis affects over 15 million people in the United States and is estimated to cost over $3.8 billion annually. Approximately 650,000 fractures occur annually in the United States as a result of osteoporosis.

Symptoms

Women approaching menopause are at risk of developing osteoporosis and should consult their physician to evaluate their skeletal integrity. Some doctors dispute the value of this type of diagnosis. Discuss its advantages with your doctor.

Osteoporosis that begins at or during menopause may often go undetected for years. Unfortunately, the first symptom of the disease is often discovered when a minor fall causes a fracture. Typical sites for these fractures are above the wrist and the top of the femur. Fractures of one or several vertebrae can also occur and result in a progressive loss of height and a curvature of the spine. In these cases, compression of the spinal cord may cause chronic pain. Osteoporosis can also cause a backache if it is occurring in the vertebrae.

If you develop a sudden and extremely severe attack of back pain, see your physician. A spine fracture can occur in osteoporosis and could result in paralysis.

Causes

After menopause, women are particularly vulnerable to osteoporosis due to decreased estrogen levles, which contributes to bone loss. Other possible causes of osteoporosis are lack of calcium in the diet, removal of the ovaries, Cushing's syndrome, lack of mobility, lack of sunshine, prolonged use of corticosteroid drugs, smoking, alcohol consumption, malabsorption of nutrients from food, genetic predisposition, diuretics, blood thinners, some anticonvulsants, and use of sinthroid (L-thyroxine).

Certain factors increase the risk for developing osteoporosis. Some of these are consuming alcohol and caffeine, smoking, never having been pregnant, having a fragile frame and fair skin, being underweight, sedentary lifestyle, low intake of calcium, a high protein diet, too much iron, presence of digestive disorders, early menopause, family history of osteoporosis, diabetes, chronic pulmonary disease and rheumatoid arthritis.

Conventional Therapies

Traditional treatments of osteoporosis are sometimes too late to make a significant difference. Prevention should be stressed more in the medical community and women need to educate themselves on preventative measures. Hormone replacement therapy has had some good success within the medical community and should be investigated upon reaching menopause.

Osteoporosis is diagnosed from bone x-rays, blood tests and in some cases, a bone biopsy. Unfortunately, x-rays do not usually detect the disorder until a 30 to 50 percent bone loss has already occurred. Calcitonin, a prescription drug recently approved by the FDA, can help to prevent bone loss in a large percentage of patients with osteoporosis. However, it may cause kidney stones to form. The use of estrogen replacement therapy may also be recommended by your doctor and its pros and cons should be carefully discussed. Today we know that progesterone replacement may be even more effective than estrogen. There are some natural compounds which can safely raise progesterone levels.

Dietary Guidelines

- Eat a diet high in fruits and vegetables and low in fat and animal protein. Increase your consumption of flavonoid-rich foods, such as dark colored berries and fruits.
- The current recommendation for post-menopausal women is to obtain 1,200 to 1,500 mg of calcium per day. Recommended sources of calcium are buttermilk, buckwheat, kelp, flounder, nuts, oats, cheese, whole wheat, yogurt, skim milk and sardines. Osteoporosis is more common in lactose-intolerants, possibly due to avoidance of milk products.[1]
- Some vegetables are also high in calcium but contain oxalic acid which can inhibit calcium absorption. Some of these are broccoli, kale and turnip greens. Other foods high in oxalic acid are beet greens, almonds, cashews, chard, rhubarb and spinach.
- Calcium/magnesium supplements are suggested along with dietary sources.
- Eat soy-based foods like tofu, which contain natural estrogenic activity.
- Soluble calcium is recommended.
- Eliminate soft drinks, high-protein animal foods, caffeine and alcohol. The phosphates contained in these foods can cause calcium to be excreted in excess amounts. Colas and carbonated drinks are often high in phosphoric acid and should be avoided.
- Several studies confirm that eating a diet high in meats seems to initiate more bone loss than a vegetarian approach.
- Caffeine has also been linked to calcium loss by causing the excretion of increased amounts of calcium in the urine.
- Do not eat too much fiber. A high-fiber diet can bind calcium in the stomach and limit the amount that is absorbed. Fiber in the diet is a good thing and for fiber to be a significant factor in calcium reduction, the amount of fiber would have to be abnormally high. If you do take a fiber supplement, do not take your calcium supplement at the same time.
- Avoid salt; it can cause too much calcium to be excreted in the urine. Check ingredient labels for high-salt foods.

Recommended Nutritional Supplements

PRIMARY NUTRIENTS

Take a good strong multivitamin and mineral supplement. Many recent studies have found that a deficiency in one of many nutrients can predispose the body to developing osteoporosis.

CALCIUM Calcium supplementation is crucial to prevent osteoporosis. Take your calcium supplements before going to bed. Clinical evidence suggests that it is absorbed better in the evening. Calcium can help to calm the nerves and insure a better night's rest.[2] *Suggested Dosage:* 1.5 g daily for postmenopausal women and 1 g daily for premenopausal women over 35. Use calcium citrate or other chelated forms. Several studies indicate that a high percentage of post-menopausal women are severely deficient in stomach acid which can dramatically decrease that absorption of calcium ingested.[3] Ensuring absorption is essential. If you take a supplement and it does not enter the bones, it does you no good. In these cases, calcium carbonate is not recommended as a supplement. Soluble calcium found in calcium citrate, calcium lactate and calcium gluconate is superior. Calcium citrate also appears to be less likely to cause kidney stones.

MAGNESIUM Supplementation is also essential for proper calcium assimilation and in and of itself may increase bone density.[4] *Suggested Dosage:* 500 mg daily.

VITAMIN D This vitamin enhances the ability of the body to absorb and utilize calcium in the bones.[6] In addition, people with osteoporosis may have trouble converting vitamin D to its active form.[7] *Suggested Dosage:* Take as directed; it is also beneficial to take vitamin D with a calcium supplement.

WILD YAM (CREAM OR TOPICAL FORM) An excellent source of natural progesterone due to its precursor compound diosgenin, which converts to progesterone in the body. In 1981, Dr. John Lee conducted a landmark study evaluating the effectiveness of using natural progesterone for osteoporosis.[8] His study indicated that it is the cessation of progesterone production in postmenopausal women that causes the development of osteoporosis. Contrary to current trends, progesterone replacement—not estrogen—may really be the answer to preventing and treating osteoporosis. *Suggested Dosage:* Use as directed.

FOLIC ACID Tests have found that supplements of folic acid help to reduce homocysteine concentrations in the body which interfere with proper calcium absorption and utilization in the bones.[9] *Suggested Dosage:* 2 to 3 mg daily.

VITAMIN B6 Deficiencies of this vitamin have been linked to bone disease and can have an effect even years before the onset of osteoporosis.[10] *Suggested Dosage:* 100 mg daily.

VITAMIN B12 This vitamin is involved in the proper metabolism and use of osteoblast specific proteins in bone.[11] *Suggested Dosage:* 1,000 mcg daily.

VITAMIN C WITH BIOFLAVONOIDS A depletion of this vitamin can actually contribute to the development of osteoporosis. Supplementation can help to raise serum levels of vitamin D, which contributes to calcium absorption.[12] *Suggested Dosage:* 3,000 mg daily.

GLUCSAMINE/CHONDROITIN SULFATE Special compounds found in these two natural substances work to produce collagen which holds joints together.[13] *Suggested Dosage:* Should be calculated according to weight. Use as directed.

HERBAL COMBINATION This combination includes horsetail, alfalfa, feverfew and oatstraw. *Suggested Dosage:* Four to six capsules daily.

HORSETAIL (SHAVE GRASS): Contains silica and manganese required for calcium uptake and fracture healing. It contains silica, a mineral found in bones and collagen (connective tissue).[14] Collagen is essentially the glue that holds everything together. ALFALFA: This herb is naturally high in calcium and vitamin K, which are both essential for proper bone maintenance.[15] FEVERFEW: This plant contains silicon and zinc and is also good for pain relief.[16] OATSTRAW: This herb is rich in silica which is needed for calcium assimilation.

HERBAL COMBINATION FOR ESTROGENIC ACTIVITY This combination includes wild yam, dong quai, licorice and black cohosh. *Suggested Dosage:* Four to six capsules daily.

WILD YAM: Contains natural phytoestrogenic compounds which are precursors to progesterone. Raising progesterone is thought to be just as important or even more so than boosting estrogen for osteoporosis prevention and treatment.[17] DONG QUAI: Dong quai helps to relieve the unpleasant symptoms associated with menopause.[18] Dong quai is also said to have analgesic properties. BLACK COHOSH ROOT: Black cohosh has been proven to be such an effective remedy for menopausal disorders due to its endocrine activity which mimics estrogen.[19] LICORICE ROOT: Licorice not only contains hormonal precursors but stimulates the production of estrogen.[20] This has been shown to decrease the symptoms associated with hormone fluctuation which contributes to osteoporosis.

SECONDARY NUTRIENTS

PROTEOLYTIC ENZYMES: Contribute to the better breakdown and assimilation of nutrients including calcium by boosting digestion. *Suggested Dosage:* Take as directed.

HYDROCHLORIC ACID: Should be used by anyone who suspects a deficiency. A lack of this stomach acid can result in the eventual development of osteoporosis. *Suggested Dosage:* Use as directed only if you have a deficiency.

VITAMIN K: Supplementation seems to keep more calcium in the bones rather than being excreted in the urine. *Suggested Dosage:* Use fat-soluble forms of chlorophyll which is naturally rich in vitamin K. Use as directed.

MANGANESE: This mineral is needed for proper bone development and maintenance. *Suggested Dosage:* Take as directed but not with your calcium or magnesium supplement.

ZINC: Enhances the activity of vitamin D and indirectly effects the proper metabolism of bone. *Suggested Dosage:* Take 50 mg daily.

Home Care Suggestions

◆ Keeping your body active by exercising regularly can help to minimize calcium loss which causes osteoporosis. Even if calcium is present in the body, it cannot be used properly unless exercise is present. In addition, exercise can slow the effects of osteoporosis and help to reverse some of its symptoms to some extent. A brisk daily walk is recommended. Mini-trampolines are also good in that they do not put as much impact stress on the skeletal frame. Some studies indicate that some weight-bearing exercises can also block the usual loss of calcium that occurs after menopause.

◆ Take precautions to avoid falls. Remove possible hazards such as loose rugs or electrical wires. Keep your house well-lit at night.

◆ Use a cane to avoid the possibility of falls and fractures.

◆ When you stand, use furniture, etc., to help support your body.

◆ Do not smoke, drink alcohol or consume caffeine. All three of these activities have been linked to an increase in bone loss.

◆ Use cushioned soles to prevent injury.

◆ Don't twist to pick something up off the floor.

◆ Do not ingest aluminum. Watch for aluminum content in cookware, pre-packaged foods and over-the-counter medications.

Other Supportive Therapies

ACUPUNCTURE: Can help with malabsorption and balance of energy.

MASSAGE: Deep massage with essential oils can help boost circulation to bones and increase flexibility.

HOMEOPATHIC: Tissue salts like calc flour and calc phos can be used.

Scientific Facts-at-a-Glance

Recent studies suggest that even a very small ingestion of aluminum can contribute to bone disease.[22] Another interesting link to osteoporosis is a lack of stomach acid (HCL), which impairs calcium absorption and inevitably leads to the excretion of calcium in the urine.[23]

Spirit/Mind Considerations

Osteoporosis can be a very debilitating disease and can effect women who are still relatively young. Anyone who has this condition needs to use relaxation techniques geared at creating emotional and spiritual tranquility in order to relax muscles and inhibit the disease process. Support groups of women who walk together or meet for various activities can force mild exercise while lifting the spirit as well.

Prevention

◆ Preventing osteoporosis should begin long before old age. Diet and lifestyle changes can greatly contribute to a reduced risk of developing osteoporosis.

◆ Both men and women should make sure that their calcium intake is adequate. Sources for calcium are milk and dairy products, green leafy vegetables, citrus fruits, sardines and shellfish. Calcium/magnesium supplements are recommended. It is important to remember that studies have indicated that even if high levels of calcium are ingested, if the diet is protein-rich, absorption of calcium can be impaired.

◆ Exercise regularly. Exercise helps to build bone and maintain its mass. The importance of exercise in preventing osteoporosis cannot be overemphasized. Without exercise, the bones will not absorb the calcium present in the body. Studies indicate that a sufficient amount of exercise can maintain bone strength at a normal level for an indefinite period of time. Exercise is perhaps the best antiaging factor available.

◆ Hormone replacement therapy during menopause has been shown to help prevent osteoporosis in women. It has cut fractures caused by post menopausal women by half in the United States. The possible side effects of this treatment should be carefully discussed with your physician.

◆ A diet that is adequate in protein, calcium, magnesium, phosphorus, vitamin C and vitamin D, combined with regular exercise, is the best prevention for osteoporosis.

◆ Do not smoke. Smoking accelerates bone loss in both men and women.

Doctor's Notes

We are just beginning to understand the profound role of progesterone in the development of osteoporosis. One very interesting side note is that foods and beverages that are high in phosphorus can actually leach calcium from the bones into the bloodstream as well as impairing its absorption, even if supplements are taken religiously.[21] Phosphorus is found in meat, grains, potatoes and soft drinks. If you already have osteoporosis, phosphorus ingestion can make it worse.

Additional Resources

Medications and Bone Loss
NOF
1150 17th Street, NW, STE 500
Washington, DC 20036

Endnotes

1. G. Finkenstedt, et al. "Lactose absorption, milk consumption, and fasting blood glucose concentrations in women with idiopathic osteoporosis," Br Med Jour, 1986, 292:161-62.

2. M. Horowitz, et al., "Biochemical effects of calcium supplementation in postmenopausal osteoporosis." Eur J Clin Nutr 1988, 42:775-78.

3. R. Heaney, et al., "Menopausal changes in calcium balcane performance," J Lab Clin Med 1978, 92(6):953-63. See also H. Spencer et al., "Absorption of calcium in osteoporosis," Am J Med, 1964, 37: 223.

4. Louis Branett, "The influence of calcium in the periodontal patient," J Holistic Med, 1980, 2(1):32-9. R. Rude et al., "Low serum concentrations of 1,2,5-dihydroxyvitamin D in human magnesium deficiency," J Clin Endocrinol Metab, 1985, 61:933-40.

5. F. Nielson, et al., "Effect of dietary boron on mineral, estrogen and testosterone metabolism in postmenopausal women," Fed Am Soc Exp Biol, 1987, 1(5):394-97.

6. M. Chapu,y et al., "Calcium and vitamin D supplements: Effect on calcium metabolism in elderly people," Am J Clin Nutr, 1987, 6:324-28.

7. D, Rudman, et al., "Fractures in the men of a Veterans Administration nursing home: Relation to 1,25-dihydroxyvitamin D," J Am Coll Nutr, 1989, 8(4):324-34.

8. Alan R. Gaby, M.D., Preventing and Reversing Osteoporosis. (Prima Publishing, Rocklin, California: 1994), 150. See also John R. Lee, M.D. "Osteoporosis reversal: the role of progesterone," Int Clin Nutr Rev. (1990) 10:3, 384-91 and John R. Lee, M.D., "Osteoporosis reversal with transdermal progesterone," Lancet, (1991), 336: 1327 and John R. Lee, M.D., "Is natural progesterone the missing link in osteoporosis prevention and treatment?" Med Hypotheses, 35: 316-18.

9. L. Brattstrom et al., "Folic acid responsive postmenopausal homocysteinemia metabolism," Metabolism, 1985, 34(11):1073-7.

10. P. Benke et al., "Osteoporotic bone disease in the pyridoxine-deficient rat," Biochem Med, 1972, 6:526-35.

11. R.Carmel et al., "Cobalamin and osteoblast-specific proteins," N Engl J Med, 1988, 319:70-75.

12. D. Hyams and E. Ross , "Scurvy, megaloblastic anaemia and osteoporosis," Br J Clin Pract, 1963, 17:332-40. See also W. MacLennan and J. Hamilton, "Vitamin D supplements and 25-hydroxy vitamin D concentrations in the elderly," Br Med J 1977, 2:859-61.

13. Jason Theodosakis, M.D., The Arthritis Cure, (St. Martin's Press, New York: 1997).

14. Daniel B. Mowrey, The Scientific Validation of Herbal Medicine (Keats Publishing, New Canaan, CT: 1986), 32.

15. Ibid., 1.

16. S. Heptinstall, et al., "Extracts of feverfew inhibit granule secretion in blood platelets and polymorphonuclear leukocytes," Lancet, 1985, I: 1071-74.

17. Lee, 384-91.

18. D. Zhy, "Dong quai," Amer Jour Clin Med, 1987, 15(3-4).

19. E.M. Duker, et al., "Effects of extracts from Cimicifuga racemosa on gonadotropin release in menopausal women and ovariectomized

rats," Planta Medica, 1991, 57(5): 420-24.

20. C.H. Costello, E.V. Lynn, "Estrogenic substances from plants: Glycyrrhiza," Jour Amer Pharm Soc, 1950, 39: 177-80.

21. A. Portale, "Oral intake of phosphorus can determine the serum concentration of 1,25-dihydroxyvitamin D by determining its production rate in humans," Jour Clin Invest, 1986, 77: 7-12.

22. M. Burnatowska-Heldin et al., "Aluminum, parathyroid hormone, and osteomalacia," Spec Top Endocrino Metab, 1983, 5:201-26.

23. M. Grossman, et al., "Basal and histalog-stimulated gastric secretion in control subjects and in patients with peptic ulcer or gastric cancer," Gastroenterology, 1963, 45:15-26.

PANIC DISORDER

SEE "ANXIETY"

PARKINSON'S DISEASE

Parkinson's disease is also referred to as "palsy" or "paralysis agitans." It is a degenerative disease of the nervous system. Approximately one person in 200 is affected by this disease with 50,000 new cases diagnosed in the United States each year. Elderly people are the most vulnerable to Parkinson's disease and men are more likely to be affected than women. The disease usually begins between the ages of 50 and 65. Untreated, Parkinson's disease can progress over 10 to 15 years, resulting in severe incapacity. With modern drug treatment and natural supplementation, the outlook is significantly more positive.

Symptoms

This disease will usually begin with a slight tremor of one hand, arm or leg. In this early stage the tremor is worse when the hand or limb is at rest. At this point, using these muscles will stop the shaking. As the disease progresses, both sides of the body will be affected causing weakness, stiffness, an unsure shuffling walk, an overbalanced walk, quick, tiny steps, constant hand trembling, head shaking, drooling, a pill-rolling movement of the thumb and forefinger, unblinking expression, a marked stoop and/or a gradual inability to take care of everyday demands.

When the disease is in its latter stages, intellect may become affected. During this stage, speech may be slow and handwriting illegible. Depression is also commonly apparent in victims of Parkinson's disease.

Causes

The specific cause of this disease is well-known. It is caused by an imbalance of dopamine and acetylcholine, two chemicals found in the brain. A deficiency of dopamine in certain brain cells inhibits brain messages transmitted from one cell to another. As a result, a degeneration of these nerve cell clusters occurs. This degeneration of nerve cells in the brain affects the way muscle tension and movement is controlled, causing the muscles to remain overly tense. There is some speculation that certain medications administered to the elderly, such as stelazine, can cause symptoms which may mimic Parkinson's disease.

Other factors which have been linked to the disease are viral infections, heavy metal exposure, faulty mineral metabolism, manganese poisoning, aluminum ingestion, mercury poisoning and carbon monoxide poisoning.

Drugs which can block the action of dopamine and cause symptoms associated with Parkinson's disease include haloperidol, reserpines, phenothiazines, droperidol, chlorprothizene, thiothixene, methyldopa and lithium.

Parkinson's disease can also be the result of an earlier brain infection such as encephalitis. There is some evidence that Parkinson's disease runs in families.

Conventional Therapies

There is no cure for Parkinson's disease. Medical treatment in the form of drugs can help victims of Parkinson's disease manage their symptoms and lead productive lives. While the side effects of levadopa, the primary drug for this disease are considerable, it can make a significant difference in slowing the progression of the disease and reducing its symptoms. Early on, certain exercises, special aids and support groups will be recommended. In later stages of the disease, levadopa (L-dopa), a substance which the body converts to dopamine may be initially prescribed. This drug can have severe side effects and is usually ineffective if taken alone. Other drugs used in conjunction with levadopa are bromocriptine and amantadine. Supplemental drugs called artane and cogentin are commonly used. Anticholinergic drugs such as trihexyphenidyl may be used to provide relief from tremors. Sinemet, which contains levadopa, is a drug which can help to reduce the stiffness that accompanies the disease. In rare instances, a brain operation may be indicated to reduce rigidity and tremors. This option is usually done in cases where Parkinson's disease has afflicted a young and relatively active person. Current experimentation with transplanting dopamine-secreting adrenal tissue is currently being done and may provide a much better treatment alternative in the future.

Dietary Guidelines

- Drink six to eight glasses of pure water per day. Avoid all alcoholic beverages, nicotine, caffeine, soda pop, chocolate, red meats, sugar and refined flour.
- Eat a diet high in raw fruits and vegetables and low in animal fat.
- Emphasize seeds, grains and nuts. Fresh fava or broad beans are considered a dietary source of levadopa.
- Use flaxseed and olive oils.
- Eating coldwater fish like salmon on a weekly basis is also recommended.
- If taking levadopa, limit your intake of beef, bananas, fish, liver, peanuts, potatoes, whole grains and oatmeal. These foods contain vitamin B6, which can inhibit the drug's action and potency.

Recommended Nutritional Supplements

PRIMARY NUTRIENTS

ALPHA LIPOIC ACID A very powerful antioxidant which potentiates the action of vitamin E and Vitamin C, which are both excellent free radical scavengers in the brain.[1] Researchers at the University of Rochester Medical Center found that ALA protected brain cells from certain hazardous chemicals which have been associated with Parkinson's and Huntington's diseases. *Suggested Dosage:* Take as directed.

VITAMIN E AND SELENIUM Two antioxidant compounds which have been shown to offer protection against Parkinson's by lowering its risk factor.[2] In addition, studies have shown that the progression of this disease may be slowed by supplementation of these two nutrients.[3] *Suggested Dosage:* 800 mg of vitamin E; take selenium as directed.

GRAPE SEED AND PINE BARK EXTRACT Another powerful free radical scavenger which can help collect harmful metabolites in brain tissue.[4] *Suggested Dosage:* Take as directed using a higher dose initially to achieve tissue saturation and then taper off to dosages as directed.

VITAMIN C WITH BIOFLAVONOIDS Open trials using vitamin C as an antioxidant in the early stages of Parkinson's have shown some promise.[5] Vitamin C can also help to counteract the side effects of L-dopa therapy. *Suggested Dosage:* 1,000 to 3,000 mg per day.

ESSENTIAL FATTY ACIDS Because the brain is primarily composed of unsaturated fatty acids, supplying the right kind of fatty acid compounds in diseases like Parkinson's is vital. Canadian researchers have used evening primrose oil as a clinical treatment for Parkinson's and other tremor-causing disorders.[6] *Suggested Dosage:* Two tablespoons of evening primrose oil daily.

GINKGO BILOBA Works to boost brain cell oxygenation which can help inhibit the progression of senile dementia.[7] *Suggested Dosage:* 60 to 80 mg of 24 percent ginkgo flavonglycoside product.

PHOSPHATIDLYSERINE Tests conducted on the elderly show that this compound can help alleviate depression and boost mental function.[8] *Suggested Dosage:* 100 mg with each of three meals daily.

FOLIC ACID A folic acid deficiency has been linked to the development of this disease. Folic deficiency may be associated with Parkinson's disease.[9] *Suggested Dosage:* Take as directed.

NIACIN Nicotinic acid can actually prolong elevated levels of brain dopa and dopamine in patients who were taking L-dopa as a treatment for Parkinson's disease.[10] *Suggested Dosage:* Take as directed. NADH may also be used instead of a simple niacin supplement.

VITAMIN B6 AND THIAMINE Vitamin B6 has been used in clinical trials as a treatment for Parkinson's. It can boost the production of dopamine in the brain. Together with thiamine, it helps to treat disorders of the nervous system.[11] *Suggested Dosage:* Do not take if you are using L-dopa. Ask your doctor about injections of vitamin B6.

MAGNESIUM Levels of this nutrient may be reduced in people with Parkinson's in the caudate nucleus.[12] *Suggested Dosage:* Take 750 mg daily.

L-METHIONINE This essential sulfur-containing amino acid has been used in clinical trials and it has been determined that levadopa can lower concentrations of this amino acid in the cells of the central nervous system.[13] *Suggested Dosage:* Take as directed on an empty stomach and at a different time than L-dopa medication.

L-TYROSINE A deficiency of this amino acid due to reduced food intake exists in many elderly people who do not eat properly and is important for proper brain neurotransmitter production.[14] *Suggested Dosage:* 100 mg daily. Do not take at the same time as L-dopa medication.

HERBAL COMBINATION This combination should include St. John's wort, ginkgo, hops, valerian root, skullcap, wood betony and passionflower.

ST. JOHN'S WORT: Contains hypericum which works to alleviate depression and other brain disorders by elevating certain neurotransmitters.[15] GINKGO BILOBA: Impressive antioxidant herb which also boosts vascular circulation to brain cells affording them enhanced oxygenation.[16] HOPS: Considered an herbal nerve food which also quiets the central nervous system.[17] SKULLCAP: A natural sedative which helps to calm nervous disorders and should be taken in combination with other nervine herbs.[18] VALERIAN: An antispasmodic that helps to calm tremors and promotes safe sleep without dependency or hangover-like effects.[19] WOOD BETONY: A nervine which helps to calm nerves and control the shaking typically seen in Parkinson's disease.[20]

SECONDARY NUTRIENTS

CALCIUM: Works in tandem with magnesium to calm the central nervous system. *Suggested Dosage:* 1,500 mg daily.

GABA: Helps to normalize neurotransmitter activity in the brain. *Suggested Dosage:* Take as directed.

DMAE: Helps to boost choline levels in the brain. *Suggested Dosage:* Take as directed.

DHA: A compound found in fish oil that significantly boost brain function. *Suggested Dosage:* Take as directed.

L-GLUTAMIC ACID: Supports proper nerve transmission. *Suggested Dosage:* Take as directed.

Home Care Suggestions

- Try to get exercise regularly. Water exercises are especially good.
- Get a regular massage from a qualified therapist.
- Become part of a Parkinson's disease support group.
- Make practical changes in your household such as installing bath rail supports, special wall banisters, chairs with high arms, etc.
- The benefits of acupressure or acupuncture should be investigated.

Other Supportive Therapies

ACUPUNCTURE: The earlier stage of Parkinson's disease responds well to acupuncture treatments.

MASSAGE: Gentle massage that is not too intensive can stimulate circulation to muscle tissue.

YOGA: Helps to keep muscles from becoming stiff and inflexible and promotes relaxation, which can help to control symptoms.

Scientific Facts-at-a-Glance

Many scientific studies have linked Parkinson's disease with heavy metal poisoning or with faulty mineral metabolism. Copper levels are typically high in people with the disease.[21] In addition, an excess intake of iron and manganese are thought to be contributing factors.[22] Aluminum toxicity must also be ruled out as a potential cause of this disease. Elevated levels have been found in the brain tissue of people with Parkinson's as well as Alzheimer's diseases.[23]

Spirit/Mind Considerations

Approximately one-third of people suffering from Parkinson's disease will suffer some form of dementia. The deterioration of memory and thought processes can occur in the later stages of the disease. Even in the earlier stages of the disease, the progressive debilitation that occurs can commonly cause severe depression. Learning about the disease is vital for any family member who is close to the person affected. Support groups can be helpful. Taking the time to just listen or provide practical help is very important in preventing the kind of depression that can occur in Parkinson's patients.

Prevention

- Use a powerful blend of antioxidants daily.
- Avoid ingesting aluminum.
- Avoid exposure to heavy metals such as lead, copper, iron and to high levels of carbon monoxide.
- Avoid ingesting large quantities of manganese.
- Check all medications you currently take to see if any of them interfere with dopamine production.
- Stay physically active, eat a diet high in raw vegetables and fruits and low in animal fat.
- Take essential fatty acid supplements daily.
- Use flaxseed and olive oils.

Doctor's Notes

Lifestyle factors play a significant role in determining the risk of developing Parkinson's disease in an individual. Poor diet, smoking, drinking and poor environment (occupational and otherwise) can put a person at greater risk for oxidative damage. Oxidative damage has been implicated in many chronic degenerative diseases, including Parkinson's disease, cataracts, cancer, emphysema, rheumatoid arthritis and hardening of the arteries. There is a strong belief that if this harmful oxidation did not occur, people would be better able to withstand the effects of aging and live much longer. Indeed, some animal studies have demonstrated a 45 percent increase in longevity brought about by a significant increase of antioxidants in the diet. You will notice that many of the nutrients recommended for this disease are powerful antioxidant compounds. If you have been diagnosed with Parkinson's disease, be assured that with the proper medication and supplementation, you can continue to live a quality life. Taking excellent care of yourself and using powerful blends of antioxidants can slow the progression of the disease.

Additional Resources

American Parkinson's Disease Association
116 John Street
New York, NY 10038
(212) 923-4700

Endnotes

1. Lester Packer, Ph.D., et al., "Alpha lipoic acid as as a biological antioxidant," Free Radical Biology and Medicine, 1995, 19: 227-250.

2. L. Golbe, et al., "Follow-up study of early-life protective and risk factors in Parkinson's disease," Mov Disord, 1990, 5(1):66-70.

3. J. Grimes, "Prevention of progression of Parkinson's disease with antioxidative therapy," PRG Neuropsychopharmacol Biol Psychiatry, 1988, 12(2-3):165-72.

4. R.M. Facino, et al., "Free radicals scavenging action and antienzyme activities of procyanidines from Vitis vinifera: as a mechanism for their capillary protective action," Arzneim Forsch, 1994, 44: 592-601.

5. S. Fahn, "An open trial of high-dosage antioxidants in early Parkinson's disease," Am Jour Clin Nutr, 1991, 53:380S-1S.

6. E. Critchley, "Evening primrose oil (Efamol) in Parkinsonian and other tremors: as a preliminary study," in D.F. Horrobin, ed, Clinical Uses of Essential Fatty Acids, (Eden Press, Montreal: 1982), 205-8.

7. H. Allain, et al., "Effect of two doses of ginkgo biloba extract on the dual coding test in elderly subjects," Clin Ther, 1993, 15(3): 549-58.

8. T. Cenacchi, et al., "Cognitive decline in the elderly: as a double-blind placebo-controlled multi center study of Phosphatidylserine administration," Aging, 1993, 5: 123-33. See also E. W. Funfgeld, et al., "Double-blind study with phosphaditylserine in Parkinsonian patients with senile dementia of Alzheimer's type (SDAT)," Prog Clin Biol Res, 1989, 317: 1225-34.

9. P. Clayton, et al. "Subacute combined degeneration of the cord, dementia and Parkinsonism due to an inborn error of folate metabolism," Jour Neorol Neurosurg Psychiatry, 1986, 49:920-27.

10. M. Block and R. Brandft, "Nicotinic acid or N-methyl nicotinamide prolongs elevated brain dopa and dopamine in L-dopa treatment," Biochem Med Metab Biol, 1986, 36(2):244-51.

11. A. Vainshtok, "Treatment of Parkinsonism with large doses of vitamin B6," Sov Med, 1979, 7:14-9. S. Stone, "Pyridoxine and thiamine therapy in disorders of the nervous system," Dis Nerv Sys, 1950, 11(5):131-8.

12. R. Uitti, et al., "Regional metal concentrations in Parkinson's disease, other chronic neurological diseases, and control brains," Can Jour Nerol Sci, 1989, 16(3):310-14.

13. E. Catto E, et al., "Brain monamine changes following the administration of S-adenosyl methionine (SAM)," Neuropharmacol, 1978, 2 and R. Surtees and K. Hyland K, "L-3,4-dihydroxyphenylalanine (Levadopa) lowers central nervous system S-adenosylmethionine concentrations in humans," Jour Neurol Neurosurg Psychiatry, 1990, 53(7): 569-72.

14. P. Lemoine, et al., "L-tyrosine: as a long-term treatment of Parkinson's disease," CR Acad Sci, III: 1989, 309(2): 43-7.

15. G. Harrer and H. Sommer, "Treatment of mild to moderate depression with Hypericum," Phytomedicine, 1994, !: 3-8.

16. J. Kleijnen, et al., "Ginkgo biloba for cerebral insufficiency," Bri Jour Clin Pharm, 1992, 34: 352-58.

17. Daniel B. Mowrey, Ph.D. The Scientific Validation of Herbal Medicine (Keats Publishing, Connecticut, 1986, 2. Mowrey): 164-65.

18. B.A. Kurnakov. "Pharmacology of skullcap." Farmakologastrointestinalia I Toksikologastrointestinalia. 20(6): 79-80, 1957.

19. P.D. Leathwood and F. Chauffard. "Aqueous extract of valerian reduces latency to fall asleep in man." Planta Medica. 54, 144-48, 1985.

20. Jack Ritchason, The Little Herb Encyclopedia, Woodland Publishing, Pleasant Grove, Utah, 1994, 255.

21. H. Pall, et al., "Raised cerebrospinal-fluid copper concentration in Parkinson's disease," Lancet, 2:238-41, 1987).

22. J. Zayed, et al., "Environmental factors in the etiology of Parkinson's disease," Can Jour Nerol Sci, 1990, 17(3):286091. See also T. Florence, "Neurotoxicity of manganese," Letter, Lancet, 1988, 1:363 and I. Mena, in F Bronner, J.W . Xoburn, eds., Disorders of Mineral Metabolism, (Academic Press, New York: 1981), 233-70.

23. E. Hirsch, et al., "Iron and aluminum increase in the substatia nigra of patients with Parkinson's disease: an X-ray microanalysis," Jour Neurochem, 1991, 56(2):446-55.

PERIODONTAL DISEASE

Periodontal disease refers to any disorder which affects the gums or other tissue that surrounds the teeth. Gingivitis which is an inflammation of the gums is considered an early form of periodontal disease and if left untreated, can progress to pyorrhea, which can result in serious complications. Gum disease is a common condition of middle-aged people that can often require painful and expensive dental treatment. According to some estimates, the majority of the American public is at high risk for developing periodontal disease. The average senior citizen has only five natural teeth left. Forty percent of all retired people wear dentures of some type. Men are more susceptible to periodontal disease, and it is also more common among lower social and economic groups.

Symptoms

Gingivitis is characterized by gums that are swollen, sore and bleed upon contact. In addition, the gums can appear red, soft and shiny. Pyorrhea which is an advanced stage of periodontal disease, is characterized by painful, bleeding gums, shrinking or receding gums, localized pain, swelling in the jaw region, sensitivity to hot and cold, toothaches, halitosis, bone loss in the jaw, and abscesses.

See your dentist immediately if you have gums that are shrinking away from your teeth, have an altered bite so that your teeth come together differently than they did before, find pockets of pus between your teeth, find teeth that become loose or fall out, or have gums that continually bleed and stay sore and swollen.

Causes

Gingivitis can be caused by deposits of plaque and bacteria in and around the teeth as a result of poor dental hygiene, food impaction, mouth breathing, tooth grinding, dentures that do not fit properly, faulty dental fillings which can cause gum irritations, missing teeth, tooth decay, a diet low in fibrous foods, lack of vitamin C, folic acid, calcium or niacin, chronic illness, blood diseases such as leukemia or anemia, smoking, poor nutrition, certain drugs, some glandular disorders, excessive consumption of sugar, and alcohol consumption.

Diabetics can be at much higher risk for developing gum disease due to their decreased resistance to infection. Tobacco smoking also increases the risk of gum disease. In addition, pregnant women are also more susceptible to periodontal disease.

Conventional Therapies

Most orthodox treatments are initiated long after gum disease has progressed and can only offer limited success if the disease is advanced. Often teeth are lost which results in full or partial dentures which can be troublesome. Implants offer a better alternative to dentures; however, they are costly and can only be done if bone mass permits. Initial treatment may be to prescribe an antibacterial mouthwash such as peridex and encourage good oral hygiene. In severe cases, x-rays will be taken to determine the condition of the underlying bone. Very loose teeth can be anchored, and cementum that has worn away can be replaced with synthetic material. If pus is present, it is drained through a root canal. Very meticulous cleaning of the teeth can help prevent further plaque and calculus formation. Scaling and root planing are used to accomplish this. Teeth may have to be extracted. If bone loss is extensive, dentures may be required. Antibiotics are routinely prescribed if infection is severe. Periodontal surgery may be required where deep pockets of infection have formed. A gingivectomy is a minor surgical procedure performed in a dentist's office under local anesthesia in which the gums are trimmed. After the surgery, a periodontal pack is used to cover the gums, and it remains in place for about two weeks during which healing takes place. Curettage may be required to remove any diseased lining from gum pockets, so healthy tissue can reattach itself to the tooth. Splinting is a procedure which can anchor loose teeth to ones that are still firmly planted. Osseous surgery may be necessary in advanced cases of periodontal disease to correct bone structure.

Dietary Guidelines

- Eat plenty of raw vegetables and fruits which supply sources of vitamin C and minerals and also serve to stimulate and clean the teeth and gums.
- Avoid refined sugar, white breads, pastries, soda pop, candy, gum, etc. These foods provide an excellent environment for bacterial breeding in the mouth.
- The fact that the Western diet is so high in sugar not only increases rates of tooth decay but can depress the immune system as well which can increase the risk of periodontal disease.
- Make sure your diet is high in calcium and magnesium to help prevent jawbone loss; this can have an adverse effect on the health of teeth and gums. In some studies, even those suffering from advanced periodontal disease showed improvement after taking calcium supplements. Gum inflammation and tooth mobility were both reduced.
- Blueberries are especially recommended for their high content of flavonoid. A high-fiber diet is also desirable due to the fact that fiber causes an increase in salivation.

Recommended Nutritional Supplements

PRIMARY NUTRIENTS

VITAMIN C WITH BIOFLAVONOIDS Vitamin C is excellent for bleeding gums and should be supplemented daily. Bioflavonoids are essential in maintaining collagen integrity in the gums and in boosting the immune system. A lack of vitamin C can also result in increased permeability of the gums to toxins and bacterial invasion.[1] *Suggested Dosage:* 1,000 mg daily.

CALCIUM Taking absorbable forms of calcium may actually reverse the course of periodontal disease while strengthening bone.[2] *Suggested Dosage:* 1,000 to 3,000 mg daily.

MAGNESIUM Magnesium supplements help to boost bone density and prevent bone loss associated with this disease.[3] *Suggested Dosage:* Take as directed.

VITAMIN A Low levels of this vitamin have been linked to the inflammatory changes that can initiate gum disease and deterioration—a condition which can happen more readily during pregnancy.[4] *Suggested Dosage:* Take as directed.

COENZYME Q10 The ability of this nutrient to boost oxygenation of tissue can be of great value when dealing with diseased gums.[5] *Suggested Dosage:* 25 mg twice daily (2-month minimum trial).

VITAMIN D A vitamin D deficiency can impair calcium absorption which is necessary for the maintenance of healthy gums and teeth.[6] *Suggested Dosage:* Take as directed.

VITAMIN E Clinical trials have shown that vitamin E supplementation can help to reduce inflammation not only taken internally but applied orally as well.[7] *Suggested Dosage:* 800 mg daily for three weeks (capsules open and vitamin applied locally before swallowing).

FOLIC ACID Folate mouthwashes have significant effects on well-established gingivitis.[8] *Suggested Dosage:* Take as directed.

ZINC Applying zinc mouthwashes or oral applications can help to inhibit plaque growth which contributes to tooth decay and gum disease.[9] *Suggested Dosage:* Topical application may be beneficial.

HERBAL COMBINATION This combination should contain goldenseal, gotu kola, licorice, and bilberry. *Suggested Dosage:* Take as directed; however, do not use for more than two-week periods at a time.

GOLDENSEAL: The berberine content of this herb has impressive antibacterial properties and astringent properties and boosts the immune system to fight infection as well.[10] GOTU KOLA: Exerts impressive healing properties on damaged gums.[11] LICORICE ROOT: Topical use of licorice as well as internal ingestion can have antibacterial effects.[12] BILBERRY: Stimulates circulation to the gums, calms the inflammatory response, and promotes capillary strength and healing.[13] GREEN TEA EXTRACT: Contains powerful flavonoid compounds, which inhibit inflammation, swelling and pain, and work to effectively scavenge free radicals.[14]

SECONDARY NUTRIENTS

GRAPE SEED OR PINE BARK EXTRACT: The powerful antioxidant and anti-inflammatory action of the proanthocyani-

dins contained in this compound inhibit redness and swelling typical of periodontal disease. *Suggested Dosage:* Take as directed, using higher than normal doses to begin with, for tissue saturation for one week and then taper to normal dosages.

VITAMIN B-COMPLEX: Helps with the regeneration of gum tissue. *Suggested Dosage:* 150 mg daily in divided doses with three meals.

PROTEOLYTIC ENZYMES: Boosts digestion of macronutrients and inhibits the inflammatory response. *Suggested Dosage:* Take as directed 30 minutes before each meal and use products with bromelain, papain and pancreatin.

ECHINACEA: Can be rubbed on the gums in the form of a paste. Also helps to fight infection. *Suggested Dosage:* Use as directed.

MYRRH TEA MOUTH RINSE: Myrrh has a long history in treating periodontal disease. It helps to tone the gums and remove plaque. *Suggested Dosage:* Make as a tea and use as you like.

ALOE VERA GEL: Helps to heal the mouth and gums and can reduce some plaque. Brushing with the gel is recommended. *Suggested Dosage:* Use as directed.

Home Care Suggestions

◆ Take the time to brush and floss correctly and completely. Good oral hygiene takes time and should not be rushed. Brush your teeth, gums and tongue. Use unwaxed dental floss.

◆ Use a soft, flexible toothbrush. Hard toothbrushes can actually scratch and puncture gums, and they do not get into crevices efficiently.

◆ Stimulate your gums daily with rubber devices or special wooden sticks which your dentist can recommend.

◆ Stop smoking and drinking alcohol: Both of these habits can deplete the body of nutrients required for the maintenance of healthy teeth and gums.

◆ There are several natural toothpastes available in health food stores which offer alternatives to the regular ingredients offered in standard tooth pastes. Some of these natural ingredients to watch for are sea salt, calcium bases, silica, baking soda, and myrrh.

◆ Buy oral mouthwashes that contain cetylpyridinium chloride or domiphen bromide which can help reduce plaque. Plax and Listerine are recommended.

◆ Mouthwashes that contain at least 5 percent zinc solution are also recommended for inhibiting the growth of plaque.

◆ Brush with baking soda and water to neutralize acid, eliminate bad breath and clean the teeth. A paste can also be made of water, baking soda and peroxide and left on the gums for long periods of time.

◆ Make sure to brush your gums along with your teeth. Brushing the gums helps to remove hidden food particles and stimulates good circulation which discourages disease.

◆ Rinse your toothbrush with alcohol after using. Toothbrushes can accumulate bacteria.

◆ The use of water jet devices such as a waterpic to remove food particles remains somewhat controversial among dentists. Evidence to support their effectiveness is incomplete.

◆ Have your teeth and gums cleaned by as a professional dental hygienist twice a year.

Other Supportive Therapies

MASSAGE: Gum massage with rubber covered implements or even just manually can help to stimulate circulation and enhance healing and regeneration.

HOMEOPATHY: Mercurius, Kreosotum, and Natrum mur. are all used for inflamed or soft gums and for bad breath or bleeding gums.

Scientific Facts-at-a-Glance

Studies have suggested that mercury poisoning from silver amalgams in dental fillings may cause bleeding gums, increased salivation or a consistent metallic taste. If you experience these symptoms, see you dentist and have him check your existing fillings. Some dentists will be willing to replace mercury fillings with porcelain ones.[15] This is probably a good idea anyway in that mercury fillings are a source of much controversy.

Spirit/Mind Considerations

When a person loses the desire to adequately clean and take care of their teeth, it may signal an emotional problem or the existence of depression. Learning to truly respect our bodies as receptacles for our spirits enables us to practice good habits whereby we take utmost care to preserve what we have. While regular dental checkups are invaluable, there is much we can do for ourselves in order to promote good oral health. In addition, if we feel negative about life, we are often apt to let ourselves go. Dental health is one of the first things that we can begin to neglect. If we have emotional problems that are interfering with our personal hygiene habits, we need to address them first.

Prevention

◆ Good oral hygiene is essential. Taking the time to brush and floss every day is the best prevention for gum disease.
◆ Keep toothbrushes free from bacteria by rinsing them in alcohol after each use.
◆ Keep your immune system healthy. Through proper diet, a healthy immune system can fight the infections which promote gum disease. Eat a diet high in fiber, raw fruits and vegetables and low in sugar and fats.
◆ See your dentist on as a regular basis.

Doctor's Notes

I like to use coenzyme Q10 in combination with gotu kola. A mouthwash made from grape seed extract and Wisdom of the Ages is also very effective. Gum disease is very preventable if good dental hygiene and nutrition is employed. Most cases of gingivitis are the result of poor brushing, a lack of flossing or bad dietary habits. Looking at your diet and replacing sugary junk foods with fresh fruits and vegetables can go a long way. In addition, using vitamin C, calcium, bioflavonoids and compounds like coenzyme Q10, can work to reverse gum disease. I have discovered that many of my patients have a phobia about brushing their teeth properly, hence they harm their gums. Mouth rinses which contain colloidal silver with gotu kola can help. Bilberry, gotu kola, green tree extract and grape seed or pine bark extract work to strengthen and heal the gums and have excellent natural anti-inflammatory properties. Don't forget to incorporate good nutrition as well.

Additional Resources

American Dental Association
211 East Chicago Ave.
Chicago, IL 60611
(312) 440-2500

Endnotes

1. A. Rubinoff, et al., "Vitamin C and oral health," Jour Can Dent Assoc, 1989, 55(9):705-7.
2. E. Uhrbom E and L. Jacobson, "Calcium in periodontitis: Clinical effect of calcium medication," Jour Clin Periodontol, 1984, 11(4):230-41.
3. Louis Branett, reported in H. Huggins, "The influence of calcium in the periodontal patient," Jour Holistic Med, 1980, 2(1):32-9.
4. H. Cerna, et al., "Periodontium and vitamin E and A in pregnancy," Acta Univ Palacki Olomuc Fac Med, 1990, 125:173-9.
5. Y. Iwamoto, et al., "Clinical effect of Coenzyme Q-10 on periodontal disease," in K. Folkers, Y Yamamura, Eds. Biomed and Clin Aspects of Coenzyme Q-10, vol 3 (Elsevier Biomedical Press, Amsterdam, 1981): 109-19.
6. B. Migicovsky and J. Jamieson, Jour Biochem Physiol, 1955, 33:202.
7. Y. Kimura, et al., Jour Japan Assoc Periodontol, 1977, 19:413.
8. A. Pack, "Folate mouthwash: Effects on established gingivitis in periodontal patients," Jour Clin Periodontal, 1984, 11: 619-28.
9. G. Harrap, et al., "Inhibition of plaque growth by zinc salts," Jour Periodont Res, 1983, 18: 634-42.
10. H. Amin, et al., "Berberine sulfate: antimicrobial activity, bioassay and mode of action," Can Jour Microbiol, 1969, 15(9): 1067-76.
11. A. Benedicenti, et al., "The clinical therapy of periodontal disease, the use of potassium hydroxide and the water-alcohol extract of Centella in combination with laser therapy in the treatment of severe periodontal disease," Parondontol Stomatol, 1985, 24:11-26.
12. E. Frossman, et al., "A clinical comparison of antibacterial mouth rinses: effects of chlorhexidine, phenolics, and sanguinarine on dental plaque and gingivitis," Jour Periodontol, 1089, 60(8):435-40.
13. A. Lietti, et al., "Studies on Vaccinium myrtillus anthocyanosides: vasoprotective and anti-inflammatory activity," Arzneim Forsch, 1976, 26(5): 829-32.
14. C. Ho, et al., "Antioxidant effect of polyphenol extract prepared from various Chinese teas," Prev Med, 1992, 21: 520-525.
15. R. Mateer, "Corrosion of amalgam restorations," Jour Dent Res, 1970, 49:339.

PMS

Over 2 million women in the United States suffer from PMS. For many women PMS is most severe two to five days before the menstrual period begins, however it can begin much earlier and persist until the last day of the period. Over 150 symptoms have been associated with PMS. Fortunately, today there is a wealth of information and resources on PMS.

PMS is a condition that can affect women who have menstrual cycles and usually occurs one to two weeks prior to menstruation itself. It has been linked to a number of disorders, and in severe cases can be serious in its implication for its victims and the family of those who suffer from it. Severe PMS can significantly impair the professional and personal lives of affected women. PMS involves emotional, physical and behavioral symptoms. It generally affects women between the ages of 24 and 40.

Symptoms

A whole host of symptoms can occur as a result of PMS and include cramps, bloating, depression, water retention, skin eruptions, headaches, backache, breast tenderness, food cravings, increased appetite, insomnia, fatigue, constipation or diarrhea, heart palpitations, weight gain, anxiety, fatigue, irritability, restlessness, joint pain, personality changes, outbursts of anger, and/or thoughts of suicide.

Causes

PMS is a disorder that results from a hormone imbalance. High levels of estrogen can act as a stimulant to the central nervous system producing anxiety and nervousness. Levels of progesterone help balance the effects of estrogen, but in some cases, progesterone levels decrease and hormonal balance is disrupted. Other possible causes of PMS are food allergies, low blood sugar levels, edema, yeast infections, lead poisoning, nutritional deficiencies, physical and mental stress, and thyroid dysfunction.

Conventional Therapies

PMS is difficult to diagnose and to effectively treat. The use of hormonal therapy and diuretics has significant side effects (although in very severe cases of PMS, it may be warranted). Becoming dependent on tranquilizers, sleeping pills or antidepressants is not recommended. A nutritional and herbal approach should be carefully followed before resorting to these treatments. There is no single treatment that can alleviate all the symptoms associated with PMS. Some physicians will prescribe synthetic progesterone in an attempt to obtain hormonal balance. It is usually given during the last part of the menstrual cycle. Oral contraceptives may be prescribed to inhibit ovulation. Anti-prostaglandin drugs and diuretics are also routinely used. In addition, analgesics, tranquilizers and antidepressants are used to treat PMS.

Dietary Guidelines

- Eat plenty of fresh fruits and vegetables, whole grains, cereals, legumes (beans, peas, lentils), nuts and seeds, soy-based foods like tofu, broiled turkey and chicken and fish.
- Raw almonds as a high protein snack is recommended.
- Drink plenty of water.
- If you are craving sweets like ice cream or chocolate substitute these foods with complex carbohydrates like whole grains, pasta or bagels.
- Stay away from salt, nicotine, alcohol, red meats, high-fat dairy products like butter, sugar and junk foods.
- Eating fatty foods can actually increase PMS symptoms and pain. Ingesting salt can aggravate bloating and water retention.
- Processed foods and even some boxed cereals can be high in salt. Eating high-fiber foods has been found to help clear excess estrogen from the system which can cause symptoms of PMS.
- Eliminating caffeine can also be very beneficial for PMS victims. Caffeine is a stimulant which can contribute to anxiety and nervousness. It has also been linked to an increase in breast tenderness and fibroid tumors.
- Avoid alcohol which can act as a diuretic and deplete the system of needed nutrients.

Recommended Nutritional Supplements

PRIMARY NUTRIENTS

VITAMIN A Recent studies have shown that using vitamin A during the second half of the menstrual cycle can be an effective treatment for PMS.[1] *Suggested Dosage:* Take 25,000 IU daily. CAUTION: Do not take over 10,000 IU if you suspect you might be pregnant.

VITAMIN B6 Using vitamin B6 can help with water retention and can contribute to hormonal balance.[2] *Suggested Dosage:* Take 500 mg daily for three months and assess results for you personally.

ESSENTIAL FATTY ACIDS Natural antiprostaglandin compounds which promote uterine relaxation and inhibit the response which initiates cramping and other PMS symptoms.[3] *Suggested Dosage:* Take as directed in liquid or capsule form and keep refrigerated.

CALCIUM AND MAGNESIUM Calcium helps to quiet the central nervous system and to alleviate muscle cramping. It is also good for breast tenderness. Magnesium inhibits prostaglandins and was shown in studies to calm cramps by acting as a natural muscle relaxant.[4] *Suggested Dosage:* 1,500 mg of calcium and 1,000 mg of magnesium. Use calcium lactate, gluconate or citrate and chelated magnesium. Take with vitamin B6 for better assimilation.

VITAMIN E Tests have shown that even when blood levels may appear to be normal, vitamin E supplementation may still be warranted for PMS.[5] It helps to quiet cramps and acts as a reproductive organ tonic also contributing to hormonal balance. *Suggested Dosage:* Take 300 IU daily for a two month trial period then increase to 600 IU daily if initial dosage seems ineffective.

VITAMIN B-COMPLEX Helps reduce premenstrual tension. In some instances, brewer's yeast has decreased the severity of menstrual discomfort, including depression. Some research suggests that menstruation may cause a functional deficiency of vitamin B6.[6] *Suggested Dosage:* 150 mg per day.

VITAMIN B3 (NIACIN) Impressive results from studies found that 90 percent of 80 women with serious menstrual cramps treated with niacin found relief. It is thought that niacin acts as a natural vasodilator.[7] *Suggested Dosage:* Take 200 mg per day and every two to three hours for cramps. Expect flushing and some dizziness during intensive therapy.

VITAMIN C WITH BIOFLAVONOIDS Helps to strengthen blood vessels and capillary walls in the uterine system.[8] *Suggested Dosage:* 1,500 mg daily.

IRON Clinical studies found that women with cramps who were anemic experienced a complete disappearance of menstrual pain following iron supplementation.[9] *Suggested Dosage:* Take only as directed and keep out of the reach of children.

TYROSINE AND 5-HYDROXY TRYPTOPHAN These amino acids can help to discourage depression, anxiety and food cravings by raising serotonin, which are all typical symptoms of PMS.[10] *Suggested Dosage:* Take as directed on an empty stomach with fruit juice.

ST. JOHN'S WORT AND GINKGO These naturally raise serotonin, which helps alleviate the anxiety and depression associated with PMS. *Suggested Dosage:* Take as directed.

WILD YAM (CREAM OR TOPICAL) Dr. John Lee, in his book *Natural Progesterone*, discusses the merits of using wild yam as a precursor to progesterone in the body and its beneficial effects for PMS and other female disorders. He points out that PMS is usually a result of an estrogen dominance. *Suggested Dosage:* Use cream or other topical form as directed. Rotate areas and take a break during your period.

HERBAL COMBINATION TO PREVENT MENSTRUAL CRAMPS This combination hould include boswellia, turmeric, ginger and cramp bark. *Suggested Dosage:* Take as directed.

BOSWELLIA: This herb has impressive anti-inflammatory compounds which are good for alleviating pain.[11] TUMERIC: Works to inhibit the biological processes which contribute to pain.[12] GINGER: A carminative herb which catalyzes the action of other herbs. CRAMP BARK: Also known as black haw, this herb has a long history of use as a uterine muscle relaxant.[13]

HERBAL COMBINATION TO TREAT MENSTRUAL CRAMPS This combination should include black cohosh, blue cohosh, dong quai, passionflower, red raspberry leaves, fenugreek seeds, licorice root, chamomile, black haw bark, saw palmetto berries, wild yam root, kelp and butternut root bark. *Suggested Dosage:* Four to six capsules daily. For chronic conditions and imbalances maximum dosage of six capsules per day should be taken for several months or until normal function is restored. Best if used daily throughout the month. CAUTION: Do not take these herbs if pregnant or lactating.

BLACK COHOSH ROOT: Black cohosh has been proven to be an effective remedy for painful menstrual cramps and other hormonally induced disorders and has received official recognition in Britain and Germany. Studies have shown black cohosh root to have endocrine activity with the ability to mimic estrogen.[14] BLUE COHOSH: This herb was used so extensively by Native American women, it also became known as squaw root. It is effective for menstrual cramps and PMS-related symptoms. It acts as a natural antispasmodic which helps to relax uterine muscle. DONG QUAI: There is no other herb used more widely in Chinese medicine for treatment of gynecological ailments than dong quai. Dong quai relieves menstrual cramps, corrects irregular or retarded menstrual flow, and alleviates unpleasant symptoms associated with menopause. Dong quai is said to have analgesic properties but this is probably due, in part, to its antispasmodic effect.[15] As a side note, dong quai has been used to treat anemia which can result from excessive blood loss during menstruation. PASSIONFLOWER: Many women experience anxiety prior to and during menses, and discomforts such as hot flashes when adjusting to menopause. Passionflower contributes a sedative action for anxiety and relieves spasms and cramps.[16] It has an overall calming effect. RED RASPBERRY LEAVES: Red raspberry leaves have long been used for various female afflictions during pregnancy and child birth in addition to those associated with menses. More specifically it strengthens and tonifies the uterus, stops hemorrhages, decreases excess and increases deficient menstrual flow, and relieves painful menstruation by relaxing the smooth muscles.[17] FENUGREEK SEEDS: Although fenugreek seed has been used to assist proper menstruation and promote lactation, its main role in this formula stems from its other properties. Fenugreek is a tonic, mild diuretic, and a source for mucilage which provides soothing demulcent properties. Like many other seeds, fenugreek is nutritious and restorative, strengthening those recovering from illness or imbalances. LICORICE ROOT: Licorice root is incorporated into about a third of all Chinese herbal formulas and a majority of the formulas dealing with female reproductive problems. This is an indication that it has tremendous versatility. Indeed, licorice supports the effects of all the other herbs of the formula. Licorice not only contains hormonal precursors but stimulates the production of estrogen.[18] This has been shown to decrease the symptoms associated with hormone fluctuation. CHAMOMILE: Aside from chamomile's carminative and tonic properties, this herb has gained world recognition for its anodyne (pain relieving), antispasmodic, and antianxiety properties. Chamomile has demonstrated its worth in many clinical studies, officially monographed in Britain, Belgium, France, and Germany. BLACK HAW BARK (CRAMP BARK): Historical and folkloric use as well as scientific evidence have proven this bark to be effective against muscle spasms and menstrual dysfunction, especially inconsistent estrus cycles and menstrual cramping.[19] SAW PALMETTO BERRIES: One study has shown this herb to be many times more effective than prescription anti-inflammatory medication in the treatment of pelvic congestion associated with menstrual dysfunction.[20] As an interesting side note, saw palmetto can prevent the growth of unwanted facial hair in women. WILD YAM ROOT: Wild yam root contains the steroidal saponins botogenin and diosgenin. These are precursors to cortisone and other hormones like progesterone.[21] Wild yam has antispasmodic effects and is soothing to the nerves. It is also diuretic and helps to eliminate painful urination. It is highly recommended for cramping. KELP: Kelp provides important trace elements which are often missing or deficient in Western diets. Trace elements assist with many metabolic processes in the body, without which may lead to various problems. Kelp contains algin which provides soothing benefits to the gastrointestinal tract. BUTTERNUT ROOT BARK: Butternut is a soothing laxative which helps to restore general health and sense of well-being. Its laxative effect in this formula may be too gentle for it to be obvious.

SECONDARY NUTRIENTS

NERVINE HERBS (VALERIAN, KAVA, PASSIONFLOWER, SKULLCAP AND HOPS): These herbs can safely promote muscle relaxation and sleep during painful periods. *Suggested Dosage:* Take as directed. These herbs may be taken individually or in a combination.

MELATONIN: Also helps to initiate and sustain restful sleep. *Suggested Dosage:* Take as directed starting with smaller than suggested doses and see how you react.

ZINC AND CHROMIUM PICOLINATE: Helps the body regulate prostaglandins which can cause menstrual cramps and help with stabilizing blood sugar levels. *Suggested Dosage:* Take as directed.

IRON: Helps to eliminate anemia which can result from heavy periods. Fatigue and depression can result from a low hemoglobin count which occurs in anemia. *Suggested Dosage:* Take only as directed. Keep out of the reach of children.

LECITHIN: Helps with nerve transmissions. *Suggested Dosage:* Take as directed in granule or capsule form.

CHASTE BERRY: Contributes to hormonal balance. *Suggested Dosage:* Take as directed, using standardized products.

Home Care Suggestions

- Exercise can be an invaluable tool against PMS. Take a brisk walk on a regular basis to release endorphins which are brain chemicals that ease pain and create a sense of well being. Exercise also helps to reduce breast tenderness, food cravings, water retention and depression.
- Try to keep a positive mental attitude through yoga, breathing exercises, or visualization therapy.
- Discuss PMS with your family and let them know when you are experiencing it. Keep a record of PMS on your calendar and learn to recognize it for what it is.
- Keep your stress levels as low as possible. Take walks, listen to soft music, get a massage, soak in an herbal bath, etc. Try not to schedule high stress events during times of PMS.
- Don't take diuretics that can increase stress on the body by depleting it of essential minerals.

Other Supportive Therapies

AROMATHERAPY: Rose and geranium oil can help to discourage soreness when rubbed into the breasts.

HOMEOPATHY: These remedies may include lachesis, sepia, and pusatilla (for mood changes); belladonna (for hot flashes); graphites (for loss of libido and emotional instability); cimicifuga (depression, irritability, restlessness); caulophyllum (nervous tension, anxiety, emotional instability, joint pains); and arnica (backache, tiredness, aching muscles).

ACUPUNCTURE: Can help relieve stress and anxiety and work to alleviate hot flashes and back pain.

Scientific Facts-at-a-Glance

Anyone who has chronic PMS should investigate the possibility of a vaginal yeast infection or the presence of candida, which may have gone undetected. There is significant speculation that many women suffer from yeast infections that cause a number of seemingly unrelated symptoms associated with PMS.[23]

Spirit/Mind Considerations

PMS can cause mild to severe personality changes including depression, lethargy, irritability, agitation, sleep disturbances, nervousness, short temper, violent outbursts, a withdrawal of affection and thoughts of suicide. Virtually every community has PMS support groups. Contact your local health woman's center and participate in PMS reduction programs. Counseling may also offer some benefit through self-help groups. Use meditation or relaxation exercises to manage tension.

Prevention

- Take an essential fatty acid supplement daily.
- Increasing your intake of calcium/magnesium, the B-vitamins, zinc and potassium prior to your period may also help to minimize PMS.
- Making sure that your diet is adequately supplemented with vitamins and minerals throughout the cycle also helps to control PMS.
- Taking certain herbal supplements all month long that specifically target the female reproductive system may be indicated in severe PMS.
- PMS can be avoided or minimized by eating a nutritious, well-balanced diet that is high in fiber, fresh fruits and vegetables and low in fat and sugar.

◆ Regular exercise works wonders in preventing or decreasing PMS. Walking every day can help to alleviate a number of PMS symptoms.

Doctor's Notes

Various symptoms of PMS start somewhere between day 14 of the menstrual cycle and can continue until the first or second day of menstrual flow. New research has found that stimulating or enhancing serotonin in the brain can be more effective than hormonal therapy. This explains the rationale for using drugs like Prozac and Zoloft to treat PMS. With this in mind, using St. John's wort (or a combination of St. John's wort, tyrosine and 5-hydroxy-tryptophan, along with nervine herbs like valerian or kava kava) is a good idea. These supplements should be started on day 14 of the cycle and continue through to the end of the menstrual period.

The use of phytoestrogens like the ones found in soy isoflavones and red clover is also beneficial. I recommend that all my patients increase soy-based foods in their diet, especially women who have problems with hormonal fluctuation. Using phytoestrogenic herbs like black cohosh, chaste berry and blue cohosh in combination with evening primrose oil can be very helpful. In addition, studies conducted in South America using a combination of saw palmetto and pygeum (which are typically used for prostate problems), can also be effective for relieving PMS.

More and more research suggests that PMS is caused by faulty hormonal balance coupled with nutrient deficiencies. Several clinical studies in which women were given multivitamin and mineral supplements showed that after three months of treatment, significant improvement in PMS symptoms were noted. This indicates that many women may be much more depleted of essential nutrients than previously thought, and that adequate nutrition and supplementation directly affects hormonal balance.

Additional Resources

PMS Access
PO Box 9362
Madison, WI 53715
(800) 222-4767 or (608) 833-4767

Premenstrual Syndrome Action
PO Box 16292
Irvine, CA 92713
(714) 854-4407

Endnotes

1. E. Block, "The use of vitamin A in premenstrual tension," Acta Obstet Gynecol Scand, 1960, 39:586-92.
2. J. Kleijnen, et al., "Vitamin B6 in the treatment of premenstrual syndrome: a review." Br J Obstet Gynaecol, 1990, 97(9):847-52.
3. P. Ockerman, et al., "Evening primrose oil as a treatment of the premenstrual syndrome," Recent Adv Clin Nutr, 1986, 2:404-05. See also G.E. Abraham, "Primary dysmenorrhea," Clin Obstet, Gyn, 1978, 21(1): 139-45.
4. S.Thys-Jacobs, et al., "Calcium supplementation in premenstrual syndrome: a randomized crossover trial," Jour Gen Intern Med, 1989, (3):183-9. H. Fontana-Klaiber and B. Hogg, "Therapeutic effects of magnesium in dysmenorrhea," Schweiz Rundsch Med Prax, 1990, 79 (6): 491-94.
5. C. Chuong, et al., "Vitamin E levels in premenstrual syndrome," Am Jour Obstet Gynecol, 1990, 163(5 Pt. 1): 1591-5. E. Butler and E. McKnight, "Vitamin E in the treatment of primary dysmenorrhea," Lancet, 1955, 1: 844-47.
6. M. Bergman, et al., "Vitamin B6 in premenstrual syndrome," Jour Ame Diet Asso, 1990, 90(6): 859-61.
7. A. Hudgins, "Vitamins P, C, and niacin for dysmenorrhea therapy," West Jour Surg Gyn, 1954, 62: 610-11.
8. B. Cox and W Butterfield, "Vitamin C supplements and diabetic cutaneous capillary fragility," Bri Med Jour, 1975, 3: 205.
9. N. Shafer, "Iron in the treatment of dysmenorrhea: A Preliminary report," 1965, 7: 365-66.
10. G. Abraham, "Nutrition and the premenstrual tension syndromes," J Appl Nutr. 1984, 36:103-24, 1984).
11. G. Singh, "Pharmacology of an extract of salai guggal ex Bosewellis serrata, a new non-steroidal anti-inflammtory agent, Agents Action, 1986, 18, 407-12.
12. A. Mukhopadhyay, et al., "Anti-inflammatory and irritant activities of curcumin analogues in rats," Agents Actions, 1982, 12: 508-15.
13. "New methods is pharmacognosy: chromatographic evaluation of commercial viburnum drugs," Deytsche Apot Zei, 1965, 105(40): 1371-72.
14. E.M. Duker, et al., "Effects of extracts from Cimicifuga racemosa on gonadotropin release in menopausal women and ovariectomized rats," Planta Medica, 1991, 57(5): 420-24.
15. D. Zhy, "Dong quai," Amer Jour Clin Med, 1987, 15(3-4): 1987.
16. E. Speroni and E. Minghetti, "Neuropharmacological activity of extracts from Passiflora incarnata," Planta Medica, 1988, 54(6): 488-91.
17. Mark Pederson, Nutritional Herbology, (Wendell Whitman, Warsaw, In: 1995), 145.
18. C.H. Costello, E.V. Lynn, "Estrogenic substances from plants: Glycyrrhiza," Jour Amer Pharm Soc, 1950, 39: 177-80.
19. P.H. List, et al., Hagers Hanbuch der Pharmazeutischen Praxis, vols. 2-5, (Springer-Verlag, Berlin.)
20. Rebecca Flynn, M.S., Your Guide to Standardized Herbal Products, (One World Press, Prescott, AZ: 1995), 67-69.
21. John R. Lee, M.D., Natural Progesterone: The Multiple Roles of a Remarkable Hormone, revised (BLL Publishing, Sebastopol, California: 1993).
22. A. Stewart, "Clinical and biochemical effects of nutritional supplementation on the premenstrual syndrome," Jour Repro Med, 1987, 32(6): 435-41.
23. J. Schinfeld, "PMS and candidiasis: Study explores possible link," Female Patient, July 1987, 66.

PNEUMONIA

Over 2 million cases of pneumonia are diagnosed in our country annually. Pneumonia is an inflammation of the lung which can be caused by a wide variety of bacteria, viruses and fungi. Most viral pneumonias are mild. A recently discovered form of pneumonia is legionnaire's disease, caused by a bacteria. This form of pneumonia can occur in epidemics or can be restricted to a small number of cases. Pneumonia is the sixth most common cause of death in the United States and is considered an opportunistic infection. It is a common complication of any serious illness. It occurs more often in males during infancy and old age and in people whose immune system has been compromised such as alcoholics or people suffering from aids or leukemia. Pneumonia generally lasts for two weeks. Elderly people who contract the disease often fail to respond to treatment and death can occur due to respiratory failure. "Double pneumonia" is the term used when both lungs are infected with the disease.

Symptoms

◆ Pneumonia typically causes fever, headache, malaise, chills, cough, rapid breathing, nausea, vomiting, coughing up rust-colored sputum, sweating, and chest pain.
◆ There may be a bluish tinge to the skin and, occasionally, mental confusion or delirium.
◆ The larger the infected area in the lung, the more severe the symptoms will be. After recovering from pneumonia, it is common to feel fatigued for up to 8 weeks.
◆ Contact your physician immediately if you have shortness of breath, pain upon breathing, or if you cough up blood-tinged sputum.

Causes

Pneumonia can result when bacteria, viruses, fungi or other foreign substances enter the lungs and cause inflammation. When the epiglottis, which forms a protective barrier for the lungs, becomes weakened in the event of a stroke, surgery, or during loss of consciousness or seizure, microbe invasion can occur and increase the risk of infection. Other factors that predispose one to contracting pneumonia are smoking, malnutrition, kidney failure, asthma, sickle cell anemia, certain cancers, chronic viral infections of the upper respiratory tract, complication of influenza or AIDS, inhaling poisonous gases, and taking immunosuppressive drugs.

Viruses that can cause pneumonia are the adenovirus, the syncytial virus or the coxsackie virus. Bacterial pneumonia is most often the result of the streptococcus strain. Hemophilus influenzae and legionella pneumophilia can also cause the disease.

Conventional Therapies

Bacterial infections respond well to antibiotic therapy. Lives can be saved by administering specific antibiotics for pneumonia infections; however, one must be certain that the pneumonia is bacterially caused. To determine what type of infection is present, lab tests will be ordered and sputum samples taken. Antibiotic therapy will be initiated, which can be administered orally or in injection form. For bacterial pneumonia, penicillin and erythromycin will be prescribed. For viral infections tetracycline is sometimes prescribed if subsequent bacterial infection results. Simple viral infections do not respond to antibiotics. To diagnose pneumonia, listening to the chest will be carefully done to check for the presence of fine, crackling noises. If pneumonia is present, tapping the chest will produce characteristic thud-like sounds. Chest x-rays are required to make a definitive diagnosis. In severe cases, hospitalization may be required where oxygen therapy and artificial ventilation can take place. If the lungs do not respond to conventional treatments, a bronchoscopy may be ordered to exclude the possibility of lung cancer. Six weeks after recovery, another chest x-ray should be ordered to make sure the pneumonia is totally gone.

Dietary Guidelines

◆ Drink large amounts of fluid in the form of water, vegetable juices, fruit juices (dilute in half with water), soups, broths, fresh lemon juice in water and herb teas.
◆ Avoid caffeine, nicotine, alcohol, sugar, and greasy foods.
◆ Limit your sugar consumption. Eat raw fruits and vegetables and do not eat any dairy products during the infection. These foods can promote the production of mucus.
◆ Green drinks made from juicing green peppers, parsley, spinach, etc., are also recommended. Try to eat as much garlic and onion as possible.

Recommended Nutritional Supplements

PRIMARY NUTRIENTS

VITAMIN A Essential for lung tissue regeneration and to stimulate immune function. Laboratory tests have proven that vitamin A can help restore immune function even when health has been compromised.[1] *Suggested Dosage:* 25,000 IU during the infection then reduce to 10,000 when better. Do not exceed 10,000 IU if you are pregnant.

BETA CAROTENE A powerful antioxidant compound that helps protect lung tissue from oxidative damage caused by toxic fumes, smoke or infection.[2] *Suggested Dosage:* Take as directed.

VITAMIN C WITH BIOFLAVONOIDS The earlier this vitamin is used the better. Vitamin C is considered an antimicrobial compound which has wonderful anti-inflammatory properties. It also boosts immunity and acts to scavenge dangerous free radicals caused by pneumonia infection.[3] In addition, as a recent study of elderly patients hospitalized for bronchitis and pneumonia found that even modest doses of vitamin C were beneficial.[4] *Suggested Dosage:* 10,000 mg daily in three divided doses with meals.

QUERCETIN Quercetin is a bioflavonoid which is capable of antioxidant activity and has the ability to fight against respiratory viruses.[5] *Suggested Dosage:* Take as directed. May be part of a flavonoid blend.

GARLIC A powerful infection fighter used for both viral and bacterial infections. When mice were infected with the influenza virus, garlic supplementation protected against the development of the disease.[6] Garlic can be effective in fighting a broad range of infectious microorganisms. *Suggested Dosage:* Take two capsules with each of three meals.

ZINC LOZENGES Helps to stimulate immunity and fights both the viral and bacteria infections that cause pneumonia.[7] *Suggested Dosage:* Do not take more than 100 mg of zinc per day. Use zinc gluconate products.

GOLDENSEAL Has natural antiviral and antibiotic properties from its berberine content, which can augment immune function.[8] *Suggested Dosage:* Take as directed using guaranteed potency products. CAUTION: Do not take goldenseal for more than two weeks at a time. If you are pregnant, nursing or allergic to ragweed pollen, do not use this herb.

ST. JOHN'S WORT Recent studies have demonstrated the impressive antiviral properties of the hypericin content of this herb.[9] If you have a virally caused pneumonia, this herb is of value. *Suggested Dosage:* Take as directed using guaranteed potency products.

ECHINACEA Considered an immunostimulant, echinacea has the ability to help fight infections by potentiating the action of white blood cells.[10] *Suggested Dosage:* Take as directed, using high quality products with guaranteed potency. Do not take for more than two weeks at a time.

ASTRAGALUS A Chinese herb historically used to fight infections.[12] *Suggested Dosage:* Take as directed.

HERBAL COMBINATION This combination should include echinacea, goldenseal, myrrh gum, garlic, licorice, blue vervain, butternut, and kelp. *Suggested Dosage:* Take two to four capsules with each meal.

ECHINACEA: This herb has become a staple both in Europe and the U.S. It is used to fight viral and bacterial infections, and also improves the mobility of infection-combating leukocytes (white blood cells).[13] Echinacea should not be used for longer than two weeks at a time. GOLDENSEAL ROOT: Two of goldenseal's more active compounds, hydrastine and berberine, have demonstrated effectiveness in treating bacterial and viral infections. It also stimulates

immune function and acts as an anti-inflammatory agent.[14] MYRRH GUM: Myrrh gum stimulates phagocyte activity and reduces inflammation of the mucous membrane of the lungs.[15] GARLIC: Garlic is another herb that can be considered a tonic. It is a powerful agent against infections of various types and origins. Garlic can increase the number of leukocytes (white blood cells) that help fight infections. In addition, garlic increases perspiration which further cleanses the body.[16] LICORICE ROOT: Licorice root boosts adrenal function, which augments immune defenses and also exerts anti-inflammatory and antibacterial actions.[17] Long-term use of licorice is not recommended, as it may cause weakness, electrolyte imbalances, water retention and hypertension. BLUE VERVAIN: Blue vervain has the ability to break the cycle of chronically occurring infections and helps reduce fever. BUTTERNUT ROOT BARK: Butternut improves liver function, stimulates bile production and flow, and acts as a laxative without gripping, helping the body rid itself of toxins. KELP: Kelp's function in this formula is to provide needed trace elements important in many metabolic processes in the body. These nutrients may further support the healing process and return the body to normal function.

SECONDARY NUTRIENTS

LACTOBACILLUS ACIDOPHILUS: Lack of acidolphilus leads to immune system dysfunction. *Suggested Dosage:* Take as directed first thing in the morning and before retiring. Use guaranteed bacterial count products with bifidobacteria that are not milk based. Check expiration date.

VITAMIN E: A deficiency of this vitamin has been linked to infections like pneumonia. Moreover, this vitamin works to scavenge for free radicals in the lungs. *Suggested Dosage:* 400 to 800 IU per day.

GRAPE SEED OR PINE BARK EXTRACT: Powerful compounds called proanthocyanidins help to scavenge for free radicals in the lungs and have a natural anti-inflammatory action. *Suggested Dosage:* Take as directed, although you may want to start off with a higher dosage during the infection for tissue saturation and then taper off.

CHINESE MUSHROOMS (MAITAKE, SHITAKE OR REISHI): Special compounds found in these mushrooms have proven their ability to fight infection by enhancing immune function. *Suggested Dosage:* Take as directed.

ESSENTIAL FATTY ACIDS: Studies have found that oils of evening primrose, fish and linseed have an innate antibacterial action. *Suggested Dosage:* Take as directed in liquid form (two tablespoons a day) or in capsules.

LOBELIA AND THYME: Considered natural expectorants to help move out mucus. *Suggested Dosage:* Take as directed. Lobelia can cause nausea.

Home Care Suggestions

- Coughing should not be suppressed with cough medicines. Coughing brings up sputum and mucous and should be encouraged unless it becomes too irritating.
- Apply a heating pad or hot water bottle to the chest to ease pain.
- Increase fluid intake to thin secretions in the lungs, which encourages a productive cough.

◆ Increase air moisture with a cool mist vaporizer. Make sure that bed clothes and linen are changed often to prevent chilling.

◆ Hang the top half of your body off the bed and stay that way for 5 to 15 minutes to promote mucus drainage.

Other Supportive Therapies

HOMEOPATHY: Aconite, bryonia and phosphorus are all used for different symptoms caused by pneumonia.

Scientific Facts-at-a-Glance

Today with all the emphasis we place on low-fat diets, it is fascinating to learn that too much dietary fat and an excess of cholesterol can actually increase our susceptibility to infection. Recent studies concluded that cholesterol may suppress antibody production, and that excess lipid consumption can encourage infection due to its inflammatory properties.[18]

Spirit/Mind Considerations

Pneumonia is one of a very long list of diseases that can strike when immunity is compromised by chronic stress. Taking time out to recuperate from stress is vital to preventing infectious diseases organisms from taking hold. So many cases of pneumonia are secondary infections that result as a complication of a less serious disease like the flu. If we do not deal with tension on a level we can understand, our immune defenses will be weakened and we will undoubtedly become more prone to infections like pneumonia.

Prevention

◆ Eat plenty of garlic and onion.

◆ Don't smoke or consume alcohol. Both of these habits can increase the risk for pneumonia as well as other respiratory illnesses.

◆ Keep your immune system healthy by eating nutritious foods that are high in raw fruits, vegetables, and fiber and low in sugar and meat. In addition, use certain herbal and nutritional supplements geared toward fortifying immunity.

◆ Make sure to get an adequate daily supply of vitamin C with bioflavonoids.

◆ A vaccine is now available that can offer protection against some 23 strains of pneumonia, which make up approximately 80 percent of pneumonia cases in the United States. It is recommended that everyone over 65, with their doctor's approval, should receive this vaccine along with the influenza vaccination.

Endnotes

1. Pharmacology, April, 1985, 30: 181-87.

2. N.I. Krinksy, "Antioxidant function of carotenoids," 1989, Free Rad Biol Med, 7: 627-35.

3. Annals of Nutrition and Metabolism, May-June, 1984, 28: 186-91.

4. C. Hunt, et al., "The clinical effects of vitamin C supplementation in elderly hospitalized patients with acute respiratory infections," Inter Jour of Vit Nutri Res, 1994, 64: 212-19.

5. I. Musci and B.M. Pragai, "Inhibition of virus multiplication and alteration of cyclic AMP levels in cell cultures by flavonoids," Experientia, 1985, 41: 930-31.

6. K. Nagai, "Experimental studies on the preventative effect of garlic extract against infection with influenza virus," Jpn Jour Infect Dis, 1973, 47: 321. See also N.D. Weber, et al., "In vitro virucidal effects of Allivum sativum (garlic) extract and compounds," Planta Medica, 1992, 58: 417-23. See also B. Hughes, et al., "Antimicrobial effects of Allium sativum (Garlic), Allium ampeloprasum (elephant garlic, and Allium cepa, (onion): Garlic compounds and commercial garlic supplement products," Phytother Res, 1991, 5:154-8.

7. G.A. Eby and G.R. Davis, "Reduction in duration of common colds by zinc gluconate lozenges in a double-blind study," Anti Microb Agents Chemo, 1984, 25: 20-24.

8. Y. Kumazawa, et al., "Activation of peritoneal macrophages by berberine alkaloids in terms of induction of cytostatic activity," Int Jour Immunpharmacol, 1984, 6: 587-92.

9. H. Someya, "Effect of a constituent of Hypericum erectum on infection and multiplication of Epstein-Barr virus," Jour Tokyo Med Coll, 1985, 43: 815-26.

10. Braunig B, et al., "Echinacea purpurea radix for strengthening the immune response in flu-like infections," Z Phytother 1992,13:7-13.

11. A. Amin et al., "Berberine sulfate: antimicrobial activity, bioassay, and mode of action," Can Jour Microbiol, 1969, 15(9):1067-76.

12. Y. Yang, et al., "Effect of Astragalus membranaceous on natural killer cell activity and induction with Coxsackie B viral myocarditis," Chin Med Jour, 1990, 103(4):304-7 1990.

13. B. Luettig, et al., "Macrophage activation by the polysaccharide arabinogalactan isolated from plant cell cultures of Echinacea purpurea," Journal of the National Cancer Institute, 1989, 81: 669-75.

14. T. Kumazawa, et al., "Activation of peritoneal macrophages by berberine alkaloids in terms of induction of cytostatic activity," Int Jour Immunopharmacol, 1984, 6: 587-92.

15. F. Ellingwood, American Materia Medica, Therapeutics and Pharmacognosy, Eclectic Medical Publication, Portland, Oregon: 1983.

16. B.G. Hughes and L. Lawson, "Antimicrobial effects of Allivum sativum (Garlic)," Phototherapy Res, 1991, 5: 154-58.

17. N. Abe, et al., "Interferon induction by glycyrrhizin and glycyrrhetinic acid in mice," Micorb Immunol, 1982, 26: 353-359.

18. J. Wan et al., "Invited comment: Lipids and the development of immune dysfunction and infection," JPEN J Parenter Enteral Nutr, 1988, 12(6): suppl, 43S-52S.

PREGNANCY-RELATED COMPLICATIONS

Changes in hormones, as well as weight, physiological factors, and nutrition-related conditions linked to pregnancy can cause a number of problems, ranging from minor to life threatening. During pregnancy, which usually lasts for approximately 280 days, a number of medical problems and discomforts can occur. The presence of progesterone can result in conditions like constipation. The pressure from the growing fetus places stress on the abdomen and bladder and can cause gas, heartburn and frequent urination. Increased pressure from the enlarged uterus on major blood vessels can cause feelings of dizziness. The rise in estrogen which accompanies pregnancy can also result in swelling which is usually seen in the hands and feet. These and others comprise a long list of pregnancy-related ailments.

Symptoms

Pregnancy typically causes constipation, gas and heartburn, nausea and vomiting, backache, sleeping difficulties, anemia, groin spasms, leg cramping, varicose veins, dizziness and fatigue, bleeding gums, hemorrhoids, mood changes, shortness of breath, pigmentation spots, urinary tract infections, incontinence, nosebleeds, stretch marks, sore ribs, skin disorders, sweating, frequent urination, swelling, and high blood pressure.

Serious problems associated with pregnancy are toxemia, Rh incompatibility, ectopic pregnancy, spontaneous abortion, hemorrhaging, placenta previa, placenta abrupta, or a premature rupture of the membranes which may result in premature birth.

WARNING: If you are pregnant and have any of the following symptoms, see your doctor immediately: bleeding, swelling of face and hands, persistent headache, blurred vision, a rise in blood pressure, sharp abdominal pains, early contractions, fever, or an absence of fetal movement.

Conventional Therapies

Pregnancy is a time that should be spent under the care of a qualified physician; however, the use of medication should be avoided and taken only with your doctor's approval. Doctors will routinely prescribe certain antacids, prenatal vitamins, bed rest, salt-restricted diets and specific exercises to help alleviate the many discomforts that can accompany pregnancy. Regular visits to a physician are recommended. During these visits, weight and blood pressure will be monitored. At times, blood samples will be taken to check for anemia, and iron supplements may be prescribed. Urine samples will be checked for the presence of sugar. Regular medical care can help to detect problems like toxemia that are potentially life threatening.

While prenatal care under general practitioners and obstetricians is considered very good, there is significant evidence that up to half of the Cesarean sections performed in the United States each year are not necessary. The threat of potential lawsuits is thought to be one reason for the increased number of Cesareans performed. The use of this option should be carefully discussed with your doctor and should not take place unless a threat exists to mother or baby. Contrary to some notions, vaginal births can occur after Cesarean births.

Medical Tests Routinely Used During Pregnancy

ULTRASOUND: A procedure in which sound is projected off of the developing fetus through the use of high-frequency sound waves. This test is called a sonogram and produces an outline image of the baby, placenta and other structures. The image is transmitted to a video screen where a physician can assess fetal position, the maturity of the fetus, check the heart rate, sex and placental health. There is some controversy as to the absolute safeness of this procedure. It is widely accepted that the test should not be routinely done without sufficient medical cause.

AMNIOCENTESIS: Aimed at assessing the health of the baby, a local anesthetic is used, after which a long, hollow needle is inserted into the uterus through the abdominal wall. Amniotic fluid is removed for subsequent cellular analysis. This test poses a considerable risk to both mother and baby and should be done only when an obstetrician feels it is warranted. Some possible risks are infection of the amniotic fluid, a blood exchange between mother and baby, injury to the baby, placental damage and premature labor.

NON-STRESS TEST, ESTRIOL EXCRETION STUDIES AND OXYTOCIN CHALLENGE TEST: These three tests are used to evaluate the health of the unborn baby. They are used in special cases which may involve a diabetic mother and can usually assess how well the baby will withstand the stress of labor. Discuss these tests with your obstetrician.

CHORIONIC VILLI SAMPLING (CVS): A small sample is taken of the chorionic tissue which is found on the embryonic sac to determine whether any genetic abnormalities exist. It can be done earlier than amniocentesis. Possible risks of the procedure are fetal bleeding, uterine bleeding, infections and spontaneous abortion.

Dietary Guidelines

- ◆ Eating a good nutritious diet is vital to the health of the developing baby. Statistics tell us that many women become nutrient depleted during pregnancy. While low-fat products are encouraged, unsaturated fats are needed for proper growth.
- ◆ Eat a diet high in nutrients and fiber found in whole grains, lean meats, and fresh fruits and vegetables.
- ◆ Adequate protein consumption is essential and should be obtained through eating lean meats, legumes and low-fat dairy products.
- ◆ Avoid high-sugar, high-fat foods which can lead to digestive distress and excess weight gain.
- ◆ Adding dried prunes or bran to your diet and drinking 6 to 8 glasses of water per day can also prevent consti-

pation. Raw almonds are an excellent source of protein and calcium.

- Psyllium supplements can relieve chronic constipation.
- Decrease you salt intake because salt can induce water retention, which can raise blood pressure. Watch your ingredient labels. Many processed foods are high in salt; avoid processed cheeses, bacon, chips, meats, etc.
- Do not use diuretics unless prescribed by your physician.
- Do not smoke or drink alcohol; both of these activities are extremely harmful to the developing fetus and can result in low birth weight or even retardation.
- Do not use caffeine.
- Steam and bake your foods. Fried foods can cause heartburn and gas.
- Eating small meals throughout the day can help with nausea and vomiting. Eating dry snacks upon waking in the morning can help control morning sickness.
- Foods high in potassium and calcium can help control leg cramps. Emphasize bananas, grapefruit, oranges, cottage cheese, yogurt, sardines, almonds, and green leafy vegetables.

Recommended Nutritional Supplements

If you are pregnant, do not take any herb or other nutritional supplement without the approval of your doctor. Take a good multivitamin/mineral supplement with potencies that qualify for prenatal requirements. If you add any single nutrients, tally their total dosage with what is offered in your multiple product so as to avoid any overdosing. A lack of zinc, manganese and folic acid and an imbalance of proteins have been linked to birth defects, including mental retardation.

PRIMARY NUTRIENTS

FOLIC ACID The requirement of this vitamin actually doubles during pregnancy. Supplementation of this vitamin is essential and is thought to help prevent low birth weight babies and may even play a part in preventing certain birth defects.[1] *Suggested Dosage:* 0.6 mg per day.

B-COMPLEX VITAMINS The B-vitamins are extremely important not only to insure the health of the developing baby and mother but to also help avoid the mood changes which can result from a lack of B-vitamins. Extra B6 can help alleviate morning sickness.[2] *Suggested Dosage:* Take as directed. Take 25 mg of B6 three times daily for nausea.

CALCIUM AND MAGNESIUM Adequate supplies of these minerals are required to protect the bones and teeth of the mother, help reduce the risk of eclampsia (toxemia) and hypertension, contribute to the hard structural development of the baby, help with leg cramps and even help prevent premature delivery.[3] *Suggested Dosage:* 1,500 mg of calcium and 1,000 mg of magnesium, Use calcium citrate, gluconate or lactate and chelated magnesium products.

VITAMIN C WITH BIOFLAVONOIDS Vitamin C helps to control excessive bleeding after delivery, is vital for good collagen tissue growth, and enables iron to be absorbed. It also helps promote uterine muscle strength and can effectively treat leg cramps.[4] *Suggested Dosage:* Take as directed. CAUTION: Do not take megadoses of vitamin C (more than 5,000 mg daily) when pregnant.

VITAMIN E Pregnant women are typically low in this vitamin, which helps prevent toxemia, premature birth, and even miscarriage.[5] *Suggested Dosage:* 400 to 800 IU daily.

VITAMIN K Almost half of women in test studies were found to be vitamin K deficient. This vitamin helps to control hemorrhage and, when taken with vitamin C, can be an effective remedy for nausea and vomiting that sometimes accompanies pregnancy.[6] *Suggested Dosage:* Take as directed.

VITAMIN A A lack of this vitamin has been linked to lung disease in the developing infant and low levels also seem to play a role in developing toxemia.[7] *Suggested Dosage:* Take as directed. CAUTION: Do not take more than 10,000 IU per day when pregnant.

ESSENTIAL FATTY ACIDS Consuming omega-6 fatty acids in the form of evening primrose oil, which is a source of GLA, can help to prevent pregnancy-related hypertension.[8] *Suggested Dosage:* Take as directed and keep refrigerated.

CHROMIUM This mineral helps to normalize blood sugar, and low levels in the placenta have been linked to low birth weights.[9] *Suggested Dosage:* Take as directed.

IRON Iron is essential for the development of healthy blood cells and can often become depleted in pregnant women. It is very important to get enough iron during the first trimester to help ensure an acceptable birth weight for the baby.[10] It's important to note that iron can deplete zinc stores. *Suggested Dosage:* 60 mg daily if deficient.

ZINC Needed for the proper growth of the baby and for normal delivery. Low levels of zinc are thought to contribute to abnormal labor, toxemia, low birth weight, miscarriage and central nervous system defects in the baby.[11] Because pregnant women are prone to zinc deficiencies, proper supplementation is essential. *Suggested Dosage:* Take only as directed. Do not exceed 100 mg per day.

BILBERRY Administration of this herb may be effective in preventing and treating varicose veins of pregnancy.[12] *Suggested Dosage:* Take as directed, using standardized products.

GINGER Clinical studies strongly support the use of ginger for nausea and vomiting in pregnancy, even if it is severe.[13] *Suggested Dosage:* Take as directed in capsule or tea form. Look for standardized products.

HERBAL COMBINATION FOR MORNING SICKNESS This combination should include ginger root, cayenne, licorice root, and chamomile. *Suggested Dosage:* Two to six capsules. May be used every day to prevent or treat nausea. Use maximum dosage if necessary.

GINGER: This herb can be taken as a capsule or a tea. Nutritional deficiencies such as a lack of vitamin B6 may contribute to nausea and vomiting, and pregnancy is notorious for causing nutrient depletion. Clinical studies on ginger have found it to be more effective than prescription medications.[14] CAYENNE, LICORICE ROOT AND CHAMOMILE: Cayenne, along with licorice and chamomile, is used in smaller proportions in this formula compared to ginger root, but are nevertheless important contributors in that they help treat flatulence and poor digestion through their carminative and stimulant properties.

SECONDARY NUTRIENTS

PROTEOLYTIC ENZYMES: Digestive enzymes can help boost digestion which if often impaired in pregnancy which helps prevent heartburn and indigestion and contributes to better nutrient assimilation for mother and child. *Suggested Dosage:* Take as directed 30 minutes before eating or with meals.

RED RASPBERRY LEAF TEA: Promotes uterine muscle health. This particular herb is well known for its use in pregnancy. It helps to decrease bleeding after delivery and is believed to shorten the duration of labor. *Suggested Dosage:* Take as directed.

PAPAYA, MINT, GINGER AND ALFALFA TEA: All of these are good for heartburn, nausea and indigestion. *Suggested Dosage:* Take as directed.

ALOE VERA GEL: Good for stretch marks. Use it on the abdomen and breasts before the marks appear and as a treatment for existing marks. *Suggested Usage:* Apply as desired.

SQUAW VINE: Used as a uterine tonic and stimulant. It is best taken during the last two months of pregnancy. American Indian women use this particular herb all through pregnancy to help facilitate a safe delivery. It also promotes lactation. *Suggested Dosage:* Take only as directed and with the approval of your doctor.

Home Care Suggesstions

- A mild exercise for backache involves getting on your hands and knees and arching your lower back four or five times. When you relax, do not allow your back to sag. Repeat.
- Certain stretching exercises that can be obtained from your obstetrician can help control side cramping and muscle spasms caused by the expansion of uterine muscles.
- To help avoid hemorrhoids, keep your feet and legs elevated while having a bowel movement. Do not strain and do not remain on the toilet for long periods of time.
- Warm (not hot) sitz baths can help with hemorrhoids.
- If you have trouble sleeping, arrange pillows under your stomach, placing one between your legs to give added support.

- Leg cramps can be treated with a heating pad or hot water bottle. Leg massage is also helpful.
- Do not stand for long periods of time.
- Walking is an excellent exercise while pregnant. It can help minimize back pain, increase circulation, help control swelling, promote better digestion, lessen constipation, lessen muscle cramping and promote a better night's sleep.
- If you are prone to dizziness or lightheadedness, do not get up from a sitting or lying position too quickly.
- Do not use nasal sprays or nose drops. If you have trouble with nosebleeds, use a saline solution designed to relieve dry nasal membranes.
- Stretch marks that develop on the breasts or abdomen can be treated with vitamin E and vitamin A oil. Elastin cream is also recommended. Using these types of preparation before stretch marks appear may help minimize them.
- Do not use hot tubs or saunas while pregnant. An increase in temperature can be harmful to the developing baby. It can also promote excessive sweating.
- Do not use over-the-counter laxatives unless specifically prescribed by your physician.
- Wear support hose if you have trouble with varicose veins. Special hose can be recommended by your obstetrician if the problem is severe. Put support hose on first thing in the morning before you get out of bed.
- Avoid falling; this can cause the placenta to detach, which can be fatal to the fetus.
- Do not douche when pregnant. At least one major study has linked douching with ectopic pregnancies. In addition, some of the chemicals found in douches may endanger the health of the fetus.

Other Supportive Therapies

MASSAGE: Can help boost circulation to legs and lower back. Essential oils of lavender or rosewood can be massaged into the legs during pregnancy.

AROMATHERAPY: Add two drops of lavender oil or geranium oil to a warm bath. Use very warm washcloths to cover the breasts.

HOMEOPATHY: Conium and Bryonia can ease soreness. Cracked nipples respond to Castor equi. Increase intake of vitamin E, and use it topically on the skin for stretch marks.

Scientific Facts-at-a-Glance

A new study done in Ireland indicates that pregnant women need even larger amounts of B-vitamins than previously thought. Nutritional deficiencies during pregnancy are common.[16] Pregnant women metabolize nearly 0.7 mg of folic acid daily during the second trimester of pregnancy and 0.5 mg during the third. The new advised dose of folic acid for pregnant women is 0.6 mg per day.

Spirit/Mind Considerations

Pregnancy can be a time of elation, and at the same time, cause a wide variety of emotional reactions ranging from resentment to fear. Most pregnant women are prone to mood swings and will find themselves crying for no apparent reason. The circumstances surrounding each pregnancy greatly helps to determine psychological reaction. Unwanted pregnancies can induce periods of significant depression and lethargy. In addition, a depletion of certain nutrients in pregnancy can occur if the diet is not adequate and further aggravate negative mental conditions. Taking prenatal classes is recommended to prepare for childbirth. Research at McGill University in Canada has shown that night-shift work can increase the risk for a miscarriage. Scientists speculate that night work may interrupt the 24-hour cycle of sleep and may produce possible hormonal imbalances. Stress related to working at night may also interfere with fetal development. Learn to relax and recognize stress and use measures to diffuse it.

Prevention

- The best way to prevent possible complications of preganacy is to eat right and take supplements all the way through adolescence.
- Eating disorders that plague our young women, the use of alcohol and tobacco and the elimination of whole grains and fresh vegetables from the diet can take an enormous toll.
- Become health conscious long before you become pregnant.

Doctor's Notes

Pregnancy should not be viewed as an illness. It is a perfectly normal state; however it can cause a vast array of physiological changes. In most cases, if you are supplied with all the vitamins, minerals and other nutrients you need, many pregnancy-related problems can be less severe or completely prevented. We know now just how crucial certain levels of these nutrients are for the developing baby. We also understand very clearly that using tobacco and alcohol, even in very small amounts, can result in disorders such as ADD, not to mention the risk of possible birth defects, low birth weight, or even SIDS.[15] The bottom line is to take care of yourself and the baby through nutritious diet, supplementation, proper exercise and stress management.

Endnotes

1. U. Goyal, "Effects of folic acid supplementation on birth weight of infants," Jour Obst Gyn Ind, 1980, 30: 104.

2. W. Doyl, et al, "The association between maternal diet and birth dimensions," Jour Nutr Med, 1990, 1: 9-17.

3. J. Villar and J. Repke, "Calcium supplementation during pregnancy may reduce preterm delivery in high risk populations," Amer Jour Obst Gyn, 1990, 163: 1124-31.

4. M. Hammar, et al., "Calcium and magnesium status in pregnant women: A comparison between treatment with calcium and vitamin C in pregnant women with leg cramps," Int Jour Vit Nutr Res, 1987, 57(2): 179-83.

5. J. Marks, "Critical appraisal of the therapeutic value of alpha-tocopherol," Vitami Horm, 1962, 20: 573-98.

6. R. Merkel, "The use of menadione bisulfite (vitamin K) and ascorbic acid in the trament of nausea and vomiting of pregnancy: A preliminary report," Amer Jour Obstet Gyn, 1952, 64(2): 416-18.

7. V. Hustead et al., "Relationship of vitamin A (retinol) status to lung disease in preterm infant," Jour Ped, 1984, 105(4): 610-15.

8. P. Obrien, "The effect of dietary supplementation with linoleic acid and linolenic acid on the pressor response to angiotensin I: A possible role in pregnancy-induced hypertension?" Bri Jour Clin Phar, 1985, 19(3): 335-42.

9. N. Ward, "Elemental factors in human fetal development," Jour Nutri Med, 1990, 1: 19-26.

10. Doyle, 9-17.

11. A. Hagashi et al., "A prospective survey of serial serum zinc levels and pregnancy outcome," Jour Ped Gastro, 1988, 7: 430-33.

12. G. Grismond, "Treatment of pregnancy-induced phlebopathies," Minerva Ginecol, 1981, 33:221-30.

13. W. Fischer-Rasmussen, et al., "Ginger treatment of hyperemesis gravidarum," Eur J Obstet Gynaecol Reprod Biol, 1990, 38:19-24.

14. Wl Fischer-Rasmussen, et al., "Ginger treatment of hyperemesis gravidarum," Eur Jour Gyn Repro Bil, 1990, 38: 19-24.

15. Sherry Gold, "Hyperactivity learning disabilities and alcohol," Jour Learn Dis, 1984, 17(1): 3-6.

16. L. Dostalova, "Correlation of the vitamin status between mother and newborn during delivery," Dev Pahrmacol Ther, 1982, 4: 45057.

PROSTATE DISEASE

Nearly every man will have an enlarged prostate gland if they live long enough. Already, prostate cancer is the number one cause of death among males.

Essentially, the prostate gland, unlike other glands, tends to degenerate over time. It is more prone to toxin accumulation, due in part to slow blood circulation and to its fatty, sponge-like makeup. The fact that blood flow is sluggish in the prostate area explains why antibiotic therapy for prostatitis takes so long to clear the infection.

BHP refers to a prostate condition where the gland become enlarged and diseased thereby affecting the function of the male urinary system. Prostatitis is an condition in which the prostate becomes inflamed (the symptoms of both BHP and prostatitis can be quite alike and their treatment protocols are similar).

Symptoms

Prostate malfunction can be characterized by pain or burning when urinating, dribbling urine, increased frequency of urination, fever and chills, penile discharge, abdominal pain, pain around the rectum or scrotum or in the lower back, blood or pus in the urine and impotence.

Precautions

Most men suffering from prostate trouble are experiencing nothing more than enlargement or inflammation although these same symptoms may be caused by prostate cancer. Prostate cancer, if caught early enough, is one of the most treatable forms of cancer. Call your physician immediately if you have any symptoms involving the prostate gland. It is essential to see a urologist or a similar expert to rule out the possibilty of prostate cancer, which, if unchecked, will ravage other organs, like the lower intestine, the small intestine and the reproductive organs. If you cannot urinate at all, go to the nearest emergency room. Excessive urine retention is potentially life threatening.

Causes

Prostatitis usually results from a bacterial infection that has spread to the prostate gland from the urethra or other area of the body through the blood. BPH can result from prostatic tissue that has been infiltrated with certain hormonal compounds which encourage overgrowth. It has also been linked to diet, high cholesterol levels and zinc deficiencies.

Other ways that prostatitis and other prostate conditions may develop through sexual contact; as a complication of venereal disease; from the presence of a urinary catheter; zinc deficiency; taking antihistamines and decongestants for prolonged periods of time; and exposure to pesticides and heavy metals.

Some health care professionals believe that constipation, the consumption of alcohol and a high-fat diet are connected to prostatitis. High cholesterol levels are thought to promote prostate enlargement by cholesterol metabolite accumulation within the gland itself. Lowering cholesterol levels is believed to reduce the risk of prostate disorders.

Conventional Therapies

Your physician will examine the prostate gland manually by inserting a gloved finger into the rectum. The gland will be tender to the touch and enlarged. Lab tests will be ordered to classify the infection using urine samples and urethral secretions which can be obtained through manual massage of the prostate gland.

Antibiotic treatment will be initiated with a slow recovery being more the rule than the exception. In severe cases, antibiotics will be administered intravenously. Unfortunately, the prostate gland has a poor blood supply making it difficult for antibiotic therapy to reach the area which prolongs curing the disease. Nalidixic acid is also prescribed for prostatitis. Proscar, (finasteride) is commonly used for prostate enlargement and while it can shrink the gland, it comes with unpleasant side effects such as possible impotence.

Taking Proscar can also inhibit the detection of prostate cancer. Painkillers are also routinely prescribed. If an abscess develops, surgical drainage may be required. If the infection does not respond to antibiotic therapy, an operation to drain out infected fluids may be required. It is considered fairly simple and requires a short hospital stay.

TURP (transurethral resection of the prostate) is also available for an enlarged gland but has some side effects and may not provide permanent relief. New laser techniques will eventually improve this surgery.

Dietary Guidelines

- Increase your fluid intake by drinking large quantities of purified water to stimulate urine flow before 6 p.m.
- Drinking parsley juice with apple juice is also good.
- Eat plenty of artichokes and asparagus, which act as natural diuretics and help to cleanse the prostate gland.
- Avoid saturated or trans-fatty acids found in butter, margarine, shortening, etc. Use olive oil instead.
- Lower your cholesterol levels by eating a high-fiber, low-fat diet.

Recommended Nutritional Supplements

PRIMARY NUTRIENTS

PYGEUM Pygeum is an herb that has been used in Europe to help the prostate return to a more normal state and helps to concentrate zinc in the gland. Pygeum also helps to lower prolactin, a hormone which is elevated in men with prostate disorders and it also helps eliminate excess fluid from the prostate. Numerous double-blind studies confirm the efficacy of pygeum in treating an enlarged prostate. Using pygeum resulted in a significant improvement in prostate swelling, and urinary difficulties.[1] *Suggested Dosage:* 100 to 200 mg daily in three doses for several weeks. Do not exceed recommended dosages.

PROSTAGIUM This mix of pygeum, vitamin B6, zinc and copper helps maintain a healthy prostate through its synergistic effect. *Suggested Dosage:* Take as directed.

SAW PALMETTO Saw palmetto extract (*Serenoa repens*) has undergone extensive studies with clinical trials supporting its use as a primary treatment for both short and long-term BPH. Statistics have been impressive showing a very high improvement rate in relieving almost every symptom associated with prostate enlargement after only 45 days of treatment.[2] *Suggested Dosage:* 150 mg in fat-soluble extract form taken twice a day.

NETTLE Recent studies strongly advocate using nettle with saw palmetto due to its ability to inhibit the potentially dangerous forms of testosterone which are associated with the development of prostate disease.[3] *Suggested Dosage:* Take only as directed. Not recommended for children.

ZINC Extremely important to prostate health. The gland contains a concentration of zinc ten times greater than other organs in the body. Zinc depletion has been linked to prostate disorders. Zinc gluconate in lozenge form or zinc picolinate are readily absorbed. Clinical tests support the ability of zinc to shrink the prostate and alleviate other symptoms associated with prostatitis and BPH.[4] *Suggested Dosage:* Take as directed.

L-ALANINE, L-GLUTAMINE, L-GLYCINE This trio of amino acids can help to relieve the frequency of nighttime urination.[5] *Suggested Dosage:* Take as directed.

PUMPKIN SEEDS A naturally-rich source of zinc as well as other nutritious compounds, such as essential fatty acids. *Suggested Dosage:* Take as directed.

VITAMIN B6 Helps to promote normal cholesterol metabolism, which can prevent fatty buildup in the vascular system of the prostate and fatty deposits from accumulating in the gland. *Suggested Dosage:* Take as directed.

ESSENTIAL FATTY ACIDS Vital to the healthy functioning of the prostate gland, EFAs have proven their ability to ease symptoms of BPH.[6] Evening primrose oil, sunflower, soy, borange and flaxseed oil are recommended. *Suggested Dosage:* Take as directed.

SELENIUM AND VITAMIN E Powerful antioxidant duo which helps to protect gland from tissue damage. *Suggested Dosage:* Take as directed.

B-SITOSTEROLS These compounds are phytosterols extracted from plants and used in Germany to reduce cholesterol levels. Tests have found that these plant sterols can significantly ease the symptoms of BPH.[7] Interestingly, saw palmetto, pygeum, oils containing EFAs and pumpkin seeds are all rich in phytosterols. *Suggested Dosage:* Take as directed.

HERBAL COMBINATION Also recommended is an herbal combination containing saw palmetto, cornsilk, pumpkin seeds, ginger, nettle root, kelp, burdock and parsley. Several of the herbs (or their constituents) of this blend have been the subject of a number of clinical studies for the treatment of prostatic enlargement. Side effects caused by the most popular prescription drug product makes this formula an attractive alternative, as it is more effective and virtually free of side effects when used as directed. *Suggested Dosage:* Four to eight capsules daily for several months until symptoms subside.

SECONDARY NUTRIENTS

GARLIC: Acts as a natural antibiotic to fight infection and inflammation and helps to improve vascular health by lowering bad cholesterol. High cholesterol levels are thought to contribute to prostate disease. *Suggested Dosage:* Take as directed. Deodorized forms are available.

VITAMIN A AND BETA CAROTENE: Act as antioxidants which help remove free radicals caused by inflammation. *Suggested Dosage:* No more than 10,000 IU of vitamin A each day. Take the beta carotene as directed.

PROANTHOCYANIDINS: The flavonoid content of these compounds acts as a natural anti-inflammatory agent. *Suggested Dosage:* Take as directed. Grape seed extract or pycnogenol supply these compounds.

FLOWER POLLENS: Several studies suggest that bee pollen can reduce prostate inflammation and infection. Flower pollens have been used to treat prostatitis in Europe for decades, and tests show that it is indeed effective.[7] Bee pollen is commonly used; however, it must be used carefully at first to rule out the possibility of any allergic reaction. Look for quality, freeze-dried varieties. Local pollens are always preferable. *Suggested Dosage:* Take as directed.

PANAX GINSENG: Acts as an herbal tonic for the male reproductive system and helps to decrease prostate gland swelling.[8] *Suggested Dosage:* In extract form, take 50 mg of ginsenosides or three grams of dried ginseng each day.

Home Care Suggestions

◆ Limit your fluid intake after 6 p.m. and empty your bladder before retiring.

◆ Fifteen-minute sitz baths in water that is approximately 95° F can help boost circulation.

◆ In cases of prostatitis, avoid sexual intercourse until the infection is gone. Intercourse may further irritate the prostate gland and prolong recovery.

◆ Mild exercise is recommended to increase circulation; however, riding a bicycle is not advised.

◆ Avoid exposure to very cold temperatures. Apparently, urination difficulties and retention are more common in cold climates.

◆ Try not to take antibiotics for longer than two weeks. Often, after antibiotic therapy, prostatitis recurs.

Other Supportive Therapies

ACUPUNCTURE: Pressure points located near the bladder, colon, spleen and kidney meridians can help to stimulate circulation to the prostate gland.

YOGA: The kneeling position is recommended to stimulate circulation to the prostate gland.

Scientific Facts-at-a-Glance

A recently-published academic article examining how saw palmetto works and why it should be used by physicians in their treatment protocols for prostate disease points out the fact that if may be one of the best deterrent compounds to prostate cancer available.[9] In light of this fact, all men should consider taking saw palmetto singly or in an herbal combination long before they experience prostate disease symptoms. The value of adding nettle to saw palmetto has also recently come to light for even better management of prostate disease symptoms. A 1993 study also showed that using pollen extracts (cernilton) for prostatitis resulted in some favorable results.[10]

Spirit/Mind Considerations

The effects of stress on prostate disorders is clearly underrated. Increased adrenalin, which is typical in unmanaged stress, causes both the neck of the bladder and prostate gland to react, making urination more difficult. Moreover, the link between stress and high cholesterol levels may also impact the gland. Learning to relieve stress and to find spiritual contentment helps to lower the risk of these types of degenerative diseases we normally associate with age.

Prevention

- ◆ Do not consume alcohol, coffee, tobacco, caffeine, acidic foods, or red pepper, which are considered prostatic irritants.
- ◆ Avoid becoming constipated by eating plenty of high-fiber foods and getting adequate exercise.
- ◆ Eat a diet high in zinc and take a zinc picolinate supplement once a day.
- ◆ Take a pygeum and saw palmetto supplement after the age of 55.
- ◆ Avoid becoming constipated by eating plenty of high-fiber foods and getting adequate exercise.
- ◆ Drink plenty of water. Becoming dehydrated can stress the prostate gland.
- ◆ Avoid red meats and rich foods which may be high in uric acid which is believed to cause prostate irritation.
- ◆ Prolonged jarring to the seat area which results from too much sitting, riding a horse, motorcycle or bike can increase the risk of prostate infection.
- ◆ If you are allergic and must use an antihistamine, ask your physician about taking hismanal or seldane, which do not contain antihistamines.
- ◆ Having frequent sexual intercourse can empty the prostate of secretions and promote better prostate health.
- ◆ Having a vasectomy has been linked to the incidence of prostate disorders including cancer. Some studies report the risk of prostate cancer for males who have had a vasectomy is three times greater than those who have not.
- ◆ Keep cholesterol levels normal to prevent the accumulation of cholesterol metabolites in the prostate gland.
- ◆ Avoid exposure to pesticides, heavy metals or any toxic substance.
- ◆ Take a supplement of essential fatty acids every day.

Doctor's Notes

I have found that taking pygeum and zinc together greatly enhances the ability of zinc to stay within the prostate gland. The inflammatory process which causes prostatitis and BPH is closely linked with compounds called prostaglandins.

Men who experience BPH have higher prostaglandin activity. Taking pygeum can reduce both the synthesis and activity of prostaglandins so that inflammation, swelling and enlargement are all decreased. Studies with pygeum have found that pretreating the prostate with this herbal compound can also inhibit the growth of certain tumor cells.

Saw palmetto contains specific fatty acids called steriles, which do not allow testosterone to attach to the prostate gland; this can ultimately stimulate enlargement and tumor growth. Saw palmetto also decreases the production of leukotriens which contribute to inflammation. Studies have found that saw palmetto accomplishes the same action as Proscar, the most common prescription drug for prostate diseases, without any negative side effects.

The combination of these two herbs helps to decrease prostate swelling and to inhibit the negative action of inflammatory compounds and negative-acting hormones. Make sure you purchase products with guaranteed potency when buying saw palmetto and pygeum. When chemically analyzed, some products claiming to contain saw palmetto actually contained none of the herb. This type of fraud gives good and effective natural supplements a bad reputation. Look for fat-soluble types of saw palmetto with an 80 to 90 percent sterol and fatty acid content in the extract.

Additional Resources

Prostate Information Hotline
(800) 543-9632

Endnotes

1. P. Bassi, et al., "Standardized extract of Pygeum africanum in the treatment of benign prostate hypertrophy," Minerva Urologica, 1987, 39: 45.

2. J. Braeckman, "The extract of Serenoa repens in the treatment of benign prostatic hyperplasia: A multi center open study," Current Therapy Research, 1994, 55: 776-85.

3. E. Koch and A. Biber, "Pharmacological effects of saw palmetto and urtica extracts for benign prostatic hyperplasia," Urologe 1994, 34

(2): 90-95. See also H.J. Schneider, et al., "Treatment of benign prostatic hyperplasia: Results of a surveillance study in the practices of urological specialists using a combined plant-based preparation," Fortshcr Med, 1995, 113: 37-40.

4. M. Fahim, Z. Fahim and J. Harman, "Zinc treatment for the reduction of hyperplasia of the prostate," Fed. Proc. 1976, 35: 361.

5. F. Dumrau, "Benign prostatic hyperplasia: amino acid therapy for symptomatic relief," American Journal of Ger., 162, 10, 426-30.

6. J. P. Hart and W.L. Cooper, "Vitamin F in the treatment of Prostatic Hyperplasia," Lee Foundation for Nutritional Research, Report #1, (Milwaukee, Wisconsin: 1941).

7. R.R. Berges, J. Windeler, et al., "Randomized, placebo-controlled, double-blind clinical trail of B-sitosterol in patients with benign prostatic hyperplasia," Lancet, 1995, 345: 1529-32.

8. Y. Saito, "Diagnosis and treatment of chronic prostatitis with special reference to experience with Cernilton," Clinical, Exp. Med., 1967, 44: 387-93.

9. W.S. Fahim, et al., "Effect of Panax Ginseng on testosterone level and prostate in male rats," Arch. Androl, 1982, 8: 261-63.

10. H.J. Nieferprum, et al., Phytomedicine 1994, 1:127-33.

11. E.W. Rugendorff, et al., "Results of treatment with pollen extract (Cernilton) in chronic prostatitis and prostatodynia," British Journal of Urology, 1993, 71: 433-38.

PSORIASIS

Psoriasis is a common skin disorder that is characterized by thickened patches of inflamed skin. It occurs in approximately two percent of the population of the United States and Europe. Both men and women are equally affected by psoriasis, which usually appears between the ages of 10 and 30.

The disorder results from the abnormally fast production of new skin cells. A healthy skin cell takes four weeks to complete its cycle of production, while a psoriatic cell takes less than four days. This abnormal production of cells causes skin cells to accumulate forming thick patches sometimes referred to as plaques. Psoriasis can affect large areas of the skin causing significant physical discomfort. Psoriasis may take different forms, therefore requiring specific treatment for each type. The disease is less common in the summer and can disappear for long periods of time. Psoriasis is considered a long-term disorder without a permanent cure. Most attacks of psoriasis can be well-controlled with the appropriate treatment.

Symptoms

Psoriasis generally causes the appearance of thick patches of red, inflamed skin that has a silvery scaly surface. It usually affects the elbows, knees, scalp, genitals and buttocks although it can appear in any part of the body. Toes and fingernails which are affected can developed pits and ridges. Itching can be present. Joint tenderness can also accompany psoriasis.

Discoid or Plaque Psoriasis

Characterized by thick scaly patches appear on the trunk and the limbs. The elbows, knees and scalp are particularly susceptible. In addition, the nails may become pitted or thickened and can separate from the nail bed.

Guttate Psoriasis

This type occurs most frequently in children and consists of small patches of red, inflamed skin that can develop quickly, especially following an infection.

Pustular Psoriasis

Small pustules form in this type of psoriasis and can appear anywhere on the body or can stay confined to the palms or soles of the feet.

Causes

The exact cause of psoriasis is unknown, although there is a genetic predisposition to the disorder. It results from the abnormally fast production of new skin cells with the normal rate of old skin cell removal. As a result, these new live cells accumulate and form the characteristic thick patches, which are covered with dead flaking skin. Attacks of psoriasis have been linked to emotional stress, surgery, physical illness, the faulty utilization of fat, immune dysfunction, alcohol consumption, impaired liver function, incomplete protein digestion, trauma to the skin, poison ivy, sunburn, certain drugs such as lithium and beta-blockers, food allergies, and a lack of hydrochloric acid.

Conventional Therapies

Doctors will treat new patches of psoriasis early. In mild cases of psoriasis, ultraviolet lamp exposure (phototherapy) may be helpful. Emollient creams are also routinely prescribed. For more severe cases, ointments which contain coal tar or anthralin may be recommended. Corticosteroid drugs, methotrexate, and anticancer drugs are also used.

Cyclosporine drugs have had some good results although they are not approved by the FDA for treating psoriasis. Rocaltrol is currently being tested for its potential benefits. Freezing smaller areas of psoriasis with liquid nitrogen is also being researched. Skin patches such as Actiderm can more effectively treat affected areas. Some drugs such as Legison can have significant side effects and should be discussed with your doctor. Oxsoralen-ultra, a liquid preparation is also routinely used in the treatment of psoriasis. If joint swelling is present, nonsteroidal anti-inflammatory drugs may be prescribed. Injecting cortisone directly into an old thick patch of psoriasis can help to remove it. In severe cases, intensive ultraviolet therapy may require hospitalization. Continued use of corticosteroid creams can make the skin weak and thin.

Dietary Guidelines

◆ Emphasize fish (sardines, tuna, salmon), "raw" foods, soybeans, sesame seeds and fiber.
◆ Fiber helps to reduce cholesterol levels, which have been found to be abnormally high in some psoriatic skin. Some studies suggest that psoriasis may be caused by a toxic build-up in the colon.
◆ Fish oil or primrose oil can help to inhibit arachidonic acid, which can make psoriatic lesions turn red. These oils also help to prevent skin dryness.
◆ Avoid foods that contain arachidonic acid. It is a natural inflammatory substance which can turn psoriatic patches red.
◆ Avoid alcohol; it aggravates the symptoms of psoriasis.
◆ Eliminate white sugar, white flour, processed foods and citrus fruits.
◆ Avoid tomato-based foods and caffeine.
◆ Eat plenty of raw vegetables and stay away from citrus fruits, hydrogenated and saturated fats and white sugar foods. Avoid fatty dairy products as well.

Recommended Nutritional Supplements

PRIMARY NUTRIENTS

ESSENTIAL FATTY ACIDS These have shown that supplementation with fish oils and with other oils like evening primrose and flaxseed is very beneficial in helping correct faulty lipid metabolism, which is linked to psoriasis.[1] *Suggested Dosage:* Use as directed daily. Take a vitamin E supplement with fish oil. Keep refrigerated. Use for at least eight weeks and evaluate results.

LIPOIC ACID, VITAMIN E AND SELENIUM Lipoic acid greatly potentiates the availability of vitamin E and C and glutathione in the cells and makes it possible for enhanced free radical scavenging by these agents. Selenium can also be applied topically.[2] *Suggested Dosage:* Take all three supplements as directed and in combination.

LECITHIN This nutrient contains choline which helps to metabolize lipids correctly.[3] *Suggested Dosage:* Take as directed in granule or capsulized form daily.

VITAMIN A Works to boost skin tissue regeneration and scavenges for free radicals. Its use in cases of psoriasis suggests that it may slow the disease process.[4] *Suggested Dosage:* 25,000 IU daily. If you are pregnant, do not exceed 10,000 IU per day.

ZINC Contributes to the healing of the skin through its participation in protein metabolism. A low level of zinc has been found in people with pustular psoriasis.[5] *Suggested Dosage:* 50 to 100 mg per day. Use gluconate or picolinate products.

FOLIC ACID A deficiency of this nutrient has been observed in people with psoriasis.[6] *Suggested Dosage:* Take as directed.

VITAMIN B12 Some evidence exists that supplementation through injection or oral supplements may be helpful in treating psoriasis.[7] *Suggested Dosage:* Ask your doctor about injections, although sublingual products may be just as effective.

VITAMIN D Faulty metabolism of vitamin D has been observed in people with psoriasis.[8] In addition, using vitamin D3 in topical applications on lesions has shown some promise.[9] *Suggested Dosage:* Use as directed in topical form.

GLYCOSAMINOGLYCANS These compounds, found in glucosamine sulfate, provide certain compounds that can help battle psoriatic arthritis.[10] *Suggested Dosage:* Take as directed.

HERBAL COMBINATION This combination should include burdock root, gotu kola, yellow dock, dandelion root, milk thistle seeds, Irish moss, red clover blossoms, kelp, cayenne and sarsaparilla. *Suggested Dosage:* Two to six capsules daily. For chronic conditions, use maximum dosage of six capsules per day for a prolonged period. For best results use every day.

BURDOCK ROOT: In Europe, this herb is well known for its ability to treat skin disorders.[11] This herb helps to expel toxins from the skin and blood. It promotes liver function and increases bile flow, which in turn cleanses the blood and reduces toxin production in the gastrointestinal tract, which has a direct bearing on psoriasis. It can also be used in powdered form directly on plaques. GOTU KOLA: Supported by tremendous clinical research conducted in Europe, which backed up its effectiveness in the treatment of various skin disorders associated with psoriasis, cellulitis, and even leprosy.[12] It also possesses wound healing activity and has been shown to decrease scarring.[13] YELLOW DOCK: Yellow dock root is a reputed blood purifier and has been prescribed for all types of skin problems, including psoriasis. It has also been reported to be able to clear a congested liver. Its laxative effect is well documented and supports the body's detoxifying ability.[14] DANDELION ROOT: Dandelion has a long history of use in herbal medicine. It is part of this formula for its ability to strengthen the liver, improve bile formation, regulate the bowels, purify the blood, and tonify the skin.[15] MILK THISTLE: There is probably not a person alive who could not benefit from milk thistle (also called "silymarin"). This wonderful herb cleanses, strengthens, and protects the liver and its functions and has proven itself valuable for skin disorders like psoriasis. Time-tested and proven in hospitals and clinics all over Europe, milk thistle is one of the only herbs known to treat some forms of psoriasis.[16] IRISH MOSS: Provides a demulcent and soothing source of mucilage and improves intestinal function. RED CLOVER BLOSSOM: Red clover blossoms are a reputed blood purifier and officially recognized in the United Kingdom for treatment of skin conditions such as psoriasis, eczema, and rashes. KELP: Kelp serves a similar function as Irish moss, but kelp is thought to be a blood purifier with the ability to alleviate skin problems, burns, and insect bites. CAYENNE OR CAPSICUM: Capsaicin-treated patients demonstrated significantly greater improvement in their evaluation of psoriasis and did well on their combined psoriasis-severity scores.[17] Cayenne is a also a stimulant that helps to make all the other herbs function better. Such herbs are referred to as activators. SARSAPARILLA ROOT: Sarsaparilla root has many benefits including the treatment of psoriasis and eczema. It contains saponins shown to help improve psoriasis by binding to endotoxins in the gastrointestinal tract.[18]

SECONDARY NUTRIENTS

VITAMIN C WITH BIOFLAVONOIDS: Helps to strengthen the skin and acts as a natural anti-inflammatory agent. *Suggested Dosage:* 3,000 to 5,000 mg per day.

PROTEOLYTIC ENZYMES: These compounds boost digestion of macronutrients discouraging the buildup of toxins in the gastrointestinal tract which have been linked to skin diseases like psoriasis. *Suggested Dosage:* Take as directed 30 minutes before meals and during meals.

GRAPE SEED OR PINE BARK EXTRACT: These proanthocyanidins scavenge free radicals and have potent anti-inflammatory actions. *Suggested Dosage:* Take as directed during a flare-up. However, you may want to increase dosage for better cellular saturation.

PABA: Helps to maintain skin integrity and contributes to proper skin cell regeneration. *Suggested Dosage:* Take as directed.

MYRRH GUM SPRAY: The astringent property of this herb helps to heal damaged skin. *Suggested Usage:* Use as directed.

ALOE GEL: Helps to boost healing of the skin and to minimize scarring. *Suggested Dosage:* Use high quality pure products as directed.

GOLDENSEAL: Inhibits the formation of polyamines that result from improper protein digestion and may be linked with psoriasis. *Suggested Dosage:* Take as directed using standardized products but not for longer than two week intervals at a time.

SHARK CARTILAGE: There is some evidence that the antiangiogenesis activity of compounds contained in cartilage can discourage episodes of psoriasis. *Suggested Dosage:* Take as directed. Look for pure products without fillers.

Home Care Suggestions

◆ Spend time in the sun every day. Exposure to sunlight greatly reduces the severity of psoriasis. Dry, desert climates are especially beneficial. However, protect unaffected areas with sunscreen; sunburns can actually cause psoriasis to worsen.

◆ Maintain an optimum weight. Being overweight seems to make psoriasis worse.

◆ Keeping the skin moisturized cannot be over emphasized. Apply cream onto patches of psoriasis and wrap the area in plastic overnight. Petroleum jelly can be used or Lacticare or Eucerin creams are also recommended.

◆ Zostrix, an over-the-counter cream for the treatment of shingles has been found to effectively treat psoriasis, however it has not been approved for that purpose yet and should only be used with your doctor's approval. Applying the cream results in significant burning.

◆ Cosmetic cover up ointments can help to conceal unsightly areas and should be used only with your doctor's approval.

◆ Use ginger or yarrow in bath water. Get into the bath and then add a couple of teaspoons of olive oil.

◆ Use oatmeal-based soaps which do not dry the skin.

◆ Sensitize your skin with tar before you use ultraviolet lamps or expose the are to sunlight. Apply cortisone ointments in the morning and tar ointments at night.

◆ Applying flaxseed oil or kochia oil to affected areas can help to soften the patches. Linseed oil can be taken internally also.

◆ For itching, make a wet compress of baking soda and water. Apple cider vinegar and water is also recommended.

◆ Keep stress levels to a minimum through hypnotherapy, breathing exercises, yoga, etc.

◆ Protect yourself from infection. Often a strep throat can be followed by an attack of psoriasis.

◆ Some studies indicate that acupuncture can help to control psoriasis. Discuss this with your doctor and a qualified acupuncturist.

Other Supportive Therapies

ACUPUNCTURE: Helps to manage symptoms and should complement dietary changes and stress management.

LIGHT THERAPY: Exposure to sunlight improves psoriasis,

which is usually worse during the winter months in the Northern Hemisphere.

HOMEOPATHY: Sulfur is used for itching, petroleum for dryness, and graphites for oozing sores or patches.

Scientific Facts-at-a-Glance

Food allergies are thought to play a significant role in the development of diseases like psoriasis which have no known cause.[19] If you suffer from psoriasis, rule out food sensitivities by utilizing the food elimination plan outlined in the first section of this book. Deranged digestion due to inflammatory responses to certain foods is thought to be implicated in all autoimmune diseases as well a variety of others. A lack of hydrochloric acid in the stomach may also play a role in psoriasis, once again illustrating the profound health implications of faulty digestion in disease development.

Spirit/Mind Considerations

People who suffer from psoriasis often become weary of dealing with it and will alter their lifestyle so it remains concealed. Embarrassment commonly accompanies psoriasis and those that suffer from it avoid any recreational activity in which the patches could become exposed. The effect of emotional stress is also a significant factor in causing attacks of psoriasis. It is common for someone suffering from psoriasis to have experienced a specific stressful event within one month prior to an outbreak. For this reason, hypnosis and biofeedback may be of some value as treatment options.

Prevention

- Avoid becoming sunburned.
- Keep the immune system healthy through a good, nutritious diet and avoid exposure to infections.
- Use olive and flaxseed oils.
- Control stress levels through biofeedback, exercise, and yoga.
- Eat a diet high in fish oils and fiber, and low in animal fats and sugar.
- Don't consume alcohol.
- Make sure your diet is high in zinc and lecithin.
- Take proteolytic enzymes with your meals.

Doctor's Notes

The skin is the largest and one of the most important organs of the body. The condition of the skin is often a reflection of the health of the body. Imbalances and toxic build-up due to a dysfunctional liver or improper elimination may reveal themselves in skin diseases like psoriasis. By improving the internal health of the body, the skin's functionality and appearance will be positively affected. The herbs and nutrients in this section are designed to cleanse the body by activating all its methods of elimination which include cleansing, strengthening, and supporting liver function. Longer-lasting and more wide-ranging results can be achieved by improving the diet, using flaxseed and olive oil and abstaining from chocolate, nuts and stimulants such as caffeine.

Additional Resources

National Psoriasis Foundation
6600 SW 92nd Ave. Suite 300
Portland, OR 97223
(800) 723-9166 or (503) 244-7404

Endnotes

1. V. Ziboh, "Implications of dietary oils and polyunsaturated fatty acids in the management of cutaneous disorders," Arch Dermatol, 1989, 125(2):241-5. See also A. Lassus et al., "Effects of dietary supplementation with polyunsaturated ethyl-ester lipids (angiosan) in patients with psoriasis and psoriatic arthritis," Jour Int Med Res, 1990, 18:68-73.
2. E. Broglund and A. Enhamre, "Treatment of psoriasis with topical selenium sulphide," Letter, Br J Dermatol, 1987, 117(5):665-6.
3. P. Gross et al., "The treatment of psoriasis as a disturbance of lipid metabolism," N Y State J Med, 1950, 50:2683-86.
4. M. Haddox et al., "Retinol inhibition of ornithine decarboxylase induction and gastrointestinal progression in CHD cells," Cancer Res, 1979, 39:4930-38.
5. B. Dreno et al., "Plasma zinc is decreased only in generalized pustualar psoriasis," Dermatologica, 1986, 173(5):209-12.
6. L. Fry et al., "The mechanism of folate deficiency in psoriasis," Br Jour Dermato 1971, 84:539-44.
7. R. Carslaw and J. Neil, "Vitamin B12 in psoriasis," Letter, Bri Med Jour, 1963, 1:611.
8. B. Staberg et al., "Abnormal vitamin D metabolism in patients with psoriasis," Acta Dermatol Venerol, 1987, (Stockh) 67:65-68, 1987).
9. T. Kato et al., "Successful treatment of psoriasis with topical application of active vitamin D-3 analogue, 1 alpha, 24-dihydroxycholecalciferol," Bri Jour Dermatol 1986, 115(4): 431-33.
10. Arthritis Information: Psoriatic Arthritis, (The Arthritis Foundation, Atlanta, Ga: Oct, 1995) No. 9053.
11. F. Ellingwood, American Materia Medica, Therapeutics and Pharmacognosy, (Eclectic Medical Publications, Portland: 1983).
12. T. Chakrabarty, et al., "Centella asiatica in the treatment of leprosy," Sci Culture, 1976, 42: 573.
13. J.P. Bosse, et al., "Clinical study of a new antikeloid drug," Ann Plastic Surgery, 1979, 3: 13-21.
14. H.W. Felter, The Eclectic Materia Medica: Pharmacology and Therapeutics, (Eclectic Medical Publications, Portland: 1983).
15. K. Bohm, "Choleretic action of some medicinal plants," Arzneimittel-Forsch, 1959, 9: 376-78.
16. G. Weber and K. Galle, "The liver, a therapeutic target in dermatoses," Med Welt, 1983, 34: 108-111.
17. D. Brown, Quarterly Review Of Natural Medicine, Spring 1994, 17.
18. F. Thurman, "The treatment of psoriasis with sarsaparilla compound," New Eng Jour Med, 1942, 227: 128-33
19. H. Lithell et al., "A fasting and vegetarian diet treatment trial in chronic inflammatory disorders," Acta Derm Venererol, 1983, (Stockh) 63:397-403, 1983).

RHEUMATIC FEVER

Rheumatic fever is a disease that causes inflammation in various tissues of the body. It typically develops as a complication of various infections caused by the streptococcal bacteria such as strep throat, scarlet fever, tonsillitis or an ear infection.

In developed nations rheumatic fever is considered a rare disease, although an increase of the disease has been noted in some parts of the United States.

Rheumatic fever generally affects children between the ages of 3 and 18. Rheumatic fever causes joint inflammation and can infiltrate heart tissue, causing permanent heart damage. Until recently, heart damage was involved in a majority of cases of rheumatic fever. Today, perhaps through the widespread use of antibiotics, heart disease is a less common complication. Instead, joint disease among people who have contracted rheumatic fever has become the serious problem.

Approximately one percent of teenagers show signs of heart disease associated with rheumatic fever. Ten percent of rheumatic fever cases result in chorea, which affects the brain. The incidence of rheumatic fever can increase after one occurrence.

Symptoms

Typically, the symptoms of rheumatic fever begin with a sore throat that clears up within one to six weeks; this is followed by unexplained fatigue, fever and joint pain. The symptoms of rheumatic fever can resemble arthritis and include fever, inflammation and swelling of the larger joints, skin rash, and/or aching joints (often preceded by a strep infection).

Symptoms may not appear for years. The most common heart damage involves the thickening and scarring of the heart valves, which leads to mitral insufficiency. If the damage is severe, heart valve surgery may be required. If any member of your family has these symptoms, consult your physician immediately.

Causes

Rheumatic fever typically follows a streptococcal throat infection and is thought to be caused by a dysfunction of the immune system, which is triggered by the presence of the streptococcal bacteria. In this respect, it can be considered an autoimmune disorder that is triggered in genetically susceptible people.

Conventional Therapies

Antibiotic therapy can prevent the disease or lessen its effects. Antibiotics have significant side effects that can be minimized with supplements and adequate diet. Diagnosing rheumatic fever is often difficult. It may be suspected if arthritis-like symptoms move from joint to joint.

Lab tests may indicate the presence of certain antibodies directed at streptococcal bacteria. Often the condition is not discovered until symptoms of a heart murmur are noted. An x-ray may be ordered to look for heart enlargement. Penicillin is used to kill the streptococcal bacteria that are present in the body. Aspirin is sometimes used to control joint pain and inflammation, and corticosteroid drugs may be prescribed in severe cases. The use of penicillin on an ongoing basis may be required to prevent further streptococcal infections, although this therapy comes with its downside and may even predispose an individual to infection.

Dietary Guidelines

- ◆ Keep the diet mild and light, emphasizing soups, steamed vegetables, yogurt and cottage cheese.
- ◆ Drink plenty of raw fruit and vegetable juices.
- ◆ Avoid sugar, junk foods, alcohol, caffeine, nicotine, and fatty foods.

Recommended Nutritional Supplements

PRIMARY NUTRIENTS

ACIDOPHILUS Restores friendly flora that help boost immunity. If your child has been on antibiotics, replacing lost bacteria is essential.[1] Some controversy exists over whether taking acidophilus during antibiotic therapy is effective or not. Certainly, it is warranted immediately following therapy and may be useful during also. *Suggested Dosage:* Take liberally using active culture yogurts and bifidobacteria-containing supplements. Antibiotics kill friendly bacteria which, in turn, increases susceptibility to future infections. Use milk-free products with guaranteed bacterial count, including bifidobacteria. Check expiration date.

VITAMIN A WITH BETA CAROTENE Even in 1931, studies found that a diet rich in carotenes correlated with the number of days missed by school children.[2] In addition, vitamin A boosts immunity and is especially important during periods of infection.[3] *Suggested Dosage:* 10,000 IU of vitamin A, or an age-appropriate dose, and 20,000 IU of beta carotene daily.

VITAMIN C WITH BIOFLAVONOIDS Fights infection by boosting immune function. In addition, the presence of an infection can deplete vitamin C stores.[4] *Suggested Dosage:* 1,000 mg with each of three meals, or age-appropriate dose. Use esterized or buffered products if stomach upset is a problem. Powdered ascorbic acid is practical for treating children.

ZINC Boosts immune response, which may shorten the length of the ear infection or lessen its severity. Moreover, children who suffer from zinc deficiencies are more susceptible to infection.[5] *Suggested Dosage:* Take as directed in age-appropriate doses. Do not exceed 100 mg per day for an adult. Use picolinate of gluconate products, which can be found in lozenge form.

HERBAL COMBINATION This combination should include echinacea, goldenseal root, myrrh gum, garlic, licorice root, blue vervain, butternut root, and kelp. *Suggested Dosage:* Six to twelve capsules daily. This formula should not be used for more than three weeks at a time.

ECHINACEA: In Germany, this herb is routinely used to treat infections of the head, nose and throat. Immune stimulation is a well-known property of echinacea. It stimulates the ingestion and digestion of foreign bacteria and matter by cells called phagocytes. It also improves mobility of infection combating leukocytes (white blood cells).[6] GOLDENSEAL ROOT: The berberine content of this herb is recognized by many herbalists and natural healers to have the ability to strengthen mucus linings, making it harder for pathogens to penetrate. Two of goldenseal's more active compounds, hydrastine and berberine, have demonstrated effectiveness in treating various bacterial and viral infections, especially those of the respiratory tract.[7] MYRRH GUM: Myrrh gum has some of the same properties found in echinacea and goldenseal root. Myrrh gum stimulates phagocyte activity and reduces inflammation of mucus membranes.[8] Myrrh is officially recognized in Britain, France, and Germany for its medicinal value. GARLIC: Garlic is another herb that can be considered a tonic. It is a powerful warrior against infections of various types and origins. Garlic can increase the number of leukocytes (white blood cells) which help fight infections.[9] In addition, garlic increases perspiration which further cleanses the body. LICORICE ROOT: Licorice root contributes in several important ways to this formula. It stimulates secretion of the hormone aldosterone from the adrenal cortex. This can produce a higher energy level which is usually needed when combating infections. It is also an impressive immune system booster.[10] Long-term consumption of licorice is not recommended as it may cause weakness, electrolyte imbalances, water retention and hypertension. Licorice is officially recognized for therapeutic activity in Britain, France, Germany, Belgium, China and many other countries. BLUE VERVAIN: This herb helps to break the cycle of chronically occurring infections. It has been used for colds and flu and has an ability to reduce fever. BUTTERNUT ROOT: Butternut is a laxative that is used to treat dysentery and diarrhea. It also has an ability to expel worms. Butternut improves liver function and stimulates bile production and flow. KELP: Kelp's function in this formula is to provide needed trace elements important in many metabolic processes in the body. These nutrients may further support the healing process and return the body to normal function. Kelp contains a soluble fiber, algin, which is soothing to the gastrointestinal tract and improves bowel function.

SECONDARY NUTRIENTS

COENZYME Q10: Helps to oxygenate and protect heart muscle. *Suggested Dosage:* Take as directed.
GERMANIUM: An antioxidant agent which works to boost cellular function by scavenging for free radicals. *Suggested Dosage:* Take only as directed.
ASTRAGALUS: A Chinese herb well known for its ability to enhance immune function when fighting an infection.

Suggested Dosage: Take as directed using standardized products.
L-CARNITINE AND L-METHIONINE: Work to protect heart muscle. *Suggested Dosage:* Take as directed on an empty stomach with fruit juice.
ESSENTIAL FATTY ACIDS: The omega-3 and the omega-6 fatty acids have natural antiprostaglandin properties that fight inflammation and help relieve joint pain associated with rheumatic fever. *Suggested Dosage:* Take in liquid or capsule form. If you use fish oil, take a vitamin E supplement. Keep refrigerated.

Home Care Suggestions

- Bed rest is essential to overcoming the effects of rheumatic fever.
- The suggestions listed in the "Arthritis" ailment section can help with joint pain.

Other Supportive Therapies

MASSAGE: Using essential oils with gentle massage can help alleviate joint pain.

Scientific Facts-at-a-Glance

With all of our attention on newer and more virulent strains of the strep bacteria, we need to understand that while antibiotics save lives, they must be used with prudence. Rheumatic fever is a complication of a bacterial infection typically seen in tonsillitis, ear infections or scarlet fever. If you are being treated for a bacterial infection, it is important to take the full course of antibiotics prescribed, even if you feel better; if you don't, the infection may survive. At the same time, it is also important not to take an antibiotic for infections which are viral in nature or immunity will be compromised and new strains of bacteria will mutate.

Spirit/Mind Considerations

Rheumatic fever is one of those diseases which requires bed rest and patience and can cause feelings of frustration or depression. Like mononucleosis, it is imperative to accept that resting is absolutely necessary for recovery.

Prevention

Keeping the immune system strong through supplements and proper diet is the best preventative. Because this fever often results as a complication of strep infection, fortifying our immune defenses is crucial.

Prompt treatment of streptococcal throat infections with antibiotics can effectively prevent rheumatic fever. One must realize, however, that continued use of antibiotics weakens immunity and predisposes us to new, mutated antibiotic-resistant strains of bacteria.

Doctor's Notes

Boosting immune function must be our first priority when fighting rheumatic fever. At the top of the herb list are echinacea, goldenseal, myrrh gum and garlic. The herbal formula and nutrient list provided includes substances designed to fight viral and bacterial infections, enhance and support immune response, reduce fevers, cleanse the body and improve health. This formula is meant to fight infection. With children, dietary changes are often profoundly significant in controlling infections of any type. Milk allergies and sugar sensitivities can be major contributing factors to recurring infections. Building up your child's resistance is far better than having to treat symptoms. Watch out for culprit foods and tell your doctor that you want to use antibiotics only when absolutely necessary. Whether or not you do, always supplement your child's diet with acidophilus.

Endnotes

1. G. Zoppi, et al., "Oral bacteriotherapy in clinical practice: The use of different preparations in the treatment of acute diarrhea," Euro Jour Pedia, 1982, 139: 22-24.

2. A. Bendich, "Betacarotene and immune response," Proc Nutri Soc, 1991, 50: 263-74.

3. R.D. Semba, "Vitamin A immunity and infection," Clin Info Dis, 1994, 19: 489-99.

4. J.J. Aleo and H. Padh, "Inhibition of ascorbic acid uptake by endotoxin: evidence of mediation by serum factors," Proc Soc Exp Biol Med, 1985, 179(1): 128-31.

5. I. Lombeck, et al., "Hair zinc of young children from rural and urban areas in North Rhine-Westphalia, Germany," Euro Jour Pedia, 1988, 147(2): 179-83.

6. R. Bauer and H. Wagner, "Echinacea species as potential immunostimulatory drugs," Econ Med Plant Res, 1991, 5: 253-321.

7. D. Sun, et al., "Berberine sulfate blocks adherence of streptococcus pyogenes to epithelial cells, fobronectin and hexadecane," Antimivrob Agents Chemo, 1988, 32: 1370-74.

8. Encyclopedia of Chinese Drugs, (Shanghai Scientific and Technical Publications, People's Republic of China: 1997).

9. H.P. Koch, "Garlicin, Fact or Fiction," Phytother Res, 1993, 7: 278-80.

10. Melvyn R. Werbach and Michael T. Murray, Botanical Influences on Illness, (Third Line Press, Tarzana, Ca: 1994).

SHINGLES

Shingles refers to an infection by the herpes zoster virus of the nerves that service certain areas of the skin. This is a common disorder that affects mainly people over the age of 50. The disease is characterized by the appearance of a painful rash and small, crusty blisters. Shingles can cause a significant amount of discomfort, and even after the rash disappears, pain can persist for prolonged periods of time. Doctors refer to this pain as postherpetic neuralgia. For anyone with an immune deficiency, shingles can be a serious disease with potentially dangerous complications. Shingles affects over 800,000 Americans annually and usually resolves itself within a few weeks.

Symptoms

Initial symptoms include a heightened sensitivity of certain areas of the skin, followed by pain which, until the rash appears, may be mistaken for appendicitis or pleurisy. Areas that may be affected include the chest, abdomen (especially the rib area), limbs, hands, neck, forehead and face. Within five days the rash appears and is characterized by small, slightly raised red spots that rapidly turn to tight blisters that are full of the viral organisms. The blisters are numerous, itchy and extremely painful, sometimes causing a burning sensation. These blisters will turn yellow and dry out within three days, forming flat crusts. These crusts will fall off within two weeks, leaving pitted scars. The pain which follows an attack of shingles can be quite intense and is caused by nerve damage. Pain can persist for months or even years, especially in the elderly. If shingles develops near the eye, the cornea can become affected and blindness can occur. If the facial nerve has become affected, temporary paralysis may result. Shingles can also cause depression, shooting pains, headaches, and achiness.

If you have shingles which affect the forehead, face or eye area, or are extremely painful, see a physician as soon as possible to avoid possible blindness or facial paralysis.

Causes

Shingles is caused by the varicella-zoster virus, which also causes chicken pox. In some cases, after an attack of chicken pox, some of the viral organisms survive and become dormant in certain sensory nerves. Apparently, when the immune system is compromised, they can reemerge later and cause shingles. Attacks of shingles can be triggered by emotional or physical stress, malnutrition, the use of corticosteroid drugs, certain illnesses such as lymphoma or Hodgkin's disease, and immunosuppressant or anticancer drugs.

The pain which lingers long after the rash has disappeared is believed to be caused by scarring and excess fiber on the damaged nerves.

Conventional Therapies

There is only so much that can be done to alleviate the discomfort of shingles by the medical community. Unfortunately, once the rash is established, symptomatic treatment is the only option. Analgesics are routinely given to help control pain. In some cases, antiviral drugs, such as acyclovir (zovirax), are used to help reduce the severity of the active stage of the disease and lessen nerve damage. Steroids can also be employed to reduce inflammation and pain. In addition, skin stimulation through rubbing, applying electric currents, heat, cold, and injections of local anesthetics may be recommended. In very extreme cases, the nerves are surgically cut to stop pain impulses. Injecting nerve block medications and implanting electrical devices seem to be the most effective treatments for severe chronic pain. Zovirax ointment is considered ineffective for recurrences of herpes caused skin diseases like shingles.

Dietary Guidelines

- Some nutritionists recommend going on a juice cleanse during the first three days of an attack of shingles. After that period, emphasize the following foods: fresh fruits and vegetables, whole grains, brewer's yeast and brown rice.
- Citrus juices are recommended, as well as green vegetable juices and carrot juice.
- Vegetable broths, steamed vegetables and raw salads can be eaten as the healing occurs.
- Avoid alcohol, caffeine, nicotine, white sugar, animal fats, saturated oils and white flour.

Recommended Nutritional Supplements

PRIMARY NUTRIENTS

VITAMIN B12 Clinical tests have found that supplementation with injections has been beneficial for people suffering from shingles.[1] *Suggested Dosage:* Ask your doctor about vitamin B12 injections, or take 1,000 mcg twice a day in sublingual form.

L-LYSINE This amino acid helps to facilitate healing and inhibits the spread of the disease. *Suggested Dosage:* Take 1,000 mg per day on an empty stomach with fruit juice. Do not use for more than three to six month intervals.

VITAMIN A AND BETA CAROTENE Helps enhance the immune system and aids in healing tissue. *Suggested Dosage:* Take 25,000 IU of vitamin A and 25,000 IU of beta carotene. Interestingly, a vitamin A deficiency has been linked to susceptibility of virally-caused diseases.[2]

VITAMIN C WITH BIOFLAVONOIDS High doses of this vitamin have been used to dry up the lesions typically seen with shingles.[3] Vitamin C possesses properties that work similarly to interferon in helping the immune system fight off viral infections. *Suggested Dosage:* Take up to 10,000 mg per day, using ascorbic acid or buffered products. If you experience diarrhea, decrease the dose until gastrointestinal symptoms subside.

VITAMIN E Vitamin E therapy has had some success in treating the post-herpes zoster neuralgia which can occur after the disease has passed.[4] Vitamin E also promotes healing, contributes to cell oxygenation and is an excellent antioxidant. Capsules can be opened and placed directly on sores to help minimize scarring. *Suggested Dosage:* Take 800 IU daily.

LIQUID CHLOROPHYLL Helps to purify the blood of toxins released by viral invaders. *Suggested Dosage:* Take as directed. Can be added to juice.

HERBAL COMBINATION This combination should include echinacea, St. John's wort, goldenseal, garlic, astragalus, and ginseng. *Suggested Dosage:* Take as directed. Do not use for more than three weeks at a time.

ECHINACEA: Helps to boost the immune system and has impressive antiviral properties.[5] Try to find guaranteed potency liquid extracts. ST. JOHN'S WORT: The hypericin content of this herb has powerful antiviral actions against the herpes strain.[6] GOLDENSEAL: A natural antibiotic herb which contains berberine compounds that are beneficial for severe itching and stimulate immune defenses as well.[7] GARLIC: The sulphur-containing compounds found in garlic have proven their ability to kill viruses in several clinical studies.[8] ASTRAGALUS: This Chinese herb has impressive antiviral properties.[9] GINSENG: This herb builds stamina and helps to boost immunity.[10]

SECONDARY NUTRIENTS

HOPS, KAVA AND VALERIAN: Can be used to promote sleep and calm the nerves. *Suggested Dosage:* Take as directed for the appropriate age of the child.

CALCIUM/MAGNESIUM: Helps to facilitate the uptake of vitamin C and has a calming effect on the nervous system. *Suggested Dosage:* Take 1,500 mg of calcium and 1,000 mg of magnesium daily using calcium citrate, gluconate or lactate and chelated magnesium.

ZINC: This mineral takes part in virtually all immune functions. *Suggested Dosage:* Take 100 mg daily. Do not exceed this dose. Gluconate or picolinate products are recommended.

COENZYME Q10: Provides extra oxygenation to nerve cells and scavenges for free radicals as well. *Suggested Dosage:* Take as directed.

CAPSAICIN OINTMENT: This preparation can provide some pain relief; however, it should not be applied until the blisters are gone. *Suggested Dosage:* Use as directed. NOTE: Initial application can cause burning and redness, which subsides with continued use.

PAU D'ARCO TEA: Helps cleanse the blood and strengthen the liver, which, in turn, strengthens the immune system. Can be used in lotion form also on the affected areas. *Suggested Dosage:* Take as directed.

LADY'S SLIPPER: This herb is considered an herbal tonic for nerve endings. *Suggested Dosage*: Take as directed.

CHINESE MUSHROOMS: These botanicals have strong antiviral properties. *Suggested Dosage*: Take as directed.

Home Care Suggestions

- ◆ Calamine lotion is suggested by some professionals. Add a little rubbing alcohol to it to promote drying. Make sure not to buy Caladryl, which contains antihistamines that can cause an allergic reaction in some people.
- ◆ Avoid becoming hot and sweating; this can aggravate pain and itching.
- ◆ Soft ice packs can be applied to painful areas while the rash is present and after the rash has gone.
- ◆ There is some indication that taking acetaminophen analgesics can actually prolong shingles. Use other nonsteroidal, anti-inflammatory medications such as ibuprofen.
- ◆ Do not touch or scratch the blisters. Bathe in herbal baths such as comfrey or ginger; wet compresses also work well.
- ◆ Domeboro compresses can help dry out the blisters. Use several times a day and for 15 minutes at a time.
- ◆ If the lesions become infected, hydrogen peroxide can be applied directly to them. Polysporin or erythromycin are antibiotic ointments that are better than Neomycin and Neosporin.
- ◆ Avoid stress: take leisurely walks, practice yoga, biofeedback, breathing exercises, etc.
- ◆ Zostrix, a topical cream, can be used for pain and itching but should not be applied until the blisters are gone. Applying this preparation to the rash will cause extreme pain. Some people suffering from shingles feel that ointments and creams can sometimes further irritate the skin. Experiment with topical preparations. Nutriderm lotion is recommended after the blisters have dried and some zinc based ointments may prove beneficial.
- ◆ Using Chinese essential oils on the blisters can provide pain relief.

Other Supportive Therapies

AROMATHERAPY, HOMEOPATHY, AND ACUPUNCTURE: Qualified practitioners can help to treat individual symptoms of shingles. Acupuncture can also be an effective treatment for the post-herpetic syndrome which can cause considerable pain after the infection has passed.

Scientific Facts-at-a-Glance

Some studies have found that people with shingles have low levels of a naturally occurring purine nucleotide called AMP (adenosine monophosphate).[11] Using this compound in gel form has met with some success; however, it is not available in the United States.

Spirit/Mind Considerations

We must keep in mind that shingles is an opportunistic infection in that although it remains dormant within the body, it only becomes active during times of physical or emotional stress.

Chronic stress or prolonged periods of stress play a profound role in the development of shingles. For this reason, if we are prone to herpes infections, we need to be particularly attentive to our stress management skills. Massage, relaxation and meditation must be utilized in order to take the burden of stress off or our immune systems. Having shingles is a miserable experience and causes a great deal of stress in and of itself. If you have experienced this disease then you know how important it is to fortify both your mind and spirit.

Prevention

- ◆ Supplement your diet with plenty of vitamin C and garlic to fight infection and boost immunity.
- ◆ Get plenty of rest and regular exercise.
- ◆ Avoid using nicotine or alcohol, both of which can decrease immunity.
- ◆ In all likelihood, a weakened or compromised immune system probably caused your shingles; therefore, keeping your immune system healthy is the best prevention of all. Good immunity requires a diet that is high in vitamins and minerals and low in fat and empty carbohydrates.
- ◆ If you know you are a carrier of the herpes virus or have compromised immunity, use immune fortifying herbal formulas at the first sign of an infection.
- ◆ Take a strong multivitamin/mineral supplement daily.

Doctor's Notes

Shingles is caused by a herpes virus that has remained dormant in nerves and is activated in times of stress or when immunity has become compromised. It is often misdiagnosed as tendinitis, pleurisy or other painful conditions before its characteristic rash appears. If a person knows that they have herpes zoster, taking St. John's wort and echinacea can sometimes prevent the rash from appearing. Shingles and related conditions can be very painful, especially in places where the rash was present. Injections of vitamin B12 can help to reduce the irritation from the rash and promotes healing. Acupuncture laser treatments can also shorten the duration of shingles and its post-herpetic pain. I remember a 45-year-old female who had developed shingles on her lower jaw and chin. The lesions had been active for about four days when she came in. Laser acupuncture using a 5-milliwatt laser was used to stimulate acupuncture points and to treat the sores. Each lesion was given a 10 to 15 second treatment. I also placed her on St. John's wort and echinacea and gave her an injection of vitamin B12. After the second treatment the lesions were markedly improved, and after a week, they were all but gone. Zovirax, a prescription medication, can be helpful in reducing the length of shingles. If you choose to use Zorvirax, combine it with St. John's wort and echinacea. This reduces the chance of post-herpetic neuralgia. Because our immunity weakens with age, taking a good strong multivitamin and mineral supplement along with extra vitamin A is highly recommended. Of course, managing stress plays a profound role in immunity. Prolonged periods of stress such as a divorce, job loss, or taking care of an elderly person can also predispose us to diseases like shingles. Taking astragalus and ginseng can help to prevent stress-related diseases.

Additional Resources

Herpes Resource Center
P.O. Box 13827
Research Triangle Park, NC 27709
(919) 361-8488

Endnotes

1. A. Fupta and H. Mital, "Cyanocobalain (vitamin B12) in the management of herpes zoster," Indian Pract, 1967, 20(7): 457-59.

2. Michael T. Murray, ND, Encyclopedia of Nutritional Supplements, (Prima Publishing, Rocklin, CA), 24.

3. M. Zureick, "Treatment of shingles and herpes with vitamin C intravenously," Jour des Praticiens, 1950, 64:586. See also A. Bendich, "Vitamin C and immune response," Food Techol, 1987, 41: 112-14.

4. S. Ayres and R. Mihan, "Post-herpes zoster neuralgia: Response to vitamin E therapy," Arch Dermatol, 1973, 108: 855-56. See also Plastic and Reconstructive Surgery, June, 1982, 69: 1029-30.

5. R. Bauer, and H. Wagner, "Echinacea species as potential immunostimulatory drugs," Econ Med Plant Res, 1991, 5: 253-321.

6. G. Lavie, et al., "Antiviral pharmaceutical compositions containing hypericin or pseudohypericin," European Patent Application, 87111467, 8-8-87, European Patent Office.

7. M. Sabir and N. Bhide, "Study of some pharmacologic actions of berberine," Indian Jour Physiol Pharm, 1971, 15: 111-132.

8. D. Weber, et al., "In vitro virucidal effects of allium sativum (garlic) extract and compounds," Planta Medica, 1992, 58: 417-423.

9. Y. Yang, et al., "Effect of Astragalus membranaceous on natural killer cell activity and induction with Coxsackie B viral myocarditis," Chin Med Jour, 1990, 103(4): 304-7.

10. B. Bohn, et al., "Flow-cytometric studies with Eleutherococcus senticosus extract as an immunomodulatory agent," Arzneimittel-Forsch, 1987, 37: 1193-96.

11. S. Sklar, et al., "The treatment of prevention of neuralgia with adenosine monophosphate," JAMA, 1985, 253(10): 1427-30.

SINUSITIS

Sinusitis is an inflammation of the mucus membranes of the sinuses. It commonly affects the frontal and maxillary sinuses. Sinusitis usually occurs as a complication of a cold or other viral infection of the nose or throat. It is usually caused by a subsequent infection of bacterial origin. When the sinuses become obstructed from a cold, allergy, dental problems, or related conditions, mucus flow is impeded and bacterial invasion can take place. Sinusitis is common; however, some people never get it. Those that do sometimes have it for weeks on end.

Symptoms

In an acute sinus infection, symptoms usually consist of nasal congestion and discharge which will usually come from one nostril only. Other possible symptoms include a sensation of heaviness around the eyes and behind the nose, a nasal speaking tone, tearing, fever, chills, frontal headaches, pain in the cheekbones, tenderness and swelling over the sinus area, a nonproductive cough, a musty odor, bad breath, or a bad taste in the mouth.

In chronic sinusitis, a post-nasal drip may be present; however, pain is usually absent. In the cases of chronic sinusitis, permanent mucosal damage can occur.

A sinus infection requires prompt medical attention. See your doctor if you have pain which radiates from your sinuses to the area of the eyes or beneath the forehead. You may also have a fever or develop bad breath or have a bad taste in your mouth. If left untreated, a sinus infection can lead to serious complications.

Some experts believe that the notion of a sinus headache is more of a myth than truth. Persistent headaches due to chronic sinus problems or allergies are usually considered rare. A true sinus headache will feel worse if you bend or lean over.

Causes

Sinus infections occur when a sinus outlet is obstructed by a swelling of the nasal lining. Air and mucous build-up can cause an increase in pressure and be a perfect environment for bacterial invasion. Bacterial sinusitis is typically caused by an upper respiratory tract infection such as the common cold or influenza. Allergies can also predispose one to sinus infections. Other factors which can result in sinusitis are underlying dental infections, sudden changes in pressure (which can occur in flying, swimming and diving), smoking, fumes, foreign bodies in the nose, nasal polyps, damage to the nasal bones, asthma, nasal deformities such as a deviated septum, and presence of various bacteria. Sensitivity to birth control pills or to aspirin can also cause the sinuses to close and predispose one to infection.

The notion that a dysfunctional colon can cause the build up of toxins in the system which result in retaining mucosal secretions which subsequently become infected has received more scientific attention recently. Avoiding constipation through the proper diet is a factor that should not be overlooked.

Conventional Therapies

Sinusitis is difficult to distinguish from a cold. Nose, ears, throat and teeth will be examined. In some cases, an x-ray may be ordered. Antibiotic therapy will be initiated if a bacterial infection is present. Some doctors point out that removing the nasal obstruction through decongestants or surgery will sometimes clear up the infection.

Over-the-counter nasal decongestants in both pill and spray form will be recommended, along with the application of heat and steam. The overuse of these products can produce a rebound effect, which aggravates nasal congestion. In rare instances, puncturing the sinuses may be necessary to relieve pain and pressure. Irrigating the infected sinus passages is also routinely done. Surgical options exist for chronic sinusitis and involve a surgical procedure in which the infected tissue is removed to facilitate permanent nasal drainage. If a deviated septum is causing the problem, it can be surgically corrected. Antibiotics should not be used unless a bacterial infection is present.

Dietary Guidelines

- Eliminate dairy products and wheat, both of which can cause nasal congestion and mucus production.
- Avoid alcoholic beverages. Fermented alcohol can actually clog up nasal passages. A short fruit juice fast (two days) is initially recommended.
- Use plenty of orange, grapefruit, lemon, pineapple or grape juice.
- After the two days, add plenty of raw vegetables, and broths.
- Drink plenty of fluids. Sipping hot herb teas or broths can help facilitate mucus flow.
- Eating hot peppers and cajun spices can initiate mucus flow.
- Horseradish has also been a traditional treatment for sinus congestion.

Recommended Nutritional Supplements

PRIMARY NUTRIENTS

GARLIC Compounds found in garlic are potent antiviral agents and have shown through animal and human studies that they can protect against influenza virus infection.[1] *Suggested Dosage*: Take two capsules with each of three meals.

VITAMIN A AND BETA CAROTENE Helps to lessen inflammation of mucus membranes and acts as an immune system booster. Clinical studies have shown that vitamin A supplementation can reduce the incidence of colds in children and improve resistance to influenza in the elderly.[2] *Suggested*

Dosage: 25,000 IU daily for the duration of infection. CAUTION: Pregnant women should not take over 10,000 IU daily. Take 15,000 IU of beta carotene daily.

VITAMIN C WITH BIOFLAVONOIDS Some studies suggest that vitamin C significantly lessens the symptoms of an upper respiratory infection. Double-blind trials have shown that using 1 to 2 grams a day lessens the severity and duration of a rhinovirus.[3] In addition, quercetin, a bioflavonoid, may actually inhibit the replication of RNA and DNA viruses.[4] *Suggested Dosage*: 10,000 mg daily divided out in equal doses taken with each of three meals. If you cannot tolerate pure ascorbic acid, use buffered forms or calcium ascorbate varieties.

ZINC GLUCONATE LOZENGES These can be dissolved under the tongue and should be taken at the first sign of a cold or flu. Zinc has been found to cut down not only upper respiratory infections, but also the duration of these infections. Studies confirm zinc's ability to potentiate the action of macrophages, organisms that stick to and destroy pathogenic microorganisms. This is why some experts believe taking zinc at the onset of an infection can prevent its progression.[5] *Suggested Dosage*: One lozenge every four hours for no more than a week. Do not take more than 100 mg daily.

ECHINACEA Clinical studies have shown that supplementing with echinacea can strengthen the immune response to infections.[6] In addition, echinacea reduces susceptibility to colds and minimizes their symptoms, which could have an impact on sinusitis.[7] *Suggested Dosage*: Take as directed, using guaranteed potency or standardized products. Do not use for more than two-week intervals at a time.

ASTRAGALUS AND SCHIZANDRA Used by the Chinese to reduce the incidence and length of a cold. Tests have proven the ability of these herbs to fight viral infections.[8] *Suggested Dosage*: Take as directed.

ST. JOHN'S WORT The hypericin content of this herb has some impressive antiviral actions and should be utilized for virally caused upper respiratory infections.[9] *Suggested Dosage*: Take as directed, using guaranteed potency or standardized product.

GOLDENSEAL Contains natural berberine compounds that fight infection. *Suggested Dosage*: Take as directed using standardized products. CAUTION: This herb should not be used for more than two weeks at a time or if you are pregnant or nursing.

HERBAL COMBINATION This combination should include pleurisy root, wild cherry bark, slippery elm bark, plantain, mullein leaves, chickweed, horehound, licorice root, kelp, ginger root, and saw palmetto berries. *Suggested Dosage*: Four to eight capsules daily. For chronic conditions it is best to use maximum dosage of eight capsules per day for a prolonged period of three to six weeks or until symptoms subside.

PLEURISY ROOT: The English word *pleurisy* comes from the French word *pleurisis*, which means "lung trouble," indicating a primary use for this herb. This root has been used for other respiratory problems which produce mucus. Pleurisy root also helps to cleanse the body of toxins through mild diuretic effects and its ability to promote perspiration.[10] WILD CHERRY BARK: Wild cherry bark has the ability to relax the respiratory nerves. Wild cherry bark also improves the stomach, digestion, and appetite which may provide a secondary healing benefit to people suffering from upper respiratory infections like sinusitis.[11] SLIPPERY ELM BARK: Slippery elm bark has a reputation as a medicine for inflamed mucus membranes. The inner bark is known for its demulcent, diuretic and emollient properties attributable to its high mucilage content. This bark cleanses, heals, and strengthens and is particularly effective for inflammatory irritation associated with sore throats.[12] PLANTAIN: Plantain is similar to slippery elm bark in that it too contains mucilage. Plantain is used as an expectorant and is especially good for those suffering chronic catarrhal problems. It is also beneficial for hoarseness and sore throats. It seems to be able to help almost all respiratory problems.[13] MULLEIN LEAVES: Mullein leaves also contain high amounts of mucilage. It is considered to be a good remedy for inflamed tissue found in the lungs, throat and nose. Mullein leaves were officially recognized as a treatment for respiratory disorders and allergic reactions in the *National Formulary* until 1936.[14] CHICKWEED: Chickweed is an expectorant. It also has mild laxative effects which will contribute to the cleansing and healing process and has been used to treat stubborn respiratory infections such as tuberculosis.[15] HOREHOUND: Horehound is an excellent remedy for upper respiratory tract infections. Its activity is thought to be attributed to a volatile oil found in the herb called marubiin. Horehound helps to cleanse the body of toxins through its diuretic properties and ability to promote perspiration.[16] LICORICE ROOT: Licorice root has received official recognition in Britain, Germany, France, and Belgium for its ability to assist with various respiratory infections.[17] It shares some of the same properties as other herbs of this formula in cleansing and healing through its mild diuretic and laxative properties. CAUTION: Licorice should not be taken for more than three consecutive weeks and should be avoided by anyone with diabetes, high blood pressure or kidney disease. KELP: Kelp's direct application in this formula is in assisting with bronchitis, emphysema, and asthma. However, indirectly kelp provides a very rich storehouse of nutrients which can assist with the healing process. GINGER ROOT: Ginger root makes the other herbs more effective. It is also believed to be able to "warm" the body, which can help to expedite immune function in the same way as a natural fever does.[18] SAW PALMETTO BERRIES: Saw palmetto berries are useful in the treatment of mucus causing infections. The berries are recognized for their diuretic properties, thereby contributing to the overall cleansing action of this formula.

SECONDARY NUTRIENTS

ACIDOPHILUS: Helps to replenish friendly bacteria stores in the intestine that help fight infection. *Suggested Dosage:* Take as directed, using milk-free products with guaranteed bacterial count. Check expiration date.

TRACE SILVER INTRANASAL SPRAY: Helps to fight infection topically. *Suggested Dosage:* Use as directed.

COMFREY AND FENUGREEK: Helps control mucus production by liquefying it and expediting its expulsion from the body. *Suggested Dosage:* Take as directed using guaranteed potency or standardized products.

LICORICE COUGH DROPS OR TEA: Helps to soothe irritated throats and helps to relieve coughs. *Suggested Dosage:* Take as directed, using pure licorice and not artificial licorice. Do not take pure licorice products if you have kidney disease, hypertension, or diabetes.

CHAMOMILE TEA: Helps to promote rest and bring down a fever. *Suggested Dosage:* Take as directed.

Home Care Suggestions

◆ Avoid using decongestant nasal sprays, such as Afrin, over a long period of time. Over-the-counter nasal sprays are among the most addictive drugs around. They can also damage the nasal lining and impair the normal function of nasal cilia and membranes. Nasal sprays can cause a rebound effect in which nasal congestion returns with more swelling and pressure than was originally present.

◆ Using these sprays sparingly in the early stage of a sinus infection can help to facilitate drainage.

◆ Using Sudafed, Sine-aid, Sinarest, or Drixoral are recommended by some physicians, but should not be taken if driving, operating machinery or if heart or kidney disease is present.

◆ Nasal saline sprays designed to moisten the nose can be purchased or made at home by mixing 1/4 teaspoon of salt with 1/4 teaspoon of baking soda in a glass of warm water. The saline will not clear up congestion.

◆ Swabbing the sinus passages with oil of bitter orange can help relieve swelling and promote drainage.

◆ Make a tea of bayberry bark or goldenseal and bring it to a simmer, inhaling the vapors.

◆ Use a menthol or eucalyptus pack over the sinus membranes.

◆ Rubbing Chinese essential oils on the nose can relieve congestion (do not use near the eyes).

◆ Use a cool mist vaporizer to add humidity to the air.

◆ Certain yoga exercises can help to drain fluids and decrease congestion. Neck and eye exercises, corpse pose and shoulder stand are recommended.

◆ Exercise can help to clear sinus passages by releasing adrenaline. Avoid swimming.

◆ If you smoke, stop. Chronic sinusitis is often related to smoking.

◆ Get plenty of rest. Stay in bed if necessary to get the kind of rest required to fight infection.

◆ Applying moist hot packs to the nasal area can facilitate drainage.

◆ Alternating soft ice packs and hot packs can also bring relief.

◆ Do not blow your nose too forcefully. Gently blow your nose after you have used steam inhalation or a decongestant. Blowing one nostril at a time is recommended. It can prevent a buildup of pressure in the ears. Gently sniffling helps to drain the sinuses and should be encouraged.

◆ Raise the head of the bed or sleep with extra pillows. Lying flat can increase pressure in the nasal passages and cause more discomfort.

Other Supportive Therapies

ACUPUNCTURE: This therapy, combined with herbal supplementation, can significantly improve chronic sinus conditions.

Scientific Facts-at-a-Glance

Over 25 percent of chronic sinus infections are due to underlying dental infections. Before going on and off of antibiotics indefinitely, take a trip to the dentist and have your teeth checked thoroughly. A tooth can actually be infected without presenting any obvious symptoms. Having a chronic tooth infection can also tax the immune system and cause fatigue and other symptoms. One recent experiment took an abscessed tooth that a person had lived with for months and placed it under the skin of a laboratory animal. The animal died within 48 hours.

Prevention

◆ Use good dental hygiene and take care of tooth problems promptly to avoid developing sinusitis as a complication of dental disease.
◆ Keep your colon functioning well by eating plenty of foods that are high in fiber, raw fruits and vegetables and avoiding fatty junk foods, rich dairy products, white sugar and white flour. The notion that poor intestinal function can cause the production of mucus and lead to subsequent infection should not be dismissed.
◆ If you have a cold or the flu and your sinuses swell, use decongestants so that they do not remain obstructed for long periods of time.
◆ Try to control allergies so that nasal mucosa are not constantly irritated and blocked. Irrigating the nose on a regular basis with saline solutions can help remove allergens that cause irritation.
◆ Build up your immune system with proper diet and supplementation.
◆ Try not to weaken your immunity by taking antibiotics regularly.
◆ Stay away from foods that cause allergic reactions and other allergens.
◆ Do not use over-the-counter nasal sprays.

Doctor's Notes

I have discovered that many people who believe they have sinusitis are actually suffering from a frontal headache. Frequently these people use antibiotics for lack of a better treatment, which will offer them no benefit at all. If you are consistently on and off antibiotics for symptoms of sinusitis, you need to insist that an x-ray be taken to confirm the presence of an infection. If you do have chronic sinusitis, you may want to aggressively pursue some natural treatments. I remember Laura, a 17-year-old who was actually scheduled for sinus surgery, but her mother insisted that she come in for acupuncture treatment as a last resort. After six treatments she was 90 percent free of her symptoms. She also used an herbal formula called Nasal Tabs.

If a person is battling chronic sinus infections, it is a sign that their immune system is not functioning optimally. Taking a short course of echinacea therapy can help boost immune defenses. In addition, using a strong multivitamin/mineral supplement on a permanent basis can help to maintain immunity. Making sure to get enough selenium, zinc and calcium is vital. Astragalus, one of my favorite Chinese herbs, can greatly contribute to enhanced immunity. Schizandra in combination with Chinese mushrooms is also good. I've also used some of the "green foods" like wheat grass to treat chronic infection. Intranasal sprays, which consist of trace silver, have also worked well on occasion.

Endnotes

1. K. Nagai, "Experimental studies on the preventative effect of garlic against infection with influenza virus," Jpn Jour Infect Dis, 1973, 47: 321.
2. C.B. Pinnock, et al., "Vitamin A status in children who are prone to respiratory tract infections," Aust Pedia, 1986, 22(2): 95-99. See also M. Chavance, et al., "Nutritional support improves antibody response to influenza in the elderly," Bri Med Jour, Letter, Nov. 9, 1985, 1348-49.
3. A.B. Carr, "Vitamin C and the common cold: Using identical twins as controls," Med Jour Aust, 1981, 2: 411-12.
4. T.N. Kaul, et al., "Antiviral effect of flavonoids on human viruses," Jour Med Virol, 1985, 15: 71-79.
5. P.J. Fraker, et al., "Zinc requirement for macrophage function: Effect of zinc deficiency on uptake and killing of a protozoan parasite," Immunology, 1989, 68: 114-19.
6. B. Braunig, et al., "Echinacea purpurea radix for strengthening the immune response in flu-like infections," Z Phytother, 1991, 13: 7-13.
7. D. Shoneberber, "The influence of immune-stimulating effects of pressed juice from Echinacea purpurea on the course and severity of colds: The results of a double-blind study," Forum Immunologi, 1992, 8: 2-12.
8. Z.Y. Yang, et al., "Effect of astragalus membranaceous on natural killer cell activity and induction with Coxsackie-B viral myocarditis," Chin Med, 1990, 103(4): 304-07.
9. H. Someya, "Effect of a constituent of hypericum erectum on infection and multiplication of Epstein-Barr virus," Jour Tokyo Med, 1985, 43: 815-26.
10. C.F. Millspaugh, American Medicinal Plants (Dover Publications, New York: 1974), 540-41.
11. T.R. Brendle and C.W. Unger, "Folk medicine of the Pennsylvania Germans: The non-occult cures," in Proceedings of the Pennsylvania German Society, 1935, Vol. XLV, II: Norristown, Pennsylvania German Society.
12. H.H. Smith, Ethnobotany of the Ojibwa Indians, 1932, Bulletin of the Public Museum, Vol. IV, 3: Milwaukee.

13. M. Matev, et al., "Clinical trial of a plantago major preparation in the treatment of chronic bronchitis," Vutreshni Bolesti (Sofia), 1982, 21(2): 133-37.

14. P.S. Benoit, et al., "Biological and phytochemical evaluation of plants: XIV, Anti-inflammatory evaluation of 163 species of plant," Lloydia, 39(2-3): 160-171.

15. F.K. Fitzpatrick, "Plant substances active against mycobacterium tuberculosis," Antibiotics and Chemotherapy, 1954, 4(5): 528-36.

16. M.O. Karryev, et al., "Some therapeutic properties and phytochemistry of common horehound," Izvestiia Akad Nauk Turk SSSR, Seria Biol, 1976, 86-88.

17. D.M. Anderson and W.G. Smith, "The antitussive activity of glycyrrhetinic acid and its derivatives," Journal of Pharmacy and Pharmacology, 1961, 13: 36-96-404.

18. C.J.K. Henry and S.M. Piggott, "Effect of ginger on metabolic rate," Hum Nutr Clin Nutr, 1987, 41(c): 89-92.

SKIN DISORDERS

SEE "ECZEMA" AND "PSORIASIS"

SLEEP DISORDERS

SEE "INSOMNIA"

SPRAINS/STRAINS

While it may be confusing, there is a difference between a sprain and a strain. A strain occurs when a muscle is stressed beyond its capability, due to putting excess weight on the muscle or over using it. Strains are also referred to as pulled muscles. Strains typically occur in the hamstring, quadricep muscles of the thigh, groin muscles and shoulder muscles. A sprain results when a ligament which connects bone to muscle is stretched to the point of tearing. In this case, the soft tissue which surrounds the joint may become inflamed. Strains and sprains are treated much the same way except in strains heat can be initially applied to promote healing. In the case of a severe sprain, treatment should be the same as for a fracture or a broken bone. Any joint can become sprained and the severity of that sprain depends on the extent of the ligament tear. Knees, ankles and fingers are especially susceptible to injury. Most people will refer to any painful joint injury as a sprain, though that may be technically incorrect. The majority of strains and sprains heal within two weeks.

Symptoms

Pain and tenderness in the joint area are typical, although the joint will usually still function to some extent. Other symptoms include bruising, swelling, which usually occurs quickly due to bleeding into the tissue surrounding the joint, and in severe cases, a deformed appearance. CAUTION: If pain and swelling persist for over two days, see your physician immediately to eliminate the possibility of a fractured or broken bone.

Causes

Muscles can become overstretched during vigorous exercise. Sprains also commonly occur when dancing, playing tennis, soccer, hiking, or during downhill skiing. Sprains commonly occur from unexpected movements or twisting motions typical of a fall or athletic injury. If the demands placed on a muscle are excessive, a ligament tear results. Strains are milder than sprains and usually result in a muscle that contracts and becomes stiff and painful. Strained or pulled muscles commonly result when lifting a heavy weight.

Conventional Therapies

Most strains and sprains can be treated at home; however, in severe cases, casting may be required. The debate between the use of cold vs. hot therapy is still ongoing, with varying opinions on the value of both. In cases of severe sprains, an x-ray will be taken to rule out a fracture, and the joint may be casted. Watching for swelling is important if casting has occurred, which may impair circulation. Analgesics may be prescribed for pain and in extreme cases, nonsteroidal anti-inflammatory drugs may be recommended. Occasionally, surgery may be required to repair badly torn ligaments. In these cases, subsequent physical therapy will be recommended to restrengthen the joint and restore mobility.

First Aid for Sprains

- Do not use the injured part.
- Elevate the affected area using pillows or a sling.
- Apply a cold pack to the areas to reduce pain and swelling for several hours.
- After 24 hours, heat may be applied.
- Support the joint involved with an elastic bandage and do not put any weight on the area for at least two days.

First Aid for Strains

- Use heat on the strained area with a heating pad or hot water bottle for 15 minutes several times a day.

Dietary Guidelines

- Drink plenty of pineapple juice immediately after the injury. Pineapple has an enzyme called bromelain which helps with bruising and can promote healing.
- Juice your own fresh fruits and vegetables and eat plenty of raw foods with live enzymes.

Recommended Nutritional Supplements

PRIMARY NUTRIENTS

VITAMIN C WITH BIOFLAVONOIDS Tests have confirmed that ascorbic acid boosts healing due to injuries and that citrus bioflavonoids can actually reduce recovery time by minimizing inflammation.[1,2] *Suggested Dosage*: 5,000 mg daily.

COENZYME Q10 May protect against exercise-induced muscle injury by boosting muscle cell oxygenation and acts to scavenge for free radicals released in injured tissue.[3] *Suggested Dosage*: 50 to 100 mg daily.

GLUCOSAMINE SULFATE Supplements of this compound help to heal and regenerate the cartilage matrix and prevent the formation of arthritis in joint injuries.[4] *Suggested Dosage*: Take as directed according to weight.

BROMELAIN Administration of this enzyme extracted from pineapple may speed healing of contusions, sprains, hematomas and other soft tissue injuries.[5] *Suggested Dosage*: Take as directed.

BILBERRY Using this herb which is rich in anthocyanicides may reduce capillary permeability which will result in much less bruising in injured tissue.[6] *Suggested Dosage*: Take as directed using standardized guaranteed potency products.

GINKGO BILOBA This herb helps to boost muscle tissue oxygenation and may also discourage edema which can result from tissue injury.[7] *Suggested Dosage*: Take as directed using standardized products.

GRAPE SEED OR PINE BARK EXTRACTS The proanthocyanidins of these extracts are potent free radical scavengers and powerful anti-inflammatory agents which treat swelling and pain.[8] *Suggested Dosage*: Take as directed; however, during the first four days of the injury, take a larger dose to ensure tissue saturation and then taper off.

CALCIUM/MAGNESIUM Helps boost the regeneration and repair of connective tissue. *Suggested Dosage*: Take 1,500 mg of calcium and 750 mg of magnesium. Use calcium citrate, lactate or gluconate and chelated forms of magnesium.

HERBAL COMBINATION This combination includes devil's claw, yucca, alfalfa leaf and seed, wild yam root, sarsaparilla root, kelp, white willow bark, cayenne, horsetail, and chickweed. *Suggested Dosage*: Four to six capsules daily. For extreme cases it is best to use maximum dosage of six capsules per day for a longer period of time.

DEVIL'S CLAW: The secondary roots of this plant have a rich history of use as an anti-inflammatory and analgesic.[9] YUCCA: Yucca has a similar action to that of devil's claw. It reduces histamine production and, as a result, inflammation and pain may be alleviated. The constituents of yucca which are bioactive are saponins.[10] ALFALFA LEAVES AND SEEDS: Alfalfa leaves and seeds provide a rich nutrient source to help the body to return to a healthy state.[11] WILD YAM ROOT: Other common names for wild yam root include rheumatism root and colic root, suggesting its use as an antirheumatic and digestive aid. Its antirheumatic property is primarily thought to be attributed to its cortisone precursor diosgenin. As diosgenin is converted to cortisone, anti-inflammatory activity results, and the patient may notice a reduction of pain.[12] SARSAPARILLA ROOT: Sarsaparilla, used as a food flavoring in the United States, is officially recognized in Germany and the United Kingdom for its antirheumatic and anti-inflammatory properties. Historically, this herb has been used to treat gout and rheumatism and is classified as a tonic and blood purifier.[13] KELP: Kelp, like alfalfa, is a dense source of nutrients, particularly trace elements which can improve the body's nutrition. WHITE WILLOW BARK: White willow bark has been used for over a thousand years to relieve pain. Salicin, aspirin's forerunner, was discovered to be white willow's active constituent. Apart from its ability to assist with pain, salicin reduces inflammation, but unlike aspirin it will not thin the blood or irritate the stomach. CAYENNE: Cayenne stimulates circulation and makes the other herbs more effective. Cayenne's hot principle, capsaicin, is also a noted analgesic and can be applied in topical ointment form. HORSETAIL: The main action of this herb is to strengthen and regenerate connective tissues. Connective tissue (found abundantly in joints) is destroyed by inflammation. Silica is vital in regenerating connective tissue and horsetail is one of the richest known sources of silica.

SECONDARY NUTRIENTS

VITAMIN B-COMPLEX: Important for any tissue repair and helps the body cope when under stress due to trauma. *Suggested Dosage*: 100 mg daily.

POTASSIUM AND SILICON: Helps to promote calcium absorption and contributes to connective tissue repair and strength. *Suggested Dosage*: Take as directed.

ZINC: Promotes tissue repair and boosts immunity during periods of stress. *Suggested Dosage*: 50 mg daily.

ARNICA: This herb comes from the high mountains of western North America and is a traditional remedy used for bruising and sprains. Use it externally in cream or tincture form to decrease bruising and discoloration. Arnica can be purchased in some drug stores and in herb shops. Do not take internally. *Suggested Usage:* Use as directed for topical use only.

Home Care Suggestions

◆ Soak the affected area in comfrey tea and take internally for its healing properties. Comfrey encourages cell growth in the connective tissues and the bones.

◆ Apple cider vinegar compresses are also good to help reduce swelling and pain.

◆ With a strain, which does not swell or bruise, apply a hot water bottle or heating pad to the area for 15 minutes several times per day.

◆ Do not place any weight on the injured area.

◆ Let pain be your guide to activities. If it hurts don't do it.

◆ If you suspect a sprain which is identified by swelling and bruising, rest the joint by elevating it to drain fluids and apply ice packs to reduce swelling.

◆ An elastic bandage can be used to wrap a sprain and provide support, but make sure that it is not so tight as to impair circulation. The ace bandage should be firm but not tight. There should not be any purple or bluish color to the area. Do not stretch the bandage as you wind it on. The stretchiness is for mobility purposes. Wrap the bandage as you would a roll of gauze.

◆ Turmeric and hot water can be combined to form a paste that can be applied to the sprained or bruised area with a gauze dressing to reduce swelling. Clay poultices can accomplish the same thing.

◆ A paste made from five egg whites, cayenne pepper, and thyme leaves can be applied on a gauze bandage to the sprain to promote circulation.

Other Supportive Therapies

HYDROTHERAPY: Treat affected area with a cold compress or icepack, then elevate and rest injured joint.

HOMEOPATHY: Arnica 6c and Ruta grav. 6c are routinely prescribed for injuries.

AROMATHERAPY: Add oil of sweet marjoram and rosemary to water and soak affected body part from 10 to 15 minutes. Cold compresses can also be made from essential oil decoctions.

MASSAGE: Can be gently applied to muscles around the injured portion to stimulate circulation.

ACUPUNCTURE: This form of therapy can help relieve pain.

OSTEOPATHY OR CHIROPRACTIC: Either of these may be helpful if the injury is serious enough to warrant periods of immobility.

Scientific Facts-at-a-Glance

New information on *Ginkgo biloba* tells us that it has the ability to boost vascular circulation and oxygenation to heart muscle as well as other muscles. Much like coenzyme Q10, it can help to counteract the kind of oxygen starvation which can occur during periods of strenuous exercise. Because sprains and strains commonly occur during athletic activities, it only stands to reason that using these supplements prior to exercise may help to protect the muscles from injury.

Spirit/Mind Considerations

Any injury brings with it a certain degree of emotional shock. It is important to recognize this post-trauma reaction and to deal with the depression or anxiety which may accompany it. Immobilization or having to use crutches requires a new mind set or frustration and nervousness will result. Let your body have the time to heal and don't fight it. Take advantage of the healing time by reading more or just learning to visit or relax. Insisting on trying to maintain your previous workload or schedule can result in a great deal of stress and stress impedes the healing process.

Prevention

◆ Stretching before exercising and staying flexible are important preventative measures; staying fit is probably the best deterrent to sprains and strains.

◆ Use good, supportive shoes that fit well during athletic activities.

◆ Walk or jog in well lit areas to avoid falling in divots and hidden ruts.

◆ Strengthening weak muscles through proper exercise can help avoid strains and sprains.

◆ Don't overdue when exercising and avoid violent twisting motions.

◆ Use elastic supports around areas susceptible to injury such as ankles or knees.

Doctor's Notes

A common result of sprains and strains is the inflammation which causes swelling and pain. The blend of herbs and nutrients listed is designed to alleviate the symptoms of inflammation and pain and also to provide a rich nutrient base to help the body's healing process and return the body to normal function. While immobilization has been preached as the best policy for injuries of this type, new attitudes recommend returning to activity sooner under controlled situations. The ability of nutrients like bromelain to reduce swelling should not be underestimated. Bilberry has some remarkable vascular effects, as does grape seed extract. Unfortunately, most doctors will freely mention Tylenol or Advil for pain but rarely recommend using bioflavonoids and proteolytic enzymes as natural anti-inflammatory agents with no side effects.

Endnotes

1. G. Gey, et al., "Effect of ascorbic acid on endurance performance and athletic injury," JAMA, 1970, 211(1): 105.
2. R. Cragin, "The use of bioflavonoids in the prevention and treatment of athletic injuries," Med Times, 1962, 90: 529-30.
3. Y. Shimomura, et al., "Protective effect of coenzyme Q-10 on exercise-induced muscular injury," Biochem Biophys Res Commun, 1991, 176: 349-55.
4. D. Bohmer, et al., "Treatment of chondrorpathia patellae in young athletes with glucosamine sulfate," in N. Bach, L Prokop, and R. Suchert, eds., Current Topics in Sports Medicine (Proc World Congress of Sports Med, Vienna: 1982).
5. S. Taussig and S. Batkin, "Bromelain, the enzyme complex of pineapple (Ananas comosus) and its clinical application," An Update, Jour Ethnopharmacol 1988, 22: 191-203.
6. E. Mian, et al., "Anthocyanosides and the walls of micro vessels: further aspects of the mechanism of action of their protective effect in syndromes due to abnormal capillary fragility," Miverva Med, 1977, 68(52): 3565-81.
7. G. Lagrue G et al., "Idiopathic cyclic edema: The role of capillary hyper permeability and its correction by Ginkgo biloba," Presse Med, 1986, 15(31): 1550-53.
8. R.M. Facino, et al., "Free radicals scavenging action and anti-enzyme activities of procyanidines from Vitis vinifera: A mechanism for their capillary protective action," Arzneim Forsch, 1994, 44: 592-601.
9. L.R. Brady, et al., Pharmacognosy, 8th ed. (Lea and Gebiger, Philadelphia: 1981, 480).
10. R. Bingham, et al., "Yucca plant saponins in the management of arthritis," Jour Applied Nutrition, 1975, 27: 45-50.
11. M.R. Malinow, et al., "Effect of alfalfa saponins on intestinal cholesterol absorption in rats," Amer Jour Clini Nutri, 1977, 30: 2061-67.
12. H.W. Feller, The Eclectic Materia Medica, Pharmacology and Therapeutics (Eclectic Medical Publications, Portland Oregon: 1983, first published in 1922).
13. Kiangsu Institute of Modern Medicine, Encyclopedia of Chinese Drugs, 2 vols. 1977, Shanghai, People's Republic of China.

STRESS

Unfortunately, stress is a normal part of our lives. While stress is not necessarily bad, individual reaction to stress can produce undesirable and detrimental results, such as prolonged states of anxiety. Stress-related medical and emotional problems have dramatically increased over the last few decades and testify to the fast paced, demanding lives that most of us lead. The fact that Valium and Tagamet have been among the most widely prescribed drugs in the world indicates that stress related disorders exist in epidemic proportions. The emotionally distressed state that occurs in stressful situations can lead to illness and emotional dysfunction. We now know that stress precipitates many diseases.

Symptoms

Stress related ailments include the following:

- ulcers
- high blood pressure
- headaches
- neck aches
- loss of appetite
- asthma
- hives
- impotence
- TMJ syndrome
- colitis
- heartburn
- backaches
- diarrhea
- dizziness
- skin rashes
- heart palpitations
- hair loss
- lowered immunity

It is important that you seek medical help if you are experiencing the following symptoms:

- blackouts or dizzy spells
- overwhelming anxiety/panic
- racing pulse or palpitations
- trembling
- hives
- chronic pain

Some other more serious diseases thought to be associated with prolonged stress or anxiety are:

- angina
- cancer
- diverticulosis
- menstrual irregularities
- migraine headaches
- pancreatic disease
- autoimmune diseases
- Crohn's disease
- heart disease
- impotence
- rheumatoid arthritis

During periods of prolonged stress, the body can react by increasing adrenalin production. This increases heart rate, shuts down digestion and results in elevated blood pressure and faster breathing. In addition, fats, cholesterol and sugars can be released from body stores. Internalizing stress can keep the mind agitated and throw the nervous system off. A number of biological changes can be initiated by stressors.

Causes

None of us can completely escape stress. To some extent it defines our lives and pushes us to excel or produce. When it remains unmanaged, however, it can kill. Stress can be the by-product of several things which become a routine part of some life styles. These include death of a loved one, financial problems, alcoholism, job related pressures, deadlines, problematic family relationships including marital discord, difficult in-laws, teenagers, etc. Stress and anxiety can result from crowded environments, high traffic areas, loneliness, medical concerns, divorce and single parenting, PMS, and over-scheduling one's life. Long-term stress is typical of care givers of the elderly, or physically or mentally handicapped. When the body fails to manage stress, various physical and mental symptoms can result.

Conventional Therapies

Medical science usually approaches the management of stress with drug therapy. While in severe cases, tranquilizers, antidepressants and sleeping pills may be indicated, often these therapies are counter-productive and have negative side effects. Managing stress through good diet, exercise, relaxation techniques and counseling is certainly preferable than to become dependent on drugs. The most common drugs used to treat stress are the benzodiazepines which include valium, librium, xanax and ativan. Because insomnia typically accompanies anxiety, sleeping pills are also routinely prescribed. Triazolam (Halcion) is a benzodiazepine most commonly used as a sedative. Antidepressants such as Prozac and Zoloft are also used to relieve anxiety.

Dietary Guidelines

- Eat whole grain foods with plenty of fiber to keep blood sugar levels stable and to supply energy.
- Concentrate on eating raw foods with live enzymes and cut down on dairy products.
- Eat a good nutritious breakfast and don't eat a heavy meal before going to sleep. If you can't eat food in the morning, try a good protein supplement powder that can be blended with milk or juice.
- Avoid alcohol, caffeine and nicotine. These in and of themselves can create stress on the body and the emotions. Coffee, tea, chocolate, and caffeine drinks can really alter mind states and increase levels of internal stress.
- Avoid eating white sugar products, heavily spiced foods, colas, fried foods, MSG, and high-fat junk foods. These foods can heighten the stress response.
- The adrenal glands are directly responsible for our reaction to stressors. Proper diet helps to keep these glands functioning properly.

Recommended Nutritional Supplements

PRIMARY NUTRIENTS

VITAMIN B-COMPLEX The 17 vitamins that belong to this category are considered stress vitamins and are essential for maintaining good mental health and the proper function of the nervous system.[1] A deficiency in just one of the B-vitamins has been linked to various mental disorders including schizophrenia. Depression and anxiety should be treated with B-vitamin supplementation. *Suggested Dosage*: Take as directed using sublingual products or ask your doctor about injections.

PANTOTHENIC ACID This nutrient is important for healthy adrenal gland function which is vital to coping with stressors.[2] It is also considered a natural antidepressant that can reduce anxiety and help promote sleep. *Suggested Dosage*: 500 mg per day.

CALCIUM/MAGNESIUM These two minerals work to quiet the central nervous system and are often low in people suffering from chronic stress. A lack of these nutrients can cause a whole host of emotional and mental problems. Calcium also contributes to high blood pressure control which can be a factor in people under stress.[3] *Suggested Dosage*: 1,500 mg of calcium and 750 mg of magnesium. Use calcium citrate, gluconate or lactate and chelated magnesium.

VITAMIN E, SELENIUM AND LIPOIC ACID Help to protect the glands and to effectively scavenge for free radicals which are caused by adrenal overload. Lipoic acid potentiates the action of vitamin E, creating a powerful antioxidant effect.[4] *Suggested Dosage*: Take each supplement as directed together.

VITAMIN C WITH BIOFLAVONOIDS Helps to stimulate adrenal function which may become impaired during prolonged periods of stress. These compounds also fortify immunity.[5] *Suggested Dosage*: 3,000 to 5,000 mg daily.

GINKGO AND ST. JOHN'S WORT These herbs work to boost serotonin and oxygen in the brain which discourages depression and enhances mental ability. St. John's wort has also been used for sleep disorders which are commonly seen in people under stress. Ginkgo research has found that even PMS mental stress can be relieved with supplementation.[6] *Suggested Dosage*: Take as directed using standardized products.

MELATONIN This compound has been used to realign sleeping patterns and to promote rest and relaxation.[7] *Suggested Dosage*: Start off with half of the recommended dose and see how you react. Do not take more than advised dosages.

PASSIONFLOWER, KAVA, VALERIAN AND SKULLCAP These natural herbal tranquilizers are not habit forming, but can prompt relaxation and sleep and work to counteract feelings of nervousness or anxiety.[8,9,10,11] *Suggested Dosage*: Take as directed using one or a combination of the herbs. Look for standardized or guaranteed potency products.

HERBAL COMBINATION This combination includes sarsaparilla root, Siberian ginseng, astragalus, fo-ti, gotu kola, saw palmetto, licorice root, kelp, alfalfa, ginger root and stillingia. *Suggested Dosage*: Four to eight capsules daily. Can be used continuously as a general tonic.

SARSAPARILLA: This herb is known to contain hormone precursors that are believed to help balance hormone function in both genders. It has gained official recognition in Germany and the United Kingdom as a general tonic. SIBERIAN GINSENG: Siberian ginseng has a clinically demonstrated ability to block the effects of stress. Ginseng is also good for stimulating energy production in the body. Many nervous system disorders are effectively treated with Siberian ginseng. Studies confirm its ability to boost coping skills under stress.[12] ASTRAGALUS: This very prominent Chinese herb strengthens and readies the body's immune function which is often weakened by stress. Astragalus will not stimulate the immune system to action, but prepares it so when an immune response is required it functions at a higher level.[13] FO-TI: Fo-ti contains very powerful antioxidants which can be useful in treating many common maladies and has traditionally been used to promote longevity. Fo-ti improves kidney function and contains antiaging antioxidants which may actually contribute to longevity.[14] GOTU KOLA: Gotu kola has been used in ayurvedic medicine as a central nervous system tonic. Studies have shown it to improve mental function including memory and ability to learn.[15] Gotu kola improves circulation which can help the body to cope in stressful situations. It is also considered an antifatigue herb. SAW PALMETTO: For men, saw palmetto berry is best known for its ability to protect and maintain a healthy prostate. For women, it decreases ovarian and uterine irritability and relieves painful periods. It appears to have a hormone balancing effect for both genders. LICORICE ROOT: Licorice root in any herbal formula helps to modulate and strengthen activity of other herbs that are present and to strengthen the adrenal glands which can become exhausted during periods of chronic or prolonged stress.[16] KELP: Kelp is a plant from the sea that contains many nutrients beneficial to the body's metabolic processes. It can help normalize thyroid function and hypertension and contains algin which is soothing to the GI tract. ALFALFA: Alfalfa, like kelp, is very nutritious and much of its benefit can be attributed to this property. It can stimulate the appetite and has no equal as a spring tonic. GINGER ROOT: Ginger root improves and maintains a healthy digestive system. Perhaps no other herb has such broad applications or performs as well as ginger. Ginger improves circulation and makes the other herbs of this formula more effective. STILLINGIA: Stillingia, like sarsaparilla, is described as an alterative which restores proper body function. Stillingia has been used in many ways to treat such diverse conditions as cancer and eczema and is added here for its overall therapeutic effect.

SECONDARY NUTRIENTS

LECITHIN: Helps protect nerve fibers by promoting proper lipid metabolism and assimilation. *Suggested Dosage*: 2,000 mg with meals. Use capsules or granules.

L-TYROSINE AND 5-HYDROXY-TRYPTOPHAN: Two amino acids that help to reduce stress and promote sleep by raising levels of serotonin in the brain. *Suggested Dosage*: Take as directed on an empty stomach with fruit juice.

GABA AND INOSITOL: These nutrients act as a natural tranquilizer and contribute to normal brain function. *Suggested Dosage*: 500 mg of GABA twice daily and 50 mg of inositol.

ZINC: Helps calm and control feelings of nervousness while boosting immune function. *Suggested Dosage*: Take 50 mg per day. Do not exceed 100 mg per day total.

Home Care Suggestions

- Exercise regularly. The importance of exercise in relieving stress cannot be over valued. Walking, jogging, taking an aerobics class, etc., can release endorphins in the brain, creating a sense of well-being and providing a release for tension.
- Get away from urban areas and let nature work its magic on your nerves.
- Take long, warm baths; spa use is also beneficial.
- Listen to soothing music when driving through traffic.
- Learn yoga techniques to control breathing, relax muscles and to meditate. Transcendental meditation can be of great benefit in relieving tension.
- Don't wear tight or uncomfortable clothing or shoes.
- Keep your environment cool rather than too warm.
- Learn to see the humor in life and laugh heartily and often.
- The conscious regulation of breathing can be an invaluable technique for achieving relaxation. Exhale completely through your mouth slowly. Inhale through your nose to the mental count of four. Hold your breath for a mental count of seven. Exhale slowly and completely through your mouth to a mental count of eight. Repeat the cycle three more times. This particular exercise can act as a natural tranquilizer.
- Avoid taking any over-the-counter or prescription drug you don't need. Several drugs can cause agitation and anxiety. Over-the-counter antihistamines can cause extreme restlessness and depression.
- Get a regular professional massage. Massage therapy is wonderful to ease tension and soothe the nerves. A good massage is relatively inexpensive and can work wonders.
- Leave job-related stresses at work and make a commitment to leave work promptly.
- Don't be afraid to say no. Stay in charge of your life and your calendar. It is better to under-schedule than to overdo it.
- Avoid listening to the news, the radio or reading the newspaper if these activities produce stress or anxiety.
- Don't react to irritating comments from others. Avoid political or religious topics that make you feel volatile.

◆ Unplug the telephone during dinner or in the evening and invest in some soothing music.

◆ Make sure you set a strict bedtime for children so you can count on some quiet evening time for yourself.

◆ Involve yourself in a hobby or group activity.

◆ Try hypnotherapy, yoga, biofeedback or music therapy to relax and meditate. Deep breathing exercises are very good for relieving tension.

◆ Pray and regularly attend a worship service.

◆ Make your bedroom a restful quiet place where you can relax and unwind.

◆ Get professional counseling if you need the extra coping skills.

Other Supportive Therapies

RELAXATION TECHNIQUES: The best stress treatments are those that help you learn how to cope. Good examples are yoga and meditation.

BIOFEEDBACK: Stress-related conditions can be helped by recognizing how your body responds to stress. Treatment involves using a biofeedback machine and is normally given by a psychologist.

MASSAGE: Lavender or basil oil are recommended for intensive massage for relaxation.

AROMATHERAPY: Neroli oil is considered an antidepressant that helps to combat feelings of anxiety or tension.

Scientific Facts-at-a-Glance

The ability to visualize or imaging is thought to help relieve stress.[17] Putting your head back, closing your eyes and imagining yourself on the shores of a tropical paradise or walking through a lush garden can help to restore feelings of serenity and contentment, and dispel tension. We are just beginning to understand the power of the mind in matters of physical control. This biofeedback technique can work if you take the time to use it properly.

Spirit/Mind Considerations

Counseling one on one or in support groups can be a great value if coping with stress becomes too difficult. Psychotherapy doesn't make life easier, but it can provide coping skills and relaxation techniques and provide a controlled setting in which to unload emotional baggage. Under periods of prolonged stress, one can become anxious, fearful, angry or depressed. Stress can induce the following symptoms: irritability, short temper, insomnia, over or under eating, panic attacks, forgetfulness, crying or a decline in productivity. Gleaning from spiritual powers can also be very helpful. Prayer can be very effective in not only calming us down, but by giving us spiritual strength to cope as well. Look to greater powers when dealing with stress and utilize all of the helps available. Life was never meant to be easy but it can be much more enjoyable if stress is not allowed to build up.

Prevention

◆ Keep all necessary nutrients supplied by taking a strong multivitamin/mineral supplement daily.

◆ A nutritious diet, regular exercise and the ability to recognize stress indicators can contribute to preventing anxiety.

◆ Learning to relax is vital. Today there are a number of ways to control stress and lessen its detrimental effects. Some of these are biofeedback, yoga, music therapy, self hypnosis, breathing exercises, music therapy and stretching exercises. Taking time every day to relax has become essential to the maintenance of good mental and physical health.

◆ Try to get the amount of sleep you need.

◆ Consider a personality assessment to help you understand what causes you stress and how to best deal with it individually.

◆ Many of the suggestions found in the "Home Care" section of this chapter are also stress-preventative.

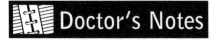 **Doctor's Notes**

Stress is responsible for numerous and varied health problems. How it affects a person is based partly on their previous health history, genetics, and how they view the stress they are under. Because the causes of stress are varied and multiple, it is important that people who have an unknown cause of fatigue or other symptoms visit their physician to obtain a base line laboratory test, so they can be sure that their stress is not caused by hypothyroidism, anemia, candida, or some of the other disorders that can be determined by a blood test. Nevertheless, the majority of people with fatigue have absolutely normal blood studies. Therefore, iron or thyroid therapy holds no promise for such people, and stress must be addressed. This herbal formula is an invaluable tool in treating nonspecific fatigue that may be caused by underlying stress or other undiagnosed factors. This formula is ideal as a general tonic as it has the ability to improve just about all aspects of health especially stamina and endurance. For more information on stress, immune and adrenal function, refer to the stress section in Part 1 of this book.

Additional Resources

American Mental Health Foundation
1049 Fifth Avenue
New York, NY 10028
(212) 737-9027

Endnotes

1. Robert H. Garrison and Elizabeth Somer, The Nutrition Desk Reference, (Keats Publishing, New Canaan, CT: 1985), 203.

2. Ibid., 53

3. J.R. Sowers, et al., "Calcium and hypertension," Jour Lab Clin Med, 114: 338-48.

4. L. Packer, et al., "Alpha-lipoic acid as a biological antioxidant," Free Rad Biol, 1995, 19: 227-50.

5. A. Bendich, "Vitamin C and immune response," Flor Tech, 1987, 41: 112-14.

6. A. Tamborini and R. Taurelle, "Value of standardized Ginkgo biloba extract in the management of congestive symptoms of premenstrual syndrome," Rev Fr Gyn Obst, 1993, 88: 447-57. See also H. Schubert, and P. Halama, "Depressive episode primarily unresponsive to therapy in elderly patients: efficacy of Ginkgo biloba in combination with antidepressants," Geria Forsch, 1993, 3: 45-53.

7. S.P. James, et al., "Melatonin administered in insomnia," Neuropsychopharmacol, 1990, 3: 19-23. See also A.B. Dollins, et al., "Effect of pharmacological daytime doses of melatonin on human mood and performance," Psychopharmacol, 1993, 112: 490-96.

8. V. Schellenberg, et al., "Quantitative EEG monitoring in phyto- and psychopharmacological treatment of psychosomatic and affective disorders," Schizophrenia Res, 1993, 9(2,3): Abstract

9. W.E. Scholine and H.D. Clausen, "On the effect of d,l-kavain: experience with neuronika," Med Klin, 1977, 72: 1301-06 and D. Lindenberg and H. Pitulę-Scholdel, "D,l-kavin in comparison with oxazepam in anxiety disorders: A double-blind study of clinical effectiveness," Forschr med, 1990, 108: 49-50, 53-54.

10. U. Boeters. "Treatment of autonomic dysregulation with valepotriates (valmane)," Muenchener Medizinische Wochenschrift, 37, 1873-1876, 1969. V. Kempinskas. "On the action valerian." Famakologii I Toksikologiia, 4(3): 305-309, 1964. See also R. Klich and B. Gladbach. "Childhood behavior disorders and their treatment." Medizinishce Welt, 26(25): 1251-1254, 1975.

11. B.A. Kurnakov, "Pharmacology of skullcap," Farmakologiia I Toksikologiia, 20(6): 79-80, 1957.

12. C. Hallstrom, et al., "Effect of ginseng on the performance of nurses on night duty," Comp Med East and West, 1982, 6: 277-82.

13. Z.Y. Yang, et al., "Effect of astragalus membranaceous on natural killer cell activity and induction with Coxsackie-B viral myocarditis," Chin Med, 1990, 103(4): 304-07.

14. S. Cheung, et al., "Polygonum multiflorum thumb," Chinese Medicinal Herbs of Hong Kong, 1980.

15. R. Appo, et al., "The effect of Centella asiatica on the general mental ability of mentally retarded children," Ind Jour Psy, 1977, 19: 54-59.

16. N. Abe, et al., "Interferon induction by glycyrrhizin and glycyrrhetinic acid in mice," Microb Immunol, 1982, 26: 353-359.

17. B. Brown, Stress and the Art of Biofeedback (Harper and Row, New York: 1977).

STROKE

Strokes are caused by a reduction in blood flow to a particular area of the brain. Lack of blood subsequently leads to oxygen starvation of brain cells and resulting tissue death. Strokes cause a significant amount of disability and death in the United States although they are half as common as they were 25 years ago due to better high blood pressure control. Strokes commonly strike older people between the ages of 60 and 80. Many of the risk factors for a heart attack apply to strokes as well. Strokes are more prevalent in people who have diabetes and a high cholesterol count. As in the case of heart attacks, the damage from a stroke can vary with each individual. In mild strokes, full recovery is common. Moderate strokes will usually leave some permanent effect ranging from a minor speech impediment to total paralysis. Damage is determined by the location and extent of the stroke. One hundred seventy thousand strokes per year are fatal. Approximately 50 percent of stroke cases experience a full or partial recovery occurs within a few months. About 5 percent will require long term institutional care.

Symptoms

Frequently, a stroke is preceded by a number of warning signs brought on by temporary spells of impaired brain function caused by brief reductions in blood flow. These may include

- temporary weakness
- fainting
- loss of memory
- paralysis
- loss of vision
- difficulty speaking
- numbness
- clumsiness
- blurred vision
- dizziness
- loss of hearing
- disorientation

These warning signs are called TIAs (transient ischemic attacks) and last a short time due to a temporary blockage of blood. Headaches are uncommon with strokes. A full blown stroke may cause

- a loss of consciousness
- paralysis on one side of the body
- the inability to speak
- double vision
- memory impairment
- confusion
- numbness

NOTE: Unlike the warning symptoms of a heart attack, these will persist for at least 24 hours or longer. If you notice any of the above warning signs of a stroke, contact your doctor or a hospital immediately. Anticlotting agents may be prescribed to prevent the onset of a stroke. Any unexplained fainting, dizziness, paralysis or visual or hearing disturbances need immediate medical attention.

Causes

Blood clots make up half of all strokes. Arteriosclerosis, high blood pressure, a cerebral embolism, and cerebral hemorrhage can all result from a stroke. Coronary artery disease (atherosclerosis) is the most common cause of stroke. Blood flow to the brain can be obstructed by arteries that have progressively narrowed by the rupture of a blood vessel or by the lodging of a clot or piece of plaque within an artery. Factors that increase the risk of having a stroke include the following:

- diabetes
- irregular heart beats
- a recent heart attack
- high blood cholesterol
- high blood pressure
- obesity
- damaged heart valves
- smoking
- birth control pills

NOTE: A person with even a moderate elevation in blood pressure runs six times the risk of experiencing a stroke than someone with normal blood pressure.

Conventional Therapies

Stroke patients need the kind of care that often requires hospitalization. Unfortunately medical science cannot cure strokes. Adapting a healthy lifestyle can go a long way to prevent strokes. For impaired mobility following a stroke, proper physical therapy is essential to keep muscles from withering. Brain scans, such as CT scanning, can now pinpoint the exact location of a stroke and rule out the possibility of a brain tumor, abscess or subdural hematoma. A carotid arteriogram which is a special x-ray of the arteries may be required to assess if surgery to prevent further strokes may be possible. Other tests that are standard are chest x-rays, ECG, and MRI.

Keeping the patient well nourished through intravenous feedings, and nasogastric tubes, preventing infection and bedsores and keeping the limbs mobile will constitute the primary medical goals in treating a stroke patient. To prevent the accumulation of fluid within the brain, corticosteroid drugs may be used. Controlling high blood pressure and keeping the blood thin can be achieved using drugs and in rare occasions, surgical repair of a damaged artery or manually removing a clot may be possible. Physical therapy is imperative in stroke patients who have lost the use of a limb. Vocal therapy can help to retrain vocalization skills and pronunciation. Using sensitive ultrasound screening can detect atherosclerotic lesions which are considered silent predictors of stroke. This procedure can locate potentially dangerous changes in the carotid artery which could result in a stroke. Angioview 600 ultrasound machines have only become available within the last two years.

Dietary Guidelines

- Avoid all animal fats, butter, ice cream, white sugar, white flour, greasy fried foods, high fat cheeses, and red meats.
- Eat fish, white meats, such as skinless turkey or chicken breast and drink plenty of fluids.
- Eat a diet high in fiber, including whole grains such as oat, wheat, barley, millet, buckwheat, cornmeal and brown rice.
- Eat plenty of raw fruits and vegetables.
- Add significant amounts of onion and garlic to your diet.
- Do not consume alcohol, nicotine or caffeine.
- Use flaxseed and olive oil and do not use hydrogenated fats found in most vegetable margerines.

Recommended Nutritional Supplements

PRIMARY NUTRIENTS

PHOSPHADITYL CHOLINE Increases acetylcholine levels in the brain which directly impact memory function. Clinical data suggests that elevating acetylcholine in the brain may improve memory.[1] *Suggested Dosage*: 10 to 20 g daily. Use high quality preparations.

PHOSPHADITYL SERINE This compound is one of the primary phospholipids found in brain tissue and plays an important role in brain function. Animal and human studies have found that supplementing this nutrient can improve age-related changes in brain chemistry.[2] *Suggested Dosage*: 300 mg divided out in three doses with meals.

GINKGO BILOBA Clinical studies are supportive of this herb's ability to reverse mental deterioration associated with cerebrovascular insufficiency.[3] It can also help prevent or decrease the dementia and edema which often follows a stroke. *Suggested Dosage*: 60 mg of 24 percent extract taken two to three times a day.

VITAMIN B12 AND FOLIC ACID A distinct depletion of these vitamins have been found in people with dementia and other brain-related disorders.[4] *Suggested Dosage*: 1,000 to 2,000 mg daily of B12 which can also be administered in injections. Folic acid supplements should be taken as directed.

LECITHIN Lecithin contains choline which stimulates the production of acetylcholine and may help with overall brain function while it works to lower cholesterol levels and treat depression as well.[5] *Suggested Dosage*: 100 mg three times daily with meals. Use granules or capsulized varieties of lecithin.

OMEGA-3 FATTY ACIDS Taking fish oil helped to normalize brain prostaglandins, boosted cerebral blood flow and decreased swelling in laboratory test animals.[6] *Suggested Dosage*: Take as directed with a vitamin E supplement.

VITAMIN B6 AND FOLIC ACID A lack of B6 has been closely linked with a number of neurological disorders including depression and schizophrenia. Elderly people can easily become deficient in both these nutrients. In addition, taking adequate doses of B6 and folic acid can reduce the risk of cardiovascular disease which is a major cause of stroke.[7] *Suggested Dosage*: 50 to 100 mg of B6 per day. Sublingual forms or injections are available.

CHROMIUM Recent studies have found that people who are suffering from vascular disease have a tendency to have low chromium levels.[8] *Suggested Dosage*: Take as directed, using picolinate or GTF products.

POTASSIUM We are just beginning to understand the role of this mineral in the case of a stroke. It is important to make sure that you have adequate levels of potassium (which can become depleted if you take high blood pressure medication or diuretics).[9] *Suggested Dosage*: Take as directed.

MAGNESIUM Keeping magnesium levels up can help to treat the preliminary symptoms of toxemia which can result in a stroke.[10] *Suggested Dosage*: Take 1,000 mg per day with calcium. Use chelated products.

ST. JOHN'S WORT, GOTU KOLA AND GINKGO These herbs have proven their ability to counteract the effects of cerebrovascular insufficiency by boosting blood flow which enhances mental function while raising brain serotonin levels.[11] *Suggested Dosage*: Take each herb as directed, using guaranteed potency products.

VITAMIN E Helps transport oxygen to brain cells and scavenges for free radicals which can cause brain tissue damage. *Suggested Dosage*: 800 IU to 1,200 IU per day.

VITAMIN C WITH BIOFLAVONOIDS Helps to strengthen blood vessels and scavenge for free radicals. *Suggested Dosage*: 5,000 to 10,000 mg daily.

HERBAL COMBINATION This combination includes peppermint leaves, Siberian ginseng, gotu kola, kelp, rosemary leaves, damiana leaves, and butternut root bark. *Suggested Dosage*: Two to four capsules daily. In severe cases, a person may consume up to 12 capsules daily.

PEPPERMINT LEAVES: Peppermint has some general applications which will improve overall health and works to boost the action of the other herbs in this formula. SIBERIAN GINSENG: Siberian ginseng is considered to be an adaptogen, a substance with the ability to normalize systems of the body, irrespective of the direction, deficiency or excess of the pathologic state. Ginseng combats mental fatigue and reduces serum cholesterol which can help prevent a recurring stroke.[12] GOTU KOLA: Ayurvedic doctors use this herb as a central nervous system tonic and to improve mental stamina and enhance memory. Clinical studies performed in Europe show gotu kola has the ability to increase circulation to brain tissue.[13] KELP: Kelp's high concentration and broad range of trace elements are most likely the reason kelp is considered essential for the nervous system and normal brain function. The algin in kelp binds with cholesterol and toxins to remove them from the body. ROSEMARY LEAVES: Rosemary helps maintain a healthy nervous system. It assists in combating stress and improves circulation especially in the elderly who may be experiencing chronic poor circulation. Long-term use improves a bad memory. Rosemary contains powerful antioxidants which can reduce damage caused by free radicals released after a stroke. DAMIANA LEAVES: Germany's drug regulatory board suggests the use for damiana to include "fortification and stimulation in cases of overwork, mental stress, and nervous debility, and for enhancement and maintenance of mental and physical efficiency." BUTTERNUT ROOT BARK: Butternut root bark has been included in this formula as a laxative to cleanse toxins from the body and to improve health.

SECONDARY NUTRIENTS

GERMANIUM: Oxygenates brain cells and acts as an antioxidant agent. *Suggested Dosage*: Take as directed.

DHA: This compound which is found in fish oils can be taken alone to boost mental function and brain activity. *Suggested Dosage*: Take as directed.

CAPSICUM: Helps to clean veins and strengthen artery walls and boosts vascular blood flow. *Suggested Dosage*: Take as directed using pure products with a meal.

HAWTHORN: Works to regulate high blood pressure and prevent hardening of the arteries. *Suggested Dosage*: Take as directed using guaranteed potency products.

Home Care Suggestions

◆ The positive and supportive attitude of those who are care givers for the stroke patient is the one most important factor in facilitating recovery. Patience is required for the relearning of speech and movement.

◆ Take advantage of the community rehabilitation organizations. Contact your hospital or health centers for sources.

◆ You may need to have ramps and handrails installed in strategic places during the recovery process. If you are in a wheelchair, often just changing the hinges on a door can allow for a complete swing of the door, allowing the wheelchair to move freely.

◆ Keep your environment barrier free.

◆ Put grab bars near the toilet and tub areas.

◆ Get rid of throw rugs, big floor pillows, boxes, stools and furniture that gets in the way.

◆ Supervised swimming is an excellent exercise for recovering stroke victims and can provide valuable physical therapy.

◆ Board games can help to sharpen mental skills.

◆ Working at the computer can be an invaluable way to increasingly develop hand eye coordination.

◆ Social workers and physical therapists can make home visits. Make sure they are accredited and check Medicare coverage policies.

◆ Keep yourself looking good. Make sure you dress nicely and keep your hair clean and attractive.

SUGGESTIONS FOR THE CAREGIVER

◆ Encourage the stroke survivor to do things independently, but keep your expectations realistic.

◆ Keep family life structures, with meals at the same times, sleep schedules, activities, etc.

◆ Watch for signs of depression and be a constant source of encouragement. Talk to a stroke survivor often, even if his or her response is limited.

◆ Learn some basic sign language skills to facilitate communication.

Other Supportive Therapies

ACUPUNCTURE: Specific treatments can be very helpful in controlling pain and boosting nerve and muscle function.

Scientific Facts-at-a-Glance

The merits of both *Ginkgo biloba* and St. John's wort should not be overlooked for anyone dealing with a stroke or ischemic episodes. Both of these botanicals have some remarkable properties which are only now beginning to surface. Ginkgo not only boosts oxygenation but can actually improve the viscosity of the blood in patients who have already had a stroke.[14] Moreover, St. John's wort can help to boost serotonin levels which works to treat the depression that inevitably occurs after a stroke.

Spirit/Mind Considerations

One of the worst complications of a stroke is the depression that can follow. The very nature of paralysis or speech impediments can initiate feelings of despair. In most cases this depression passes and is treatable. Being aware that this is a normal reaction in a stroke patient helps both the stroke victim and his or her family deal with the event in a more productive manner. Emotional support at this time is vital to recovery. Stroke patients require a great deal of patience while they relearn old skills. Feelings of anger and frustration are normal following a stroke, but a positive attitude can greatly enhance recovery.

Prevention

◆ Keep your weight within optimum levels by eating right and exercising daily. Aerobic exercise is recommended.

◆ Women who smoke should not use birth control pills which can increase the risk of a stroke due to the formation of blood clots.

◆ Taking folic acid and vitamin B6 supplements in greater than RDA recommended doses has been found to reduce the risk of cardiovascular disease.

◆ Keep blood cholesterol low by eating a high fiber, low fat diet. Have your cholesterol levels checked often. Diet is the single most important factor for the prevention of atherosclerosis which is a leading cause of stroke. Avoid eggs, animal meats, ice cream and butter.

◆ Keep your salt intake low. In some people, a salt sensitivity can cause blood pressure elevation.

◆ Don't smoke or drink alcohol. Smoking causes spasms in the artery walls.

◆ Control the stress levels in your life through daily relaxation techniques.

◆ Low doses of aspirin taken daily may help to prevent a stroke if you are at high risk. If you are at high risk for a stroke, other anticoagulant drugs may be prescribed indefinitely. Discuss these options with your doctor.

◆ Bypass operations which re-route blood flow which had been impeded by an obstructed artery can prevent stokes.

◆ Surgery in which blood vessels are re-positioned to supply the brain with adequate oxygen can decrease one's risk for stroke. Another operation done under a local anesthetic is able to open up a roughened section of the carotid artery and clean out any deposits that may have accumulated.

◆ Keep your blood pressure within the normal range. Have it checked frequently. High blood pressure facilitates the formation of plaque in the arteries and increases the risk that a weak artery will burst, which can cause a stroke. High blood pressure medication may be necessary.

Doctor's Notes

I once treated a 65-year-old male who had suffered a stroke, which left him with decreased sensation in his right leg. In addition, he had a very painful condition in the left side of his face diagnosed as a tic disorder. This patient had seen two neurologists and was placed on medication that did nothing to improve his facial pain or other symptoms. Upon evaluation, it was noted that his pain seemed to center around a medial nerve branch affecting his eye and cheekbone area. I started him on gotu kola and St. John's wort, along with acupuncture treatments. After the fourth treatment two weeks later, the patient started to notice marked improvement in his facial pain. In time he began to go two weeks between treatments with little or no pain. As the acupuncture treatments tapered off, I suggested that he remain on the gotu kola and St. John's wort supplements for 4 to 6 months before stopping. His story is a good example of the efficacy of using acupuncture and herbal therapy combined.

Additional Resources

Evergreen Stroke Association
9423 Southeast Thirty-Sixth St.
Mercer Island, WA 98040

Courage Stroke Network
3915 Golden Valley Road
Golden Valley, MN 55422

Caregiver Support
Children of Aging Parents
2761 Trenton Road
Levittown, PA 19056

Barrier Free Environments
P.O. Box 30634
Water Garden Highway 70 West
Raleigh, NC 2762280.

Endnotes

1. D.J. Canty and S.H. Zeisel, "Lecithin, and choline in human health and disease," Nutr Reviews, 1994, 52: 327-339.

2. T. Crook, et al., "Effects of phosphaditylserine in Alzheimer's disease," Psychopharmacol Bull, 1992, 28: 61-66. See also E. W. Funfgeld, et al., "Double-blind study with phosphaditylserine in Parkinsonian patients with senile dementia of Alzheimer's type (SDAT)," Prog Clin Biol Res, 1989, 317: 1235.

3. B. Hofferberth, "The efficacy of Egb761 in patients with senile dementia of the Alzheimer type: A double-blind, placebo-controlled study on different levels of investigation," Human Psychopharmacol, 1994, 9: 215-22.

4. M.G. Cole and J.F. Prichal, "Low serum vitamin B 12 in Alzheimer-type dementia," Age Aging, 1984, 13: 101-05. See also G.M. Craig, et al., "Masked vitamin B 12 and folate deficiency in the elderly," British Journal of Nutrition, 1985, 54: 613-19.

5. J. Levine, et al., "Double-blind, controlled trial of inositol treatment of depression," Amer Jour Psy, 1995, 152: 792-94.

6. K. Black, et al., "Eicosapentaenoic acid: Effect on both brain prostaglandins, cerebral blood flow and edema in ischemic gerbils," Stroke, 1984, 15(1):65-69.

7. R. Clarke, et al., "Hyperhomocysteinemia: an independent risk factor for vascular disease," N Engl J Med, 1991, 324(17): 1149-55.

8. G. Huang, et al., "Hair chromium levels in patients with vascular diseases," Biol Trace Elem Res, 1991, 29: 133-7.

9. C. Lee, et al., "Dietary potassium and stroke," Letter, N Engl. J Med, 1988, 318(15): 995-96.

10. M. Sadeh, "Action of magnesium sulfate in the treatment of preeclampsia/eclampsia," Stroke, 1989, 20(9):1273-75.

11. G. Lagrue, G et al., "Idiopathic cyclic edema: The role of capillary hyper permeability and its correction by Ginkgo biloba," Presse Med, 1986, 15(31): 1550-53.

12. D. H. Zhou, "Preventative geriatrics: an overview from traditional Chinese medicine," American Journal of Chinese Medicine, 1982, 10(1-4): 32-39.

13. R. N. Chopra, Indigenous Drugs of India, 2nd ed. (Arts Press, Calcutta: 1933).

14. "Hemorrhological findings in patients with completed stroke and the influence of Ginkgo biloba extract," Clin Hemor, 1985, 5: 411-20.

SUNBURN

While considered a relatively harmless condition, sunburn can cause serious immediate damage as well as predispose the skin to premature wrinkling or the later development of melanoma (skin cancer). Sunburn can occur even on cloudy days; therefore, we must consider the dangers of ultraviolet rays when we participate in outdoor activities and take the necessary precautions for ourselves and our families.

Symptoms

Sunburn, like other skin burns, can be classified in degrees of severity. If your skin only becomes reddened by sun exposure, then you have a first degree sunburn. If the skin is red, tender, hot and then forms water-filled blisters, the sunburn is considered second degree. In cases where the skin is damaged beyond the first layer, immediate medical attention should be sought or infection and scarring can occur. Most sunburns cause redness, swelling, tenderness, warmth, itchiness, blisters, eventual peeling of surface skin layer, and stiffness or tightness of skin.

Causes

Sunburn is caused by excess exposure to the ultraviolet rays of the sun or an artificial ultraviolet source, such as a sun lamp or tanning bed. The longer the exposure to harmful ultraviolet rays, the more severe the burn. Factors that determine the tendency to sunburn include

- skin pigment type
- altitude and atmosphere
- time of day
- reflection of the light from water, sand or snow

The midday sun is considered the most damaging, although sunburn can occur before and after this time. Cloudy days, with indirect sunlight, can also cause sunburn and precautions must be taken to protect the skin even when the temperature does not feel warm. NOTE: Some acne medications, such as Retin-A, can cause enhanced sun sensitivity, and proper precautions should be taken to protect the skin. Using St. John's wort internally may also cause photosensitivity (abnormal sensitivity to ultraviolet light) or light sensitivity.

Conventional Therapies

Most cases of sunburn do not require medical attention, although your physician may recommend using wet cold compresses. If your sunburn is severe, your doctor should assess its seriousness. Antibacterial ointments, dressing and even hospitalization may be required if the burn is extensive enough. The use of IV fluids to prevent dehydration and shock and to guard against infection may be warranted in these cases.

Dietary Guidelines

♦ In the case of second and third degree burns, the diet should be high in both protein and calories for tissue regeneration.

♦ In addition, plenty of fluids should be consumed.

♦ Protein drinks can supplement a diet high in raw vegetables, fruits, cereal and nuts.

♦ Citrus fruits, potatoes and broccoli are good sources of vitamin C, which aids the healing process.

♦ In order to heal properly from a serious burn, diets should be higher than normal in calories that should be obtained from good, nutritious sources rather than empty calorie junk foods.

Recommended Nutritional Supplements

PRIMARY NUTRIENTS

POTASSIUM Potassium can be lost from sun exposure and burning and should be replaced as soon as possible. *Suggested Dosage:* Take as directed using chelated products that are food based. Eating more potassium-rich foods like bananas is also recommended.

VITAMIN A AND BETA CAROTENE Play a major role in the regeneration of epithelial and mucosal surfaces of the skin.[1] In addition, both of these compounds act as powerful free radical scavengers which in the case of tissue destruction caused by sunburns is especially useful.[2] *Suggested Dosage:* 50,000 IU of vitamin A and 25,000 IU of beta carotene until healing is sufficient, then drop to 25,000 IU of vitamin A and 10,000 IU of beta carotene.

ZINC Promotes tissue healing by stimulating immune function and by also acting as an antioxidant to inhibit inflammation.[3] *Suggested Dosage:* 75 to 100 mg per day in divided doses. Do not exceed 100 mg per day. Use picolinate varieties.

SELENIUM AND GERMANIUM Two excellent antioxidants which help to minimize tissue oxidants which can result from sunburn. Selenium helps to boost the level of glutathione peroxidase which helps to inhibit the production of prostaglandins and leukotrienes which cause inflammation and pain.[4] *Suggested Dosage:* Take as directed.

VITAMIN E Can be taken internally and used externally to minimize scarring if the sunburn is first or second degree in its severity. Clinical studies have found that vitamin E supplementation enhances tissue regeneration.[5] *Suggested Dosage:* Take as directed.

VITAMIN C WITH BIOFLAVONOIDS Helps in healing processes and can reduce inflammation. A wash made with powdered vitamin C and water can be applied externally. Laboratory tests on mice with burns found that ascorbic acid supplementation retarded the transformation of tissue from second to third degree burns.[6] *Suggested Dosage:* Take as directed.

ESSENTIAL FATTY ACIDS These vital acids contain compounds that affect prostaglandin synthesis. Prostaglandins, when combined with arachidonic acid, cause swelling, pain and inflammation.[7] *Suggested Dosage:* Take as directed.

GOTU KOLA Extracts of this herb have had remarkable results treating burns caused by scalding, explosions or electrical shock. Taking the herb internally and applying it topically resulted in less skin shrinkage and swelling.[8] *Suggested Dosage:* Take as directed and make poultices out of teas or extract and apply externally.

ST. JOHN'S WORT OIL Helps to heal first or second degree burns due to its ability to speed tissue healing and prevent infection.[9] *Suggested Dosage:* Use as directed on burn. Oil-based products are preferable.

GLYCOSAMINOGLYCANS A natural anti-inflammatory that contributes to the regeneration of connective tissue.[10] *Suggested Dosage:* Take as directed. You may need to take this for at least six weeks if your burn is severe enough.

PABA Clinical tests have found that PABA (para amino benzoic acid) can help to boost skin healing and decrease inflammation.[11] *Suggested Dosage:* Take as directed.

HERBAL FORMULA This herbal combination contains burdock root, gotu kola, yellow dock, dandelion root, butcher's broom. *Suggested Dosage:* Two to six capsules daily.

BURDOCK ROOT: If there was ever an herb to promote healthy skin through internal cleansing, burdock is it. Burdock root's cleansing power is multifaceted. It has a diaphoretic action (promotes perspiration) which expels toxins from the skin and blood. GOTU KOLA: Gotu kola is supported by tremendous clinical research performed in Europe. It possesses wound-healing properties and has been shown to decrease scarring.[12] YELLOW DOCK: Yellow dock root is a reputed blood purifier and has been prescribed for all types of skin problems, including burns. Its laxative effect is well documented and supports the body's detoxifying ability as it heals. DANDELION ROOT: The dandelion, a common yard weed, has had a long history of use in herbal medicine. It is part of this formula for its ability to strengthen the liver, improve bile formation, regulate the bowels, purify the blood, and tone the skin. In the case of serious burns, the body must remove toxins and metabolites.[13] BUTCHER'S BROOM: This herb helps to facilitate tissue healing, works to detoxify the blood and is a natural astringent.

SECONDARY NUTRIENTS

TEA TREE OIL: Used externally for milder burns, this preparation helps to control pain and expedite healing. It can mix with sebaceous gland secretions and actually penetrate the epidermis and has antiseptic properties as well.[14]

TRACE MINERALS (LIQUID): Use directly on the sunburn to prevent infection and speed healing.

MYRRH OR GOLDENSEAL POWDER: Can be used to dust a first or second degree burn. It is also available in spray form.

WHITE OAK BARK: Contains tannic acid, which helps promote healing of skin. Can be used as a compress made from tea.[15]

ALOE VERA: Has healing properties and can reduce scarring with topical application.[16]

Home Care Suggestions

- Apply cold water, not ice water, to the sunburn in the form of moist compresses.
- Taking a baking soda bath can be soothing. Use one box per tubful of water.
- Using aloe vera gel after cold water treatment has been administered and the sunburn has started to heal is considered beneficial by some experts. Keeping a live plant nearby provides fresh juice which can be continually applied for days after the sunburn has occurred.
- Over-the-counter analgesics may help with pain and include aspirin or acetaminophen.
- Do not break open blisters that may appear with a second degree burn.
- Anesthetic creams or sprays are not recommended for sunburns because they inhibit healing.
- The use of butter, Vaseline or other cream ointments is generally discouraged.
- In the case of minor sunburns, creams such as neosporin or bacitracin are not thought to be very effective.
- Avoid cortisone-based creams or ointments. These can actually increase the risk of infection.

Other Supportive Therapies

HOMEOPATHY: Hypericin (active ingredient of St. John's wort) can be mixed with pure water and used as a topical application on a sunburn.

HYDROTHERAPY: Water treatments helps to remove loose or dead skin. Cool water baths can be soothing to sunburns.

Scientific-Facts-at-a-Glance

The notion that the weakening of the ozone layer of the earth's atmosphere has contributed to more skin cancer, DNA mutations or even sunburn has recently come to light. It has been theorized that because of "holes" in the ozone, we are more prone to skin damage from these rays than we would have been decades ago. The use of hats and sunscreen is considered absolutely essential by some experts who believe that our exposure to ultraviolet rays will continue to escalate as the atmosphere becomes more compromised.

Spirit/Mind Considerations

A sunburn can very aptly spoil a time which was meant to achieve rest, relaxation or rejuvenation. Many a honeymoon has been ruined by underestimating the power of the sun to damage unprotected skin. If you find yourself in this rather unfortunate predicament, see the humor in it and become the wiser for it.

Prevention

- Keep out of sunlight during the hottest parts of the day.
- Wear protective hats and sunscreen when exposed to the sun.
- Build up your exposure to the sun gradually so that your skin becomes acclimated and does not initially burn.
- Protect your face and other parts of your body from the reflective rays of the sun when near water, snow or sand.

Doctor's Notes

Any sunburn that causes significant damage needs to be evaluated by someone that is familiar with treating burns. First and second degree burns, identified by simple redness of the skin or mild blisters, can easily be treated at home. In sunburns where the skin is intact or has superficial blisters, applications of liquid trace minerals can be used for pain and healing. Poultices can be made from gotu kola decoctions or extract and placed directly over the burn. Taking gotu kola and butcher's broom orally can also speed healing. Applying lavender oil diluted in olive oil can help decrease pain and speed healing. Often we only think to treat a sunburn externally. There is much nutrient support needed to augment the healing process, to ward off infection, replace fluids and electrolytes and promote new tissue regeneration. Certain supplements discussed in this section can greatly enhance and speed the healing of sunburns while minimizing scarring. The herbal and nutritional supplements listed in this section are designed to cleanse the body by activating all its methods of elimination which include cleansing, strengthening, and supporting liver function. This formula will assist not only with sunburn, but applies to a wide range of skin disorders, including eczema, cellulitis, acne, psoriasis, burns, and insect bites.

Additional Resources

National Burn Victim Foundation
32-34 Scotland Road
Orange, NJ 07050
(201) 676-7700

Endnotes

1. R.D. Semba, "Vitamin A, immunity and infection," Clin Info Dis, 1994, 19: 489-99.
2. N.I. Krinsky, "Antioxidant function of carotenoids," Free Rad Biol Med, 1989, 7: 637-35.
3. J.V. Haley, "Zinc sulfate and wound healing," Jour Surg Res, 1979, 27(3): 168-74.
4. L.J. Hinks, et al., "Trace element status in eczema and psoriasis," Clin Exp Derm, 1987, 12: 93-97.
5. G.W. Burton and M.G. Traber, "Antioxidant activity, biokinetics, and bioavailability," Annu Rev Nutr, 1992, 10: 357-82.
6. C.R. Spillant, "The beneficial effects of ascorbic acid in murine burns," Clin Res, 1983, 31: A690.

7. Michael T. Murray, N.D., Encyclopedia of Nutritional Supplements (Prima Publishing, Rocklin CA: 1996) 252-53.

8. J.A. Gravel, "Oxygen dressings and asiaticosides in the treatment of burns," Laval Med, 1965, 36: 413-15.

9. C. Hobbs, "St. John's wort, Hypericum perforatum," Herbalgram, 1989, 18-19: 24-33.

10. Y. Vidal, et al., "Articular cartilage pharmacology: in vitro studies on glucosamine and non-steroidal anti-inflammatory drugs," Pharmacol Res, Comm, 1978, 10(6): 557-69.

11. C.J.D. Zarafonetis, et al., "Paraaminobenzoic acid in dermatitis herpetiformis," Arch Dermatol Syphiolo, 1951, 63: 115-32.

12. T. Kartnig, "Clinical applications of Centella asiatica (L)," URB Herbs Spices Med Plants, 1988, 3: 146-73.

13. F. Susnik, "Present state and knowledge of the medicinal plant Taxicum officinale," Med Razgledi, 1982, 21: 323-28.

14. P.M. Altman, "Australian tea tree oil," Aust Jour Pharm, 1988, 69: 276-78.

15. Mark Pedersen, Nutritional Herbology (Wendell W. Whitman Co., Warsaw, IN: 1994) 169.

16. D. Grindlay and T. Reynolds, "The aloe vera leaf phenomenon: A review of the properties and modern use of the leaf parenchyma gel," Jour Ethnopharmacol, 1986, 16: 117-51.

TEMPOROMANDIBULAR JOINT SYNDROME (TMJ)

This syndrome consists of pain and a variety of other symptoms that are thought to result from a malfunction of the temporomandibular joint and the muscles that operate the joint. Approximately 10 million Americans suffer from TMJ, although this condition is often misdiagnosed and subsequently mistreated. It is frequently blamed for a very wide and somewhat absurd list of symptoms.

Causes

The most common cause of true TMJ syndrome is the spasm of muscles that control chewing. Factors that can bring about these spasms are teeth grinding or a misaligned bite, which continually place stress on these muscle groups. Other possible causes of TMJ are

◆ injuries to the jaw, head or neck
◆ impacted wisdom tooth
◆ emotional stress
◆ nail biting
◆ chewing the inside of the cheek
◆ the presence of osteoarthritis
◆ disc degeneration

Symptoms

Symptoms are usually more severe in the mornings and can include

◆ frequent headaches
◆ tender jaw muscles
◆ facial pain
◆ pain around the ear
◆ ringing in the ears
◆ toothaches
◆ eye pain
◆ neck pain
◆ clicking or popping jaw joint
◆ difficulty opening the mouth
◆ jaws that can get locked or feel as if they have become unhinged
◆ pain upon yawning or chewing
◆ fluttering sound in the ears

CAUTION: If you cannot eat properly, brush your teeth or are suffering severe headaches, see your physician or dentist. Be careful when dealing with a diagnosis of TMJ. Get a second opinion from a reputable dentist or orthodontist before embarking on an expensive therapeutic plan for treatment.

Conventional Therapies

TMJ has become a widespread condition that can often be mistreated by dentist, chiropractors and physicians. The treatments can be costly and are sometimes not particularly effective. The use of splints or surgery should be considered only as last resorts. Arthroplasty surgery has had limited success when the meniscus or disc needs replacement. Breaking the jaw to realign the bite is a major operation and involves a significant amount of trauma, pain and discomfort period. Relaxation techniques, and proper diet should be employed first and other treatment options assessed. A combination of moist heat and muscle relaxants may be tried initially. If symptoms persist, a bite splint may be prescribed which fits over the teeth to prevent clenching or grinding. An arthroscope, in which dye is injected into the joint and then is viewed with a fluoroscopy, may be required to examine the joint. If the bite needs correction, an orthodontic appliance may be indicated and in severe cases, jaw surgery may be required to properly align the teeth and jaws. Nonsteroidal anti-inflammatory drugs such as naprosyn, ibuprofen and aspirin are routinely prescribed for TMJ pain. In some cases, a cortisone injection will be administered directly into the temporomandibular joint to relieve inflammation and pain.

Dietary Guidelines

- Avoid foods that stress the body, such as candy, colas, potato chips, pies and rich pastries, fried and fatty foods, and red meats.
- Stay away from caramels or other sticky foods that can stress the jaw joints.
- Eat nutritious foods that do not stress the jaw joint, such as steamed vegetables, soft fruits, fruit and vegetable juices, whole grain cereals and breads, fish, skinless turkey and chicken, yogurt, low-fat cottage cheese, and soups.
- Do not chew gum or bite on hard candy.

Recommended Nutritional Supplements

PRIMARY NUTRIENTS

GLUCOSAMINE SULFATE/CHONDROITIN SULFATE A very effective combination of compounds that relieves pain and inflammation while encouraging the regeneration of joint cartilage. Double-blind studies confirm that these two supplements are actually more effective than ibuprofen if taken long term.[1] *Suggested Dosage*: Take both supplements as directed over a four- to six-week period.

CALCIUM/MAGNESIUM Both of these minerals are essential for bone strength and inhibit muscle spasms. Calcium can help prevent bone loss in the jaw as well.[2] *Suggested Dosage*: 1,000 mg of each per day. Use chelated forms for maximum absorbability. Calcium citrate, gluconate and aspartate are recommended.

SILICON Improves the assimilation of calcium and is needed for the proper function of an enzyme which participates in the synthesis of collagen in bone and cartilage tissue.[3]

Suggested Dosage: Take as directed. NOTE: The herb horsetail is naturally rich in silicon.

VITAMIN B12 Increases the absorption of calcium and is vital to the production of healthy muscle fiber. *Suggested Dosage*: Take as directed.

MARINE LIPIDS The compounds contained in fish oils or the omega-3 fatty acids have potent anti-inflammatory properties.[4] *Suggested Dosage*: Take as directed. Using vitamin E along with fish oils is also recommended.

DL-PHENYLALANINE This amino acid form helps with pain relief. Studies have shown that it can be effective for chronic pain even when standard medications have failed.[5] *Suggested Dosage*: Take as directed on an empty stomach with fruit juice.

MALIC ACID Participates in muscle cell metabolic processes which helps muscles to use glucose properly. This compound which is part of the Krebs's cycle in the body is thought to reduce the severity of symptoms associated with muscle pain especially when combined with magnesium.[6] *Suggested Dosage*: Take as directed with magnesium supplement.

GRAPE SEED OR PINE BARK EXTRACT A powerful antioxidant and natural anti-inflammatory compound which helps to inhibit the inflammatory response and scavenges for free radicals which can cause muscle pain or damage.[7] *Suggested Dosage*: Take as directed. You may initially want to start with a higher dose to saturate cells and then taper down to less. NOTE: If injury has caused TMJ and inflammation is present, refer to the chapter on arthritis for a recommended herbal combination.

HERBAL COMBINATION This combination intended for stress-related TMJ includes valerian root, hops, skullcap, passionflower, dandelion root, chamomile, marshmallow root, and hawthorn berries. *Suggested Dosage*: Two to four capsules daily. CAUTION: This formula should not be used when driving or operating heavy equipment or with conditions of low blood pressure.

VALERIAN ROOT: Compounds found in this herb interact with brain receptor sites to promote relaxation.[8] There are literally dozens of pharmaceutical and tea preparations throughout Europe which employ its tranquilizing benefits. HOPS: Hops has a calming effect on the nervous system which helps with insomnia and restlessness, particularly that associated with anxiety.[9] SKULLCAP: This plant has proven itself useful for sleep disorders, nervous conditions, tremors, and muscle spasms. Skullcap is officially recognized in Europe. Its uses there include sedation, as well as for epilepsy, hysteria, and nervous tension.[10] PASSIONFLOWER: This herb is widely used in Europe as a sedative and to treat common nervous conditions including nervous headaches and restlessness.[11] It is officially recognized in Britain, Belgium, France and Germany and has been listed in the *National Formulary* of the United States. DANDELION ROOT: Dandelion root plays a supportive role in this formula, even though it has no sedative or antianxiety action. It does have a mild laxative effect which helps cleanse the body and return it to a more normal state of health.[12] Quite often, conditions like TMJ are the result of anxiety. CHAMOMILE: This herb has been the subject of a tremendous amount of chemical, scientific, and pharmacological research. Chamomile supports the overall properties of this formula, and is a natural anti-inflammatory agent.[13] MARSHMALLOW: Marshmallow is accepted in Britain, Belgium, France, and Germany as an emollient and demulcent.[14] Marshmallow root does not have any muscle-relaxing action, but also plays a supporting role in this herbal formula. HAWTHORN BERRIES: Hawthorn berries have been used as a mild tranquilizer as well as an antispasmodic.[15] Interestingly, hawthorn berries have been incorporated in many European natural sedative formulas.

SECONDARY NUTRIENTS

VITAMIN B-COMPLEX WITH EXTRA PANTOTHENIC ACID (VITAMIN B5): This duo helps to control nervousness and stress that are directly linked with TMJ. *Suggested Dosage*: Take both as directed.

L-TYROSINE: An amino acid that helps to promote sleep and fight depression and anxiety. *Suggested Dosage*: Take as directed on an empty stomach with fruit juice.

VITAMIN C WITH BIOFLAVONOIDS: Vital to maintain the health of connective tissue and enable the body to cope with stress. *Suggested Dosage*: Take 3,000 to 5,000 mg daily.

GENTIAN: Works to relieve joint inflammations. *Suggested Dosage*: Take as directed, using standardized products.

DEVIL'S CLAW: A powerful botanical anti-inflammatory agent. *Suggested Dosage*: Take as directed, using standardized products.

Home Care Suggestions

- Don't try to hold the phone between your head and chin.
- Don't wear a heavy shoulder bag that can throw the alignment of your body off.
- Don't bite into an apple, corn on the cob, or eat sticky, chewy candies like caramels: these can throw your jaw joint into a lock. Avoid hard to chew foods such as bagels and don't chew gum.
- Don't sleep on your stomach—it puts pressure on one side of your face and can push your jaw joint out of alignment. Using a cervical pillow can encourage sleeping on your back and promote the relaxation of jaw muscles.
- Don't lie on your back and prop your head up at a sharp angle to watch T.V.
- If you are clenching your teeth due to emotional stress, make time for relaxation. Wear a splint if you need to break the habit of grinding or clenching the teeth and keep a record of the times when you engage in the behavior.
- Cut food into small, easy-to-chew pieces and eat slowly.
- Don't let yourself yawn too wide.
- Apply soft ice packs to the jaw area that hurts. Moist heat is also recommended although cold seems to be more beneficial.

- Try biofeedback and controlled breathing exercises to promote relaxation and reduce tension.

Other Supportive Therapies

ACUPUNCTURE: This therapy is good for pain relief and to loosen tight muscles.

HYDROTHERAPY: Alternating hot towels and an ice pack on the painful area offers immediate relief.

AUTOGENIC TRAINING: This therapy involves special exercises that can successfully relieve muscle tension in the jaw.

PHYSICAL THERAPY: Using TENS, which is the use of nerve stimulating machines, the jaw muscles can be relaxed and pain minimized.

HOMEOPATHY: Specific remedies for teeth grinding include cina, santoninum, phytolacca, zinc, and arsenicum alb.

Scientific Facts-at-a-Glance

Data now supports the fact that a significant number of headaches, including migraines, are really symptoms of TMJ. In addition, people who suffer from TMJ have more tension headaches than the general population and vice versa. This suggests that a certain type of person is susceptible to stress-induced TMJ and that many people who suffer from tension headaches, may have TMJ.[16]

Spirit/Mind Considerations

TMJ is often a stress-related disorder. The development of TMJ symptoms can be caused by an individual's ability to cope with stress. Stress management in combination with supportive therapy can help to control nervous habits which compound TMJ. Many of us unknowingly clench our jaws when we are tense. Learning to recognize cues like this can help us to relax our jaw through controlled breathing.

Prevention

- Learn to relax and manage tension every day.
- Eat well-balanced meals that can fortify the body to manage stress more effectively.
- Don't use alcohol, tobacco or caffeine. These substances can increase stress and also deplete the body of essential nutrients.
- Don't chew gum for long periods of time.
- Don't clench or grind your teeth or move your jaw from side to side.
- Don't sleep on your stomach.
- Protect your jaw joints from injury by not opening your mouth too wide or biting down on hard candies.

Doctor's Notes

While I have seen several cases of TMJ that were the direct result of trauma such as an automobile accident, people who chew gum and have a misaligned bite can also develop symptoms. Certain personality types seem more prone to TMJ and include those individuals who are characteristically nervous and usually grind their teeth at night (bruxism) or unconsciously clench their jaw during the day. TMJ is associated with pain in the jaw joint which is usually localized just in front of the ear. Headaches associated with this pain can develop on the side of the face affected.

TMJ can affect one or both jaw joints. Again, determining the cause of the problem rather than just addressing its symptoms is preferable. In cases where stress is thought to be the culprit, using antianxiety herbs such as valerian and kava can be useful. I like to add magnesium supplementation for extra relaxation. If the cause of TMJ is due to physical injury, then inflammation will need treatment. Anti-inflammatory herbs and nutrients are recommended and include devil's claw, tumeric, boswellia, and ginger. If a misaligned bite is at fault, you will need to work with your dentist to correct the problem. TMJ syndrome is often associated with trigger points in the neck of face muscles (chewing muscles). A chiropractic exam from someone who is familiar with this disorder can also be useful. Our clinic uses a combination of chiropractic treatment, articular therapy or ear acupuncture and regular acupuncture along with a complement of herbs and nutrients.

Keep in mind that several other disease processes can mimic TMJ. One of the most common is a pain syndrome in which the muscles around the shoulders and neck become inflamed and trigger pain is areas distant from the source. There are times when a trigger point in one of the chewing muscles will simulate TMJ. Neck muscles can produce the same phenomenon. People who have pain in their face (the number of these people is on the increase) need to have their neck and shoulder muscles examined before embarking on a course of treatment for TMJ that totally misses the true cause.

Additional Resources

American Dental Association
211 East Chicago Ave
Chicago, IL 60611
(312) 440-2500

Endnotes

1. A.L. Vaz, "Double-blind clinical evaluation of the relative efficacy of ibuprofen and glucosamine sulfate in the management of osteoarthritis of the knee in out-patients," Current Med Res Opinion, 1982, 8: 145-49.

2. J.F. Aloia, et al., "Calcium supplementation with and without hormone replacement therapy to prevent postmenopausal bone loss," Annal Intern Med, 1994, 120: 97-103.

3. Robert Garrison and Elizabeth Somer, The Nutrition Desk Reference (Keats Publishing, New Canaan, Connecticut: 1990), 82.

4. Biochemical Pharmacology, 1986, 35 (5): 779-85.

5. N.E. Walsh, et al., "Analgesic effectiveness of D-phenylalanine in chronic pain patients," Arch Phys Med Rehabil, 1986, 67(7): 436-39.

6. G. Abraham, "Management of fibromyalgia: Rationale for the use of magnesium and malic acid," Jour Nutri Med, 1992, 3: 49-59.

7. B. Schwitters and J. Masquelier, OPC in Practice: Bioflavonols and Their Application (Alpha Omega, Rome: 1993).

8. T. Mennini, et al., "In vitro study on the interaction of extracts and pure compounds from Valeriana officinalis roots with GABA, Benzodiazepine, and barbiturate receptors in rat brain," Fitoterapia, 1993, 54(4): 291-300.

9. Michael T. Murray, The Healing Power or Herbs, 2nd ed. (Prima Publishing, Rocklin, CA: 1992), 371.

10. K.L. Reichelt, et al., "Gluten, milk proteins and autism: Dietary intervention effects on behavior and peptide secretion," Jour Appl Nutr, 1990, 42(1):1-11.

11. N. Sopranzi, et al., "Biological and electroencephalographic parameters in rats in relation to Passiflora incarnata," Clin Ter, 1990, 132(5): 329-33.

12. J.K. Bohm, "Choleretic action of some medicinal plants," Arzneimittel-Forsch, 1959, 9: 376-78.

13. Della, Loggia R., et al., "Evaluation of the anti-inflammatory activity of chamomile preparations," Planta Med, 1990, 56:657-8.

14. "Marshmallow" The Lawrence Review of Natural Products: Facts and Comparisons, 1991, St. Louis.

15. S. Uchida, et al., "Inhibitory effects of condensed tannins on angiotensin converting enzyme," Jap Jour Pharmacol, 1987, 43:242-5.

16. P. Watts, et al., "Migraine and the temporomandibular joint: The final answer," Bri Dent Jour, 1986, 170-73.

TOOTH GRINDING

Bruxism is a clinical term for simple tooth grinding, which can involve rhythmic grinding and tooth clenching. Tooth grinding commonly occurs while sleeping, and people who do it are rarely aware of the practice. If tooth grinding is severe or occurs over an extended period of time, gum and tooth damage can occur. In addition, jaw problems may also develop.

Symptoms

- consistent tooth grinding
- loosened teeth
- receding gums
- misaligned bite
- jaw problems

Causes

While certain personalities may seem more prone to tooth grinding, it is viewed as a habit which usually reflects stress and tension. Tooth grinding can also be caused by

- teeth that are sensitive to heat and cold
- blood sugar changes
- anxiety and unresolved fears
- crooked teeth that compel biting down
- food allergies
- vitamin or mineral deficiencies

NOTE: For decades, the notion that having worms caused a child to grind the teeth was widely circulated. While it may be true that a person with parasites grinds their teeth, there is no scientific evidence that the two conditions are related.

Conventional Therapies

If the problem persists, a type of splint or tooth guard can be worn both during the day and while sleeping. While this is not considered a cure, it can discourage the practice because the plastic surface of the oral appliance is much smoother than the teeth, making it more difficult to achieve any kind of pressure or friction.

Dietary Guidelines

- Avoid caffeine in any form, such as soft drinks, chocolate, coffee, tea and some medications. People who are prone to anxiety will sometimes also be sensitive to caffeine. It only makes good sense to avoid stimulants of any kind.
- Do not eat white sugar and highly sweetened foods. Experiencing sporadic fluctuations in blood sugar can in itself create feelings of anxiety and stress the adrenal glands.
- Eat complex carbohydrates, such as whole grains, and avoid empty-calorie junk foods and cold cereals.

- Try to add more protein to your diet instead of concentrating on high carbohydrate foods.
- Try to rule out food allergies by keeping a careful record of what you eat and the incidence of attacks.
- Do not take any drugs that you absolutely do not need. Look for correlations between any drug you might be taking and anxiety attacks. Some drugs which are considered to have tranquilizing side effects can actually agitate the nervous system of some people. Certain decongestants, codeine preparations, cough medicines, etc. can have this effect.
- Do not consume alcohol.

Recommended Nutritional Supplements

PRIMARY NUTRIENTS

VITAMIN B COMPLEX All of the B-vitamins are vital to the proper functioning of the nervous system and the maintenance of mental health. Strong supplementation of the B-vitamins can improve brain function and help in reducing anxiety and stress.[1] Take extra vitamin B1, B6 and B12. *Suggested Dosage:* Take as directed. Use sublingual forms where possible.

VITAMIN C WITH BIOFLAVONOIDS Important for healthy adrenal gland function which can become overworked during periods of anxiety. During periods of prolonged stress, the adrenal gland may become overworked, increasing the need for vitamin C. Taking high doses of this vitamin has been linked to increased stress resistance.[2] *Suggested Dosage:* 1,000 mg with each meal.

CALCIUM/MAGNESIUM Has a calming effect and helps to decrease feelings of nervousness. *Suggested Dosage:* Take as directed, using chelated gluconate or citrate products.

L-TYROSINE An amino acid which can help alleviate symptoms of stress and also promotes sleep.[3] *Suggested Dosage:* Take as directed on an empty stomach in the morning with fruit juice. CAUTION: Do not use if you are taking beta-blocker drugs or suffer from high blood pressure.

MELATONIN Promotes relaxation and sleep and has been used to treat mental disorders such as depression and the type of insomnia that accompanies anxiety.[4] *Suggested Dosage:* Take only as directed, starting with very small amounts. Not recommended for pregnant or nursing mothers.

VALERIAN ROOT A safe and nonaddictive tranquilizing herb which has proven its efficacy in treating anxiety disorders and promoting more restful sleep.[5] Valerian works especially well in combination with passionflower. *Suggested Dosage:* Take as directed only. CAUTION: May cause drowsiness.

KAVA Kavain, the major bioactive compound found in kava, has proven its effectiveness in clinical trials with patients who suffered from anxiety disorders and was compared to Valium without side effects.[6] *Suggested Dosage:* Take as directed.

GINKGO BILOBA Improves brain cell oxygenation and has proven antidepressive effects.[7] *Suggested Dosage:* Take as directed, using guaranteed potency products.

HERBAL COMBINATION This combination should contain valerian, passionflower, wood betony, ginger, hops, skullcap, chamomile, and blessed thistle. *Suggested Dosage:* Four to eight capsules daily.

VALERIAN: Valerian is probably the most widely used botanical in Europe for nervous tension, anxiety and insomnia. In fact, the herb is found in dozens of drugs and teas. Interestingly, valerian is calming and relaxing in cases of nervous tension and anxiety while at the same time improving alertness and ability to concentrate.[8] PASSIONFLOWER: This herb effectively works to combat stress, nervous tension, anxiety, and restlessness, which can all contribute to tooth grinding. It contains small amounts of serotonin which act to calm the brain.[9] CAUTION: Do not use if you are pregnant or nursing. WOOD BETONY: Wood betony has been well appreciated and prescribed for hundreds of years by old and new world physicians for treating nervous and sleep disorders, with particular application for tension headaches.[10] It also acts as a cleansing tonic to the blood and certain organs of the body. Along with valerian, wood betony is mildly carminative or settling to the GI tract. GINGER ROOT: Eating disorders and digestive disturbances often accompany nervous tension and anxiety. A better herb than ginger cannot be found to treat digestive disorders. Ginger assists almost every aspect of digestion. It stimulates saliva and bile production; prevents nausea, gas and bloating; improves peristalsis by toning the intestinal muscle; and optimizes friendly intestinal flora. HOPS: Hops is widely cultivated in North and South America, England, Germany and Australia for use in beer production. It has been so used for over a thousand years. Perhaps for just as long, hops has been used medicinally to treat restlessness, anxiety and sleep disorders.[11] Hops is officially recognized in Britain, Belgium, France and Germany. SKULLCAP: Skullcap has proven itself useful for sleep disorders, nervous conditions, tremors, and spasms. It has the ability to calm an excited nervous system.[12] In earlier years it enjoyed official recognition in the *United States Pharmacopeia* and the *National Formulary*. Skullcap is still officially recognized in Europe to treat epilepsy, hysteria, nervous tension and insomnia. CHAMOMILE: While chamomile has been modestly employed in this country as a tea and in other health preparations, it does not even approach the success found in western and eastern Europe, especially Germany, where it is considered to be a panacea or cure-all. Chamomile has been extensively researched where it has demonstrated usefulness in sleep and digestive disorders. BLESSED THISTLE: Blessed thistle plays a supporting role in this formula. It helps activate a sluggish liver and correct stomach and digestive problems, flatulence and tension headaches. It further supports the body's cleansing and detoxifying systems by promoting perspiration and removing excess fluids.

SECONDARY NUTRIENTS

ESSENTIAL OILS OF LAVENDER, FRANKINCENSE OR JASMINE: These can be rubbed on the temples or other areas of the body to induce relaxation prior to bedtime. *Suggested Dosage:* Use as directed.

L-GLUTAMINE: Works to gently tranquilize the central nervous system. SUGGESTED DOSAGE: 1,500 mg divided into three doses, taken on an empty stomach with fruit juice.

PANTOTHENIC ACID: Helps to nourish the brain and is essential for brain cell health and stress control. *Suggested Dosage:* Take as directed.

Home Care Suggestions

◆ As much as possible, avoid stress. Learn stress management and relaxation techniques.

◆ Find support groups that provide a forum for sharing feelings and contributing to overcoming stress through a network of mutual sharing and counseling. Your local mental health organization will have a number of support groups that you can contact.

◆ Exercise daily. Exercise is a wonderful outlet for pent-up tension or anxiety. Choose something you enjoy and learn to express your emotional fears in a constructive physical way, such as jogging, swimming, racquetball, etc. If you feel you cannot leave your home, get home exercise equipment or use exercise videos.

◆ Get a regular massage for its relaxation value, and if you feel an attack coming on, have your companion give you a deep shoulder and neck massage.

◆ Investigate therapies such as self-hypnosis, breathing exercises, music therapy, and biofeedback. Any of these may offer valuable advice on how to control the mind and subsequently stop the habit of tooth grinding.

◆ Aromatherapy may have some real benefit for anxiety-related disorders like bruxism. Sniffing certain aromas can have the immediate affect of calming and relaxing the nerves and creating a feeling of well-being. Some of the smells which typically produce a state of happiness are cookies or bread baking, cinnamon and ginger. Use these just prior to going to bed.

◆ If you suspect a mineral deficiency, have a hair analysis done; these are the most effective tests.

Other Supportive Therapies

MEDITATION: Learning to meditate can help to dispel feelings of anxiety or tension while teaching you to focus on only what you want to think about. Mind control is an integral part of learning to deal with feelings of uncontrolled anxiety or panic.

VISUALIZATION: The ability to visualize sleep without tooth grinding and put the mind into a relaxed state can help with anxiety. In addition, bringing to mind certain pleasant images when you first close your eyes to go to sleep can help to achieve better rest.

CONTROLLED BREATHING: This discipline is invaluable for achieving relaxation amid stress and can be perfected with a little practice. Do it as you lay down just prior to closing your eyes for the night.

AROMATHERAPY: Certain fragrances like lavender can help to dispel stress and promote a tranquilizing effect. Aromatic oils can be kept by the bedside.

BIOFEEDBACK: Tell yourself over and over before you close your eyes that you will not grind your teeth.

Scientific Facts-at-a-Glance

Since we know that stress impacts our physical bodies and can disrupt our neurochemistry, we are well aware of the fact that anxiety can manifest itself even during periods of sleep. People who experience frightening nightmares on a regular basis which often involve intense fear, can also be prone to tooth grinding. Children who are very sensitive about their performance at school may tend to grind their teeth at night, especially when they face higher levels of stress. It is also true that a deficiency in the B-vitamins can cause all sorts of abnormal emotional states, implying that what we eat profoundly affects our brain chemistry and our ability to cope during the day and to sleep well at night.

Spirit/Mind Considerations

Learning to recognize how we handle stress is vital to overcoming habits like tooth grinding. Like nail biting, this practice may be an inadvertent attempt by our body and mind to release pent up stress. Both habits are counterproductive and may even cause physical harm if taken to the extreme. Believing that meditation, visualization or even suggestion can help us to control behaviors we may not be aware of is the first step. If you have ruled out nutrient deficiencies, then look at tooth grinding as an indication that you may be more stressed than you assumed. Use essential oils, massage, self-talk, etc., to achieve complete relaxation before you fall asleep and leave your problems on the nightstand.

Prevention

- ◆ Eat nutritionally, get exercise and learn to control your thoughts through biofeedback.
- ◆ Manage stress and learn to relax by setting aside a certain portion of each day for relaxation techniques.

Doctor's Notes

Discouraging consistent tooth grinding or bruxism may require a trip to the dentist for the creation of an oral appliance that will protect your teeth and jaw and make grinding more difficult. Because this disorder has been linked to anxiety and is known to increase during periods of stress, using nervine herbs combined with other supplementation and counseling may be very beneficial. Valerian, chamomile, kava, hops and skullcap are excellent calming herbs which promote good and restful sleep without the side effects of sedative drugs. These herbs may be taken as a combination or as separate supplements. Make sure to look for guaranteed-potency products. In addition, taking magnesium is also recommended. One to two drops of lavender oil in a fourth of a cup of warm water sipped twice a day can be helpful. Lavender can also be used on the skin, over the temples, or on areas where the skin is thin for absorption.

Other essential oils that are beneficial include frankincense and jasmine.

Endnotes

1. L. Christiansen, et al., "Impact of a dietary change on emotional distress," Jour of Abn Psychol, 1985, 94: 565-79.
2. A. Kallner, "The influence of vitamin C status on the urinary excretion of catecholamines in stress," Human Nutr Clin Nutri, 1983, 37: 447-52.
3. G.E. Abraham, "Nutrition and the premenstrual tension syndromes," Jour App Nutri, 1984, 36: 103-24.
4. S.P. James, et al., "Melatonin administered in insomnia," Neuropsychopharmacology, 1990, 3: 19-23. See also A.B. Dollins, et al., "Effect of pharmacological daytime doses of melatonin on human mood and performance," Psychopharmacol, 1993, 112: 490-96.
5. V. Schellenberg, et al., "Quantitative EEG monitoring in phtyo- and psychopharmacological treatment of psychosomatic and affective disorders," Schizophrenia Res, 1993, 9(2,3): Abstract.
6. W.E. Scholine and H.D. Clausen, "On the effect of d, l-kavain: experience with neuronika," Med Klin, 1977, 72: 1301-06 and D. Lindenberg and H. Pitule-Scholdel, "D, L-kavin in comparison with oxazepam in anxiety disorders: A double-blind study of clinical effectiveness," Forschr med, 1990, 108: 49-50, 53-54.
7. H. Schubert, P. Halama, "Depressive episode primarily unresponsive to therapy in elderly patients: Efficacy of Ginkgo biloba in combination with antidepressants," Geria Forsch, 1993, 3: 45-53.
8. U. Boeters. "Treatment of autonomic dysregulation with valepotriates (valmane)," Muenchener Medizinische Wochenschrift, 1969, 37, 1873-1876. V. Kempinskas. "On the action valerian." Famakologii I Toksikologiia,1964, 4(3): 305-309. See also R. Klich and B. Gladbach. "Childhood behavior disorders and their treatment." Medizinishce Welt, 26(25), 1251-1254, 1975.
9. Rebecca Flynn, M.S., Mark Roest, Your Guide to Standardized Herbal Products (One World Press, Prescott Arizona: 1995), 61.
10. Daniel P. Mowrey, The Scientific Validation of Herbs, (Keats Publishing, New Canaan, Connecticut: 1986), 193. T.V. Zinchenko and I.M. Fefer. "Investigation of glycosides from betonica officinalis," Farmatsevt A-Zhurnal, 1962 17(3): 35-38.
11. Mowrey, 164-65.
12. B.A. Kurnakov, "Pharmacology of skullcap," Farmakologiia I Toksikologiia, 20(6): 79-80, 1957.

ULCERS

After many years of misunderstanding ulcers and what causes them, we are discovering new and fascinating facts about them. An estimated five million Americans suffer from ulcers—peptic, duodenal and gastric. With drug therapy, peptic ulcers usually heal within eight weeks. The chances of an ulcer recurring without continuing treatment is between 60 and 70 percent. Gastrointestinal ulcers can occur at any age. An ulcer is an open sore that forms on the skin or any mucus membrane such as the lining of the stomach. It may be shallow or deep and is characterized by pain and inflammation. Most ulcers are found within the upper digestive tract and are comprised of peptic, duodenal and gastric ulcers. Ulcers usually initially form in the duodenum, which is the first section of the small intestine. They may also occur in the stomach lining itself.

Symptoms

Only around 50 percent of all people who suffer from stomach ulcers have obvious symptoms. Symptoms of a duodenal or peptic ulcer typically include a gnawing burning sensation below the breastbone that is relieved by eating food but then recurs two to three hours after a meal. Other possible symptoms include the following:

◆ heartburn
◆ intense pain
◆ passing dark stools
◆ vomiting, especially dark vomit
◆ nausea

NOTE: If an ulcer bleeds for a prolonged period of time, anemia can result. CAUTION: If you spit up blood that looks like coffee grounds, or have dark tar-like stools, contact your doctor immediately. These symptoms may indicate gastrointestinal bleeding and should be immediately addressed. Bleeding ulcers can be serious enough to be life-threatening. A perforated ulcer—when an ulcer perforates through the abdominal wall, spilling its contents into the abdominal cavity—is a medical emergency.

Causes

Stomach ulcers occur when the mucus lining that normally protects the stomach from the caustic effects of stomach acid breaks down. While the effects of stress are debated, stress definitely causes an increase in the production of stomach acid and a decreased blood flow to the stomach. The belief that too much acid causes ulcers is now questioned. The underlying causes of stomach ulcers seem to involve factors that permit damage to the mucus membrane by the acid present. Certain corrosive prescription drugs such as nonsteroidal anti-inflammatories can increase the risk of developing ulcers by damaging the mucus membrane. Damage may also result from cigarette smoke, a genetic predisposition (people with type-O blood have a higher rate of duodenal ulcers), and the possibility of bacterial infection. The notion that stress and anxiety can compromise the immune system, thus allowing for the development of bacteria that can cause ulcers, is also accepted by some health care professionals. Irregular, hurried meals have also been associated with ulcer formation. Some studies have also linked food allergies with peptic ulcers. Recently, evidence has pointed to the presence of bacterial infection as a possible cause of peptic ulcers. As a result, antibiotic treatment has produced some encouraging results. Discuss this option with your physician.

Conventional Therapies

New drugs can help heal ulcers and significantly reduce their discomfort; however, they have a tendency to recur. In most cases, even without treatment, ulcers will heal themselves within six weeks. Unfortunately, medical science does not effectively get at the root of tissue susceptibility to ulceration. Consequently, the rate at which ulcers recur is high. Most doctors fail to teach their ulcer patients lifestyle modifications that will minimize their chances of further ulcer development. Diagnosis of an ulcer is confirmed by an x-ray and by viewing the lesion directly through a gastroscopy, in which a tube is threaded through the mouth into the intestinal tract. A barium swallow and x-ray are usually done to examine the stomach lining.

Lab tests to assess stomach acid content and a bowel movement analysis may be done to check for internal bleeding. Sucralfates (carafate) is recommended by some physicians as the best drug choice in treating ulcers. It produces a thick paste that protects the ulcerated tissue. Because it coats the stomach so efficiently, Sucralfates succeeds in healing 80 percent of ulcers within the first six weeks of treatment. Other drugs routinely prescribed are H2 blockers (Tagamet, Zantac, Axid, Pepcid) which suppress the production of stomach acid. Antispasmodics may also be used. Prostaglandin drugs can now be used to treat ulcers caused by anti-inflammatory drugs. For peptic ulcers drugs that block the effects of histamine which causes inflammation are used. Sucralfates and other ulcer healing drugs are also prescribed and create a protective barrier over the ulcer allowing for healing. Antacid drugs are also commonly prescribed. Once the peptic ulcer is healed, maintenance drugs may be prescribed. A fairly new drug, Misoprostol, is currently being used in several other countries for the treatment of peptic ulcers.

If the ulcer does not heal after eight weeks of treatment, an operation to remove the portion of the stomach that contains the ulcer may be advised. Antibiotics combined with traditional ulcer medications are being used to treat patients with *H. pylori* infection.

Dietary Guidelines

◆ White sugar and flour may increase the production of stomach acid.
◆ Eat frequent, smaller meals. Up to six meals a day are recommended. The presence of food can help to neu-

tralize stomach acid, therefore don't go for long periods of time without eating.

- ◆ Avoid the following foods: dairy products (drinking milk or cream was recommended in the past to control acid but can actually aggravate the production of stomach acid), fatty foods, soda pop, caffeine, and alcohol.
- ◆ High-fiber diets are recommended for their therapeutic use. Fiber promotes mucin secretion and delays gastric emptying.
- ◆ Coffee (in any form) must be strictly avoided.
- ◆ Avoid taking large doses of vitamin C. This can create more stomach acid.
- ◆ Taking iron supplements is not recommended if you have an ulcer. Iron is a gastric irritant.
- ◆ Potatoes and almond milk are recommended for their acid-neutralizing properties.
- ◆ Barley helps rebuild the lining of the stomach.
- ◆ Foods that are recommended include low-fat yogurt, avocados, bananas, squash, yams, steamed broccoli, and carrots.
- ◆ Blue grapes are widely used in Europe to treat ulcers.
- ◆ Okra powder acts as a demulcent to stop inflammation.
- ◆ Papaya fruit contains enzymes that promote good digestion and heal the stomach lining.
- ◆ Persimmons help to facilitate healing of the stomach lining and whey powder contains compounds that help heal ulcerated tissue.

Recommended Nutritional Supplements

PRIMARY NUTRIENTS

VITAMIN A Vitamin A supplementation has proven its ability to combat the development of duodenal ulcers which are caused by an excess of acid.[1] In addition, using it can actually boost the healing of gastric ulcers.[2] *Suggested Dosage:* 25,000 to 50,000 IU. Do not exceed 10,000 IU if pregnant.

VITAMIN E Consistently using this vitamin can protect the gastric mucosa against ulceration.[3] *Suggested Dosage:* 800 IU daily.

CALCIUM Taken in the form of carbonate after meals and before retiring in the evening can help to prevent the formation of ulcers.[4] *Suggested Dosage:* 1,500 to 2,000 mg daily.

MAGNESIUM This mineral actually has the ability to neutralize stomach acid if taken after meals and before going to bed.[5] *Suggested Dosage:* Take 30–60 mg one hour after each meal and at bedtime. Use chelated products.

ZINC Some clinical data supports the use of zinc as a therapeutic agent in the treatment of peptic ulcers.[6] Zinc boosts the healing process and fortifies immunity. *Suggested Dosage:* 100 mg daily. Use zinc picolinate or gluconate in lozenge form.

VITAMIN B6 In clinical studies this nutrient has shown that it can protect against the type of ulcers thought to be caused by stress.[7] *Suggested Dosage:* Take as directed.

VITAMIN C WITH BIOFLAVONOIDS Studies have confirmed that using relatively large doses of ascorbic acid can actually boost healing.[8] *Suggested Dosage:* Take 1,000 to 3,000 mg prior to each meal and at bedtime. For gastric upset, try 1,500 mg of ascorbic acid in water.

L-GLUTAMINE Tests using glutamine supplements found that it was effective in treating peptic ulcers by enhancing healing.[9] *Suggested Dosage:* Use 100 mg one hour before each meal and at bedtime.

S-METHYL METHIONINE (VITAMIN U) This compound is found in trace amounts in certain raw foods, particularly cabbage. It enhances the healing of damaged mucus membranes.[10] *Suggested Dosage:* Take as directed.

ESSENTIAL FATTY ACIDS Both the omega-3 and the omega-6 acids help to control leukotriene production in the gastric mucosa, which can contribute to ulcerated lesions.[11] Moreover, people whose diets are high in omega-6 fatty acids, obtained from oils like flaxseed, have a lower rate of peptic ulcer disease.[12] *Suggested Dosage:* Take as directed using a liquid blend and keep refrigerated.

FIBER SUPPLEMENT Studies indicate that low fiber intake correlates with increased duodenal ulcers.[13] In addition, clinical trials found that guar gum significantly boosted the rate of healing for peptic ulcers and contributed to their prevention.[14] *Suggested Dosage:* Use first thing in the morning and before retiring. Use products with guar gum, pectin and psyllium.

BILBERRY The powerful anthocyanosides found in this herb have proven their ability to expedite the healing process in ulcers and to help prevent their recurrence.[15] *Suggested Dosage:* Take as directed using standardized products.

LICORICE ROOT Unquestionably, the flavonoid derivatives of this herb have significant antiulcer properties and promote healing of the gastric mucosa.[16] *Suggested Dosage:* Take as directed, using guaranteed potency products.

RHUBARB This familiar plant can help to reduce gastric ulcer bleeding.[17] *Suggested Dosage:* Take in powdered form as directed.

HERBAL COMBINATION This combination should contain astragalus, schizandra, goldenseal root, licorice root, papaya leaves, gentian root, myrrh gum, Irish moss, fenugreek seeds, ginger root, and aloe vera gel. *Suggested Dosage:* Two to four capsules daily.

GOLDENSEAL ROOT: Goldenseal has been used to restore the mucus lining of the GI tract and keep it from being easily disrupted by strengthening the cross linking of proteins in the mucus. Its berberine content is effective in treating the majority of gastrointestinal infections which may be at the root of ulcers.[18] LICORICE ROOT: Licorice has been recognized for its anti-inflammatory activity which can help in cases of gastric ulcers. It can inhibit the formation of inflammatory prostaglandins which promote ulceration.[19] PAPAYA LEAVES: Both papaya fruit and leaves are a source of papain which is a mixture of protein digesting enzymes. Studies have found that it can enhance the digestion of wheat gluten and inhibit its inflammatory response in the gastrointestinal tract.[20] GENTIAN ROOT: Gentian enjoys widespread use particularly in Europe as a digestive aid. It increases saliva and is believed to increase secretion of gastric juices.[21] Its anti-inflammatory effects are helpful with gastric-related disorders. It is considered a bitter tonic. MYRRH GUM: Myrrh gum is used to heal the gastric mucosa of the intestinal tract. Myrrh gum is carminative, reduces gas and bloating, and calms the stomach. It also is a mild laxative.[22] IRISH MOSS: Irish moss is rich in trace mineral nutrients. It also contains large amounts of mucilage which soothes and protects the GI tract from excess acid.[23] FENUGREEK SEEDS: As much as 40 percent of the weight of fenugreek seeds is mucilage. Mucilage is a gelatin-like substance usually made up of proteins and polysaccharides which heals the irritated intestinal tract lining and helps to hold water. It also prompts pancreatic secretion which boosts digestion.[24] GINGER ROOT: Ginger is one of the best herbs for the treatment of digestive disorders. Ginger prevents nausea, gas, bloating, and vomiting. Ginger root is not a laxative, but it will tonify the intestinal muscle and provides a source of proteolytic enzymes to aid digestion.[25] ALOE VERA GEL: Aloe vera gel is a clear jelly-like material called mucilage. Aloe has been successfully employed in treating irritated mucus membrane. It also reduces putrefaction in the intestinal tract, and increases friendly bacteria like acidophilus.[26] NOTE: If you have any gripping with aloe, add more ginger. This herb is usually part of combinations and if used alone may cause cramping.

SECONDARY NUTRIENTS

CABBAGE JUICE: Promotes healing of the mucus membranes. Freshly juiced cabbage is best. *Suggested Dosage:* Take as directed on an empty stomach before each meal. Cabbage juice or powder may be hard to find and can be made at home in a juicer.

VITAMIN K: Helps to control bleeding. *Suggested Dosage:* Take as directed.

GARLIC OIL: A natural antibiotic that also promotes healing. *Suggested Dosage:* Take on an empty stomach before each meal as directed. Be careful not to take an excess or burning may result.

CATECHIN: Tests have shown this compound to be of value in preventing and treating postoperative stress ulcers. *Suggested Dosage:* Take as directed.

TURMERIC AND CAYENNE: Helps to boost healing and fight infection. *Suggested Dosage:* Take as directed starting off with very small doses of cayenne and working up.

TRACE SILVER: Helps to fight the bacterial infection that causes gastric ulcers to form. *Suggested Dosage:* Take only as directed.

Home Care Suggestions

◆ Taking over-the-counter antacids can provide some relief and helps to promote healing; however, long-term use of these preparations may cause diarrhea or constipation.

◆ Some studies suggest that calcium carbonate antacids (Tums, Alks-2) may actually produce a rebound effect of gastric acid secretion. The prolonged use of sodium bicarbonate antacids (Rolaids, Alka-Seltzer, Bromo-Seltzer) may cause metabolic imbalances.

◆ The type of antacids most frequently recommended for ulcers are aluminum-magnesium compounds (Maalox, Mylanta, Digel) and these may cause a depletion of calcium and phosphorus and contain aluminum which may be toxic.

◆ While some doctors are skeptical that stress can cause ulcers, there is enough credible evidence that the connection is a valid one. People who live in high stress cities have a greater incidence of ulcers. Keep stress levels controlled through biofeedback, visualization therapy, yoga, controlled breathing, exercise, etc.

◆ The majority of ulcers will heal on their own with bed rest and proper diet.

◆ Pepto-Bismol contains bismuth, which can kill bacteria that invade the stomach and are thought to cause ulcers. If the theory that bacteria cause stomach lining vulnerability to ulcers is valid, this approach may be worth trying.

◆ Slow down your pace of living, including the speed in which you eat and drink. Don't eat under stress.

◆ Stop smoking. Smokers are twice as likely to get ulcers as nonsmokers. Smoking also inhibits ulcer healing and increases your chances of having recurring ulcers.

◆ Avoid taking aspirin and ibuprofen. These medications along with other nonsteroidal anti-inflammatory drugs should not be taken by anyone suffering from an ulcer. They can cause further deterioration of the stomach lining. Acetaminophen is recommended.

◆ Keep your immune system strong with proper supplementation, stress control and diet.

Other Supportive Therapies

HOMEOPATHY: Arsenicum alb. and nux vomica are traditionally used for gastric ulcers.

MEDITATION: This practice helps to diffuse stress which is still a major causal factor in the development of gastric ulcers.

Scientific Facts-at-a-Glance

For years, people with ulcers were told to drink milk to calm down excess acid production. We know now that milk should definitely be avoided as it only has a very transient acid neutralizing effect and actually prompts a subsequent rise in stomach acid.[27] The question of controlling excess acidity is a complex one. Concerning ulcers, it is vital that we discover why the lining of the gastrointestinal tract is vulnerable to acid damage in the first place. Interestingly, bismuth, which is the main ingredient in medicines like Pepto-bismol, taken four times daily 20 minutes before meals and at bedtime for six to eight weeks can help to kill the *H. pylori* bacteria which has been implicated in the development of some gastric ulcers.[28] It is important to consider, however, why certain people are vulnerable to the *H. pylori* bacteria and others are not.

Spirit/Mind Considerations

Despite the fact that the stress connection to gastric ulcers has been doubted by some medical doctors, the link is unquestionably valid. High-stress jobs, relationships, and certain personality traits do increase the risk for developing ulcers. This association may not be due to the increase of stomach acid which can result under times of stress but rather, in lowering immunity and susceptibility which can cause a vulnerability in the stomach lining to ulceration. Now that we know a possible bacteria may be causing ulcers, the role of immunity is even more crucial. Learning to relax and cope with every day stressors is vital to decreasing one's risk of developing ulcers.

Prevention

- Keep your immune system healthy by eating nutritiously and supplementing your diet with garlic capsules which fights both bacterial and viral infection.
- Taking daily supplements of zinc has a protective effect against the formation of ulcers.
- Stress in all its forms is unquestionably a contributing factor to ulcers. Reduce stress through daily relaxation times using music therapy, stretching, yoga, biofeedback, exercise, etc. Change jobs or locations if stress is severe.
- Don't smoke. Smoking greatly increases your risk for developing ulcers as well as a whole other host of serious diseases. Smoking constricts the blood vessels that supply nourishment to the stomach lining.
- Eat regular meals and don't overeat.
- Avoid alcohol, which can result in stomach lining irritation.
- Avoid taking corticosteroids, ibuprofen, aspirin, indomethacin, prioxicam, and naproxen for long periods of time.

Doctor's Notes

Treatments for ulcers have undergone dramatic changes over the last few years. When I went to medical school, I can remember attending a conference in which Tagamet was announced as the new ulcer therapy of choice. I also recall that some of my colleagues who were going into gastroenterology expressed concern that now ulcers would be cured and they would be left with no one to treat. The introduction of Tagamet almost prompted them to change their specialty. While it is true that medications such as Tagamet, Pepsid AC and Zantac have made a dramatic change in the treatment of peptic ulcers, ulcers persist. We now know that recurring ulcers can be caused by the bacteria *H. pylori*. There is even some speculation that contaminated food may be the source of this bacteria. Doctors use strong doses of erythromycin, tetracycline and ampicillin to kill this bacteria in combination with standard ulcer medications. Yet questions still remain. For some people, even when the bacteria has been eradicated, they still have problems. The question is: Why do these people have the bacteria in the first place? I am convinced that stress may once again emerge as a major player. I believe Type-A personalities who are continually stressed out are unable to fight off bacteria, and are therefore more susceptible to ulcers than other people. Licorice root has a good track record for healing ulcers and controlling their symptoms. If recurring ulcers are a problem, use herbs with natural antibiotic activity such as goldenseal. Cayenne used initially in small doses and then increased can exert both an antibacterial and healing effect. Turmeric may also help heal ulcers and kill bacteria at the same time.

Endnotes

1. T. Mahmood, et al., "Prevention of duodenal ulcer formation in the rat by dietary vitamin A supplementation," JPEN J Parenter Enteral Nutr, 1986, 10(1): 74-7.
2. E. Patty, et al., "Controlled trial of vitamin A in gastric ulcer," Letter, Lancet, 1982, 2: 876.
3. T. Yoshikawa, et al., "Vitamin E and gastric mucosal injury induced by ischemia reperfusion," Am J Clin Nutr, 1991, 53: 210S-4S.
4. J. Mcguigan, et al., "Peptic ulcer and gastritis," in J.D. Wilson, Harrison's Principles of Internal Medicine, Twelfth Edition, (McGraw-Hill Book Company, New York: 1991).
5. Ibid.
6. J. Banos, et al., "Zinc compounds as therapeutic agents in peptic ulcer," Methods Find Exp Clin Pharmacol, suppl 11, 1989, 1: 117-22.
7. E. Lindenbaum, et al., "Effects of pyridoxine on mice after immobilization stress," Nutr Metab, 1974, 17: 368-74.
8. C. Debray, et al., "Treatment of gastro-duodenal ulcers with large doses of ascorbic acid." Semaine Therapeutique (Paris), 1968, 44: 393-8, 1968).
9. W. Shive, et al., "Glutamine in treatment of peptic ulcer," Texas State J Med, 1957, 53: 840-3.
10. S. Szabo, G. Vargha, "Unhtersuchung de Wirkungswiese des sogenannten 'vitamin U' mit histochemischen Reaktionen," Arzneimittel Forsch, 1960, 10: 23-8 (in German).
11. C. Rogers, et al., Role for leukotrienes in the pathogenesis of hemorrhagic mucosal lesions induced by ethanol or HCL in the rat," Gastroenterolgy, 1986, 90: 1797. See also S. Szabo, "Diet, ulcer disease, and fish oil," Letter, Lancet, 1988, 1: 119.
12. D. Hollander and A Tarnawski, "Dietary essential fatty acids and the decline in peptic ulcer disease—a hypothesis," Gut, 1986, 27: 239-42.
13. G. Gimeno, et al., "Antiulerogenic properties of bran rice oil in rats," Revista Español, 1989, 75(3): 225-30.
14. A. Rydning, et al, "Prophylactic effect of dietary fiber in duodenal ulcer disease," Lancet, 1982, 2: 736.
15. A. Criston and M. Magistretti, "Anti-ulcer and healing activity of Vaccinium myrtillus anthocyanosides," Il Farmaco, 1986, 42(2): 29-43.
16. K. Yamamoto, et al., "Gastric cytoprotective anti-ulcerogenic actions of hydroxychalcone in rats," Planta Med, 1992, 58(5): 389-93.

17. H. Zhou and D. Jiao, "312 cases of gastric and duodenal ulcer bleeding treated with 3 kinds of alcoholic extract rhubarb tablets," Chung Hsi I Chieh Ho Tsa Chi, 1990, 10(3): 150-1, 131-2 (in Chinese).

18. Y. Kaneday, et al., "In vitro effects of berberine sulfate on the growth of Entamoeba histolytica, Giardia lamblia and tricomanons vaginalis," Ann Trop Med Parasitol, 1991, 85: 417-25.

19. E. Okimasa, et al., "Inhibition of phospholipase A2 by glycyrrhizin, an anti-inflammatory drug," Acta Med Okayama, 1983, 37: 385-91.

20. M. Messer, C.M. Anderson and L. Hubbard, "Studies on the mechanism of destruction of the toxic action of wheat gluten in celiac disease by crude papain," Gut, 1964, 5: 295-303.

21. H. Glatzel and K. Hackenberg, "Roientgenological studies of the effect of bitters on digestive organs," Planta Medica, 1967, 15(3): 223-32.

22. F. Ellingwood, American Materia Medica, Therapeutics and Pharmacognosy, (Eclectic Medical Publication, Portland, Oregon: 1983).

23. W. Szturma, "Method for treating gastro-intestinal ulcers with extract of herb cetaria," US Patent 4150123, issued April 17, 1979.

24. G. Ribes, et al., "Effect of fenugreek seeds on endocrine pancreatic secretions in dogs," Annals of Nutrition and Metabolism, 1984, 28: 37-43.

25. E.H. Thompson, et al., "Ginger rhizome: A new source of proteolytic enzyme," Journal of Food Science, 1973, 38(4): 652-55.

26. J. Bland, "Effect of orally-consumed Aloe vera juice on human gastrointestinal function," Natural Foods Network Newsletter, August, 1985.

27. A.F. Ippoliti, et al., "The effect of various forms of milk on gastric-acid secretion," Intern Med, 1976, 84: 286-89.

28. C. McNulty, et al., "Susceptibility of clinical isolates of Campylobacter pyloridis to 11 antimicrobial agents," Antimicrob Agents Chemother, 1985, 28: 837-38.

URINARY TRACT INFECTIONS

SEE "BLADDER INFECTIONS"

VAGINITIS

Vaginitis refers to an inflammation of the vagina which can result from a variety of causes. Vaginal infections are commonly caused by the fungus *Candida albicans* (yeast infections). Most vaginal infections result from a change in the vaginal environment which can be due to a number of factors. Vaginitis is commonly experienced by women and accounts for approximately 7 percent of all visits to gynecologists.

Symptoms

◆ burning
◆ irritation
◆ itching in the vaginal area
◆ vaginal discharge with or without a foul odor

NOTE: In vaginitis, a discharge may or may not present. The discharge can be an abnormal color. Painful urination or intercourse may also be present. In some instances, vaginitis may be a symptom of a more serious condition such as a chronic inflammation of the cervix or a sexually transmitted disease. Pelvic inflammatory disease can sometimes cause symptoms thought to be vaginitis and requires immediate medical treatment. Chlamydia, gonorrhea and syphilis may produce similar symptoms and need prompt medical attention.

Causes

Vaginal infections result from a variety of microbial invaders. A common fungus which normally inhabits the vagina can cause yeast infections. The use of antibiotics can increase the risk of this type of vaginal infection by killing good bacteria which keep it controlled.

High blood sugar found in diabetics can greatly increase the risk of vaginal yeast infections. Sugar from the urine can help to feed the infection. Increased risk for yeast infections has also been linked to using birth control pills, although low dose pills seem less prone to do so. Pregnancy can also increase the risk of vaginitis. Other factors linked to vaginal infections include

◆ high stress levels
◆ prolonged use of corticosteroids
◆ regular douching which disrupts normal pH
◆ tampon use
◆ wearing nylon tights
◆ hormonal changes associated with menstruation
◆ lack of estrogen

- chemical irritants
- allergens or the presence of foreign bodies
- injuries caused by physical agents, trauma or sexual activity

NOTE: After menopause, the lining of the vagina can become dry and thin, making it more susceptible to inflammation.

Conventional Therapies

In some cases, to clear up vaginitis doctors will recommend antibiotics, the use of which can actually trigger or worsen some vaginal infections. In addition, while prescribed or over-the-counter preparations are usually effective at clearing up vaginitis, inexpensive douches and home self-care techniques are often effective. Your doctor may want to do a laboratory analysis of vaginal discharge to confirm the presence of a vaginal infection. Nystantin (mycostantin, nilstant) and imidazole creams or suppositories are routinely prescribed. Varieties of this treatment include miconazole (Monistat), terconazole (Terazol), clotrimazole (Gyne-lotrimin, Mycelex), and econazole. All of these are thought to be equally effective in treating a yeast infection. Mycelex-G is also routinely used to treat vaginal infections. In cases of post-menopausal vaginitis, estrogen supplements may be recommended. Ketoconazole (Nizoral) has also been prescribed in pill or cream form for the treatment of fungal infections of the vagina. Using vaginal creams or douching prior to the lab test can make microscopic analysis difficult.

Dietary Guidelines

Frequently the internal environment of the vagina can reflect the condition and health of the entire body. The right kind of diet is important in enabling the body to keep infection under control. Interestingly, food allergies have been strongly associated with yeast infections.

- Eat plenty of live culture, low-fat yogurt.
- Avoid a high-sugar diet along with alcohol, chocolate, fermented foods, cheeses, other diary products, mushrooms, citrus fruits and gluten foods.
- Eat oat bran instead.
- Do not eat any yeast and keep carbohydrates low until the infection is controlled.
- Avoid vitamin supplements that are yeast based.
- The use of artificial sweeteners can increase the likelihood of yeast infections.
- Eat soy-based foods like tofu for natural estrogenic action.
- Avoid taking iron supplements while the infection is active. Iron can feed certain bacteria.

Recommended Nutritional Supplements

PRIMARY NUTRIENTS

ACIDOPHILUS LIQUID OR CAPSULES Replenishes the friendly bacteria in the vagina needed to fight infection. The lacto-bacillus variety has been found to be the most effective.[1] *Suggested Dosage:* Take as directed.

GARLIC The compounds in garlic have proven antifungal properties that has been shown to be effective against some antibiotic resistant organisms.[2] *Suggested Dosage:* Take as directed.

VITAMIN A AND BETA CAROTENE Necessary to maintain the health of the vaginal mucosa and boost the immune system.[3] *Suggested Dosage:* Take as directed.

VITAMIN B COMPLEX This nutrient can be deficient in women with recurring vaginitis. In addition, a lack of estrogen can increase the need for vitamin B6.[4] *Suggested Dosage:* Take as directed.

VITAMIN C WITH BIOFLAVONOIDS Important for immune system health in fighting any infection. These compounds help to stop the spread of infection and have been useful in reducing the frequency and severity of herpes infections. Vitamin C can also help to heal mucus membranes in the vagina.[5] *Suggested Dosage:* Take as directed.

VITAMIN E Can be used externally for itching. A lack of vitamin E in the diet can compromise immunity.[6] *Suggested Dosage:* Take as directed.

ZINC PICOLINATE In some studies, zinc has been shown to be toxic to vaginal yeast infections. A lack of zinc can also weaken the immune system, which can predispose one to infection. Topical zinc can also be used for itching.[7] *Suggested Dosage:* Take as directed.

HERBAL FORMULA This herbal formula contains goldenseal root, witch hazel leaves, plantain, myrrh gum, pau d'arco, slippery elm bark, blue cohosh root, uva-ursi leaves, juniper berries. *Suggested Dosage:* Four to eight capsules daily. For chronic conditions it is best to use maximum dosage of eight capsules per day for prolonged period of four to six weeks or until symptoms are gone. However, it should not be used for more than three months without at least a two-week break.

GOLDENSEAL ROOT: Goldenseal root has a long history of use for vaginitis. Goldenseal root exerts a positive effect upon the mucus lining by creating stronger cross links between the mucosal proteins, making it much more difficult to disrupt the protective lining.[8] WITCH HAZEL LEAVES: Vaginal yeast can produce inflammation and irritation, which often results in the common symptom of itchiness. A secondary benefit of witch hazel leaves is their ability to shrink the blood vessels that are near the surface of the vaginal wall, preventing the yeast from penetrating the capillaries.[9] PLANTAIN: Witch hazel and plantain enjoy a common bond because they both have been used together in formulas to help with hemorrhoids, bleeding, inflammation and irritation. Plantain's diuretic action helps to return the body to a more normal state of health, and its mucilage content soothes mucus membranes.[10] MYRRH GUM: This herb has powerful antiseptic action, particularly with mucus membranes such as those which line the vaginal canal. Myrrh is also said to possess a mild laxative effect. This helps with the elimination of toxins produced by the yeast and speeds recovery.[11] PAU D'ARCO: The constituents of pau d'arco which provide benefit are a class of compounds called naphthoquinones. These naphthoquinones are highly effective against *Candida albicans*, the perpetrator of vaginal yeast infections, and act as anti-inflammatory agents for the vaginal mucosa.[12] SLIPPERY ELM: Slippery elm's action is more directed toward maintaining a healthy mucus lining. Slippery elm's benefits include healing and restoration. It helps to alleviate vaginal irritations and itching.[13] BLUE COHOSH: Its ability to help with vaginitis is due to its antimicrobial property and indirectly due to its soothing effect on the nerves. UVA-URSI: Scientific studies have demonstrated that a constituent in uva-ursi called arbutin is responsible for uva-ursi's antiseptic properties, with particular application for the urinary tract and the vagina.[14] Uva-ursi constitutes one of the most documented herbal medicines of today. JUNIPER BERRIES: Juniper berries and myrrh gum provide carminative and aromatic activity which stimulates circulation. Juniper berries used with uva-ursi acts as a diuretic to reduce the congestion of the pelvic region.[15]

SECONDARY NUTRIENTS

TEA TREE OIL: After diluting this oil, it can be used in douche form to fight infection and sooth irritated tissue. Four to five drops can be placed on a tampon and inserted. *Suggested Usage:* Use as directed.

WHITE OAK BARK: Works as an astringent to fight vaginal infection. *Suggested Dosage:* Take as directed. Use standardized products.

PHELLODENDRON (HUANG BAI): A Chinese herb with impressive antifungal properties. *Suggested Dosage:* Take as directed using standardized products.

CAPRYLIC ACID: Helps fight infection and works to normalize pH in the vaginal canal. *Suggested Dosage:* Take as directed.

Home Care Suggestions

- Warm sitz baths, using herb teas, apple cider vinegar or Epsom salts can help relieve itching and burning.
- Don't use dusting powders. Powder trapped in the vaginal area can promote infection.
- During a vaginal infection don't use commercial douches, contraceptive foams or jellies, and feminine deodorant sprays. These substances can further disrupt the natural chemical balance of the vagina.
- If the itching is intense, over-the-counter preparations like benadryl or cortaid can help. Don't use these before going to the doctor for an examination.
- Tampons can be saturated with boric acid or acidophilus and placed in the vagina for treatment.
- Avoid sexual activity during treatment to avoid reinfection and reduce irritation.
- Douching with acidophilus solutions diluted with warm water has had remarkable results in fighting yeast infections. Adding garlic oil to the douche has also been recommended. CAUTION: Placing yogurt in the vagina is discouraged if there is a chance of bacterial infection. In this case, the presence of yogurt can cause the infection to proliferate.
- Wear white, cotton underwear to promote the circulation of air. Avoid plastic, polyester and leather fabrics which can trap in heat and moisture, providing a perfect environment for bacterial proliferation.
- Underwear can be sterilized by soaking it in bleach for 24 hours.
- Cleanse the vaginal area thoroughly with a cotton swab soaked in Calendula succus to remove the bacterially saturated discharge.

Other Supportive Therapies

HYDROTHERAPY: Bathe the vagina in a warm saline to soothe inflammation. Tea tree oil diluted in a glycerine or oil base can help to eliminate vaginal dryness.

HOMEOPATHY: Treatment can include Natrum mur., Sepia, or Argentum nit.

Scientific Facts-at-a-Glance

One would rarely make the link between vaginal yeast infections and allergies. There is, however, some clinical data suggesting that allergies can predispose the vaginal canal to infection. Women who suffer from recurring vaginal infections due to *Candida albicans* infection need to look in to the possibility that food or other allergens are playing a contributing role.[16] Once again, the role of stress or emotional trauma must be addressed here. Women will often confess that they seem much more prone to getting a yeast infection during periods of high stress or emotional conflict. The impact of anxiety or frustration on the immune system is profound, to say the very least. Because women play so many roles and expect so much of themselves, they can easily let themselves become run down. Opportunistic bacteria and fungi will take advantage of compromised immunity and begin to flourish. Take care to leave time to relax and to unwind.

Spirit/Mind Considerations

Unquestionably, women who let themselves get run down or try to handle too much stress can become susceptible to yeast infections. Again the immune system comes into play here. Because women are notorious for doing too much for their family and others, they need to address issues of stress and relaxation. Moreover, dealing with chronic vaginitis can be extremely annoying and create a great deal of tension. While the availability of over-the-counter yeast killing creams makes it more convenient to kill infections, the root of the problem must be found. Eating sugary foods on the run, a lack of sleep, dieting and constant conflict can wreak havoc with the natural flora that protect the vagina from infection.

Prevention

- Eat a diet that is low in sugar and high in fiber and fresh vegetables and fruits.

- Avoid artificial sweeteners because they have been linked to a higher incidence of yeast infections.
- During periods, wear pads at night rather than tampons.
- Take acidophilus culture after meals.
- Don't wear nylon underpants. Use white, cotton underwear which discourages the growth of infection.
- Avoid wearing tight fitting clothing that inhibits air circulation, especially overnight.
- Wear pantyhose that have cotton crotches.
- Double rinse underwear to prevent chemical irritation from detergents.
- Keep the immune system healthy through diet, exercise. Vitamin and mineral supplementation, if necessary, can help prevent vaginal infections. Don't smoke, drink alcohol or use caffeine.
- Use a natural lubricant during intercourse to prevent irritation. Mineral oil, egg whites, petroleum jelly and plain yogurt are recommended. Baby oil contains perfume which may prove irritating.
- Don't use spermicides as a contraceptive option. These can increase your risk of vaginal infections.
- Use unscented, uncolored toilet paper to avoid any chemical irritation.
- Don't use chemical douches which disrupt the normal alkaline/acid balance of the vagina and can increase the risk of bacterial invasion.
- Avoid the prolonged use of antibiotics if possible.

Doctor's Notes

Vaginitis or more particularly vaginal yeast infections are a growing problem in America today. One of the contributing factors is the widespread use of antibiotic therapy for such things as urinary tract infections, colds, sore throats, and eye infections. Some women who contract a vaginal yeast infection after using antibiotic therapy often conclude that the yeast infection was much worse than the condition for which they originally used the antibiotics. Many areas of the body, such as the gastrointestinal tract and the vaginal canal, are covered by a thin mucus lining. This mucus lining serves as a defense mechanism to keep bacteria, yeasts and viruses from being able to reach vulnerable tissues and cells. Antibiotic therapy can cause a disruption in the normal flora that exists in the body, not only in the gastrointestinal tract but also in the vaginal canal, allowing yeast to grow unchecked. This proliferation causes a disruption of the mucus lining. This chemical change allows unhealthy organisms to attack the tissues. Another significant factor in yeast infections is a diet rich in refined carbohydrates, which tends to lower the immune response and produce an environment conducive to yeast growth. This herbal formula and nutrient list helps to fight yeast infections and to restore the mucus lining in the vaginal canal.

Endnotes

1. E.B. Collins and P. Hardt, "Inhibition of Candida albicans by Lactobacillus acidophilus," Jour Dairy Sci, 1980, 63: 830-32.
2. R. Fromtling and G. Bulmer, "In vitro effect of aqueous extract of garlic (Allium sativum) on the growth and viability of Cryptococcus Neoformans," Mycologia, 1978, 70: 397-405.
3. Michael T. Murray, N.D., Encyclopedia of Nutritional Supplements, (Prima Publishing, Rocklin, CA), 24.
4. A. Sharaf and N. Gomaa, "Interrelationship between the vitamins of the B-complex group and estradiol," Jour Endo, 1974, 62: 241-44.
5. C. Debray, et al., "Treatment of gastro-duodenal ulcers with large doses of ascorbic acid," Semaine Therapeutique, 1986, (Paris) 44:393-8.
6. L. Stephens, "Improved recovery of vitamin E treated lambs that have been experimentally infected with intertracheal chlamydia," Bri Vet Jour, 1979, 135: 291-93.
7. S. Greenberg, et al., "Inhibition of chlamydia trachomatis growth by zinc," 1985, 27: 953-57.
8 Y. Kaneday, et al., "In vitro effects of berberine sulfate on the growth of Entamoeba histolytica, Giardia lamblia and tricomanons vaginalis," Ann Trop Med Parasitol, 1991, 85: 417-25.
9. H. Felter, The Eclecta Materia Medica, Pharmacology and Therapeutics, (Eclectic Medical Publications, Portland, Oregon: 1983).
10. M. Matev, et al., "Clinical trial of a plantago major preparation in the treatment of chronic bronchitis," Vutreshni Bolesti (Sofia), 1982, 21(2): 133-37.
11. F. Ellingwood, American Materia Medica, Therapeutics and Pharmacognosy (Eclectic Medical Publication, Portland, Oregon: 1983).
12. H. Gershon and L. Shanks, "Fungitoxicity of 1,4-naphthoquinones to Candida albicans and Trichophyton mentagrophytes," Can Jour Micro, 1975, 21: 1317-21.
13. H.H. Smith, Ethnobotany of the Ojibwa Indians, 1932, Bulletin of the Public Museum, Vol. IV, 3: Milwaukee.
14. A. Leung, Encyclopedia of Common Natural Ingredients, (John Wiley and Sons, New York: 1980), 316-17.
15. E. Racz-Kotilla and G. Racz, Farmacia, 1971, 19: 165.
16. N. Kudelco, "Allergy in chronic monilial vaginitis," Med Times, 1971, 29: 266-67.

VARICOSE VEINS

Varicose veins is the condition in which veins have become distended due to a weakness in the vessel walls or a malfunction of the one-way valves which allow for a backflow of blood. As a result, blood pools in superficial veins, causing them to become stretched and swollen. This disfiguring condition usually occurs in the legs. More than 40 million Americans suffer from varicose veins with women outnumbering men four to one. Most varicose veins do not require medical attention. They are commonly troublesome but rarely disabling. In severe cases, varicose veins can cause skin ulcers which are slow to heal and need immediate medical treatment.

Symptoms

Varicose veins become bluish, bulging and are often accompanied by dull, nagging pains. The most usual site is at the back of the calf or on the inside of the leg anywhere between the ankle and the groin area. Varicose veins may also form around the anus, which can ultimately cause hemorrhoids. They may also cause

- swelling
- leg sores
- leg cramping
- a feeling of heaviness
- veins which are tender to the touch
- itchiness
- brown discoloration of the skin near the ankles
- eczema of the skin near the veins

Spider veins, which are very common, especially in the thigh area, are considered harmless. Skin ulcers can form around serious varicose veins and will need medical attention.

Cutting or bruising the skin around varicose veins can cause a great deal of blood flow and will also require medical treatment. In severe cases, inflammation of the vein walls can result, which can lead to the formation of blood clots or thrombophlebitis.

NOTE: Feelings of heaviness or pressure can increase for some women just prior to and after menstruation.

CAUTION: See your doctor immediately if you have varicose veins that are unusually painful or exhibit red lumping that does not decrease when you elevate your legs. This might indicate the presence of a blood clot. If varicose veins are cut or ruptured around the ankle area, blood loss can be substantial. Apply finger pressure to the area and elevate it. Get medical attention immediately.

Causes

Commonly a lack of circulation can cause varicose veins to form. Certain conditions can create a lack of proper circulation causing veins to respond by dilating and twisting. Age increases the risk of this condition as the skin becomes less elastic which lessens vein support. Other causal factors include the following:

- pregnancy
- sitting for prolonged periods of time with legs crossed
- obesity
- the use of garters or tight clothing
- standing for long periods of time.
- genetic predisposition
- low-fiber diet

NOTE: Chronic constipation that causes straining during bowel movement can not only cause anal varicose veins (hemorrhoids), but has also been linked to the formation of varicose veins in the legs.

Conventional Therapies

Varicose veins are difficult to treat. Surgery is sometimes successful; however, it can be uncomfortable and disappointing. Prevention is the best approach to varicose veins and involves an awareness of genetic susceptibility and life style adaptations. The role of diet has been downplayed in the case of this disorder and may prove more significant than previously thought.

Most physicians will use elastic tourniquets on your legs to indicate which of the veins are damaged. Because varicose veins leak, they will stand out when blood flow is constricted. A venography can further assess the performance of leg veins. This is done by injecting dye in a varicose vein and watching its progress through the circulation with an x-ray. Thermography records the temperature of various parts of the leg in order to produce a heat map to pinpoint the exact location of weak valves. Injecting varicose veins with sclerosing agents (sclerotherapy) and wrapping them firmly for a few days can help to control inflammation and will eventually cause other veins to take the place of the ones treated. This is usually done on an outpatient basis and involves two to three visits. If the varicose veins are located in the thigh area, this procedure is usually unsuccessful. Stripping the veins first may be recommended in this instance. In severe cases of varicose veins, surgical removal may be advised. Bulging, discolored veins may cause pain and skin ulcers. In these cases, the veins are removed by stripping them through a small incision under a general anesthetic. This operation usually requires a week's stay in the hospital and a gradual increase in activity.

Dietary Guidelines

Varicose veins are seldom seen in areas of the world where high-fiber diets are the rule. Some health care professionals believe that the Western diet, which is high in refined carbohydrates and fat and low in fiber, contributes to the development of varicose veins.

- Emphasize a diet high in fiber and rich in legumes, fresh fruits and vegetables, and grains.
- Emphasize blueberries and citrus fruits.
- Avoid fatty foods and refined carbohydrates.

- Eat plenty of fish, fiber and raw fruits and vegetables.
- Don't eat margarine, animal fats, red meat, ice cream, pastries or other rich foods.
- Decrease your salt intake—salt can cause swelling in people who are salt sensitive.

Recommended Nutritional Supplements

PRIMARY NUTRIENTS

GRAPE SEED OR PINE BARK EXTRACT The oligomers in these compounds work to reduce capillary fragility which cause the veins to bulge or even leak in varicose veins.[1] *Suggested Dosage:* Take as directed.

FIBER SUPPLEMENT Research suggests that Americans suffer from a vegetable-depleted diet that can predispose us to thin veins and constipation. Studies find that people who are vegetarians have a much lower incidence of varicose veins than control groups.[2] *Suggested Dosage:* Use first thing in the morning and before going to bed. Look for psyllium-based products.

VITAMIN C WITH BIOFLAVONOIDS Promotes better blood circulation and promotes vein wall strength and integrity and discourages the formation of blood clots. Studies with vitamin C and hesperidin have found that a lack of these nutrients causes pain in the limbs and increased capillary fragility.[3] *Suggested Dosage:* 3,000 to 5,000 mg per day.

BILBERRY The anthocyanacides in this herb work to discourage vein weakness and actually protect veins against bulging.[4] *Suggested Dosage:* Take as directed using standardized products.

GINKGO BILOBA Ginkolides work to scavenge free radicals, boost peripheral circulation and can even help to correct capillary dysfunction.[5] *Suggested Dosage:* Take as directed using guaranteed potency standardize extracts or capsules.

HORSE CHESTNUT Horse chestnut seeds have a long folk history of use in the treatment of varicose veins and hemorrhoids. The active component is escin (syn. aescin).[6] *Suggested Usage:* Can be applied externally as a powder mixed with water on a cloth.

COENZYME Q10 This nutrient boosts cellular oxygenation and helps to enhance blood flow while it scavenges for free radicals.[7] *Suggested Dosage:* 100 mg daily.

ESSENTIAL FATTY ACIDS Both the omega-3 and omega-6 fatty acids help keep veins flexible and reduce inflammation which causes swelling and pain. *Suggested Dosage:* Take as directed. Take a vitamin E supplement if you take fish oil.

BROMELAIN Helps to increase fibrinolytic activity of the blood which can reduce risk of clot formation. Bromelain may also help to prevent the hard and lumpy skin that is found around varicose veins. NOTE: Studies found that using bromelain before varicose vein surgery prevented the formation of clots and excess bruising.[8] *Suggested Dosage:* Take as directed. Chewable products are available.

GREEN TEA The anthocyanidins in this supplement have excellent antioxidant actions, decrease inflammation and help control venous weakness. *Suggested Dosage:* Take in either capsule or tea form. Look for standardized products with guaranteed potency.

HERBAL COMBINATION This herbal combination contains cayenne, butcher's broom, kelp, gentian root, ginger, blue vervain and gotu kola. *Suggested Dosage:* Two to six capsules daily. This formula may be used every day to help maintain healthy circulation.

CAYENNE: Cayenne or capsicum is particularly noted for improving peripheral circulation and can also help stop or prevent hemorrhaging and the formation of clots.[9] Since cayenne is a reputed pain reliever, it may have particular application for problematic circulatory pain, like that produced by phlebitis or varicose veins. BUTCHER'S BROOM: This herb has an impressive history for its ability to prevent blood clots and shrink blood vessels, particularly in the legs.[10] People with varicose veins can experience a pooling of blood in their legs. Butcher's broom works to push the blood back into the upper part of the body improving circulation throughout. KELP: Kelp has a reputation of cleansing the blood vessels and preventing atherosclerosis. In those people who are iodine deficient, kelp can increase the metabolic rate which indirectly affects circulation in a positive way. GENTIAN ROOT: Gentian has been used in folk remedies to treat blood disorders. Gentian's real strength in this formula is its ability to help maintain a healthy liver and spleen which effects both the blood and digestion. GINGER ROOT: Ginger enhances the actions of the other herbs in this formula and, through its circulatory effect, hastens the delivery of the actives to the sites where they are needed. BLUE VERVAIN: Blue vervain helps the blood properly clot when an injury occurs and helps to keep blood vessels more pliable. GOTU KOLA: Many studies support the use of this herb for varicose veins due to its ability to strengthen the connective tissue that surrounds the veins, giving it more structure, hence better blood circulation. Eighty percent of people who used gotu kola in clinical trials obtained significant improvement in circulation.[11]

SECONDARY NUTRIENTS

LECITHIN: A fat emulsifier that aids in facilitating good circulation. *Suggested Dosage:* Take in either capsules or granules as directed.

ZINC: Aids in cell healing and is especially good if varicose ulcers have developed. *Suggested Dosage:* Take 50 mg per day using picolinate or gluconate products.

VITAMIN E: Improves circulation and can help control feeling of heaviness in the legs. *Suggested Dosage:* 400 IU per day.

VITAMIN K: Helps to control bleeding and clot formation. *Suggested Dosage:* Take as directed.

ST. JOHN'S WORT OIL: Can be rubbed into varicose veins. *Suggested Dosage:* Use as directed.

Home Care Suggestions

◆ Witch hazel compresses can facilitate circulation and help control discomfort.
◆ Exercise regularly to improve circulation. Walking every day for 15 minutes is excellent.
◆ Avoid sitting or standing for long periods of time.
◆ Elevate your legs several times a day to promote better blood flow.
◆ Taking aspirin every day can help with discomfort and increase the mobility of blood. Discuss this option with your doctor.
◆ Raise the foot of your bed several inches above the head to facilitate better blood flow. Do not do this if you have any breathing difficulties or a history of heart trouble.
◆ Avoid putting unnecessary stress or weight on the legs by crossing them or lifting heavy objects.
◆ Wear support hose which are specially fitted to each individual and can be ordered through medical supply houses. Put on the hose first thing in the morning.
◆ Daily sitz baths can help with discomfort.
◆ If you cut a varicose vein, elevate your leg immediately and apply pressure. Get medical attention if the bleeding does not stop.

Other Supportive Therapies

YOGA: Practicing the yoga shoulder stand is recommended to facilitate better circulation. Yoga breathing exercises can also help relieve varicose vein pain.
MASSAGE: For varicose veins, a gentle massage on the legs toward the heart can be beneficial.

Scientific Facts-at-a-Glance

Because animals do not suffer from varicose veins, health experts have concluded that their cause may be related to the specific lifestyle and diet of human beings. Because we no longer eat the fibery vegetables and fruits that our ancestors did, there is speculation that we are not receiving enough of the kind of phytochemicals which boost venous strength that we should. The anthocyanidins are such compounds and are found in berries and other fruits. Venous weakness may well be linked to diets high in cooked foods and low in live enzymes and specific compounds which contribute to venous integrity.

Spirit/Mind Considerations

Tight clothing, especially jeans, knee socks, snug-fitting boots or waist-cinching belts, not only contribute to the formation of varicose veins, but add to mental stress as well. Because elevating the legs is so important when treating varicose veins, it would do all of us some good to take that time to meditate, pray or just unwind. Guided imagery which focuses on visions of increased circulation to strengthened veins may also be helpful.

Prevention

◆ Don't wear tight shoes, garters, knee highs or girdles.
◆ Don't smoke: Smoking can contribute to circulatory disorders and the development of blood clots.
◆ Keep your weight down. Obesity significantly contributes to the development of varicose veins by putting extra pressure on soft walled veins which require an increased blood flow.
◆ Exercise regularly to promote good blood flow
◆ Try to rest your legs by elevating them often if you must stand or sit for long periods of time.
◆ Make sure your diet is high in vitamin C which contributes to blood vessel strength.
◆ Wear support hose or compression stockings if you are at risk for varicose veins.
◆ Avoid constipation which can cause straining and put pressure on the lower circulatory system.

Doctor's Notes

Varicose veins run in families, although they are often made worse by pregnancy or weight gain. Spider veins will often respond well to butcher's broom which can be taken internally and used as a poultice as well. Generally, I like to use butcher's broom, gotu kola, and bilberry combined with the proanthocyanidins found in grape seed extract or green tea. Losing weight and not standing on hard surfaces like cement for extended periods can reduce symptoms and severity. Circulation can be impeded by various factors, including plaque deposits in the arteries, abnormal clotting and platelet aggregation, cardiac dysfunction or failure, and conditions of shock. This herbal formula along with the nutrients listed works to improve circulation and to strengthen the integrity of the venous system.

Endnotes

1. G. Lagrue, Olivier-Martin F., Grillot A., "A study of the effects of procyanidol oligomers on capillary resistance in hypertension and in certain nephropathies."
2. J.W. Dickerson, Journal of the Royal Society of Health, 1985, 195: 191.
3. J. Beiler, "Biochemistry of the synergists: Ascorbic acid and hesperidin," Exp Med Surg, 1955, 12: 563-69. See also R. Paris, "Effects of diverse flavonoids upon capillary permeability," Jour Ann Pharm Fran, 1964, 22: 489-93. See also B.D. Cox and W.J. Butterfield "Vitamin C supplements and diabetic capillary fragility," British Med Jour, 1975, 3: 205.
4. E. Mian, et al., "Anthocyanacides and the walls of micro vessels: Further aspects of the mechanism of action of their protective effect in syndromes due to abnormal capillary fragility," Miverva Med, 1977, 68(52): 3565-81.
5. G. Lagrue, et al., "Idiopathic cyclic edema: The role of capillary hyper permeability and its correction by Ginkgo biloba extract," Presse Med, 1986, 15(31): 1550-3.
6. G. Hitzenberger, "The therapeutic effectiveness of chestnut extract," Wien Med Wochenschr, 1989, 139(17):385-9 (in German).
7. K. Folkers and Y. Yamamura, Eds., Biomed and Clin Aspects of Coenzyme Q-10, vol. 4, Amsterdam, Elsevier Science Publishers, 1984: 369-73.

8. J. Durrant, "Prevention of hematoma in surgery of varices," Praxis, 1972, 61: 950-51.

9. J. Wang, "The antiplatelet effect of capsaicin," Thrombosis Res, 1984, 36: 497-507.

10. G. Rudofsky, "Improving venous tone and capillary sealing: Effect of a combination of Ruscus extract and hesperidin methyl chalcone in healthy proband in heat stress," Frotschr Med, 1989, 107(1): 52, 55-58.

11. C. Allegra, et al., "Centella asiatica extract in venous disorders of the lower limbs: comparative clinico-instrumental studies with placebo," Clin Ther, 1981, 99: 507-13.

VISUAL DISORDERS

This section addresses macular degeneration, diabetic retinopathy and retinosis pigmentosa. (For cataracts and glaucoma, see separate alphabetical listings.)

Eye infections, eyesight limitations, or bloodshot, tired eyes plague us all from time to time. The types of eye disorders discussed in this section, however, refer to more serious conditions that are often brought on by disease processes that do not originate in the eye itself. Vision loss is frequently linked to diseases such as diabetes and hypertension. Diabetes can lead to the bursting of blood vessels in the retina, causing blindness. Hypertension can eventually cause a thickening of the blood vessels located in the interior of the eye which can cause compromised vision or even blindness. Malnutrition can also be a significant contributor to diminished vision or eye disease.

MACULAR DEGENERATION

This disorder involves the gradual degeneration of the macula, the portion of the retina responsible for detailed vision. Macular degeneration is the leading cause of blindness in the U.S. and Europe and usually occurs in people over the age of 50. A loss of sight can occur very suddenly or slowly; peripheral and color vision are usually unaffected. Two types of macular degeneration exist: atrophic (dry) and exudative (wet). The wet variety involves the degeneration of the macula accompanied by bleeding or the leaking of fluid from the tiny blood vessels located under the retina. This loss of fluid leads to the building up of scar tissue and a subsequent loss of vision.

Symptoms

- loss of vision
- observed scarring upon examination

Causes

Macular degeneration is probably the result of free radical damage similar to that which induces cataracts. Factors that predispose a person to developing macular degeneration include

- aging
- atherosclerosis
- hypertension
- environmental toxins
- heredity

Conventional Therapies

In the majority of cases, the disorder is considered untreatable. But, if optical examinations detect the leaking vessels early enough, they can be removed or cauterized, a difficult process that can easily damage healthy retinal tissue. This procedure is costly and poses a significant risk.

DIABETIC RETINOPATHY

Diabetic retinopathy occurs when tiny blood vessels and capillaries rupture within the retina and leave behind a deposit. The subsequent initiation of an abnormal network of new blood vessels occurs and causes a slow and progressive loss of vision. Diabetic retinopathy is one of the most common causes of blindness and is a risk for most insulin dependent diabetics. It affects seven million Americans annually and causes 7,000 cases of blindness per year.

Symptoms

This eye condition can occur without much warning and symptoms do not usually present themselves until the disease is well established.

Causes

High blood sugar levels cause the creation of mutated proteins that damage the retina of the eye.

Conventional Therapies

If you have diabetes, make sure you get an annual eye exam. This will increase the chance of detecting this disorder in its early stages. Laser surgery may help to seal off leaky blood vessels and help to inhibit the further loss of sight.

RETINITIS PIGMENTOSA

Retinitis pigmentosa is an inherited eye disease that affects approximately one out of every 3,700 people. It is characterized by the presence of an inherited metabolic flaw that slowly and progressively destroys retinal cells, eventually resulting in blindness.

Symptoms

- loss of night vision (in adolescence)
- loss of peripheral vision
- blindness

Causes

Retinitis pigmentosa causes a degeneration of the rods and cones of the retina in both eyes. This disease is considered genetic; however, its presence may not be detected until puberty or even middle age. The disorder causes pigment to proliferate throughout the retina, causing a loss of vision.

Dietary Guidelines

- Eat plenty of raw cabbage, broccoli, carrots, cauliflower, yellow vegetables, green vegetables, and sunflower seeds.
- Fresh, raw fruits are recommended but their fructose content must be taken into account when on a carbohydrate-restricted diet.
- Eliminate sugar and white flour from your diet and switch to olive oil and non-hydrogenated fats.
- Do not eat rancid oils or fats as they can cause free radical damage.
- Eat fish and lean meats, soy-based foods and drink plenty of water.
- Increase your consumption of legumes, flavonoid-rich berries such as blueberries, blackberries and cherries, and foods rich in vitamins E and C.

Recommended Nutritional Supplements

PRIMARY NUTRIENTS

VITAMIN A WITH BETA CAROTENE According to some experts, doses of vitamin A are thought to slow the loss of sight by a significant margin. Topical applications in the form of eyedrops may also be helpful.[1] Beta carotene helps to boost vitamin A production in the body and also acts as a free radical scavenger. *Suggested Dosage:* 50,000 IU of vitamin A daily. If you are pregnant, do not exceed 10,000 IU daily. When taking doses this high, use emulsion products. Take 100,000 IU of beta carotene daily.

VITAMIN C WITH BIOFLAVONOIDS Vitamin C helps improve the fluid output of the eye and lowers intraocular pressure. It also helps to promote healing and reduce inflammation. Bioflavonoids such as rutin can protect the eye against free radical damage.[2] Taking vitamin C and bioflavonoids can help to decrease one's risk of developing eye disease.[3] *Suggested Dosage:* 6,000 mg taken in divided doses daily.

ZINC This mineral plays an important role in any disorder of the eye and boosts immune response to infection. Zinc supplementation has been linked to decreased loss of vision in eye diseases like macular degeneration.[4] *Suggested Dosage:* Take as directed.

BILBERRY The anthocyanidins contained in this herb work as excellent antioxidant agents and can enhance visual performance as well.[5] NOTE: Clinical studies have shown that taking bilberry extract, eating fresh blueberries and taking *Ginkgo biloba* extract with zinc can help halt the loss of vision.[6] *Suggested Dosage:* Use a 25 percent anthocyanidin content product and take 200 mg daily.

GRAPE SEED OR PINE BARK EXTRACT Clinical tests with proanthocyanidin oligomers have found that they can enhance the retinal function of the eye and also protect retinal tissue.[7] *Suggested Dosage:* Take as directed.

GINKGO BILOBA The ginkgolides in this herb boost blood flow to the macula and retina and work to scavenge for damaging free radicals in the eye. Clinical studies have shown that ginkgo treatment can achieve significant beneficial effects in cases of macular degeneration.[8] *Suggested Dosage:* Take as directed.

BUTCHER'S BROOM AND CAYENNE (CAPSICUM) These herbs enhance blood flow and can help to prevent the ischemia that can contribute to both of these eye diseases. *Suggested Dosage:* Take as directed using guaranteed potency products.

LUTEIN This nutrient is found in several fresh fruits and vegetables and can help to prevent the process of macular degeneration if taken early enough. *Suggested Dosage: Take as directed.*

SHARK CARTILAGE The antiangiogenesis compounds in cartilage may help to prevent or even stop macular degeneration by inhibiting the proliferation of blood vessels that eventually cause blindness. Scientists who have observed the ability of shark cartilage to stop the creation of blood vessels believe that it can prevent the course of retinopathy and may also affect neovascular glaucoma in the same way.[9] *Suggested Dosage:* Take one gram per 15 lbs. of body weight daily. Look for pure, bulk powders—they are more practical than capsulized powders.

HERBAL COMBINATION This combination contains eyebright, goldenseal root, red raspberry leaves, dandelion root, fennel seeds, and slippery elm bark. *Suggested Dosage:* Four capsules daily (should be taken orally, not used topically). May be used regularly.

EYEBRIGHT: Eyebright has been found to be useful in a number of different eye disorders, including eye strain, bloodshot eyes, conjunctivitis, irritations, and dry or weeping eyes. Eyebright is also noted for its astringent qualities that help to shrink tissues and blood vessels. This may help in treating bloodshot eyes. GOLDENSEAL ROOT: Goldenseal root is considered a powerful tonic herb. Its two primary benefits for the eyes are its ability to fight infections and improve the health of mucus membranes. Its berberine content makes it an impressive antibacterial agent for eye infections since it can inhibit streptococci growth.[10] RED RASPBERRY LEAVES: Red raspberry leaves have astringent qualities that may be used to reduce the size of vessels in bloodshot eyes, especially if conditions are chronic. Red raspberry leaves are soothing and healing to mucus membranes. DANDELION ROOT: Dandelion stimulates the body's various cleansing and waste removal systems. It is mildly laxative and improves bowel function, stimulates urine flow, and promotes mild perspiration. Dandelion is an excellent liver tonic and improves digestion by causing an increase in bile secretion. By improving liver health, conditions of jaundice can be overcome. FENNEL SEEDS: The medicinal applications of fennel include digestive disorders such as gas, bloating and colic. Perhaps its main application in this formula is to improve digestion and the effectiveness of the other herbs. It has also been found beneficial in treating eye inflammation, conjunctivitis and blepharitis (inflammation of the edge of the eyelid). SLIPPERY ELM BARK: This herb contains copious amounts of a very nutritious mucilage. It is soothing, demulcent, and mildly laxative to the GI tract. Slippery elm benefits many mucus membranes, including the conjunctiva.

SECONDARY NUTRIENTS

SELENIUM: When taken with vitamin E and lipoic acid, this compound is an impressive free radical scavenger that helps to prevent the retina from damage. *Suggested Dosage:* 400 mcg daily.

LIPOIC ACID: This supplement greatly potentiates and extends the antioxidant action of vitamin E, vitamin C

and glutathione in eye tissue. *Suggested Dosage:* Take as directed.

VITAMIN E: A deficiency of vitamin E has been associated with the deterioration of the retina. In addition, using it therapeutically has resulted in a 90 percent improval rate in test groups with macular degeneration. *Suggested Dosage:* Take 800 IU daily.

TAURINE: This amino acid is released from the retina after light exposure and its depletion may be linked with retinal deterioration. *Suggested Dosage:* Take as directed on an empty stomach with fruit juice.

Home Care Suggestions

- ◆ If you wear glasses, wear clear spectacles that have been treated to keep out ultraviolet rays. This helps protect against damage from ultraviolet exposure.
- ◆ Never use hair dyes containing coal tar on the eyelashes or eyebrows; doing so can cause injury or blindness. Although coal-tar dyes are legal, marketing them for the eyebrows and eyelashes is not.
- ◆ Be careful when using drugs, whether prescription or over-the-counter. Some may cause eye problems.
- ◆ Eat plenty of raw vegetables.
- ◆ Keep blood sugar levels well monitored and controlled.
- ◆ Have a thorough eye exam every six months.

Other Supportive Therapies

HYDROTHERAPY: Home hydrotherapy treatment offers stimulation and involves using hot and cold face towels over the eyes.

HOMEOPATHY: Belladonna 30c is sometimes recommended.

Scientific Facts-at-a-Glance

Recent studies have found that elevated levels of copper can be very toxic to the retina and can accelerate its destruction.[11] Checking copper levels may be desirable.

Spirit/Mind Therapies

As is the case with any degenerative disease, the impact of unmanaged stress must be considered. Stress seems to accelerate any disease process. Meditation, visualization and learning to truly relax should be viewed with the same respect as any other medication prescribed or recommended for these visual disorders. If blindness is inevitable, every resource should be tapped to retain productivity and usefulness. Today, visually impaired individuals can be extremely independent and continue to function as they did prior to their visual impairment.

Prevention

- ◆ Faithfully take vitamin A, beta carotene and vitamin E supplements daily.
- ◆ Take an additional antioxidant array that includes lipoic acid.
- ◆ Eat plenty of raw vegetables.

◆ Be wary of drug use. Drugs that can cause damage to the retina or other eye parts include adrenocorticotropic hormone (ACTH), allopurinol, anticoagulants (such as heparin and warfarin), aspirin, corticosteroids, chlorpropamide, diuretics, antihistamines, digitalis, indomethacin (indocin), marijuana, nicotinic acid or niacin (if used for long periods), streptomycin, sulfa drugs, and tetracycline.

Doctor's Notes

The macula is the part of the retina that makes 20/20 vision possible. Anyone who suffers from macular degeneration will find it increasingly difficult to read, do needlework or any other activity involving detail. Research tells us that vegetables containing lutein may help to inhibit the development of this condition. The very best treatment for macular degeneration is prevention. Eating a variety of vegetables throughout life is probably one of the best preventative measures we can take. If you begin to experience initial symptoms, take 6 to 20 milligrams of lutein in supplemental form daily. Add herbs that boost circulation such as butcher's broom, *Ginkgo biloba* and cayenne. Bilberry is also excellent. It is also very important to make sure that your zinc intake is adequate. Nutrition-based supplements should contain 25 to 50 milligrams for daily use. You may want to take zinc as a separate, single supplement. Retinitis pigmentosa is an inherited disease and causes some degree of blindness in 100 percent of the people that it affects. There are several measures that can help. The supplements listed in this section all help to inhibit macular degeneration. If any sign of an eye infection develops, herbs with natural antibiotic action such as echinacea should be employed. In the case of viral infections like eye shingles, St. John's wort is recommended.

Additional Resources

National Eye Institute (NEI)
National Institutes of Health
Building 31, Room 6A32
31 Center Drive, MSC 2510
Bethesda, MD 20892-2510
(301) 496-5248

Retinitis Pigmentosa Foundation
11350 McCormick Road
Executive Plaza One, Suite 800
Hunt Valley, MD 21031-1014
(800) 683-5555

National Association for the Visually Handicapped
3201 Balboa Street
San Francisco, CA 94121
(415) 221-3201

Endnotes

1. R. Rengstorrff, "Topical treatment of external eye disorders with preparations containing vitamin A," Practical Optometry, 1993, 4: 163-65.

2. T. Organisciak, et al., "The protective effect of ascorbate in retinal light damage of rats," Invest Ophthalmol Vis Sci, 1985, 26(11): 1580-8.

3. S. Bouton, "Vitamin C and the aging eye," Arch Int Med, 1939, 63: 930-45.

4. D. Newsome, et al., "Oral zinc in macular degeneration," Arch Opthamol, 1988, 106: 192-98.

5. E. Gloria and A. Perla, "Activity of anthocyanosides on absolute visual threshold," Ann Otta Clin Ocul, 1966, 92: 595-605.

6. L. Caselli, "Clinical and electroretinographic study on activity of anthocyanosides," Arch Med, 1985, 37: 29-35.

7. C. Corbe, et al., "Light vision and chorioretinal circulation: Study of the effect of procyanidolic oligomers," Jour Fre Opthamol, 1988, 11: 453-60. See also C. Corbe, et al., "Light vision and chorioretinal circulation: Study of the effect of procyanidolic oligomers," Jour Fr Opthamol, 1988, 11(5): 453-60.

8. D. Lebuisson, et al., "Treatment of senile macular degeneration with Ginkgo biloba extract: A preliminary double-blind drug versus placebo study," Presse Med, 1986, 15: 1556-58.

9. I.W. Lane and L. Comac, Sharks Don't Get Cancer (Avery Publishing, Garden City, New York: 1993).

10. F. Hahn, "Berberine," Antibiotics, 1976, 3: 577-88.

11. B. Siverstone, et al., "Zinc and copper metabolism in patients with senile macular degeneration," Ann Opthalmol, 1985, 17(7): 419

WARTS

Warts (verrucae) are contagious growths that are found on the skin or mucus membranes. There are over 30 types of the papilloma virus that cause warts to develop. Warts are located on the uppermost layer of the skin and their appearance is modified according to their positioning on the body. Warts can be spread by picking, biting, touching, shaving, trimming or in the case of genital warts, through sexual contact. The peak incidence of warts is from the ages of 10 to 19, with 70 percent of all warts occurring between the ages of 10 and 39. An estimated 16 percent of the population suffers from warts, with girls being more susceptible than boys. What may look like a wart after the age of 50 is probably a raised age spot. The incubation period for warts can be anywhere from one month to 18 months. Warts appear to be less common in tropical areas of the world. Warts can be quite resistant to treatment and often recur.

Symptoms

COMMON WARTS: These are firm, round or irregular, sharply defined growths that can become up to one-quarter inch in diameter. They usually have a rough surface and appear in areas that are prone to injury such as the hands, knees, face and scalp. These types of warts are commonly seen in children.

FLAT WARTS: These are flat, flesh colored growths that occur on the wrists, the backs of the hands and sometimes the face. They may also itch.

DIGITATE WARTS: These warts are dark in color and have finger like projections.

FILIFORM WARTS: These warts are long and slender growths, usually found on the eyelids, armpits or the neck and commonly infect overweight, middle-aged people.

PLANTAR WARTS: Found on the soles of the feet, these warts become flattened due to the weight of the body. They can cause considerable discomfort.

GENITAL WARTS: These are pink, rough, irregular growths that extensively infect the genitals of both men and women. They can spread to the anus, groin, vagina and scrotal areas. They are sexually transmitted and are considered highly contagious. The incubation for genital warts is three months or more. The virus can spread without the knowledge of the carrier. Unlike the other warts mentioned, these require prompt medical attention. Some evidence indicates that warts that infect the cervix may predispose a woman to cervical cancer. Genital warts in young children may be a sign of sexual abuse. Anyone who has warts in the genital area or develops what appears to be a wart after the age of 45 should see a physician as soon as possible. Genital warts require medical attention and wart-like growths after age 54 may indicate a more serious skin condition. Warts on the face should not be treated at home. A woman who has had genital warts should receive regular cervical pap smears to check for the presence of cancer.

Causes

The papilloma virus causes the formation of warts. There are over 35 varieties of this particular virus. Children who suffer from allergies and dermatitis seem more prone to have warts. Going barefoot or wearing improper footwear has been linked with the development of plantar warts. In addition, having damp feet may also cause plantar warts. Interestingly, those that handle meat have a higher incidence of warts, implying that meat may carry the wart causing virus. Taking some drugs such as tetracycline has been linked to developing warts, although there is no scientific basis for this connection. Warts are spread by direct contact from combs, razors, swimming pools, or locker room floors. People who suffer from diseases that compromise their immune systems such as AIDS, or leukemia may become more susceptible to warts. Emotional stress has also been connected to increased vulnerability to developing warts.

If a wart enters a cut or an opening around the cuticle it is referred to as a periungual wart and can be particularly difficult to treat. Use an antibiotic cream on the area and cover it to discourage further injury or inflammation.

Conventional Therapies

Warts can be easily removed, but they have a tendency to recur. No form of medical treatment is 100 percent effective. If liquid nitrogen or other toxic chemicals are not skillfully applied, healthy tissue can be damaged and scarring is possible. The advantage of medical treatment over some home remedies is the time factor. Doctors can treat warts quickly, (although those treatments are not without pain or discomfort). Approximately half of all warts, with the exception of plantar and genital warts, will disappear in six to 12 months without any specific treatment. The application of liquid nitrogen (cryosurgery) by which the warts are frozen and subsequently fall off is common. As the frozen wart thaws, a blister forms and lifts the wart off the skin. Most physicians will choose liquid nitrogen as the most effective and least expensive treatment. Cantharidin liquids or plasters can also be used to create a blister on the wart.

Fulguration, in which heat is used to destroy warts, can also be effective. This approach is more frightening for children than using liquid nitrogen. Genital warts are usually removed by surgery or by the application of podophyllin which acts like liquid nitrogen. Injecting alpha interferon directly into warts has had some success; however, the treatment may be impractical and too expensive when a large number of warts are present. Injecting or applying bleomycin to warts has also produced some good results but is still considered inferior to the methods listed above. A product called the Trans-ver-sal patch is an adhesive patch that releases a continuous dose of medication and is available with a prescription. It is considered more effective than over-the-counter patches.

Dietary Guidelines

Warts are controlled and attacked by the body's immune system. Some people are naturally resistant to warts.

◆ Keep the immune system healthy through a diet high in vitamins and minerals and low in fat and empty calories.

◆ Get off of junk food and eat plenty of raw fruits, vegetables, and whole grains.

◆ Avoid red meat and use only low-fat dairy products.

◆ Use safflower or olive oil.

◆ Get sufficient rest.

◆ Increase your intake of sulfur-containing foods such as eggs, citrus fruits, asparagus, garlic and onions. Sulfur-containing amino acids contribute to the development of antibodies that fight the polyoma virus group. Desiccated liver tablets are high in this amino acid and can be taken daily.

Recommended Nutritional Supplements

PRIMARY NUTRIENTS

GARLIC In vitro tests have conclusively shown that the allicin content of garlic combined with its sulfuric compounds kills a variety of viral organisms.[1] *Suggested Dosage:* One capsule with each meal. Garlic extracts can also be applied locally.

ST. JOHN'S WORT This herb has impressive antiviral properties and is even under investigation for its effect on HIV. Hypericn, its primary bioactive compound, keeps viruses from replicating.[2] *Suggested Dosage:* Take as directed using guaranteed potency products. Use St. John's wort oil directly on the warts daily.

ECHINACEA This herb is well known for it antibacterial and antiviral properties. Various clinical studies have demonstrated that it can inhibit viral organisms in cell cultures.[3] *Suggested Dosage:* Take as directed using guaranteed potency products.

ZINC Zinc supplementation boosts virtually every aspect of immunity. Zinc sulfate paste can also be used externally on the warts.[4] *Suggested Dosage:* Use zinc picolinate lozenges as directed; however, do not exceed more than 100 mg of zinc per day.

VITAMIN C WITH BIOFLAVONOIDS Ascorbic acid has potent antiviral properties. It should be taken both internally and applied as a paste to the wart. *Suggested Dosage:* 3,000 to 5,000 mg daily. Make a paste with ascorbic acid powder and water and apply to warts daily.

VITAMIN A This vitamin is required for the proper formation of epithelial and mucus membranes. Applying vitamin A oil directly to warts has proven successful for some people. *Suggested Dosage:* Take 25,000 IU of vitamin A daily. Do not exceed 10,000 IU if pregnant.

VITAMIN E Vitamin E can be applied externally to warts. It helps to normalize skin tissue and prevent scarring.

Impressive results have been obtained through this method and it is definitely worth trying. *Suggested Dosage:* 400 to 800 IU daily.

WISDOM OF THE AGES This is a special product made from grape seed extract which can be applied directly to the wart. *Suggested Dosage:* Use as directed.

HERBAL COMBINATION This herbal combination contains St. John's wort, Siberian ginseng, astragalus, shiitake and reishi mushrooms, schizandra, and licorice root. *Suggested Dosage:* Four to eight capsules daily.

ST. JOHN'S WORT: One of the most impressive properties of this herb is its ability to fight viral infections. It can interfere with viral replication which is what makes warts spread.[5] SIBERIAN GINSENG: Siberian ginseng has the ability to increase important T-lymphocytes of the helper variety to fight viral infections. Double-blind studies have confirmed the ability of this herb to improve and normalize immune system actions.[6] ASTRAGALUS: This Chinese herb has been shown to increase phagocytosis and interferon production. This herb can stimulate the production of interferon and has been used for centuries by the Chinese to enhance immune function and has recently been used externally on warts.[7] SHIITAKE AND REISHI MUSHROOMS: These mushrooms have been scientifically studied and shown to stimulate interferon production and increase helper T-lymphocytes. These mushrooms contain powerful immunostimulating polysaccharides.[8] LICORICE ROOT: Animal studies have shown licorice to enhance the production of interferon and macrophage (a large phagocyte) activity and inhibit viruses.[9] Licorice should not be used by anyone with high blood pressure, kidney disease or who is taking digitalis.

SECONDARY NUTRIENTS

L-CYSTEINE: This amino acid is required for normal and healthy skin processes. *Suggested Dosage:* Take as directed on an empty stomach with fruit juice.

BLACK WALNUT AND GOLDENSEAL: Both of these herbs have strong antiviral properties and can be taken as capsules and applied externally in paste form. *Suggested Dosage:* Take as directed using standardized products.

TEA TREE OIL: Apply externally to warts. Tea tree oil has antifungal and antiviral properties *Suggested Dosage:* Use as directed.

Home Care Suggestions

◆ Applying the juice of white cabbage to the warts is an old traditional treatment.

◆ Crushing an aspirin and applying it to the wart which is subsequently covered with a piece of cellophane tape may be effective but should not be attempted by anyone with an aspirin sensitivity or allergy.

◆ Compound W or Vergo are nonprescription wart medications that can be applied at home. They are salicylic acid compounds and work by softening and dissolving the wart. These preparations have had mixed results. If a wart is unusually large, these preparations are sometimes ineffective. Mediplast is a medicated pad which sticks directly on the wart. Careful sizing of this product is necessary to prevent injury to surrounding skin. Coat surrounding healthy tissue with petroleum jelly for added protection.

- Applying a crushed garlic clove to the wart and bandaging it for at least 24 hours has been successful for some people. A blister will usually form and the wart will fall off within five to seven days.
- Apply castor oil or any sweet oil (wheat germ oil) to the warts several times a day and use an emery board to slough off dead skin. This same treatment can also soften corns and callouses.
- Exposure to heat can sometimes cure warts either through sunlight or by soaking the wart in very hot water for 30 minutes several times per week.
- A salt paste applied to the wart with a cotton ball taped to the wart can also help to dissolve the growth.
- If you have genital warts wear cotton underwear and keep the area as dry as possible.
- Put a drop of iodine on the wart every night. This particular treatment has been quite successful.
- There is a strong belief that taking time to visualize away your warts by imagining them shrinking and disappearing has produced some remarkable results and should be attempted. Visulaize for two to five minutes a day.
- Applying fresh banana skin daily and taping it to warts is a method of treatment used in Israel. This softens the wart and it can eventually be scraped off.
- Putting adhesive tape (waterproof) directly on warts for a week, exposing the wart to air for 12 hours and then reapplying the tape for another week may cause them to disappear within four to six weeks. In some cases, treating one wart in this manner has inhibited the growth of surrounding warts, which were not treated.
- Soak a cotton ball in fresh pineapple juice or bromelain powder and tape over the wart to eventually dissolve it.

Other Supportive Therapies

HYPNOTHERAPY, AUTOSUGGESTION, AND VISUALIZATION: Warts can sometimes be mentally visualized away with these techniques.

Scientific Facts-at-a-Glance

Dr. Andrew Weil has written some interesting thoughts on why warts can, in some instances, disappear virtually overnight. In his book, *Health and Healing*, he cites the incredible power of suggestion as a very real tool in curing warts that have not responded to physical therapies. Because warts can disappear with visualization therapy or even placebo treatments, he reiterates the very real notion of mind-mediated healing and why burying a potato under a tree during a full moon might cure warts. He admonishes medical science to pay attention to this phenomenon when treating other diseases like cancer.

Spirit/Mind Considerations

In spite of scientific skepticism, warts seem to have an unquestionable psychological connection. The power of suggestion, visualization therapy and hypnosis have cured warts in a number of people. The use of placebos in treating warts is remarkably successful and indicates that warts are particularly susceptible to mental influence. Psychoneuroimmunology is based on the premise that mental phenomena can affect immune function and is particularly applicable to the treatment of warts.

Prevention

- Keep your shoes dry by airing them out and changing them frequently. Use leather or canvas shoes that breathe. Vinyl shoes can trap moisture and cause sweating.
- Use Lysol in bathrooms, etc. This as well as using bleach can kill viruses and bacteria.
- Take a daily dose of vitamin C to maintain a healthy immune system.
- Keep your immune system healthy by not smoking and drinking alcohol and by eating a nutritious high-fiber, low-fat diet.
- Do not have sexual intercourse with a partner who has genital warts.
- Wear cotton socks, don't go barefoot and keep feet dry and in well fitted shoes to prevent plantar warts. Never go barefoot in public places like swimming pool areas, locker rooms, or health clubs. This also helps to avoid contracting athlete's foot.

Doctor's Notes

Wisdom of the ages, made from grape seed extract, can be used directly on warts. It has an antimicrobial action that may help in some cases. Most warts are outgrown and may be genetically predetermined in some individuals. If you choose to have warts frozen or burned off, make sure you are using the services of a doctor who is skilled so that scarring doesn't result, especially if the warts are in the eye area.

Endnotes

1. N.D. Weber, et al., "In vitro virucidal effects of Allivum sativum (garlic) extract and compounds," Planta Medica, 1992, 58: 417-23.
2. G. Lavie, et al., "Hypericin as an inactivator of infectious viruses in blood components," Transfusion, 1995, 35: 392-400.
3. A. Wacker and W. Hilbig, "Virus inhibition by Echinacea purpurea," Planta Medica, 1978, 33: 89-102.
4. S.W. Wang, et al., "The trace element zinc and aphthosis: The determination of plasma zinc and the treatment of aphthosis with zinc," Rev Stomatol Chir Maxillofac, 1986, 87(5): 339-43.
5. A. James, "Common dermatologic disorders," CIBA Clinical Symposia 1967, 19(2): 38-64
6. B. Bohn, et al., "Flow-cytometric studies with Eleutherococcus senticosus extract as an immunomodulatory agent," Arzneimittel-Forsch, 1987, 37: 1193-96.

7. H. Yunde, et al., "Effect of radix astragalus on the interferon system," Chinese Medical Jour, 1981, 94: 35-40.

8. F. Fukucuoka, "Polysaccharide extract active against tumors," Chem Abstracts, 1971, 74:324-25.

9. N. Abe, et al., "Interferon induction by glycyrrhizin and glycyrrhetinic acid in mice," Microb Immunol, 1982, 26: 353-359.

WEIGHT CONTROL

SEE "OBESITY"

WRINKLES

Trying to stop the inevitable tread of time on our skin may be seen as an exercise in futility. But there are some things we can do to protect our skin. Wrinkles are a natural part of the aging process, despite our continual efforts to eliminate them. They develop due to the gradual wearing away of the epidermis, the outermost layer of skin which is comprised of dead tissue.

Causes

Contrary to popular belief, wrinkles are not caused by dehydration or dry skin. Frowning and squinting do cause wrinkling by constantly stretching the dermis. Free radicals are innately involved in the deterioration of our skin. Other factors associated with an increased risk for wrinkling are smoking, radiation damage from sun exposure, scrubbing the skin with caustic or harsh substances, sleeping on your side or stomach, a lack of vitamins and minerals, and drinking alcohol.

Wrinkles are permanent features of aging skin because they originate from the dermis, which is deeper than the epidermis. After the age of 25 the cells in the dermis begin to die off and become smaller. Skin begins to lose some of its elasticity and resiliency. Any shrinkage of tissue in the dermis causes a wrinkle in the epidermis. The dermis becomes stiffer as we age. The more the dermis is stretched, the greater the risk for developing wrinkles. Because the face and its muscles are so active, it can be the site of significant wrinkling.

Face lifts, eye lifts, chemical peels, etc., can have dramatic results—but they come with a significant amount of discomfort and some risk. These operations have become extremely popular over the last decade, and when done by a skillful surgeon can be quite satisfying.

Chemical peels and dermabrasion are not considered as successful as face lifts although in some cases, the improvement is substantial. The use of Retin-A and alpha-hydroxy acids in cosmetic forms produce limited results. While fine lines created by sun exposure may be affected, significant wrinkles which are the natural result of aging are not.

Conventional Therapies

Alpha-hydroxy washes and Retin-A (an acne preparation), have become extremely popular over the last few years as a treatment for wrinkles. There is significant controversy over the validity of using Retin-A for this purpose. Retin-A comes with an array of side effects that may discourage its use for this purpose. Most doctors agree that Retin-A does little for wrinkles that appear with age. But they agree that Retin-A is a good treatment for wrinkles that develop from exposure to the sun.

Chemical face peels (chemosurgery) is a procedure which uses carbolic acid or alpha-hydroxy acid that is up to 70 percent concentrated. It is used for acid face peels which remove the outermost layer of skin. Some burning of the skin results and smoother skin develops as healing occurs. The procedure involves a significant amount of discomfort and causes scabbing to form. The scab will fall off after about 10 days, exposing a new layer of unblemished skin. A red or dark color to the skin can persist but usually returns to normal after several weeks. Sun exposure is prohibited for six months.

Dermabrasion involves using a special tool to sand the surface of the skin located in wrinkled areas which have been previously anesthetized. This procedure leaves areas of raw pink surfaces that will need approximately two weeks to heal. The procedure is simple and usually takes around 30 minutes.

Face lifts can now be done on an outpatient basis, although some situations still require a short hospital stay. The operation can be done under local or general anesthesia. It usually takes somewhere between two to four hours. Incisions are made under the hairline and around the ears and any fatty tissue present is removed. The neck skin is subsequently tightened. Often a chemical peel or eyelid surgery accompanies this procedure. The face will remain bandaged for several days following the surgery. After two and a half weeks, swelling goes down and the incisions are significantly healed enough to socialize. Laser surgery is now available for treating fine lines and has had some good success.

Dietary Guidelines

◆ Eat a diet high in raw fruits and vegetables, lean meats and low-fat dairy products, whole grains and drink plenty of pure water. A diet that is high in saturated fats has been linked to the development of dry skin.
◆ Use polyunsaturated and monounsaturated oils.
◆ Add essential fatty acids to your diet through omega-3 oils. Good oils include safflower, sunflower, corn, sesame, pumpkin seed, olive, canola, flaxseed, almond and hazelnut.
◆ Avoid shortening, animal fats, hydrogenated oil and coconut oil.

Recommended Nutritional Supplements

PRIMARY NUTRIENTS

ESSENTIAL FATTY ACIDS Tests have shown that supplementation with fish oils and with other oils, like evening primrose and flaxseed, is very beneficial in helping nourish the skin.[1] *Suggested Dosage:* Use as directed daily. Take a vitamin E supplement with fish oil. Keep refrigerated.

LIPOIC ACID, VITAMIN E, AND SELENIUM Lipoic acid greatly potentiates the availability of vitamins E and C and glutathione in the cells and makes it possible for enhanced free radical scavenging by these agents. Selenium can also be applied topically.[2] *Suggested Dosage:* Take all three supplements as directed and in combination.

LECITHIN This nutrient contains choline which helps to metabolize lipids correctly, vital for proper skin cell metabolism.[3] *Suggested Dosage:* Take as directed in granule or capsulized form daily.

VITAMIN A Works to boost skin tissue regeneration and scavenges for free radicals. It has even been used to slow the progression of skin diseases.[4] *Suggested Dosage:* 25,000 IU daily. CAUTION: If you are pregnant, do not exceed 10,000 IU per day.

ZINC Contributes to the healing of the skin through its participation in protein metabolism.[5] *Suggested Dosage:* 50 to 100 mg per day. Use gluconate or picolinate products.

MYRRH EXTRACT This herb is considered a good herbal skin conditioner. *Suggested Usage:* You can find this in spray form or make your own decoction.

JOJOBA OIL Used for generations by the American Indians to condition skin and improve its quality. It has a similar structure to natural sebum found in the skin. *Suggested Usage:* Use as directed.

REDMOND CLAY A traditional herbal treatment for toning the treating the skin. *Suggested Usage:* Use as directed.

ALOE VERA Helps to heal any cell damage to the skin and can be used in gel or lotion form. *Suggested Usage:* Use as directed.

SECONDARY NUTRIENTS

HONEY FACIALS: These can help to make the skin soft and supple. *Suggested Usage:* Smooth pure raw honey on the face and let it stay for 15 minutes. Then rinse off with cool water and a washcloth.

DRIED PEPPERMINT LEAF TEA: Makes for a wonderful facial rinse that is recommended for dry skin. *Suggested Usage:* Use one pint of strained tea and add to a pint of apple cider vinegar.

LAVENDER AND THYME: These are antiseptic herbs that stimulate the skin. *Suggested Usage:* Essential oils diluted in glycerin can be used or facial rinses can be made from decoctions.

Home Care Suggestions

◆ Frequently, the claims of high-priced wrinkle creams are not what they're touted to be. Before you spend a fortune, do a little homework and compare ingredients and percentages of certain chemical substances in a number of brands. Often the price tag depends on the brand name rather than its contents.

◆ Use a good moisturizer daily. While moisturizing your skin will not stop wrinkles from forming, it can significantly improve the texture of the skin, making it appear smoother.

◆ Whipping up some egg whites into a meringue-like texture and applying it to your face for 30 minutes can help to temporarily tighten the skin. The effect only lasts for about an hour or two.

◆ Avoid sun exposure. Cells from young skin that have been exposed to too much sun look the same as cells that are old and have naturally wrinkled. Unprotected sun exposure can unquestionably cause premature aging. The midday sun is the most damaging. Avoid direct exposure between the hours of 10 a.m. and 3 p.m. Use strong sun screens with high SPF factors if you must be in the sun. Apply these 30 minutes before exposure and reapply after swimming. Highly reflective surfaces such as water, sand, and concrete can cause considerable sun damage by intensifying its effect on skin cells.

◆ Tanning booths can contribute to skin damage just as much as real sunshine.

◆ Don't smoke—smokers have significantly more wrinkles than nonsmokers and age faster. Smoking decreases the body's oxygen supply which can contribute to reduced blood circulation to the face which causes more epidermal damage. The very act of smoking causes the face to contract in strange ways which may also contribute to the formation of creases and lines.

◆ Don't drink alcohol—drinking can cause facial swelling, which stretches the skin, thereby causing wrinkling. Alcohol can also rob your body of essential nutrients that promote healthy cell function in the skin.

◆ Wear hats and sunglasses to prevent squinting, frowning and sun damage.

◆ Use mild soaps and cleansers that will not dry out or remove oils that help to keep the skin supple and well nourished. Soaps such as Neutrogena are considered benign and gentle enough not to disrupt the normal balance of the skin.

◆ Train yourself to sleep on your back. Sleeping on your side or stomach can create a number of unnatural creases on the face. Bunching up your pillow and nestling your face in it can scrunch up facial tissue and create lines.

◆ Use a humidifier in your home if you live in an arid climate. While moisture will not prevent or cure wrinkles, it can minimize their noticeability.

◆ Treat yourself to facial massages that increase circulation and stimulation.

◆ Keep yourself at an optimal weight. Becoming overweight and then losing fat can create sagging wrinkled skin.

◆ Exercise regularly. Exercise can increase circulation to skin cells and improve overall oxygenation. People who exercise routinely have better overall elasticity and density to their skin. Exercise also gives skin that wonderful healthy glow.

◆ Manage stress through relaxation techniques and learn to feel happiness and joy. People under tension frown and develop unattractive ridges and furrows. Laugh lines are unquestionably preferable.

Other Supportive Therapies

YOGA: The shoulder stand and yoga mudra practices are recommended for wrinkle control.

Scientific Facts-at-a-Glance

The notion of replacing hormones such as DHEA in the body may one day help to reverse the aging process.

Spirit/Mind Considerations

The way we look undoubtedly affects how we feel. Having a face lift or other cosmetic procedure can greatly increase one's self-esteem and confidence level. However these surgeries will not guarantee your happiness. If extensive wrinkles and sagging skin are making you want to withdraw and significantly bother you, check out local plastic surgeons who are board certified and talk to patients who have had procedures done. Evaluate your situation and if finances permit, one of these procedures may significantly improve your psychological outlook. Just remember that having your face changed can in and of itself be emotionally traumatic and may require a period of adjustment which should be discussed in length with your plastic surgeon.

Prevention

◆ Protect your skin from the sun by using protective clothing and sunscreen.

◆ Do not use tobacco, alcohol or caffeine.

◆ Eat plenty of raw fruits and vegetables daily.

◆ Take a strong multivitamin, antioxidant and multimineral complex daily.

Doctor's Notes

The skin is the largest and one of the most important organs of the body. It performs many vital functions, including cleansing toxic substances from the body, keeping the body's temperature in check, and providing a barrier to pathogenic bacteria and viruses. The condition of the skin is often a reflection of the health of the body. Imbalances and toxic buildup due to a dysfunctional liver or improper elimination may reveal themselves in the skin as eczema, psoriasis, rashes, acne, dermatitis, or a number of other disorders. By improving the internal health of the body, the skin's functionality and appearance will be positively affected. The nutrients listed are designed to cleanse the body by activating all its methods of elimination which include cleansing, strengthening, and supporting liver function. Longer-lasting and more wide-ranging results can be achieved by improving the diet and abstaining from chocolate, nuts and stimulants such as caffeine. While wrinkling is an inevitable part of aging, it is quite remarkable how much better our skin can look and hold up if it is properly nourished, cared for and protected.

Endnotes

1. V. Ziboh, "Implications of dietary oils and polyunsaturated fatty acids in the management of cutaneous disorders," Arch Dermatol, 1989, 125(2): 241-5. See also A. Lassus, et al., "Effects of dietary supplementation with polyunsaturated ethyl-ester lipids (angiosan) in patients with psoriasis and psoriatic arthritis," Jour Int Med Res, 1990, 18: 68-73.

2. E. Broglund and A. Enhamre, "Treatment of psoriasis with topical selenium sulphide," Letter, Br J Dermatol, 1987, 117(5): 665-6.

3. P. Gross, et al., "The treatment of psoriasis as a disturbance of lipid metabolism," N Y State J Med, 1950, 50: 2683-86.

4. M. Haddox, et al., "Retinol inhibition of ornithine decarboxylase induction and GI progression in CHD cells," Cancer Res, 1979, 39: 4930-38.

5. B. Dreno, et al., "Plasma zinc is decreased only in generalized pustular psoriasis," Dermatologica, 1986, 173(5): 209-12.

YEAST INFECTIONS

SEE "VAGINITIS"

APPENDIX A

Resource Information

Resource Information for Natural Health Organizations

Acupuncture

American Association for Acupuncture and Oriental Medicine
4101 Lake Boone Trail
Suite 201
Raleigh, North Carolina 27607 USA

New Zealand Register of Acupuncturists Inc.
PO Box 9950
Wellington 1
New Zealand
Tel/Fax: 64 4 476 8578

Aromatherapy

Academy of Aromatherapy and Massage
50 Cow Wynd
Falkirk, Sterlingshire FK1 1PU
Great Britain
Tel: 44 1324 612658

Biofeedback

Association for Applied Psychophysiology and Biofeedback
10200 West 44th Avenue Apt 304
Wheat Ridge, Colorado 80033-8436 USA
Tel: (303) 422-8894
Fax: (303) 422-8894

Herbalism

American Herbalists Guild
PO Box 1683
Sequel, California 95073 USA

National Herbalists Association of Australia
Suite 305
BST House
3 Smail Street
Broadway, New South Wales 2007
Australia
Tel: 61 2 211 6437
Fax: 61 2 211 6452

School of Herbal Medicine/Phytotherapy
Bucksteep Manor
Bodle Street Green
Near Hailsham, Sussex BN27 4RJ
Great Britain
Tel: 44 1323 833 812/4
Fax: 44 1323 833 869

Holistic Medicine

American Holistic Health Association
PO Box 17400
Anaheim, California 90017-7100 USA
Tel: (714) 779-6152 or 777-2917

American Holistic Medical Association
4101 Lake Boone Trail
Suite 201
Raleigh, North Carolina 27607 USA
Tel: (919) 787-5181
Fax: (919) 787-4916

British Holistic Medicine Association
Trust House
Royal Shrewsbury Hospital South
Shrewsbury, Shropshire SY3 8XF
Great Britain
Tel: 44 1743 26115
Fax: 44 1743 353637

Holistic and Creative Therapy Association
2A Burston Drive
St Albans, Herts AL2 2HR
Great Britain
Tel: 44 1727 674567

Holistic Health Foundation
2 De La Hay Avenue
Plymouth, Devon PL3 4HH
Great Britain
Tel: 44 1752 671 485
Fax: 44 1345 251759

Association of Holistic Healing Centers
109 Holly Crescent
Suite 201
Virginia Beach, Virginia 23451 USA
Tel: (804) 422-9033
Fax: (804) 422-8132

Canadian Holistic Medical Association
491 Eglinton Avenue West
Apt 407
Toronto, Ontario M5N 1A8
Canada
Tel: (416) 485-3071

International Association of Holistic Health Practitioners
5020 West Spring
Mountain Road
Las Vegas, Nevada 89102 USA
Tel: (702) 873-4542

Homeopathy

American Foundation for Homeopathy
1508 S. Garfield
Alhambra, California 91801 USA

American Institute of Homeopathy
1585 Glencoe Street Suite 44
Denver, Colorado 80220-1338 USA
Tel: (303) 321-4105

Foundation for Homeopathic Education and Research
2124 Kittredge Street
Berkeley, California 94704 USA

Homeopathic Council for Research and Education
50 Park Avenue
New York, New York 10016 USA

Australian Federation for Homeopathy
PO Box 806
Spit Junction, New South Wales 2088
Australia

Australian Institute of Homeopathy
21 Bulah Heights
Berdraw Heights, New South Wales 2082
Australia

Institute of Classical Homeopathy
24 West Haven Drive
Tawa, Wellington
New Zealand

British Homoeopathic Association
27A Devonshire Street
London W1N 1RJ
Great Britain
Tel: 44 171 935 2163

Centre d'Etudes Homeopathiques de France
228 Boulevard Raspail
75014 Paris, France

International Foundation for Homeopathy
2366 Eastlake Avenue East
Suite 301
Seattle, Washington 98102 USA

National Center for Homeopathy
801 North Fairfax Street
Suite 306
Alexandria, Virginia 22314 USA

Hydrotherapy

Aquatic Exercise Association
PO Box 1609
Nokomis, Florida 34274 USA
Tel: (813) 486-8600

UK College of Hydrotherapy
515 Hagley Road
Birmingham B66 4AX
Great Britain
Tel: 44 121 429 9191
Fax: 44 121 478 0871

Hypnotherapy

American Association of Professional Hypnotherapists
PO Box 29
Boones Mill, Virginia 24065 USA
Tel: (703) 334-3035

American Guild of Hypnotherapists
2200 Veterans Boulevard
New Orleans, Louisiana 70062 USA

National Society of Hypnotherapists
2175 North West 86th
Suite 6A
Des Moines, Iowa 50325 USA
Tel: (515) 270-2280

National Register of Hypnotherapists and Psychotherapists
12 Cross Street
Nelson, Lancs BB9 7EN
Great Britain
Tel: 44 1282 699378
Fax: 44 1282 698633

Massage

International Massage Association
3000 Connecticut Avenue
NW Apt. 102
Washington, DC 20008 USA
Tel: (202) 387-6555
Fax: (202) 332-0531

National Association of Massage Therapy
PO Box 1400
Westminster, Colorado 80030-1400 USA
Tel: (800) 776-6268

Skilled Touch Institute of Chair Massage
584 Castro Street Suite 555
San Francisco, California 94774-2588 USA
Tel: (415) 861-4746
Fax: (415) 861-0443

Society of Clinical Masseurs
PO Box 483
9 Delhi Street
Mitchum 3131
Victoria, Australia
Tel: 61 3 874 6973

Academy of Aromatherapy and Massage
50 Cow Wynd
Falkirk, Sterlinghire FK1 1PU
Great Britain
Tel: 44 1324 6126598

London College of Massage
5 Newman Passage
London W1P 3PF
Great Britain
Tel: 44 171 323 3574
Fax: 44 171 637 7125

American Massage Therapy Association
820 Davis Street
Suite 100
Evanston, Illinois 60201-4444 USA
Tel: (708) 864-0123
Fax: (708) 864-1178

Associated Bodyworkers and Massage Professionals
28677 Buffalo Park
Evergreen, Colorado 80439-7947 USA
Tel: (303) 674-8478
Fax: (303) 674-0859

International Association of Infant Massage
PO Box 438
Elma, New York 14059-0438 USA
Tel: (716) 652-9789
Fax: (716) 652-9790

Naturopathy

American Association of Naturopathic Physicians
PO Box 20386
Seattle, Washington 98102 USA
Tel: (206) 323-7610

American Naturopathic Medical Association
PO Box 19221
Las Vegas, Nevada 89132 USA
Tel: (702) 793-9067

Canadian Naturopathic Association
205, 1234, 17th Avenue
South West, PO Box 4143
Station C
Calgary, Alberta
Canada
Tel:1 413 244 4487

Australian Natural Therapists Association
(ANTA)
PO Box 308
Melrose Park
South Australia 5039
Australia
Tel: 61 8 371 3222
Fax: 61 8 297 0003

British College of Naturopathy and Osteopathy
Frazer House
6 Netherhall Gardens
London NW3 5RR
Great Britain
Tel: 44 171 435 6464
Fax: 44 171 431 3630

Nutritional and Diet Therapy

American Association of Nutrition Consultants
1641 East Sunset Road,
Apt B177
Las Vegas, Nevada 89119 USA
Tel: (709) 361-1132

American Dietetics Association
216 West Jackson Boulevard
Apt. 800
Chicago, Illinois 60606-6995 USA
Tel: (800) 877-1600

British Nutrition Foundation
High Holborn House
524 High Holborn
London WC1V 6RQ
Great Britain
Tel: 44 171 404 6504
Fax: 44 171 404 6747

College of Natural Therapy
133 Gatley Road
Garley, Cheadle
Cheshire SK8 4PD
Great Britain
Tel: 44 161 491 4314
Fax: 44 161 491 4190

Shiatsu Therapy

American Association of Oriental Medicine
(AAOM)
433 Front Street
Catasauqua, Pennsylvania 18032 USA
Tel: (610) 266-1433
Fax: (610) 264-2768

American Shiatsu Association
PO Box 718
Jamaica Plain, Massachusetts 12130 USA
Tel: (617) 236-5867

Chi Kung School at the Body Energy Center
PO Box 19708
Boulder, Colorado 80308 USA
Tel: (303) 442-2250
Fax: (303) 442-3141

International Chi Kung/Qigong Directory
PO Box 19708
Boulder, Colorado 80308 USA
Tel: (303) 442-3131
Fax: (303) 442-3141

World Academic Society of Medical Qigong
No.11 Heping Jie Nei Kou
Beijing 100029
China

Australian Traditional Medicine Society Limited
ATMS
PO Box 1027
(mailing)/12/27 Bank
Street (office), Meadowbank
New South Wales 2114
Australia
Tel: 61 2 809 6800

Shiatsu Therapy Association of Australia
PO Box 1
Balaclava, Victoria 3183
Australia
Tel/Fax: 61 03 530 0067

College of Integrated Chinese Medicine
19 Castle Street
Reading, Berks RG1 7SB
Great Britatin
Tel: 44 1734 508880
Fax: 44 1734 508890

Register of Chinese Herbal Medicine
PO Box 400
Wembley, Middox HA9 9NZ
Great Britain
Tel: 44 181 904 1357 or
1 216 842 8042

Osteopathy and Chiropractic

American Academy of Osteopathy
3500 DEPauw Boulevard
Suite 1080
Indianapolis, Indiana 46268 USA
Tel: (371) 879-1881
Fax: (317) 879-0563

American Association of Colleges of Osteopathic Medicine
6110 Executive Boulevard, Apt 405
Rockville, Maryland 20852 USA
Tel: (301) 468-0990

American Osteopathic Association
142 East Ohio Street
Chicago, Illinois 60611 USA
Tel: (312) 280-5800
Fax: (312) 280-3860

**Chiropractors and Osteopaths
Registration Board of Victoria**
PO Box 59
Carlton South Victoria 3053
Australia
Tel: 61 3 349 3000
Fax: 61 3 349 3003

NSW Chiropractors and Osteopathic Registration Board
PO Box K599
Haymarket, New South Wales 2000
Australia
Tel: 61 2 281 0884
Fax: 61 2 281 2030

General Register and Council of Osteopaths
56 London Street
Reading, Berks RG1 4SO
Great Britain
Tel: 44 1734 576585
Fax: 44 1734 566246

Stress Therapy

Association of Stress Therapists
5 Springfield Road
Palm Bay
Cliftonville, Kent CT9 3EA
Great Britain
Tel: 44 1843 291255

Transcendental Meditation
Maharishi Foundation of New Zealand
3 Adam Street
Greenlane
Auckland 1105 New Zealand
Tel: 64 9 523 3324

Maharishi Vedic College
PO Box 81
Bundoora 3083
Victoria, Australia
Tel: 61 3 9467 8911

Transcendental Meditation
Freepost
London SW1P 4YY
Great Britatin
Tel: 44 990 143733

Maharishi University of Management
Fairfield, Iowa 52557 USA
Tel: (515) 472-1134

Maharishi Vedic College
500 Wilbrod Street
Ottawa, Ontario K1N 6N2
Canada
Tel: (613) 565 2030

Yoga

BSK Iyengar Yoga National Association of the US
8223 West Third Street
Los Angeles, California 90088 USA
Tel: (213) 653-0357

International Association of Yoga Therapists
109 Hillside Avenue
Mill Valley, California 94941 USA
Tel: (415) 383-4587
Fax: (415) 381-0876

Sivananda Yoga Vedanta Center
243 West 24th Street
New York, New York 10011 USA

Sivananda Yoga Vedanta Centre
5178 St Lawrence Boulevard
Montreal, Quebec H2T 1R8
Canada

Unity in Yoga International
PO Box 281004
Lakewood, Colorado 80228 USA

Unity Yoga International
7918 Bolling Drive
Alexandria, Virginia 22308 USA

Israeli Yoga Teachers Association
c/o PO Box 48087
Tel Aviv 61480
Israel

APPENDIX B
Glossary

Achlorhydria: The absence of hydrochloric acid in the stomach.

Acetylcholine: A neurotransmitter compound involved in nerve cell transmissions.

Absorption: The process in which dietary nutrients are absorbed through the intestinal tract into the bloodstream. Malabsorption occurs when nutrients are not properly absorbed and nutritional depletion can result.

Acetic Acid: A weak acid that comprises the active ingredient of vinegar.

Acute Illness: An illness or condition that suddenly appears and may cause significant symptoms that usually last for a limited time.

Adrenal Glands: A pair of glands, one located on top of each kidney, that manufacture stress hormones such as epinephrine (adrenaline) and cortisol.

Adrenaline: A hormone secreted by the adrenal glands that facilitate the release glycogen stores in the liver, the contraction of muscles, and increased blood supply in response to stressful situations.

Alkaline: A chemical substance known as a base that neutralizes an acid to form a salt. Baking soda is an example of an alkaline substance. Alkaline compounds have a greater pH than baseline levels.

Allergy: An inappropriate immune system response to what are normally benign substances.

Allopathic: A term referring to conventional or orthodox medicine.

Amino Acid: Any one of 22 nitrogen-containing organic acids that comprise protein molecules.

Anabolic Compound: A substance that contributes to the building up of living tissue.

Analgesic: A substance that works to relieve or ease pain. Aspirin is an analgesic.

Anemia: A deficiency of the iron-carrying molecules in the blood.

Angina: Also known as angina pectoris, this condition is characterized by sporadic chest pain with difficulty breathing. It is typically initiated by exertion and due to cardiovascular disease.

Antacid: A substance that neutralizes acid in the stomach, esophagus, or the initial section of the duodenum.

Antibiotic: A substance which can destroy or inhibit the growth of microorganisms such as bacteria.

Antibody: A protein molecule manufactured by the immune system that can incapacitate specific invading pathogens or other foreign substances.

Antigen: A substance or organism that, when introduced into the system, initiates the creation of an antibody.

Antihistamine: A compound that inhibits the action of histamines by binding to histamine receptors.

Antioxidant: A compound that inhibits or actually stops the action of destructive oxidants. Examples of antioxidants are vitamin E, lipoic acid, selenium, and vitamin C.

Arrhythmia: Irregular or skipped heartbeat.

Arteriosclerosis: A circulatory condition caused by a thickening of the walls of the arteries that serves to inhibit proper blood flow.

Artery: A blood vessel through which blood is pumped from the heart to all other body systems.

Ascorbate: A mineral salt of vitamin C. Ascorbates are less acidic than pure ascorbic acid and are better assimilated.

Ascorbic Acid: An organic acid commonly known as vitamin C.

Atherosclerosis: The most prevalent kind of arteriosclerosis, caused by the accumulation of fatty deposits or plaque in the linings of arteries.

Autoimmune Disorder: Any condition in which the

immune system attacks the body's own tissues due to immune malfunction. Multiple sclerosis, rheumatoid arthritis, and systemic lupus erythematosus are all examples of autoimmune diseases.

Bacteria: Single-celled microorganisms that can cause disease or infection. Friendly bacteria are found in the body and contribute to better digestion and immunity, among other functions.

Basal Metabolic Rate: The amount of energy needed for internal cellular functions when the body is at rest. This rate is expressed per unit of time and per square meter of the body surface area.

Benign: A word used to refer to a group of growing cells that are not considered cancerous.

Beta Carotene: Substance the body uses to make vitamin A.

Bile: A yellowish substance released by the liver to boost the breakdown of lipids or fats in the digestive system.

Bioflavonoids: Belonging to the family of flavonoids, these compounds contribute to the absorption of vitamin C and are also known as vitamin P.

Biopsy: Surgically removing tissue for further laboratory diagnosis.

Blood Count: Laboratory test in which a sample of blood is examined and the white and red blood cells are counted.

Blood-Brain Barrier: A part of the brain that prevents some substances, especially water-soluble ones, from passing through brain blood vessels to brain tissue itself.

Bronchi: The two primary branches of the trachea (windpipe) that lead to the lungs.

Buffer: A substance that maintains the proper acid/alkaline ratio in the body.

Calcitonin: A hormone released by the thyroid gland that inhibits the release of calcium from the bones.

Capillaries: Tiny blood vessels that allow for the exchange of nutrients and wastes from the bloodstream.

Carbohydrate: Term referring to one of several organic substances of plant origin that are composed of carbon, hydrogen and oxygen, and serve as the primary source of energy for the body.

Carcinogen: An agent that is capable of inducing cancerous changes in cells and/or tissues.

Carotene: A yellow-orange pigment that converts into vitamin A in the body. Alpha, beta and gamma forms exist.

Cell: A microscopic organic unit consisting of a nucleus, cytoplasm, and a cell membrane. All living tissue is comprised of cells.

Cellulose: An indigestible carbohydrate substance usually located in the outer layers of fruits and vegetables.

Chelation: A chemical process where a larger molecule or group of molecules encases a mineral atom making it more absorbable in the human body.

Chelation Therapy: A therapy that involves the ingestion of specific compounds that will chelate in the body, thus causing the removal of toxic compounds such as lead or other heavy metals. Chelation therapy can also remove calcium-based plaque from blood vessels.

Chiropractic: A therapeutic discipline founded on the belief that ailments can be caused by spinal misalignments (subluxations). Certain manipulations are used to bring the spine into proper alignment.

Chlorophyll: Pigment that gives green plants their color and participates in plant respiration. It can be taken as a supplement.

Cholesterol: Cholesterol is a type of lipid compound found only in animal foods such as eggs, organ meats, meat, chicken, fish, dairy products, and in foods made with animal ingredients. It is never found in plants or plant-based foods. Ingesting an excess of cholesterol-rich foods is associated with elevated blood levels of cholesterol and the increased risk of developing cardiovascular disease. Cholesterol in the right amounts is essential to life.

Chronic Illness: Any disorder that continues to persist over an extended period of time.

Citric Acid: An organic acid found in citrus fruits.

Cocarcinogen: Any agent or substance that acts with another to cause malignancies.

Coenzyme: A molecule that works closely with an enzyme, enabling it to complete its series of chemical reactions in the body.

Cold Pressed: A term referring to dietary oils that are extracted without the use of heat.

Complete Protein: A food that contains all eight essential amino acids.

Complex Carbohydrate: A dietary source of carbohydrate, also known as a polysaccharide, whose sugar is broken down more slowly due to the presence of fiber.

Contusion: A bruise caused by blood vessels bleeding under the skin.

Convulsion: A seizure in which the uncontrollable contraction of muscles occurs from an abnormal release of electrical activity in the brain.

Cruciferous: A term that means "cross-shaped," and is used to refer to a particular group of vegetables, including broccoli, Brussels sprouts, cabbage, cauliflower, turnips, and rutabagas. These vegetables contain indoles thought to prevent the formation of certain cancers.

Deamination: Removal of the nitrogen part of an amino acid.

Dementia: A disorder where the impairment of brain function causes a deterioration of memory, language ability, personality, etc. Dementia can be caused by many different factors.

Dermis: The layer of skin that lies directly beneath the epidermis.

Detoxification: A process using fasting, herbs or other nutrients to rid the body of toxic substances.

Diuretic: A substance that can boost urine flow and enhance the excretion of fluids through the kidneys.

DNA (deoxyribonucleic acid): Found in the cell nucleus, this acid contains the cell's genetic codes and determines its eventual form and function.

Edema: A term describing the retention of fluid in body tissues.

EEG (electroencephalogram): A clinical test used to measure and chart brain wave activity.

EPA (eicosapentaenoic acid): A fatty acid found primarily in coldwater fish that has a number of desirable therapeutic actions.

Electrolyte: A soluble salt compound that can be excreted in body fluids and make up the circulating form of most minerals. These salts can conduct electrical impulses and are necessary for proper muscle contraction.

Enteric Coated: A term that describes a tablet or capsule that has been coated to ensure that it does not dissolve in the stomach. In this way the tablet's medicinal value can be applied to the intestines instead.

EKG (or ECG): Electrocardiogram. A test that charts heart function by graphing the conduction of electrical impulses with every beat.

Embolus: A loose residue particle, a blood clot, or an air bubble that circulates through the bloodstream and may become lodged in a blood vessel.

Emulsion: A combination of two liquids that normally do not mix, such as oil and water.

Endocrine System: The system of glands that secrete hormones into the bloodstream.

Endorphin: One of many brain chemicals that suppresses pain by binding to opiate receptors.

Enzyme: One of several protein catalysts that initiates or actually speeds up chemical reactions in the body without being consumed in the process.

Epidermis: The outer layer of the skin.

Epstein-Barr Virus (EBV): Virus known to cause infectious mononucleosis and has been implicated in other conditions associated with compromised immunity.

Erythema: Reddening of skin tissue.

Essential: A term for any compound that the body cannot manufacture and must be obtained through the diet.

Essential Fatty Acid (EFA): Fatty acids that the body cannot synthesize, such as linoleic and linolenic acids.

Fat Soluble: A substance that dissolves in lipid compounds.

Fatty Acid: Any one of several organic acids that comprise fats and oils.

Fasting Blood Sugar (FBS): Measures the level of glucose present in a blood sample taken at least eight hours after the ingestion food.

Fiber: The indigestible part of plants that acts to sweep the intestines of toxic substances and promote good elimination.

Flatulence: Excessive amounts of gas in the gastrointestinal tract.

Flavonoid: Any of a significant group of crystalline compounds found in certain plants.

Free Radical: An atom or group of atoms that is considered chemically unstable due to the fact that it has at least one unpaired electron. These atomic structures can cause cellular damage and are found in carcinogens, pollutants, etc.

Free Radical Scavenger: A substance that removes, destroys or inhibits the detrimental action of free radicals on a cellular level. Antioxidants are free radical scavengers.

Fructose: A simple sugar also known as fruit sugar. Honey is approximately 50 percent fructose.

Fungus: A class of organisms that includes yeasts, mold, and mushrooms and lives on a host.

Gamma Linolenic Acid (GLA): An omega-3 fatty acid.

Gastritis: A condition characterized by an inflammation of the stomach lining.

Gastrointestinal: A term pertaining to the stomach, small and large intestines, colon, rectum, liver, pancreas, and gallbladder.

Gingivitis: An inflammation or infection of the gums.

Globulin: A protein found in the blood that contains disease-fighting antibodies. Gamma-globulin is sometimes given to anyone who may have a weakened immune system.

Glucose Tolerance Factor (GTF): A compound containing chromium that works to aid insulin in regulating blood sugar levels.

Glucose Tolerance Test: A test that measures the body's reaction to blood sugar and is commonly used as a diagnostic tool for hypoglycemia and diabetes. Oral glucose solutions are taken and blood sugar levels are monitored for up to four hours.

Gluten: A protein found in many grains, including wheat, rye, barley, and oats, that causes flour to bind and may also cause allergies in certain people.

Glycogen: A form of glucose stored in the liver and muscle tissue.

Hair Analysis: The process by which hair is analyzed for the presence of toxic metals and essential minerals. The analysis reflects body concentrations of these metals over an extended period of time.

HDL Cholesterol: Cholesterol found in high density lipoproteins. HDL is composed of fats and protein and it transports lipids in the blood. High HDL levels are linked with a reduced risk of cardiovascular disease.

Hemicellulose: An indigestible carbohydrate found in plant cell walls that absorbs water.

Hemoglobin: The iron-containing red pigment found in red blood cells. Its purpose is to transport oxygen.

Hemorrhage: Profuse or abnormal bleeding that is usually difficult to control.

Herbal Therapy: The use of herbs or herbal combinations for healing or detoxification.

Histamine: A compound released by the immune system that contributes to the inflammatory response in human cells. It causes the dilation of small blood vessels, allowing fluid to leak from the tissue.

Hydrogenation: A chemical process used to turn liquid oils into more solid forms by bombarding molecules with hydrogen atoms. Hydrogenation destroys nutrients and also creates undesirable compounds called transfatty acids that are not found in nature.

Hyperglycemia: High blood sugar levels often linked to diabetes.

Hypertension: High blood pressure—usually seen as readings over 140/90 when resting.

Hypoallergenic: A term describing substances that do not usually induce allergic reactions.

Hypoglycemia: Low blood sugar. Can be brought on by the use of too much therapeutic insulin in cases of diabetes or may be caused by carbohydrate metabolism malfunction.

Hypotension: Low blood pressure.

Hypothalamus: An area of the brain that regulates many aspects of metabolism, including body temperature and appetite.

Idiopathic: A term describing a disease or disorder with no known cause.

Immune System: A complex body system that functions to single out and destroy foreign substances or microorganisms that enter the body. The liver, spleen, thymus, bone marrow, and lymphatic system all play profound roles in immunity.

Immune Globulin: A protein that functions as an antibody in the immune system. Immune globulins are synthesized by specific white blood cells and found in body fluids and on mucus membranes.

Incubation Period: The period of time between the exposure to an infectious agent and the development of symptoms, during which the infection takes hold.

Indoles: A group of compounds found in cruciferous vegetables that have been linked with a reduced risk of developing cancer.

Infection: The invasion of body tissue by parasites, bacteria, viruses or fungi.

Inflammation: A cellular reaction to illness or injury characterized by swelling, warmth, and redness.

Insulin: A hormone produced by the pancreas that regulates blood sugar levels.

Interaction: A reaction that occurs when two or more substances affect each other or end up creating another totally different substance.

Interferon: A protein produced by cells when exposed to viral infection that prevents viral reproduction and helps protect nearby cells from infection.

Intolerance: In dietary terms, the inability to digest a particular food causing a whole host of physiological responses.

Ischemia: A condition where body tissues become oxygen-starved due to blocked or decreased blood flow. Ischemia in the brain may cause a stroke and in the heart, a heart attack.

IU (International Unit): A measure based on an accepted international standard that refers to potency rather than amount or weight. Vitamins A and E are measured this way.

Lactase: An enzyme that converts lactose into glucose and galactose. It is necessary for the digestion of milk and milk products.

Lactic Acid: Found in certain foods, including some fruits, and sour milk. Anaerobic exercise produces lactic acid in the muscles which causes subsequent soreness.

Lactobacilli: Any of a number of bacterial species capable of converting lactose (milk sugar) into lactic acid through the process of fermentation. Lactobacilli are found in the bowel and are also called "friendly" bacteria because they aid in digestion and fight certain disease-causing microorganisms. *L. acidophilus* and *L. bifidus* are common forms of supplemental acidophilus.

LDL Cholesterol: Cholesterol comprised of low-density lipoproteins—molecules comprised of fats and protein that carry cholesterol through the bloodstream. A high LDL level is undesirable and has been associated with an increased risk of developing cardiovascular disease.

Lethargy: An overwhelming sensation of fatigue, lack of energy or drowsiness.

Leukotrienes: Inflammatory compounds created when oxygen interacts with polyunsaturated fatty acids.

Limbic System: A group of brain structures that transmit the sensation of pain and create a reaction to it.

Linoleic Acid: An essential polyunsaturated fatty acid found in safflower oil and other vegetable oils.

Lymph: A clear fluid derived from blood plasma that circulates through the body in the lymphatic system. Lymph is collected from tissue to provide cellular nourishment and collect waste materials for excretion.

Lymphocyte: A type of white blood cell found in lymph, blood, and other specialized tissues that plays a vital role in the immune system. B-lymphocytes are primarily responsible for antibody production and T-lymphocytes attack invading organisms.

Macrobiotics: A special dietary approach to treating disease or maintaining health that consists of foods designed to balance the body's energy states. Whole grain cereals, millet, rice, soups, vegetables, and beans are commonly used.

Malignant: Refers to cells or groups of cells that are considered cancerous.

Mammography: An x-ray examination of breast tissue.

Menopause: The cessation of menstruation caused by a decrease in the production of female sex hormones. Usually occurs after age 45.

Microgram: A unit of mass or weight equal to one millionth of a gram (a gram is equal to approximately 1/28 of an ounce).

Milligram: A measurement of weight equivalent to one thousandth of a gram (a gram is equal to approximately 1/28 of an ounce).

Monounsaturated Fat: A type of fat that has only one location for the addition of a hydrogen atom. Olive, canola oil and peanut oil are monounsaturated oils.

MRI (Magnetic Resonance Imaging): A technique in which radio waves and a strong magnetic field are used to produce detailed images of internal structures. Used for diagnosis.

Mucus Membranes: Membranes that line the cavities and canals of body systems. The mouth, nose, vagina and stomach contain mucus membranes.

Neuropathy: A series of symptoms caused by nerve damage or malfunction which causes tingling or numbness followed by gradual muscle weakness.

Neurotransmitter: A chemical that serves to transmit nerve impulses from one nerve cell to another. Examples include acetylcholine, dopamine, norepinephrine, and serotonin.

Omega-3 Fatty Acids: Fatty acids found in fish oils and gamma linolenic acid that have been linked with a reduced risk of heart disease, cancer, arthritis, etc.

Omega-6 Fatty Acids: Fatty acids found in oils like flaxseed that have anti-inflammatory properties.

Organic: Term used to describe foods grown without the use of synthetic chemicals, such as pesticides, herbicides, and hormones.

Oxidation: A cellular chemical reaction where oxygen reacts with another compound, causing a chemical change that usually results in deterioration.

Oxidized LDL Cholesterol: LDL cholesterol that has been damaged by free radicals. It is suspected of accelerating the development of atherosclerosis even more than LDL molecules.

Parasite: An organism that lives on or in another organism (a host).

Pituitary: A gland found at the base of the brain that secretes a number of different hormones which regulate growth and metabolism and impact other endocrine glands.

Placebo: A substance that causes no pharmacological reaction. Placebos are used in studies to compare results with an active substance.

Plaque: An abnormal hardened deposit in body vessels, tissues or organs linked to a degradation of health. Plaque can accumulate in arteries, on teeth, and in brain tissue.

Prognosis: A health prediction concerning the most likely course a disease may take.

Prostaglandins: A group of hormone-like substances formed from polyunsaturated fatty acids that cause the contraction of smooth muscle and the dilation or contraction of blood vessels. They are directly involved in the inflammatory response.

Protein: Nitrogen-based organic compounds comprised of amino acid combinations that make up the basic elements of all animal and vegetable tissues.

Radiation Therapy: A type of therapy that uses ionizing radiation—including Roentgen rays, radium or other radioactive substances—to destroy specific areas of tissue. It is most often used in cancer or hyperthyroidism.

RAST: A blood test measuring levels of specific antibodies produced by the body's immune system that is commonly used to test for allergic reactions.

Refined: Describes grain that has had the coarse or fibrous parts of the plant removed. In wheat, for example, the chaff, the bran and the germ are discarded, leaving only the endosperm or high carbohydrate inner core for consumption.

Remission: A reversal or cessation of the symptoms and progress of a certain disease.

Retinoic Acid: A term referring to vitamin A acid. A type of retinoic acid is the active ingredient found in the acne medication called Retin-A.

Retrovirus: A type of virus that has RNA as its core nucleic acid and contains an enzyme called reverse transcriptase that allows it to replicate its RNA into the DNA of infected cells.

RNA (Ribonucleic Acid): A protein found in plant and animal cells that carries coded genetic information from DNA to protein-producing cell structures called ribosomes.

Sebum: The oily secretion produced by glands in the skin.

Secondary Infection: An infection that develops after a primary infection due to reduced immunity.

Seizure: A sudden convulsion that causes the contraction of voluntary muscles and is usually caused by an interruption in brain electrical activity.

Stroke: An attack in which the brain is deprived of oxygen due to blocked blood flow.

Sublingual: Medications or supplements designed to be placed under the tongue for absorption through the mucus membranes.

Syndrome: A group of symptoms that cumulatively characterize a disorder of unknown origin.

Synergy: The interaction between two or more substances that potentiates their action.

Systemic: Pertaining to the entire body.

T-Cell: A type of lymphocyte created by the immune system that plays a crucial role in maintaining health and fighting disease.

Thrombus: An obstruction in a blood vessel usually caused by the presence of a clot.

Topical: Term referring to the surface of the body only.

Transfatty Acids: Artificial polyunsaturated fats created during the process of hydrogenation when making margarine or shortening. These acids have been linked with heart disease.

Tumor: An abnormal mass of tissue which is either benign (non-cancerous) or malignant (cancerous).

Type-A Personality: A person who tends to be impatient, short-tempered and aggressive. These people tend to run a higher risk of developing cardiovascular disease.

Type-B Personality: A person who is generally relaxed, mellow and patient, and may be less vulnerable to stress-related illnesses.

Vascular: Pertaining to the circulatory system.

Vein: A blood vessel that returns blood from body tissues to the heart.

Venom: A poisonous or toxic substance produced by an animal, such as certain snakes and insects.

Virus: Disease-causing structures that are not considered living organisms composed of a protein coat and core of DNA and/or RNA. Viruses cannot reproduce on their own and must replicate inside cells. They are not affected by antibiotic therapy.

Water-Soluble: Capable of dissolving in water.

Western Diet: A diet, characteristic of Western societies, notoriously high in fat, refined carbohydrates and processed foods, and low in dietary fiber.

Yeast: A type of single-celled fungus that most commonly infects the mucus membranes of the mouth, vagina, or gastrointestinal tract.

Index

Abortion 64
Abrasions 69, 90
Abscess 61, 65, 75
Acetaminophen 37
Acetylcholine 70
Aches 50, 74, 92, 94
Acidity 59
Acidophilus 6, 13, 20-21, 57, 59-61, 63, 65, 70-75, 81
Acne 33, 41, 59, 61, 63-64, 68, 71, 73, 81, 84-85, 89-90, 92, 94, 97-100
Acupressure 7, 91
Acupuncture 7, 9, 13, 20, 50-53, 58, 91-92, 94, 389
ADD 11, 16, 18, 22, 24-26, 28, 45-46, 48, 59, 84, 87
Addiction 6, 24, 26, 51, 70, 93-4
Additives, food 23-24
AIDS 28, 42, 59, 62, 71, 75, 77, 81, 84, 87-89, 92, 95, 101-105
Alcohol 14-15, 20, 25-26, 29, 31, 33, 35-37, 39, 42-43, 51, 54, 70, 74
Alcoholism 34-36, 42, 66, 71, 81, 86
Alexander technique 92
Alfalfa 59
Algin 68
Alkaloids 61, 71
Allantoin 62
Allergens 82
Allergies 6, 16, 19, 35-36, 39, 42, 46, 48, 57, 59, 62, 65, 69, 72, 76-77, 81-82, 84-85, 87-88, 91-94, 106-110 ·
    food 21-23
Allicin 65, 78
Allyl sulfides 88
Aloe vera 59
Alpha lipoic acid 81
Alternative therapies (see "Medicine, alternative")

Aluminum 13, 17, 23, 38, 41, 45, 314
Alzheimer's 41, 47, 66, 81, 84, 88, 110-114
Amino acids 41-43
    deficiencies of 42
    individual 42
Ammonia 20, 42
Amphetamines 26, 85
Anemia 19, 34-36, 39, 42, 59, 61-65, 71, 77, 81, 83-84, 87, 89-90, 93-94
Angina 28, 67, 84, 114-118
Anorexia 60, 72, 93
Antacids 12, 15, 34, 38-39
Anti-inflammatory 37, 44, 59-61, 64-66, 68-72, 77-78, 85-87, 89, 91
Antibiotic 20, 33-5, 55-56, 61-62, 64-65, 67-68, 70-71, 73-74, 76, 80-81, 88, 282
Antibodies 32, 47
Antidepressants 35, 37, 51, 75, 88
Antioxidant 6, 12-13, 27, 33-34, 37, 39-40, 42, 44-45, 49, 60, 62, 64, 66, 73-74, 81, 83-84, 86-88, 90
Anxiety 22, 28, 35, 39, 42, 49, 51-52, 62, 68, 71, 74, 76, 91-95, 119-122
Aphrodisiac 63, 65, 67-68
Appendicitis 19
Aromatherapy 91, 389
Arrhythmias 45, 67
Arsenic 45
Art therapy 92
Arteriosclerosis (see also "Coronary heart disease") 34, 36, 61, 64-65, 67, 73, 87-88
Arthritis 123-127
Aspartame 14, 25-26
Aspirin 28, 34-35, 37, 65
Asthma 22-24, 35, 39, 45, 47, 59, 62-63, 65-66, 69-72, 75-77, 81-84, 89, 91-95, 128-131

Astragalus 59
Atherosclerosis (see also "Coronary heart disease") 34, 36-37, 64, 67, 70, 78, 81, 83
Athlete's foot 132-134
Attention Deficit Disorder (ADD) 134-136
Autism 137-139
Autogenic training 92
Autointoxication 6, 16, 19-20
Ayurveda 67, 92
AZT 62
B-vitamins 25, 30, 33, 37, 39, 59-70, 72-77, 81
Bach flower remedies 92
Back pain 22, 94-95, 140-142
Bad breath 143-144
Barbituates 34, 51
Bates method 92
Bedwetting 67-68, 71, 145-147
Bee pollen 81
Bee propolis 81-82
Bee stings (see "Insect bites")
Beef 14, 20, 83-84
Belching 16
Bentonite 82
Berberine 66, 71
Beta carotene 13, 33, 37, 44-46, 48, 64, 90
Bifidobacteria 13
Bilberry 59
Biochemic tissue salts 92
Bioenergetics 92
Biofeedback 7, 51, 91-92
Bioflavonoids 37, 43-45, 82
Biorhythms 92-93
Biotin 36
Birth defects 36, 56
Black cohosh 60
Black walnut 60
Bladder 34, 55, 58-60, 62-63, 67-68, 70-71, 73, 76-77, 89

infections of 147-50
Bleeding 37, 39, 45, 55, 64, 82
Blessed thistle 60
Blindness 33, 60
Blisters 90
Bloating 16, 61, 72
Bloodstream 16, 20, 30-31, 38, 85
Blue-green algae 82
Blueberry 60, 67
Boils 9, 60-61, 64, 70, 73, 77, 90, 151-152
Bones 38, 45, 58, 67, 73, 85, 93
Boron 38
Bovine cartilage 82
Bowen technique 93
BPH (Benign prostatic hypertrophy) (see "Prostrate disease")
Brain 14, 22, 25-26, 42, 45, 49-50, 66-67, 71, 76, 84-85, 87-88
Bran 17-20, 26, 30, 40, 42, 86
Breasts 12, 17, 19, 24, 27, 34, 39, 43, 50, 68, 85-90
  breast feeding 28, 37, 57, 60-61, 63-64, 70-71, 73, 84
Breathing, controlled 93
Bronchitis 63-65, 69-70, 72-76, 93-94, 153-156
Buchu 60
Buckthorn 60-61
Bulimia 156-158
Burdock 61
Burns 29, 34, 59, 62, 64, 70, 81, 85, 90, 93, 159-162
Bursitis 35, 59, 62, 73, 83, 87, 163-166
Butcher's broom 61
Cabbage 17, 21, 25, 27, 36, 38, 88
Caffeine 6, 11, 14-15, 25-26, 34-37, 67, 85, 292-93
Calcium 38
Calories 12, 28-29, 31, 50, 66
Cancer 166-173
Canker sores 59-61, 64, 90, 174-176
Capillaries 22, 59, 61, 72
Capsules 13, 27, 42, 57, 59, 82-86, 89-90
Capsulize 84
Capsulized 21, 43, 57, 81-84, 86-88
Carbohydrates types of 30-31
Cardiovascular system 12, 14, 16-19, 28, 31, 34, 39-41, 44-45, 48-50, 56, 58, 60, 62-63, 65, 67, 71, 73, 76, 84-85, 87-89, 93-94, 371-74
Carotenoids 81, 87
Carpal tunnel 34-35, 176-179
Cascara sagrada 61
Cat's claw (uña de gato) 61
Cataracts 34-35, 37, 64, 81-82, 85, 89, 179-181
Catnip 61

Cell salts 82
Cervicitis 67
Cervix 73, 89
Cetyl myristoleate (CMO) 6, 9, 83
Chamomile 62
Cheeses 14, 29, 36, 41, 81, 89
Chicken pox 182-183
Chiropractic 7, 50, 52, 54, 91-92, 94
Chitosan 6, 28, 82-83, 86
Chlorella 6, 39, 82-83
Chlorine 34, 45
Chlorophyll 6, 20-21, 34, 59, 71, 82-83, 89
Chocolate 18, 22
Cholesterol 12, 16-20, 24, 27, 31, 34-38, 42, 59, 64-69, 74, 81-88
Choline 36
Chondroitin 6, 13, 83, 86
Chondrus 23
Chromium 38
Chronic fatigue system 184-187
Circulatory system 50, 60, 64-69, 73, 91, 93-95
Cirrhosis 36, 62, 69, 81
Citrin 28-29, 83, 87
Cleansing, colon 20-21
Cocaine 26
Coenzyme Q10 84
Coffee 18, 26, 29, 33, 35-36, 54, 70
Cognitive therapy 93
Cold, common 37, 48, 58, 61, 64-66, 68-70, 72-74, 76-77, 81, 87, 93-94
Colic 61, 63-65, 72, 92-94, 188-189
Colitis 17, 19, 25, 34, 59, 65, 68-70, 72, 75, 82, 87, 89, 190-193
Collagen 39, 41-42, 87
Color therapy 93
Comfrey 62
Congestion 22, 60-61, 63-65, 69-70, 76-77, 81, 91-92
Conjugated linoleic acid (CLA) 83
Conjunctivitis 64, 67
Constipation 13, 16-17, 19-21, 54, 59-61, 63, 66, 70, 74-75, 77, 81-82, 85-86, 91, 93-94
Contraceptives 34-37
Convalescence 42, 72
Cooking 25, 31, 35, 37, 44, 58, 85
Copper 39
Cornsilk 62
Coronary heart disease 194-198
Corticosteroids 69
Cortisol 25, 50, 88
Cortisone 33, 37, 77
Couch grass 62
Coughs 60, 62, 65, 69-70, 73-77, 81, 92
Cramp bark 63
Cramps, menstrual 63-64, 69, 73, 75, 93, 287

Cranberry 63
Cranial osteopathy 93
Creatine 6, 84
Creosol 20
Crohn's disease (see "Colitis")
Culver root 63
Cystitis 60, 62, 76, 93
Cysts (see also "Fibrocystic breast disease") 76, 90
Damiana 63
Dandelion 63
Dandruff 41, 90
Dementia 66, 81, 84, 87
Depression 12, 22, 24, 34-36, 39, 42, 49-50, 52, 54, 63, 66-68, 70, 73, 75, 88-89, 91-94
Dermatitis (see also "Eczema") 36, 90
Dessicated liver 84
Devil's claw 63
DHEA 6, 13, 28, 66, 84-85, 88
Diabetes 14, 16-17, 21, 24, 30-31, 33-35, 38-42, 45, 59-60, 62, 65-71, 73-74, 76, 81-82, 84, 87, 89-90, 92, 94-95
Diarrhea 16-17, 20, 25, 34-37, 39-41, 59-61, 63, 65-67, 70, 72-73, 75-76, 81-82, 84, 86, 93-94, 198-202
Digestion 6, 13, 15-17, 21, 28, 30, 39, 57, 61, 65, 70, 72, 81, 83
Dihydortestosterone 74
Diuretic 40, 62-63, 67, 72, 74, 76
Diverticulitis 70, 93, 202-205
Dizziness 23, 36, 39, 64, 93
DMAE 6, 85
DMSO 6, 85
DNA 27, 30, 43, 82, 87-88
Docosahexaenoic acid (DHA) 6, 84-85, 89
Dong quai 64
Dosages 13, 15, 28, 34, 38, 41, 57, 61, 69, 71-75, 81, 85-86, 89
Dramamine 65
Drug overdose 12, 33-34, 39
Drugs, over-the-counter 12, 17, 38, 55-57, 65, 75, 85
  side effects of 56
Dysmenorrhea (see also "Menstrual cramps") 70
Ear infection (see "Earache")
Earache 37, 48, 65, 93, 206-209
Eating Disorders (see "Bulimia")
Echinacea 64
Eczema 35-36, 60-61, 63, 66, 68, 71, 85, 89-94, 209-212
Edema 22, 37, 44, 62-64, 71
EFAs (essential fatty acids) 48
Elastin 42
Electrolyte 16, 40, 60, 62, 68, 72, 76

Emphysema 62-63, 65, 69, 72, 89
Endocrine 39, 68, 74, 78, 89
Endometriosis 213-216
Enemas 7, 82, 91
Enteritis 72, 89
Enzymes, digestive 6, 13, 15-16, 18, 27-29, 32-33, 41, 45, 55, 60, 65-66, 70, 72, 74-75, 85
EPA 45, 85
Epilepsy 14, 34-35, 39, 42, 67, 69, 73-74, 85, 92, 216-220
Epstein-Barr (see also "Chronic fatigue syndrome) 94
Estrogen 24, 27, 33-36, 45, 59-60, 74, 76, 87-88, 283, 288-89
Exercise 48-50
    depression and 49
    stress and 49-50
    weight control and 50
    menopause and 285
Exhaustion 63, 69, 89, 92-93
Exoskeleton 89
Expectorant 69, 72, 75
Expression therapy 93
External visualization 93
Eye problems (see also "Cataracts") 378-81
Eyebright 64
Eyesight 32, 55, 58, 59, 64, 66, 71, 84, 87, 92
Faith 48, 52
Fasting 6, 21, 27, 54, 91, 93
Fats 6, 14-16, 19, 26-27, 30-32, 36, 38, 42-43, 82-83, 85, 87
    types of 32
Fats, monounsaturated 27, 31-32
Fats, polyunsaturated 31-32, 34, 85
Fennel 64
Fenugreek 65
Fever 36, 60-61, 63, 65, 67-74, 76, 91-93, 220-223
Feverfew 65
Fiber 16-20
    types of 16-18
Fibroadenomas 223
Fibrocystic breast disease 223-227
Fibroids 76, 90
Fibromyalgia 47, 62, 76, 90, 92, 94, 227-231
Fingernails 68, 91
Flatulence 60, 66, 72
Flavonoids 37, 43-44, 65, 68, 71, 79, 82, 88
Flora, intestinal 19-20, 55, 66, 83
Flotation therapy 93
Flu 37, 48, 61, 64-65, 73, 77, 81, 87
Fluoride 39-40, 45-46, 59
Folic acid 15, 36, 40, 48, 63, 66, 68-69, 73-76, 81
Folic acid 36

Fractures 12, 62, 70
Free radicals 27, 42-45, 60, 65, 69, 82, 86-87, 90
    cancer and 43
Fruits 14-17, 19-20, 22, 24-27, 29-31, 36-40, 44, 46, 48, 73, 82, 88
Gall disease ("see Gallstones")
Gallbladder 16, 21, 34, 36, 58, 60-61, 63, 66, 69, 74, 77
Gallstones 16-17, 19, 34, 59, 61, 69, 71-73, 79, 93, 231-234
Garlic 65
Gastrointestinal system 16, 25, 57, 62, 64-67, 69-70, 75, 82, 89
Genitourinary tract 72, 74
Germanium 13, 39, 70
Gestalt therapy 93
Ginger 65
Gingivitis (see also "Periodontal disease") 70, 75, 90
Ginkgo biloba 66
Ginseng, Siberian 66
GLA 6, 85-86
Glands 14, 25, 39, 41-42, 46-47, 50, 60, 64-66, 68, 72-73, 87
Glaucoma 35-36, 64, 83, 89, 92-93, 234-237
Glucomannan 66
Glucosamine sulfate 86
Glutathione 86
Gluten 17, 32
Goiter 19, 41
Goldenseal 66
Gotu kola 67
Gout 237-240
Grains 15-20, 22, 24-26, 30-32, 34-36, 38-41, 46, 48
Grape seed extract (see also "Pycnogenol," "Proanthocyanidins," and "Pine Bark Extract") 86-87
Guarana 67
Gums 16-17, 25, 37, 85-86
Gymnema 67
Hair 32, 35-36, 39, 41, 58, 67, 70, 92
Halitosis (see also "Bad breath") 71
Hangnail 56
Hawthorn berry 67, 197
HDL (high density lipoprotein) 24, 31
Headaches (see also "Migraine headaches") 22-23, 25, 34-35, 42, 45, 60, 65, 67-71, 74-76, 85, 87, 90-95
Heart (see "Cardiovascular system")
Heart attack 241-245
Heart disease (see "Coronary heart disease")
Heartburn 15-16, 51, 72, 75, 82, 85,

92, 245-248
Hemoglobin 32, 39, 42
Hemophilia 37
Hemorrhaging 34, 37
Hemorrhoids 17, 19-20, 37, 59, 61-62, 66, 70, 77, 86, 89-90, 245-248
Hepatitis 35, 59, 62-63, 69, 83
Herbs (see "Medicine, herbal")
Hernia 19
Herpes 37, 42, 59-61, 64, 71, 81-82, 85, 87
High blood pressure 252-256
Histamines 22, 44, 65, 70
Histidine 23, 32
HIV 59
Ho-shou-wu 68
Homeopathy 7, 9, 54, 82, 87, 91, 93, 389
Hops 68
Hormone replacement 283
Hormones 14, 21, 28, 32, 50, 68-69, 74, 76, 84, 87-88
Horsetail 67
Hydrochloric acid 68
    deficiency of 16
Hydrocortisone 69
Hydrolysis 30
Hydrotherapy 7, 54, 93
Hydroxy citric acid (HCA) 87
Hyperactivity 22, 25, 42, 68, 71, 93-94, 134-136
Hyperglycemia 69
Hypericin 75
Hypertension (see also "High blood pressure") 19, 28, 34, 36-37, 40-41, 59-60, 62-63, 66-67, 70-71, 76, 82, 84, 88, 92
Hyperthyroidism 36
Hypertrophy 72
Hypnosis 7, 93
Hypnotherapy 93, 391
Hypoglycemia 16, 21, 24-25, 30-31, 34-35, 38, 40, 42, 60, 63, 67-69, 71, 83, 90, 257-260
Hypoglycemic 25, 67, 77-78
Hypothyroidism 33, 68
Hysteria 63, 71, 74, 76
Immune system 6, 11, 36-37, 41, 45-50, 56, 58-59, 61-62, 64, 68, 71, 81-82, 84, 87-88, 90
    dysfunction of 47
    nutrient deficiencies and 47-8
    diet and 48-49
    herbs and 49
Immunity 12, 21, 43, 46-50, 65-66, 69
Impotence 39-40, 63, 66, 74, 81, 89, 260-263
Incontinence 72
Indoles 27, 44, 87-88

Infants 36, 55, 61, 92, 94

Infertility 34, 36, 63, 68, 74, 76, 81, 89, 94, 263-266

Inflammatory bowel disease (see "Colitis")

Influenza (see also "Flu") 59, 62, 64, 93-94

Inhalers 91

Inositol 23, 35-36, 68-69, 87

Insect bites 267-269

Insecticides 35-36, 46

Insomnia 35, 49, 61-62, 67-71, 74, 76, 85, 88, 91-95, 269-272

Insulin 25, 31, 42, 61

Interferon 47, 64, 69

Internal visualization 93

Intestines 16, 18, 20-21, 57, 62-63, 72, 77, 86, 83, 90

Iodine 38-39, 48, 68

Iron 39

Irritability 23, 49, 51, 66, 91

Isoflavones 6, 24, 27, 72, 87-88

Jaundice 61-63, 69-71, 74

Jogging 49

Joints 28, 35, 37, 72-74, 82-83, 85-86, 89, 91-94

Juniper 68

Kava kava 68

Kelp 68

Kidney stones 273-76

Kidneys 19, 33-41, 59-64, 66-71, 73, 76, 81, 84

L-alanine 42

L-arginine 42

L-asparagine 42

L-aspartic 42

L-carnitine 42

L-citrulline 42

L-cysteine 42, 86

L-cystine 42

L-glutamic 42

L-glutamine 25, 42

L-glutathione 42

L-glycine 42

L-histidine 42

L-isoleucine 42

L-leucine 42

L-lysine 42

L-methionine 42, 86

L-ornithine 42

L-phenylalanine 42

L-proline 42

L-serine 42

L-taurine 42

L-threonine 42

L-tryptophan 42

L-tyrosine 42

L-valine 42

Lactation 35, 39, 59-60, 64-65, 69, 71, 73-75, 81, 87, 89

Laryngitis 74-75, 77

Laxatives 15, 18, 35, 40, 59, 61, 71, 74, 77

LDL 31

Lecithin 6, 36, 61, 66, 87

Legumes 15, 17-20, 30-33, 35-37, 39, 41, 46, 48

Lemon grass 69

Leprosy 61

Lesions 59

Leukemia (see also "Cancer") 61, 71, 73, 84, 88

Lice 90

Licorice 69

Light therapy 94

Lignins 16-17, 31, 88

Limonene 88

Lobelia 69

Lung 58, 60, 62, 65-66, 69, 72, 75, 77

Lupus 16, 19, 32, 34, 48, 62, 71, 82-84, 87-89, 276-79

Lycopene 87

Lymphatic system 46-47, 50, 64, 76

Lymphoma (see "Cancer")

Macrobiotic dieting 94

Magnesium 39

Magnetic/electromagnetic therapy 94

Malaise 36

Malaria 55

Malnutrition 16, 24, 29, 39, 81, 89-90

Manganese 39

Margarine 27, 31

Marshmallow 69

Massage 7, 50, 54, 91, 94

Medications 15, 21, 24, 26, 35-36, 55-56, 59, 75

Medicine, alternative 53-59, 91-95
    scientific documentation of 55
    spiritual aspects of 52
    types of 91-95

Medicine, herbal 55-59
    Chinese 58-59
    applications of 59-80

Meditation 93

Megavitamin therapy (see also "Orthomolecular therapy") 94

Melanoma 35

Melatonin 87-88

Memory 35, 42, 66-67, 73-74, 81, 84-85, 88

Meningitis 93, 280-82

Menopause 40, 49, 59-60, 63-64, 67, 76, 81, 84, 87, 89-90, 283-86, 308
    exercise and 310

Menstruation 60, 64, 73, 287

Mental health 19, 22, 25, 34-36, 42, 50-52, 84, 85, 88, 89, 91, 93

Metals 16-17, 20, 41, 46, 86

Methanol 26

Migraine headaches 22, 35, 42, 45, 65, 67, 69, 75, 92-95, 290-94

Milk thistle 69-70

Minerals 38-41 chelated 38

Miscarriage 73, 75

Molybdenum 38-39, 73

Monoamine 54

Mononucleosis 294-97

Monophosphate 36

Monosaccharide 30

Morinda citrifolia (see "Noni")

Morning sickness (see also "Motion sickness" and "Nausea") 297-99

Motion sickness 297-300

Moxibustion 94

Mucilage 17-18, 65, 70, 75, 86

Mucous membranes 64, 69-70, 72, 75-76, 86

Mucus 47, 60, 62, 64-65, 69-70, 72, 77

Mullein 70

Multiple sclerosis 300-303

Mumps 69

Muscles 15, 21-22, 28-31, 34-36, 38-40, 42, 54, 58, 60-61, 63-65, 67-68, 71, 73-74, 76-77, 84-85, 89, 91, 93-94
    strains of 346-49

Mushrooms, medicinal 88

Myotherapy 94

Myrrh 70

Nails 32, 39, 92

Nausea 36, 39, 41, 59-60, 64-65, 71-74, 86, 93, 217-300

Neck 35, 85, 92-94

Neckaches 51

Nerves 32, 60, 62, 74-76, 91

Nervous system 14, 26, 36, 38, 42, 60-63, 66-69, 71, 74, 76, 94, 276

Nervousness 39, 60, 63, 68, 70-71, 74, 94

Nettle 70

Neuralgia 64, 67, 73-74, 92

Neuritis 35

Neurotransmitters 25-26, 42, 71

Nicotine 69-70, 90

Nitrates 22

Nitrites 46

Noni 70

Norepinephrine 14, 26

Oatstraw 70

Obesity 14, 19, 24, 28, 30, 32, 35-36, 66-68, 82-84, 86-87, 90, 304-08

Oils, essential 91-92

Oregon grape 71

Organic foods 13, 17, 30, 32, 34, 38-39, 41, 60-61

Orthomolecular therapy 40

Osteoarthritis 22, 83, 86, 94

Osteopathy 7, 50, 93-94, 392

Osteoporosis 16, 24, 34, 38, 46, 70-71, 76, 90, 94-95, 308-11

Ovaries 75, 84, 89-90

Ovulation 287

Oxidants 43-45, 87, 90

Oxidation 34, 43

Oxygen 22, 28, 31-32, 43, 49

PABA 36-37, 48

Pancreas 15, 25, 68

Pancreatin 16, 85

Panic (see also "Anxiety") 91, 93, 312

Pantothenic acid 25, 35, 48, 60

Papain 16, 23, 85

Papaya 61, 65, 85

Parasites 16, 21, 45, 60-62, 65, 70-72

Parkinson's disease 35-36, 63, 76, 81, 87, 312-15

Parsley 71

Passionflower 71

Pau d'arco 71

Pauling, Linus 12, 40

Penicillin 65

Peppermint 71-72

Peptides 47

Peristalsis 61, 74

Perspiration 40-41, 51, 60-62, 73-74

Pesticides 43, 45

Phen-fen (fen-phen) 28, 56, 304

Phenols 19

Phosphorus 15, 38, 40-41, 68

Photosensitivity 75

Phytoestrogen 27, 76, 90

Phytonutrients 27, 59-60, 63, 65, 67-69, 71-77

Pine bark extract (see also "Grape seed extract," "Pycnogenol," or "Proanthocyanidins") 86-87

Pinworms 65

Pleurisy root 69, 72, 74

PMS 12, 24-25, 34, 39, 60, 62-64, 67, 73, 76, 85-88, 90-92

Pneumonia 69, 72

Pollen 6, 13, 60, 63, 66-68, 71-72, 74, 76, 81, 89

Pollution 15, 33, 37, 44

Polysaccharides 17, 30, 59, 88

Posture 92

Potassium 40

Pregnancy 34-36, 64-65, 70, 73, 75-76, 95

Pregnenolone 6, 13, 88

Preservatives, food 20, 22, 33, 44

Proanthocyanidins (see "Pycnogenol," "Grape seed extract," or "Pine bark extract") 37, 44, 59-60, 62-63, 65-77, 86-87

Progesterone 13, 15, 54, 74, 76, 80,

88, 90, 283

Prostaglandins 32, 72

Prostate health 19, 24, 27, 41-42, 45, 60, 63-66, 68, 71-74, 76, 81, 84, 87-90

Prostatitis 60, 62, 72-73

Protein 32-33

    sources of 33

Prozac 51, 54

Psoriasis 36, 59, 61, 63-64, 67, 69, 71, 73-74, 77, 82, 84-85, 87-91, 94-95

Psychiatry 12, 37

Psychotherapy 22, 49

Pumpkin seed 72

Pycnogenol (see also "Proanthocyanidins," "Grape seed extract," or "Pine bark extract") 86-87

Pygeum 72

Pyruvate 6, 9, 29, 88-89

Quassia 72

Queen of the meadow 72-73

Quercetin 44-45, 82

Radiation 35, 42-43, 46, 59, 62, 65-66, 81-83, 86

RDA (recommended daily allowance) 11-12, 15, 40

Red clover 73

Red raspberry 73

Red sage 73

Reflexology 7, 91, 94

Relaxation 7, 47, 50-51, 68-69, 73-74, 76, 91-94

Respiratory disorders (see "Asthma" and "Bronchitis")

Respiratory tract 35, 37, 62, 65-66, 69-70, 72, 76-77, 81, 84, 91, 94

Retina 84

Retinol 33

Retinopathy 61, 64, 89

Rheumatic fever 337-39

Rheumatism (see also "Arthritis") 16, 19, 22, 39, 42, 59, 62-64, 67, 73, 77, 82-4, 88, 93-95

Rheumatoid arthritis 123

Rhinitis 66, 70

Ringworm 66, 71, 90

RNA 30, 82

Rose hips 73

Royal jelly 89

Rutin 37, 44, 82

Saccharin 26, 36

Sage 74

Salicylates 65

Saliva 15, 18

Salt 13, 18, 27, 29, 39, 41, 46, 82

Saponins 70, 74

Sarcoma (see "Cancer")

Sarsaparilla 74

Saw palmetto 74

Schizophrenia 12, 22, 35, 67, 93-94

Sciatica 75, 85, 91-95

Sclerosis 20, 32, 35-36, 48, 81, 84-88, 94-95

Scurvy 37, 73

Seafood 32, 39, 41, 85

Seaweeds 18

Sedatives 34, 64, 74

Seizures 14, 25

Selenium 40

Semolina 14

Senility 35, 66-67

Senna 74-75

Serotonin 42, 70-71

Sex 40, 59

Shark cartilage 89

Shellfish 22, 34, 39, 41, 82

Shiatsu, 392

Shingles 34-35, 81, 339-42

Silicon 41

Silymarin (see also "Milk thistle") 57, 69-70, 79

Sinus 22, 92, 94

Sinusitis 37, 72, 85, 91, 93-94, 342-46

Skin disorders (see "Eczema," "Warts," "Wrinkles" and "Psoriasis")

Skullcap 74

Sleep (ing) 42, 50-51, 62, 68, 70-71, 74-76, 85, 87, 91

    medications for 56

    aromatherapy and 91

    disorders (see "Insomnia")

Slippery elm 75

Smoking 37, 69

Snakebite 69

Sneezing 21

Sodium 23, 38, 40-41, 46, 89

Soils 11, 38, 40

Sorbitol 25, 31

Soy 13, 24, 30, 33-36, 42, 88, 91

Spasms 22, 60, 63-65, 68, 72, 74-76, 91

Sperm 42, 66, 83

Spine 54, 92

Spiritualism (spiritual healing) 52, 95

Spirulina 89-90

Sprains 72, 85, 92-94, 346-49

Sprouts 27, 35, 37, 88, 90

Squaw vine 75

St. John's wort 75

Sterility 40-41

Steroids 37, 88

Stevia 90

Stimulant 29, 42, 58-59, 63, 65, 67, 70, 72, 75, 77, 85, 91-92

Stomach 12, 15-16, 20-23, 28, 33,

39, 41, 43, 51, 57-58, 60-61, 63-65, 68, 70, 72-73, 75-77, 81, 86, 90, 92
Stool 17, 20, 39, 70
Strains 56, 72, 85, 93
Stress 50-52, 349-53
  symptoms of 51
  treatments for relieving 51-52
Stroke 14, 66, 81, 85, 87, 353-57
Sucrose 30
Sugar 24-26
  cravings and 24
  hypoglycemia and 24-25
Sulfite 23
Sulfur 41, 81
Sunburn 36, 59, 81, 90, 357-60
Sunlight 34, 49, 75, 94
Sunscreen 36
Superoxide dismutase (SOD) 90
Supplementation 11-13
Supplements
  overview of nonherbal 81-90
Sweeteners 6, 21-22, 24-26, 29
  FDA and 25-26
T-cell 51, 59, 68, 88
T-lymphocytes 46
Taheebo (see "Pau d'arco)
Tai chi 95
Tannins 60, 73
Tapeworm 60
Tea 6, 21, 29, 37, 59, 65, 71-72, 90
Tea tree oil 90
Teeth 38, 45, 51, 73
Teething 92
Temporomandibular joint syndrome (TMJ) 360-63
Tension 50-51, 60, 63, 67, 74, 76, 91, 93-95
Testicle 89
Testosterone 45, 74, 88
Thalidomide 56
Thermogenesis 68, 85
Thiamine 12, 34, 41, 81
Throat 48, 56, 67, 72-73, 75, 81
Thyme 75
Thymus gland 46-47, 50, 64, 75
Thyroid 28, 39, 68, 74
TMJ 86, 94
Tobacco 29, 34-36, 41, 44, 51, 54
Tocopherol 23, 34
Tofu 14, 24, 32, 38, 87
Tonsillitis 61, 64
Tonsils 46
Tooth griding 364-66
Toothache 55, 69, 94
Toothpaste 90
Touch, therapeutic 95
Toxemia 19
Toxicity 20, 25, 32-35, 37, 42, 56, 59, 61-64, 67-76, 81-83, 87-88

Tranquilizers 22, 42, 51
Transcutaneous electrical nerve stimulation (TENS) 95
Trembling 35
Triglycerides 31-32, 35, 60
Tryptophan 32-33, 42
Tuberculosis 60, 62, 66, 70, 72-73, 76, 92
Tumors (see also "Cancer") 13, 27, 42, 45-6, 61, 67, 70-71, 73, 82, 84, 87, 89-90
Twitching 51, 74
Tyrosine 23, 29, 75
Ulcers 15, 19, 21, 33, 35-36, 41-42, 59, 61-62, 65-66, 69-72, 75, 81, 83-85, 87, 89, 92-95, 367-71
Uña de gato (see "Cat's claw")
Urea 74
Ureteritis 60
Urethra 55
Urinary tract 38, 55, 59-63, 67-69, 71, 73, 76
Urinary tract infection (see "Bladder, infections of")
Urination 60, 71
Urine 20, 32, 55, 60, 62, 68, 73, 76
Uterus 63-64, 71, 73, 76, 78, 84, 90
Uva ursi 75-76
Vagina 66, 71, 75, 90
Vaginitis 66-67, 371-74
Valerian 76
Valium 51
Vanadium 41
Vanadyl 41
Varicose veins 17, 19, 37, 60-61, 86, 375-78
Vegetables, cruciferous 27
Vegetarianism 32-33, 36
Venereal disease 61, 71
Viruses 45-47, 60, 82
Vision (see "Eyesight")
Visualization (see also "Internal visualization" and "External visualization") 6-7, 52, 91, 93, 95
Vitamin A 33
Vitamin B1 (thiamine) 34
Vitamin B12 (cyanocobalamin) 35-36
Vitamin B2 (riboflavin) 34-35
Vitamin B3 (niacin) 35
Vitamin B5 (pantothenic acid) 35
Vitamin B6 (pyridoxine) 35
Vitamin C (ascorbic acid) 37
Vitamin D 34
Vitamin E 34
Vitamin K 34
Vitamin P (bioflavonoids) 37
Vitamins 33-37
  fat-soluble 33-34
  water-soluble 34-37
Vomiting 39, 41, 69, 72

Walking 48, 50, 92
Warts 382-85
Water
  consumption of 45
  safety of 45
  fluoride and 45
  filtration systems and 45
Weight loss 27-29, 304-08
  natural products for 28-29
Whiplash 94
Wild cherry 76
Wild yam 76
  topical cream form of 90
Women's health (general) 33-36, 40, 49-50, 56, 60-62, 65-67, 70-71, 74, 76, 81, 87-89, 94
  weight loss and 28
Wood betony 76
Worms 60-61, 69, 72-75
Wounds 59, 64, 67, 70, 75, 89-90
Wrinkles, skin 385-88
X-rays 42-43
Xeronine 70
Yeast 13, 22, 35-36, 42
Yeast infections (see also "Vaginitis") 19, 24-25, 46, 60, 64-65, 71, 75, 81, 90, 371-74
Yellow dock 76-77
Yerba santa 77
Yoga 95, 393
Yogurt 18, 25, 29, 81
Zinc 11-13, 18, 33, 35-36, 38-41, 46-49, 60-61, 63-64, 67-68, 71-72, 74-75, 89-90